Nanotechnology

Volume 8

Edited by
Lifeng Chi

Related Titles

Nanotechnologies for the Life Sciences

Challa S. S. R. Kumar (ed.)

Volume 1: Biofunctionalization of Nanomaterials

2005

978-3-527-31381-5

Volume 2: Biological and Pharmaceutical Nanomaterials

2005

978-3-427-31382

Volume 3: Nanosystem Characterization Tools in the Life Sciences

2005

978-3-527-31383-9

Volume 4: Nanodevices for the Life Sciences

2006

978-3-527-31384-6

Volume 5: Nanomaterials - Toxicity, Health and Environmental Issues

2006

978-3-527-31385-3

Volume 6: Nanomaterials for Cancer Therapy

2006

978-3-527-31386-0

Volume 7: Nanomaterials for Cancer Diagnosis

2006

978-3-527-31387-7

Volume 8: Nanomaterials for Biosensors

2006

978-3-527-31388-4

Volume 9: Tissue, Cell and Organ Engineering

2006

978-3-527-31389-1

Volume 10: Nanomaterials for Medical Diagnosis and Therapy

2007

978-3-527-31390-7

Nanotechnology

Günter Schmid (ed.)

Volume 1: Principles and Fundamentals

2008

978-3-527-31732-5

Harald Krug (ed.)

Volume 2: Environmental Aspects

2008

978-3-527-31735-6

Rainer Waser (ed.)

Volume 3: Information Technology I

2008

978-3-527-31738-7

Rainer Waser (ed.)

Volume 3: Information Technology II

2008

978-3-527-31737-0

Viola Vogel (ed.)

Volume 5: Nanomedicine and Nanobiotechnology

2009

978-3-527-31736-3

Harald Fuchs (ed.)

Volume 6: Nanoprobes

2009

978-3-527-31733-2

Michael Grätzel, Kuppuswamy Kalyanasundaram (eds.)

Volume 7: Light and Energy

2012

978-3-527-31734-9

Lifeng Chi (ed.)

Volume 8: Nanostructured Surfaces

2009

978-3-527-31739-4

www.wiley.com/go/nanotechnology

G. Schmid, H. Krug, R. Waser, V. Vogel, H. Fuchs,
M. Grätzel, K. Kalyanasundaram, L. Chi (Eds.)

Nanotechnology

Volume 8: Nanostructured Surfaces

Edited by Lifeng Chi

**WILEY-
VCH**

WILEY-VCH Verlag GmbH & Co. KGaA

The Editor

Prof. Dr. Lifeng Chi
University of Münster
Institute of Physics
Wilhelm-Klemm-Str. 10
48149 Münster
Germany

Cover:
Nanocar reproduced with kind permission
of Y. Shirai/Rice University

Library of Congress Card No.: applied for

British Library Cataloguing-in-Publication Data
A catalogue record for this book is available from the
British Library.

**Bibliographic information published by
the Deutsche Nationalbibliothek**
Die Deutsche Nationalbibliothek lists this
publication in the Deutsche Nationalbibliografie;
detailed bibliographic data are available in the
Internet at http://dnb.d-nb.de.

© 2010 WILEY-VCH Verlag GmbH & Co. KGaA,
Weinheim

Cover Design   Adam Design, Weinheim
Typesetting   Thomson Digital, Noida, India
Printing and Binding   Betz-Druck GmbH,
Darmstadt

Printed in the Federal Republic of Germany
Printed on acid-free paper

ISBN: 978-3-527-31739-4

Contents

Nanotechnology, Volume 8: Nanostructured Surfaces. Edited by Lifeng Chi
Copyright © 2010 WILEY-VCH Verlag GmbH & Co. KGaA, Weinheim
ISBN: 978-3-527-31739-4

Preface

Volume 8 of the Nanotechnology Series, which focuses on nanostructured surfaces, introduces the concepts and describes the recent progress in surface nanopatterning, as well as some aspects of its application.

Surface nanopatterning has become an increasingly important part of modern science and technology, notably in areas of microelectronics, information processing and storage, nano/microfluidic devices, and biodetection. Nanostructured surfaces with fascinating functions are also a universal phenomenon in Nature, examples being the wings of butterflies and the famous Lotus leaf. The fabrication and investigation of nanostructured surfaces represent active areas of research in chemistry, physics, materials science, and biology. The methods used to fabricate nanostructured surfaces are commonly catalogued as either "top-down" or "bottom-up." In the top-down approach, the features are written directly or transferred onto a substrate, and then engraved by applying appropriate etching and deposition processes. In contrast, the concepts of self-assembly and self-organization provide an alternative means of realizing small features over large areas via bottom-up approaches, which rely on the interactions of building blocks such as molecules or nanoparticles, that assemble spontaneously into nanostructures and/or microstructures. The self-assembly and self-organization processes and the characteristics of the surface patterns can be controlled by tailoring the properties of building blocks.

Within this volume, the typical top-down approaches for nanopatterning are outlined in Chapter 1, and include photo-, electron-beam, X-ray and focused ion-beam lithography. In Chapters 2, 3 and 4, "unconventional" lithography methods are introduced, such as scanning probe microscopy (SPM) -based lithography in Chapter 2, micro-contact printing (CP) methods in Chapter 3, and nanoimprinting lithography (NIL) in Chapter 4. The latter two processes belong to a special group termed "soft lithography," where the top-down methods and bottom up methods are combined. Details of the different bottom-up approaches for creating nanostructures are presented in Chapters 5 to 8. In Chapter 5, the creation of anodized aluminum oxide (AAO) equipped with nanopores of variable diameters, ranging from a few to several hundreds of nanometers, is described. In Chapter 6, up-dated

Nanotechnology, Volume 8: Nanostructured Surfaces. Edited by Lifeng Chi
Copyright © 2010 WILEY-VCH Verlag GmbH & Co. KGaA, Weinheim
ISBN: 978-3-527-31739-4

progress in colloidal lithography based on the self-organization of monodispersed colloidal particles (polymer or inorganic particles) is outlined, while Chapter 7 presents details of the fabrication of extended metallic particle arrays and the related applications based on block copolymer micelle nanolithography. In Chapter 8, a comprehensive description is provided of pattern formation by a dynamic self-assembly during the Langmuir–Blodgett (LB) transfer of molecules onto a solid substrate. The feature sizes created when employing the methods described in Chapters 1 to 8 range typically from several hundred down to 10 nanometers. Yet, to further reduce the feature size, and to keep the structure well ordered, molecular- or supramolecular-based templates can be applied, and this topic forms the basis of Chapter 9. Finally, examples of nanostructured two-dimensional and three-dimensional systems, as well as their functions, are outlined in Chapter 10.

The collection of topics in this volume represents the current state of the art in the fabrication and application of nanostructured surfaces. Attention is focused more on unconventional methods and bottom-up approaches, as the well-established lithography methods have been introduced previously, in Volumes 3 and 4 of this series. In future, the combination of top-down and bottom-up approaches might be more fully addressed for advanced technological development and applications.

Finally, it gives me great pleasure to thank my colleagues who contributed to this volume, for their ready acceptance to participate, their high level of engagement, and their extra workload.

Münster   *Lifeng Chi*
28 January 2010

List of Contributors

Xiaodong Chen
Nanyang Technological University
School of Materials Science
and Engineering
50 Nanyang Avenue
639798 Singapore
Singapore

Lifeng Chi
University of Münster (WWU)
Institute of Physics and Center
for Nanotechnology (CeNTech)
48149 Münster
Germany

Claudia Haensch
Eindhoven University of Technology
Laboratory of Macromolecular
Chemistry and Nanoscience
P.O. Box 513
5600 MB Eindhoven
The Netherlands

Nicole Herzer
Eindhoven University of Technology
Laboratory of Macromolecular
Chemistry and Nanoscience
P.O. Box 513
5600 MB Eindhoven
The Netherlands

Stephanie Hoeppener
Eindhoven University of Technology
Laboratory of Macromolecular
Chemistry and Nanoscience
P.O. Box 513
5600 MB Eindhoven
The Netherlands

and

Ludwigs-Maximilians-University
München
Center for Nanoscience (CeNS)
Amalienstrasse 54
80799 München
Germany

Zhuoyu Ji
Chinese Academy of Sciences
Institute of Microelectronics
No. 3, Bei-Tu-Cheng West Road
Beijing 100029
China

Lei Jiang
Chinese Academy of Sciences
Institute of Chemistry
No. 2, 1st North Street, Zhongguancun
Beijing 100080
China

Nanotechnology, Volume 8: Nanostructured Surfaces. Edited by Lifeng Chi
Copyright © 2010 WILEY-VCH Verlag GmbH & Co. KGaA, Weinheim
ISBN: 978-3-527-31739-4

Nikolaos Kehagias
Catalan Institute of Nanotechnology
(ICN-CIN2)
Phononic and Photonic Nanostructures
Group
Campus de Bellaterra, Edifici CM7
08193 Barcelona
Spain

Timothy Kehoe
Catalan Institute of Nanotechnology
(ICN-CIN2)
Phononic and Photonic Nanostructures
Group
Campus de Bellaterra, Edifici CM7
08193 Barcelona
Spain

Ming Liu
Chinese Academy of Sciences
Institute of Microelectronics
No. 3, Bei-Tu-Cheng West Road
Beijing 100029
China

Theobald Lohmueller
Max Planck Institute for Metals
Research
Department of New Materials
and Biosystems
70569 Stuttgart
Germany

and

University of Heidelberg
Biophysical Chemistry
INF 253 Raum 108c
69120 Heidelberg
Germany

Jan Mehlich
University of Münster (WWU)
Organic Chemistry Institute
and CeNTech
Corrensstrasse 40
48149 Münster
Germany

Bart Jan Ravoo
University of Münster (WWU)
Organic Chemistry Institute
and CeNTech
Corrensstrasse 40
48149 Münster
Germany

Vincent Reboud
Catalan Institute of Nanotechnology
(ICN-CIN2)
Phononic and Photonic Nanostructures
Group
Campus de Bellaterra, Edifici CM7
08193 Barcelona
Spain

Günter Schmid
Universität Duisburg-Essen
Institut für Anorganische Chemie
Universitätsstrasse 5-7
45117 Essen
Germany

Ulrich S. Schubert
Eindhoven University of Technology
Laboratory of Macromolecular
Chemistry and Nanoscience
P.O. Box 513
5600 MB Eindhoven
The Netherlands

and

Friedrich-Schiller-University Jena
Laboratory of Organic and
Macromolecular Chemistry
Humboldtstrasse 10
07743 Jena
Germany

and

Ludwigs-Maximilians-University
München
Center for Nanoscience (CeNS)
Amalienstrasse 54
80799 München
Germany

Liwei Shang
Chinese Academy of Sciences
Institute of Microelectronics
No. 3, Bei-Tu-Cheng West Road
Beijing 100029
China

Clivia M. Sotomayor Torres
Catalan Institute of Nanotechnology
(ICN-CIN2)
Phononic and Photonic Nanostructures
Group
Campus de Bellaterra, Edifici CM7
08193 Barcelona
Spain

and

Catalan Institute for Research
and Advanced Studies (ICREA)
08010 Barcelona
Spain

Joachim P. Spatz
Max Planck Institute for Metals
Research
Department of New Materials
and Biosystems
70569 Stuttgart
Germany

Taolei Sun
University of Münster (WWU)
Center for Nanotechnology (CeNTech)
Heisenbergstr. 11
48149 Münster
Germany

Dayang Wang
Max Planck Institute of Colloids
and Interfaces
Research Campus Golm
14424 Potsdam
Germany

Gang Zhang
Jilin University
College of Chemistry
State Key Laboratory of Supramolecular
Structures and Materials
Changchun 130012
China

Haiming Zhang
University of Münster (WWU)
Institute of Physics
Wilhelm-Klemm-Str. 10
48149 Münster
Germany

Dingyong Zhong
University of Münster (WWU)
Institute of Physics
Wilhelm-Klemm-Str. 10
48149 Münster
Germany

Part One
Top-Down Strategy

Nanotechnology, Volume 8: Nanostructured Surfaces. Edited by Lifeng Chi
Copyright © 2010 WILEY-VCH Verlag GmbH & Co. KGaA, Weinheim
ISBN: 978-3-527-31739-4

1
Top-Down Fabrication of Nanostructures

Ming Liu, Zhuoyu Ji, and Liwei Shang

1.1
Introduction

The "top-down" approach to nanofabrication involves the creation of "nanostructures" from a large parent entity. This type of fabrication is based on a number of tools and methodologies which consist of three major steps:

1) The deposition of thin films/coatings on a substrate.
2) Obtaining the desired shapes via photolithography.
3) Pattern transfer using either a lift-off process or selective etching of the films

Compared with general chemical fabrication and processing methods, top-down fabrication techniques for the creation of nanostructures are derived mainly from the techniques applied for the fabrication of microstructures in the semiconductor industry. In particular, the fundamentals and basic approaches are mostly based on micro-fabrications. In this chapter, methods of top-down nanofabrication will be discussed, with attention being focused primarily on methods of lithography, especially optical, electron-beam, X-ray and focused ion beam lithography. A brief introduction will also be provided on how to create nanostructures using various methods of thin film deposition and etching materials. Finally, the methods for pattern transfer through etching and lift-off techniques will be discussed.

In the past, top-down fabrication techniques have represented an effective approach for nanostructures and, when complemented with bottom-up approaches during the past few decades, have led to amazing progress having been made with a variety of nanostructures. The traditional top-down technology used to create nanostructures and nanopatterns is discussed in the following sections.

1.2
Lithography

Lithography, which is also often referred to as "photoengraving," was invented in 1798 in Germany by Alois Senefelder. It is the process of defining useful shapes on

Nanotechnology, Volume 8: Nanostructured Surfaces. Edited by Lifeng Chi
Copyright © 2010 WILEY-VCH Verlag GmbH & Co. KGaA, Weinheim
ISBN: 978-3-527-31739-4

the surface of a semiconductor wafer [1–5]. Typically, it consists of a patterned exposure into some form of photosensitive material that has already been deposited onto the wafer. Many techniques of lithography have been developed during the past fifty years, by using a variety of lens systems and exposure radiation sources that have included photons, X-rays, electrons, ions, and neutral atoms. In spite of the different exposure radiation sources used in the various lithographic methods, and the instrumental details, all of these techniques share the same general approaches and are based on similar fundamentals. *Photolithography* is the most widely used technique in microelectronic fabrication, particularly for the mass production of integrated circuits (ICs) [2], and has been the driving force behind the miniaturization of such circuits since they were first produced at Fairchild and at Texas Instruments during the early 1960s [6].

1.2.1
Photolithography

Photolithography (also called "optical lithography") is simply lithography using a radiation source with wavelength(s) in the visible spectrum. It has served as the dominant patterning technology in the semiconductor industry since the IC was invented almost sixty years ago. From the onset, optical lithography has always managed to keep pace with Moore's law [7, 8], including its recent acceleration. In order to keep pace with the shrinking feature size, a steady stream of improvements in the field of resolution, image placement, and pattern transfer have been introduced time after time, and these have enabled optical lithography to hold off the challenges of the competing lithography technologies.

The key historical events in photolithography have been as follow:

- 1826: Joseph Nicephore Niepce, in Chalon, France, takes the first photograph using bitumen of Judea on a pewter plate, developed using oil of lavender and mineral spirits.
- 1843: William Henry Fox Talbot, in England, develops dichromated gelatin, patented in Britain in 1852.
- 1935: Louis Minsk of Eastman Kodak develops the first synthetic photopolymer, poly(vinyl cinnamate), the basis of the first negative photoresists.
- 1940: Otto Suess of Kalle Division of Hoechst AG, develops the first diazoquinone-based positive photoresist.
- 1954: Louis Plambeck, Jr, of Du Pont, develops the Dycryl polymeric letterpress plate.

Optical lithography is a process used in microfabrication to selectively remove parts of a thin film (or the bulk of a substrate). It involves the use of an optical technique to produce images at smaller scales, which employs light to transfer a geometric pattern from a photomask to a light-sensitive chemical (photoresist, or simply "resist") on the substrate. The steps involved in the photolithographic process include: wafer cleaning; barrier layer formation; photoresist application; soft baking; mask alignment; exposure and development; and hard-baking.

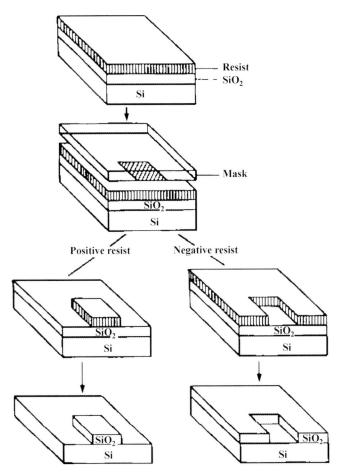

Figure 1.1 Schematic representation of the photolithographic process sequences, in which images in the mask are transferred to the underlying substrate surface.

The basic scheme of photolithography (as shown in Figure 1.1) involves three steps [9]: (i) a thin film of resist material is cast over the substrate; (ii) the substrate is then exposed to a pattern of intense light through a mask, during which time the resist material is selectively struck by the light; (iii) the exposed substrate is then immersed into the development solvent.

Depending on the chemical nature of the resist material, the photoresist is defined as either a positive or a negative type. For positive resists, the resist is exposed to ultraviolet (UV) light wherever the underlying material is to be removed. In these resists, exposure to the UV light alters the chemical structure of the resist, which causes it to become more soluble in the developing solvent than in the unexposed areas. The resist exposed under the UV light is then washed away by the developer solution. Overall, the process can be described as "whatever shows, goes away." In contrast, in the case of a negative resist, the exposed areas may be rendered less

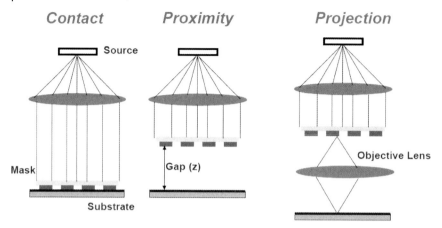

Figure 1.2 Schematic diagram of working modes of photolithography.

soluble in a certain developing solvent; this leads to the production of a negative tone image of the shadow mask, a process described as "whatever shows, stays behind."

In addition to conventional photoresist polymers, Langmuir–Blodgett films and self-assembled monolayers (SAMs) have also been used as resists in photolithography [10, 11]. In such applications, photochemical oxidation, crosslinking, or the generation of reactive groups are used to transfer patterns from the mask to the mono-layer [12, 13].

A *master mask* is necessary in the process of photolithography, and in general this is scribed using an optical method and produced by chemical etching. In this case, the light passes through the mask to define the actual structure in the material; according to the position of the mask with respect to the sample, three types of exposure lithography can be defined, namely contact, proximity, and projection lithography (see Figure 1.2).

Up until to the early 1970s, most lithography was carried out as either a contact or a close-proximity printing process, in which blue and near-UV light was passed through a photomask directly onto a photoresist-coated semiconductor substrate [14]. This apparently simple shadow imaging process has been described in many research reports and handbooks [15, 16].

1.2.1.1 Contact Printing

In contact-mode photolithography, the resist-coated silicon wafer is brought into intimate physical contact with the glass photomask. For this, the wafer is held on a vacuum chuck and the whole assembly rises until the wafer and mask make contact with each other. The photoresist is exposed to UV light while the wafer is in contact position with the mask, and this allows a mask pattern to be transferred into a photoresist with almost 100% accuracy, as well as providing the highest resolution (e.g., 1 μm features in 0.5 μm of positive resist). Unfortunately, however, the maximum resolution is seldom achieved owing to the presence of dust on the substrates and the nonuniform thicknesses of both the photoresist and the substrate. The main problem with contact printing is that debris, trapped between the resist and the mask, can damage the mask and cause defects in the pattern.

1.2.1.2 Proximity Printing

The proximity exposure method is similar to contact printing, and involves introducing a gap about 10–25 μm wide between the mask and the wafer during the exposure stage. This gap minimizes (but may not eliminate) the mask damage. Although a resolution of about 2–4 μm is possible with proximity printing, increasing the gap will reduce the resolution by expanding the penumbral region caused by diffraction. The main difficulties associated with proximity printing include the control of a small and very constant space between the mask and wafer, which can be achieved only by using extremely flat wafers and masks.

1.2.1.3 Projection Printing

Generally speaking, projection techniques have a lower resolution capability than that provided by shadow printing. However, unlike shadow printing, in projection printing the lens elements are used to focus the mask image onto a wafer substrate, which is separated from the mask by several centimeters so that damage to the mask is entirely avoided. An image of the patterns on the mask is projected onto the resist-coated wafer, which is located several centimeters away. In order to achieve a high resolution, only a small portion of the mask is imaged, and the small image field is scanned or stepped over the surface of the wafer. Projection printers that step the mask image over the wafer surface are termed "step-and-repeat" systems, and are capable of approximately 1 μm resolution.

The first widespread use of projection printing for semiconductor manufacturing was fostered by a very well-accepted family of tools from Perkin-Elmer, the so-called "Micralign" projection aligners developed during the early 1970s. For the first time, these tools allowed a higher performance pattern definition by scanning and imaging only a fractional area of the wafer at any instant. Moreover, the optical resolution and pattern overlay performances were also significantly enhanced. The technique of projection printing was further developed when a new class of projection exposure tools – typically referred to as "steppers" – was introduced during the late 1970s [17]. For the first time, the pattern definition imaging on the semiconductor wafers was performed one chip at a time, in a step-and-repeat fashion. This had profound implications not only on the requirements for the photomask but also on the precision mechanical movements needed to accurately overlay a new pattern on underlying patterns already on the wafer substrate.

1.2.1.4 Resolution Enhancement Techniques (RETs)

Various RET approaches have undergone intense investigation during the past few years, and many reports have been made worldwide at leading lithography conferences. Moreover, most of these techniques have been introduced into high-volume wafer manufacture. The RETs interact in many ways, and Smith has discussed in some detail the impact of interacting factors when designing and refining the lithography

Table 1.1 The main categories of resolution enhancement technique in current use and undergoing investigation.

Resolution enhancement technique	Type	Advantage(s)	Disadvantage(s)
Phase-shift masks	Wavefront engineering	Improves DoF and exposure latitude	High mask cost, inspection and repair difficult
Modified illumination	Wavefront engineering	Improves DoF for dense line/space feature	Less improvement for holes or isolated lines affected by lens aberrations
Optical proximity correction (OPC)	Mask engineering	Improved CD control for various patterns	Additional design data processing masks more complex and expensive
Wafer control – antireflective layers	Resist engineering	Improved CD control reduces notching	Increased cost and process complexity may complicate etch
Pupil filtering	Wavefront engineering	Improved CD control and exposure latitude	Pattern-specific capability must be designed in by lens manufacturer
Multilayer and surface imaging resists	Resist engineering	Improved CD control, resolution, including antireflective functionality	Increased process complexity and cost

CD = critical dimension.

process [18]. The main categories of RETs currently being investigated and used are listed in Table 1.1; two of these techniques – phase-shifting mask (PSM) lithography and optical proximity correction (OPC) – are discussed in the following sections.

Phase-Shifting Mask Lithography   Phase-shifting masks for optical lithography were developed by Levenson and coworkers at IBM during the early 1980s [19], although the independent development of phase shifting was also underway at the same time by Shibuya [20] and Smith [21, 22]. Phase-shifting masks are photomasks that take advantage of the interference generated by phase differences to improve the image resolution in photolithography, and exist in either alternating or attenuated forms.

Alternating Phase-Shifting Masks. In the case of an alternating PSM, a thin layer of transparent material of correct thickness is added onto the mask; this induces an abrupt change of the phase of the light used for exposure, and causes optical attenuation at desired locations. These phase masks (which are also known as "phase shifters") have produced features of −100 nm [23, 24] in photoresist. The correct thickness of the shifter is usually demonstrated by the physical thickness that provides an optical path length exactly one-half wavelength longer than the optical path length in the same thickness of air.

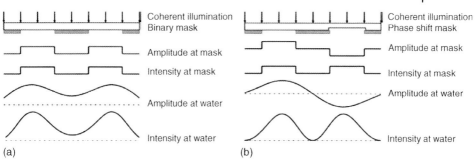

Figure 1.3 Alternating-phase shift masks. (a) Superposition of aerial image amplitudes for coherent illumination of a binary mask; (b) Superposition of aerial image amplitudes for coherent illumination of an alternating-phase shift mask.

The required phase shifter thickness is given by:

$$t = \frac{\lambda}{2(n-1)}$$

where n is the index of refraction of the shifter material. For typical conditions with $n = 1.5$, the phase shifter thickness is the same as the exposure wavelength.

The general concept of phase-shifting lithography is illustrated schematically in Figure 1.3. Phase masks may be used in both projection and contact mode photolithographic techniques, with the achievable photolithographic resolution being approximately $-\lambda/4n$, where λ is the wavelength of the exposure light and n is the refractive index of the photoresist. In fact, feature lines as narrow as 50 nm have been generated in this way [25, 26], with the resolution achieved corresponding approximately to $\lambda/5$. One improved approach to conformal near-field photolithography is to use masks constructed from "soft" organic elastomeric polymers.

Attenuated Phase-Shift Masks. Attenuated PSM lithography improves the pattern fidelity by "darkening" the edges of shapes through the destructive interference of light, using a mildly translucent photomask. Now commonly called "embedded attenuated phase masks," mask substrates are used that allow a small amount of light (∼7–10%) to penetrate the normally opaque mask regions. Terazawa and coworkers have developed a significantly different implementation of the PSM concept, which is often referred to as the embedded attenuated phase-shifting mask (EAPSM) [27]. The attenuated PSM functions with the same basic interference principles as the alternating PSM, but the details are totally different: some sketches of the attenuated PSM enhancement mechanism are shown in Figure 1.4.

Due to their simpler construction and operation – particularly in combination with optimized illumination for memory patterns – attenuated PSMs are already widely used. Although alternating PSMs are more difficult to manufacture, and this has slowed their adoption, their use is becoming more widespread. For example, the alternating PSM technique is currently being used by Intel to print gates for their 65 nm and subsequent node transistors [28, 29].

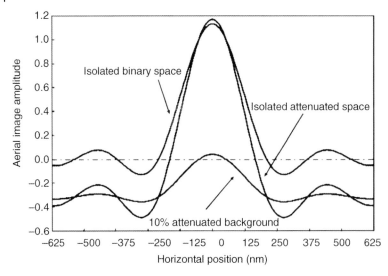

Figure 1.4 Attenuated-phase shift masks: Superposition of aerial image amplitudes for coherent illumination.

1.2.1.5 Optical Proximity Correction (OPC)

Optical proximity correction, as a photolithography enhancement technique, is frequently used to compensate for image errors caused by diffraction or process effects. The need for OPC applies mainly to the creation of semiconductor devices, the main reason for which is the limitation of light to resolve ever-finer details of patterns on the photomasks used to etch semiconductor passivation layers, and the difficulty in creating the building blocks of the transistors and other elements that constitute ICs. These projected images appeared as irregularities such as rounded corners, and with trace widths that were narrower than designed. If the diffraction effects could not be compensated, then the electrical properties of the fabricated unit would be significantly altered due to these distortions. OPC anticipates the irregularities of shape and size, and applies a corrective compensation to the photo mask images, which then produce a light beam that more closely approximates the intended shapes.

The two most common applications for OPC are line width differences between features in regions of different density (e.g., center versus edge of an array, or nested versus isolated lines), and line end shortening (e.g., gate overlap on a field oxide). In the case of the line width differences, scattering bars (subresolution lines placed adjacent to resolvable lines) or simple line width adjustments are applied to the design. For line end shortening, "dog-ear" (serif or hammerhead) features are attached to the line end in the design. OPC has a cost impact on photomask fabrication, as the addition of OPC features means more spots for defects to manifest themselves. Additionally, when using OPC the data size of the photomask layout will rise exponentially.

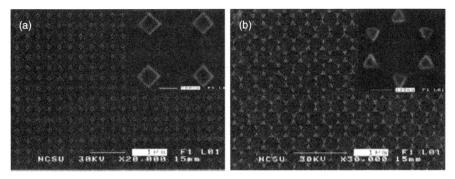

Figure 1.5 (a) Diamond shape pattern with the size of 80 nm × 80 nm and periods of 300 nm; (b) triangular shape pattern with the size is ~73 nm and periods of 159 nm.

The OPC process is started by characterizing the patterning operation and all its inaccuracies from various sources, such as the mask build, wafer exposure, etch, and so on. In the now commonplace "model-based OPC," this mathematical description of the process is used in iterative optimization routines to predistort the mask shapes to compensate for known, systematic, and modeled patterning inaccuracies.

The OPC technique improves the "effective resolution" of a patterning process by overlapping the conditions with which different feature types can be imaged accurately. Nested features typically image on-size and with the best image quality at a different exposure dose than do isolated features. However, both feature types can be imaged adequately in a single exposure by biasing the mask patterns appropriately. However, OPC does not alter the fundamental resolution limits of a lithography system.

The in-plane anisotropic nanostructures fabricated by using deep UV lithography are shown in Figure 1.5. In this case, Figure 1.5a shows an 80 nm × 80 nm (113 nm axis length) diamond-shaped pattern with a 300 nm period, while Figure 1.5b shows the triangle-shaped pattern [30].

1.2.2
Electron Beam Lithography

Electron-beam lithography (EBL; also termed E-beam lithography) involves scanning a beam of electrons in a patterned fashion across a surface covered with a resist [31]. The first EBL system was developed during the late 1960s, and was based on the principle of scanning electron microscopy (SEM). Because of its excellent high resolution and flexibility, EBL represents a specialized technique for creating the extremely fine patterns required by the modern electronics industry for use in ICs [32–35].

Typically, a EBL system consists of the following parts: (i) an electron gun or electron source that supplies the electrons; (ii) an electron column that "shapes" and focuses the electron beam; (iii) a mechanical stage that positions the wafer under the electron beam; (iv) a wafer handling system that automatically feeds wafers to the system and unloads them after processing; and (v) a computer system that controls the equipment.

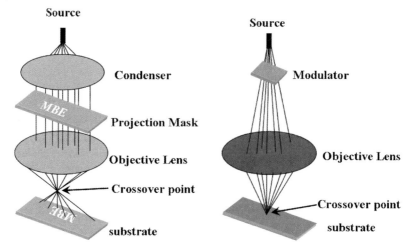

Figure 1.6 Schematic diagram of direct write and project printing.

In general, two distinct schemes are used in EBL:

- *Projection printing*, in which a relatively large-sized electron beam pattern is projected in parallel through the mask onto a resist-coated substrate by using a high-precision lens system.
- *Direct writing*, in which a small spot of the electron beam is written directly onto a resist-coated substrate, thus eliminating the expensive and time-consuming production of masks.

The principles of direct write and project printing are illustrated schematically in Figure 1.6.

EBL displays certain *advantages* over conventional photolithography techniques:

- It is capable of very high resolution, almost to the atomic level. Typically, EBL has a three orders of magnitude better resolution, although this is limited by the forward scattering of electrons in the resist layer, and back scattering from the underlying substrate.
- It is a flexible technique that can function with a wide variety of materials and an almost infinite number of patterns.

Unfortunately, however, EBL has certain *disadvantages*. Notably, it is slow in operation, being one or more orders of magnitude slower than optical lithography. Perhaps more importantly, however, it is expensive and complicated, with EBL systems costing many millions of dollars to purchase and requiring frequent servicing to maintain performance. Yet, despite these drawbacks, EBL currently represents the most powerful tool for the fabrication of features as small as 3–5 nm [36, 37].

Today, EBL is used principally in support of the IC industry, where it has three niche markets:

- In mask-making, typically the chrome-on-glass masks used by optical lithography tools. EBL is the preferred technique for masks because of its flexibility in providing a rapid turn-around of a finished part described only by a computer CAD file. The ability to meet stringent line width control and pattern placement specifications, on the order of 50 nm each, is a remarkable achievement.
- In direct writing for the advanced prototyping of ICs [38] and the manufacture of small-volume specialty products, such as gallium arsenide ICs and optical waveguides.
- For research into the scaling limits of ICs [39] and studies of quantum effects and other novel physics phenomena, at very small dimensions.

Since it is impossible to deflect an electron beam to cover a large area, in a typical EBL system mechanical stages are required to move the substrate through the deflection field of the electron beam column. Stages can be operated in a stepping mode in which the stage is stopped, an area of the pattern written, and the stage then moved to a new location where an adjacent pattern area is exposed. Alternatively, stages can be operated in a continuous mode where the pattern is written on the substrate while the stage is moving. Figure 1.7 shows SEM images of dots with a 15 nm diameter and a 35 nm pitch ($64\,mC\,cm^{-2}$) fabricated in a 30 nm calixarene resist layer on a Si substrate at 50 keV acceleration voltage [40].

1.2.3
X-Ray Lithography

X-rays with wavelengths in the range of 0.04 to 0.5 nm represent another alternative radiation source with the potential for high-resolution pattern replication into

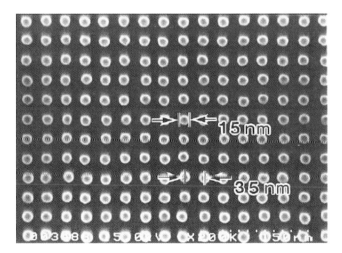

Figure 1.7 Scanning electron microscopy image of 15 nm dots at a pitch of 35 nm written in 30 nm-thick calixarene resist [40].

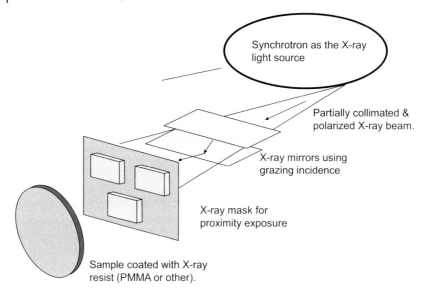

Figure 1.8 Schematic of X-ray lithography.

polymeric resist materials [41]. X-ray lithography was first shown to produce high-resolution patterns, using X-ray proximity printing, by Spears and Smith [42]. Although X-ray lithography uses the same procedure as optical lithography and EBL, an X-ray source is applied rather than using UV light or an electron beam. It would seem that X-ray lithography represents a next-generation lithography developed for the semiconductor industry, as its novel technology can be used in the same capacities as optical lithography, but with better results.

The principle of X-ray lithography is shown schematically in Figure 1.8. Basically, X-ray lithography is a shadow printing process in which patterns coated on a mask are transferred into a third dimension in a resist material, normally poly (methyl methacrylate) (PMMA). The essential ingredients in X-ray lithography include:

- A shadow mask, prepared on a thin membrane of X-ray transmitting material consisting of patterns made from an X-ray absorbing material.
- An X-ray sensitive material, which serves as the X-ray resist of high resolution and is suitable for the subsequent fabrication.
- An X-ray source of sufficient brightness in the suitable region to expose the resist through the mask.

The X-ray radiation sources represent important factors in this type of lithography, and may be generated in several ways, including: (i) by electron bombardment; (ii) by electron impact; (iii) via synchrotron sources; and (iv) as laser-generated plasmas as X-ray sources, among which synchrotron radiation sources are by far the brightest sources of soft X-rays [43–47].

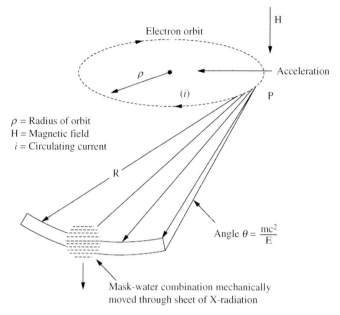

ρ = Radius of orbit
H = Magnetic field
i = Circulating current

Figure 1.9 Schematic diagram of an X-ray exposure station with a synchrotron radiation source.

Synchrotron radiation is emitted by high-energy relativistic electrons in a synchrotron or storage ring, and then accelerated normal to the direction of their motion by a magnetic field. This leads to the production of a range of electrons over the entire electromagnetic spectrum, from radiowaves to infrared (IR) light, visible light, UV light, X-rays, and gamma rays. Synchrotron or storage rings, which produce a broad spectrum of radiation stemming from the energy loss of electrons in motion at relativistic energies, have been developed primarily for experiments in high-energy physics. A schematic of an X-ray exposure station with a synchrotron radiation source is shown in Figure 1.9, where the X-ray radiation opening angle, θ, is tangential to the path of the electron describing a line on an intersecting substrate.

X-ray proximity lithography is known to provide a one-to-one replication of the features patterned on the mask, and the resolution limit of the X-ray lithography is ~25 nm [48]. The first components to be created using X-ray lithography were surface acoustic wave devices [49], and this was soon followed by bipolar [50] and metal oxide semiconductor (MOS) transistors [51]. The first sub-100 nm Si transistors were produced using X-ray lithography [52], and a velocity overshoot was observed as well as transconductances greater than $1\,\mathrm{S\,mm^{-1}}$ [53]. A wide variety of sub 100 nm quantum-effect devices have been fabricated using X-ray lithography [54], including those in which the Coulomb-blockade effect was first observed [55]; this has led to what is often referred to as the "single-electron transistor".

The SEM images of 35 nm-wide Au lines and 20 nm-wide W dots fabricated by electroplating and reactive ion etching, in combination with X-ray lithography, are shown in Figure 1.10 [56].

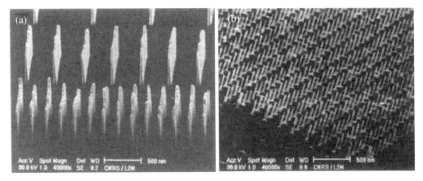

Figure 1.10 (a) 35 nm-wide Au lines grown by electroplating using a template fabricated by X-ray lithography. The mean thickness is about 450 nm, which corresponds to an aspect ratio close to 13; (b) 20 nm-wide W dots obtained after reactive ion etching of a 1250 nm-thick W layer [16].

1.2.4
Focused Ion Beam (FIB) Lithography

During the past few decades, a wide variety of nanofabrication techniques using photons, electrons, and ions have been investigated, and today focused ion-beam (FIB) technology represents one of the most promising techniques for nanofabrication, due to its great flexibility and simplicity.

Since the introduction of FIB technology to the semiconductor industry during the early 1980s, various applications have been developed for both the removal (direct ion milling, FIB chemical etching) and deposition (ion implantation, FIB chemical deposition) of a number of conductor and isolator materials, with sub-micron precision [57]. The FIB technique has also been rapidly developed into a very attractive tool for lithography, etching, deposition, and doping [58]. Because of the matching of ion and atom masses, the energy transfer efficiency of the ion beam to resist is significantly greater than with electron beams. Coupled with the fact that a focusing ion system typically operates at elevated potentials (up to 150 kV), the effective sensitivity charge per unit area of ion beams is two to three orders of magnitude higher than for electron beams, ion-beam lithography has long been recognized as offering an improved resolution [59, 60], and has also shown promise for high-resolution microfabrication [61]. When compared to EBL, FIB lithography has the advantages of a high resist exposure sensitivity, negligible ion scattering in the resist, and low back-scattering from the substrate [62].

Among the different FIB processes, direct-write milling and the dry development of FIB-implanted resists have been widely investigated for both the microfabrication and nanofabrication of advanced IC devices [63, 64].

1.2.4.1 Direct-Write Milling
The direct-write milling of the substrate by FIB represents the simplest process for pattern fabrication. In this method, the resists are eliminated and the dose of ions can be varied as a function of position on the wafer. The technique also utilizes heavy-ion

species such as Ga^+ and Au^+. Direct FIB milling has also been applied for lithography mask repair and circuit microsurgery, with resolution down to 100 nm [65]. Moreover, any opaque defects, such as any excess metal on the chromium-based masks, can simply be milled off, while clear defects can be repaired by milling a light-scattering structure (prism) into the area to be rendered opaque. FIB milling has also been applied to bilayer-structure lithography, in which a thin film of gold is usually deposited on top of the conventional resist [64].

1.2.4.2 Dry Development FIB Lithography

Dry development FIB lithography will also yield high aspect ratio structures, with nanometer resolution [63, 66, 67]. Likewise, FIB lithography may be combined with dry development processes by using the well-known top surface imaging (TSI) technique [68], which eliminates the need for wet processing and thus avoids any pattern deformation due to swelling. The limited penetration range of ions is a perfect match for the TSI processes, in which the surface of the resist is selectively manipulated by exposure to silicon-containing chemicals, so as to withstand oxygen dry development in unexposed areas [68, 69]. Other TSI processes utilize the dry development of ion-beam-irradiated resists for negative image formation in exposed areas [60, 70]. In these studies, PMMA resist regions implanted with different ion species (such as Ga^+ and Si^+) have demonstrated significant reductions in the etching rates during the oxygen reactive ion etching (RIE) process. The ion-beam-inhibited etching phenomenon can be explained on the basis of the formation of stable oxide layers during the etching process (i.e., Ga_2O_3 and SiO_2) [64]. Another explanation for etch resistance occurring in the implanted resist regions is the concept of a *physical hardening* of the resist [67]. According to this interpretation, the incident ions may break chemical bonds within the photoresist resin by sputtering the hydrogen and oxygen atoms away, which in turn results in the formation of a stable, carbon-rich "graphitized" structure.

1.3
Two-Dimensional Nanostructures: Thin-Film Deposition

Generally, the term "thin film" is applied to layers which have thicknesses on the order of microns or less, but which may be as thin as a few atomic layers. The deposition of thin films has been the subject of intensive study for almost a century, and a wide range of appropriate methods have been developed and improved. Today, electronic semiconductor devices and optical coatings are the main applications to benefit from thin-film construction. Although many excellent textbooks and monographs have been published on this topic [71–73], in this section a brief introduction of the fundamentals will be provided, and the typical experimental approaches of various well-established techniques of film deposition summarized.

Depending on the depositing process, film growth methods can be generally divided into two broad categories, namely *physical deposition* and *chemical deposition*. The former processes (often just called thin-film processes) are atomistic deposition processes in which material is vaporized from a solid or liquid source in the form of atoms or molecules, and include evaporation, molecular beam epitaxy (MBE), sputtering, pulsed laser deposition, and cathodic arc deposition. In contrast, the latter processes are based on chemical reactions that include chemical vapor deposition (CVD), plasma-enhanced chemical deposition (PECVD) and atomic layer deposition (ALD). Recently, a considerable number of novel processes that utilize a combination of different methods have been developed. This combination allows a more defined control and tailoring of the microstructure and properties of thin films. Typical processes include ion beam-assisted deposition (IBAD) and plasma-enhanced CVD (PECVD).

1.3.1
Fundamentals of Film Growth

The growth of thin films, as with all phase transformations, involves the processes of nucleation and growth on the substrate or growth surfaces. The nucleation process plays a very important role in determining the crystallinity and microstructure of the resultant films. Lattice mismatch has a marked effect on film morphology, as strain resulting from lattice mismatch contributes to the interface energy, which is a key parameter in determining the growth mode. In general, nucleation in film formation is a heterogeneous process, although the surface free energies for the substrate and film materials also influence the mode of growth. Depending on the resulting film morphology, the growth modes have been placed into three categories [74]:

- Frank–van der Merwe (FM) or layer-by-layer growth
- Volmer–Weber (VW) or 3-D island growth
- Stranski–Krastanow (SK) or 3-D island-on-wetting-layer growth.

These three basic modes of initial nucleation in film growth are illustrated in Figure 1.11.

In the FM growth mode, the interatomic interactions between the substrate and film materials are stronger and more attractive than those between the different atomic species within the film material; this results in the first complete monolayer being formed before deposition of the second layer occurs. The most important examples of layer growth mode are the epitaxial growth of single crystal films.

(a)   (b)   (c)

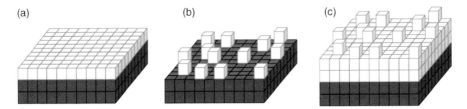

Figure 1.11   Basic modes of initial nucleation in the film growth. (a) Frank–van der Merwe mode (two-dimensional growth mode); (b) Volmer–Weber mode (Island growth mode); (c) Stranski–Krastanov mode.

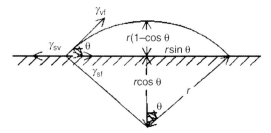

Figure 1.12 Schematic illustrating heterogeneous nucleation process with all related surface energy in equilibrium.

The VW growth mode contrasts with the FM growth mode, with the growth species being bound more strongly to each other than to the substrate; in this way, the islands that are formed initially will finally coalesce to form a continuous film. Many systems of metals on insulator substrates, alkali halides, graphite and mica substrates display this type of nucleation during the initial film deposition.

The SK growth mode occurs for interaction strengths somewhere in between FM and VW, where the layer growth and island growth are combined in intermediate fashion. This type of growth mode typically involves the stress that is developed during the formation of either nuclei or films.

When a new phase forms on a surface of another material, the process is termed "heterogeneous nucleation." The film deposition involves predominantly heterogeneous processes that include heterogeneous chemical reactions, evaporation, adsorption and desorption on growth surfaces, which in turn involves a heterogeneous nucleation at the initial stage. Provided that the growth species in the vapor phase impinge on the substrate surface, these growth species will diffuse and aggregate to form a nucleus with a cap shape, as illustrated in Figure 1.12. During formation of the thin film the Gibbs free energy and the surface energy will be increased, with the change in chemical energy, ΔG, which is associated with formation of the nucleus, given by:

$$\Delta G = a_3 r^3 \Delta u_v + a_1 r^2 \gamma_{vf} + a_2 r^2 \gamma_{fs} - a_2 r^2 \gamma_{sv}$$

where r is the mean dimension of the nucleus, Δu_v is the change of Gibbs free energy per unit volume, and γ_{vf}, γ_{fs} and γ_{sv} are the surface or interface energies of the vapor–nucleus, nucleus–substrate, and substrate–vapor interfaces, respectively. The geometric constants are given by:

$$a_1 = 2\pi(1 - \cos\theta)$$
$$a_2 = \pi \sin^2\theta$$
$$a_3 = 3\pi(2 - 3\cos\theta + \cos^2\theta)$$

where θ is the contact angle, which is dependent only on the surface properties of the surfaces or interfaces involved, and is defined by Young's equation:

$$\gamma_{sv} = \gamma_{fs} + \gamma_{vf} \cos\theta$$

The formation of new phase results in a reduction of the Gibbs free energy, but an increase in the total surface energy. The nucleus is stable only when its size is larger than the critical size, γ^* and the critical energy barrier, ΔG^*, is illustrated respectively:

$$\gamma^* = \frac{-2(a_1\gamma_{vf} + a_2\gamma_{fs} - a_2\gamma_{sv})}{3a_3\Delta G_v}$$

$$\Delta G^* = \frac{4(a_1\gamma_{vf} + a_2\gamma_{fs} - a_2\gamma_{sv})^3}{27a_3^2\Delta G_v}$$

As with the FM growth mode, the substrate is completely wetted by the depositing materials, in which case the contact angle will be equal to zero; thus, the corresponding Young's equation could be described as:

$$\gamma_{sv} = \gamma_{fs} + \gamma_{vf}$$

For island growth, the contact angle, θ, must be larger than zero. According to Young's equation, we then have:

$$\gamma_{sv} < \gamma_{fs} + \gamma_{vf}$$

In case the deposit does not wet the substrate at all, the contact angle will be 180 °C, a process which is commonly referred to as *homogeneous nucleation*.

The lattice constants of the deposit will most likely differ from those of the substrate, which commonly leads to the development of stress in the newly forming film, and a resultant island-layer growth mode. Island-layer growth involves *in situ*-developed stress, and is slightly more complicated than the above two growth modes. The thin film would proceed following the mode of layer growth initially, but when the deposit became elastically strained – due to, for example, a lattice mismatch between the deposit and the substrate – then strain energy would be developed. As each layer of the deposit continues, more stress and strain energy would be developed. Given that there is no plastic relaxation, the strain energy would be proportional to the volume of the deposit. Then, as the growth of the film continued the stress would reach a critical point and could not be released; the strain energy per unit area of deposit would then be large with respect to γ_{vf}, permitting nuclei to form above the initial layered deposit. In this case, the surface energy of the substrate would exceed the combination of both surface energy of the deposit and the interfacial energy between the substrate and the deposit:

$$\gamma_{sv} > \gamma_{fs} + \gamma_{vf}$$

1.3.2
Physical Vapor Deposition (PVD)

Physical vapor deposition (PVD) is fundamentally a vaporization coating technique that involves the transfer of material on an atomic level. The process can be described according to the following sequence of steps: (i) the material to be deposited is converted into a vapor by physical means; (ii) the vapor is transported across a region of low pressure from its source to the substrate; and (iii) the vapor undergoes condensation on the substrate to form the thin film. Typically, PVD processes are used to deposit films with thicknesses in the range of a few nanometers to thousands of nanometers. However, they can also be used to form multilayer coatings, graded composition deposits, very thick deposits, and freestanding structures.

PVD thin film technology covers a rather broad range of deposition techniques, including electron-beam or hot-boat evaporation, reactive evaporation, and ion plating. PVD techniques also include processes based on sputtering, whether by plasma or by an ion beam of some sort. PVD is also used to describe the deposition from arc sources which may or may not be filtered. In general, the methods can be divided into two groups, namely *evaporation* and *sputtering*. Evaporation refers to thin films being deposited by thermal means, whereas in sputtering mode the atoms or molecules are dislodged from the solid target through the impact of gaseous ions (plasma). Both methods have been further developed into a number of specific techniques.

1.3.2.1 Vacuum Evaporation

The formation of thin films by evaporation was first recognized about 150 years ago [75], and has since acquired a wide range of applications, notably in the past fifty years since industrial-scale vacuum techniques were developed [76]. Many excellent books and reviews have been produced describing evaporated films [77]. Vacuum evaporation (or vacuum deposition) is a PVD process in which the atoms or molecules from a thermal vaporization source reach the substrate without colliding with residual gas molecules in the deposition chamber. Vacuum deposition normally requires a vacuum of better than 10^{-4} Torr; however, even at such low pressure there will still be a large amount of concurrent impingement on the substrate by potentially undesirable residual gases that can contaminate the film. If film contamination is problematic, a high (10^{-7} Torr) or ultrahigh ($<10^{-9}$ Torr) vacuum environment can be used to produce a film with the desired purity, depending on the deposition rate, the reactivities of the residual gases and the depositing species, and the tolerable impurity level in the deposit. The evaporation of elemental metals is fairly straightforward: heated metals have high vapor pressures, and in a high vacuum (HV) the evaporated atoms will be transported to the substrate. A schematic image of a typical evaporation system is shown in Figure 1.13.

A typical evaporation system will consist of an evaporation source to vaporize the desired material, and a substrate located at an appropriate distance, facing the evaporation source. Both, the source and the substrate, are located in a vacuum chamber.

The saturation or equilibrium vapor pressure of a material is defined as the vapor pressure of that material in equilibrium with the solid or liquid surface, in a closed container. At equilibrium, as many atoms return to the surface as leave the surface, such that the equilibrium vapor pressure of an element can be estimated as:

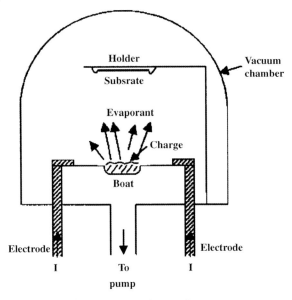

Figure 1.13   Schematic image of a typical evaporation system.

$$\ln P_e = -\frac{\Delta H_e}{RT} + C$$

where ΔH_e is the molar heat of evaporation, R is the gas constant, T is the temperature, and C is a constant.

Although most elements vaporize as atoms, some – such as Sb, Sn, C, and Se – have a significant portion of the vaporized species as clusters of atoms. For materials which evaporate as clusters, special vaporization sources (called *baffle sources*) can be used to ensure that the depositing vapor is in the form of atoms. The evaporation of compounds is more complicated, as compounds may undergo chemical reactions such as pyrolysis, decomposition and dissociation, and the resultant vapor composition may often differ from the source composition during evaporation at elevated temperatures. It should be noted that, as a material is heated, the first components to be volatilized are the high-vapor-pressure surface contaminates, absorbed gases, and high-vapor-pressure impurities.

A material vaporizes freely from a surface when the vaporized material leaves the surface with no collisions above the surface. The free surface vaporization rate is proportional to the vapor pressure, and is given by the Hertz–Knudsen vaporization equation [78, 79]:

$$\frac{dN}{dt} = C\,(2\,\pi m k T)\text{-}\frac{1}{2}\,(p^*\text{-}p)\,\text{s}^{-1}$$

where dN is the number of evaporating atoms per cm^2 of surface area, C is a constant that depends on the rotational degrees of freedom in the liquid and the vapor, p^* is the vapor pressure of the material at temperature T, p is the pressure of the vapor above the surface, k is Boltzmann's constant, T is the absolute temperature, and m is the mass of the vaporized species.

According to Raoult's law, the constituents of a mixture of elements or compounds vaporize in a ratio that is proportional to their vapor pressures; that is, a constituent with a high vapor pressure will vaporize more rapidly than a material with a low vapor pressure [78, 79]. Thus, the chemical composition of the vapor phase is most likely to be different from that in the source, although adjusting the composition or molar ratio of the constituents in the source may help in this respect. However, the composition of the source would change as the evaporation proceeds, with the higher vapor pressure material steadily decreasing in proportion to the lower vapor pressure material in the melt. As a result, the composition in the vapor phase will change. For a multi-component system, the chemical composition of evaporated film is likely to produce a gradation of film composition as the evaporant is selectively vaporized. Therefore, it is in general difficult to deposit complex films using an evaporation method.

However, vacuum deposition does have advantages in some cases:

- Line-of-sight deposition allows the use of masks to define area of deposition.
- Large-area sources can be used for some materials (e.g., "hog trough" crucibles for Al and Zn).
- High deposition rates can be obtained.
- Deposition rate monitoring is relatively easy.
- The vaporization source material can exist in many forms, such as chunks, powder, wire, and chips.
- A vaporization source material of high purity is relatively inexpensive.
- High-purity films are easily deposited from high-purity source materials, as the deposition ambient can be made as noncontaminating as is desired.
- The technique is relatively inexpensive compared to other PVD methods.

1.3.2.2 Molecular Beam Epitaxy (MBE)

Perhaps the most sophisticated PVD process is that of MBE or vapor-phase epitaxy (VPE) [80–82], which take place in either high-vacuum or ultra-high-vacuum environments (10^{-8} Pa) [83–85]. The most important aspect of MBE is the slow deposition rate (typically $<1000 \, \text{nm} \, \text{h}^{-1}$), which allows the films to grow epitaxially. The slow deposition rates require (proportionally) a better vacuum to achieve the same impurity levels as other deposition techniques. Hence, MBE can be considered a special case of evaporation for single-crystal film growth, with the highly controlled evaporation of a variety of sources in ultra-high-vacuum.

Figure 1.14 shows, schematically, a number of effusion cells aligned radially with the substrates. Since MBE is a variant of evaporation, instead of an open crucible the source material can be heated in an equilibrium source known as the Knudsen cell. In this case, an atomic beam (in the molecular flow regime; hence the name MBE) exits the cell through an orifice that is small compared to the source size. Such equilibrium sources are much more stable than open sources, because they are heated resistively or by an electron beam. In high vacuum, the evaporated atoms do not experience

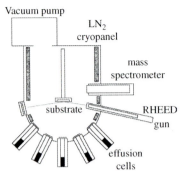

Figure 1.14 Schematic diagram of a number of effusion cells aligned radially with the substrates. LN_2 = liquid nitrogen; RHEED = reflection high-energy electron diffraction.

collisions, and therefore will take a line-of-sight route from the source to the substrate. The mean free path of atoms or molecules ($\sim$100 m) far exceeds the distance between the source and the substrate (typically $\sim$30 cm) inside the deposition chamber; therefore, the atoms or molecules striking on the single crystal substrate will result in formation of the desired epitaxial film.

Atoms arriving at the substrate surface may undergo absorption to the surface, surface migration, incorporation into the crystal lattice, and thermal desorption, but which of these competing pathways dominates the growth will depend heavily on the temperature of the substrate. At a low temperature, atoms will "stick" where they land without arranging properly, leading to poor crystal quality; however, at a high temperature the atoms will desorb (re-evaporate) readily from the surface, leading to low growth rates and a poor crystal quality. In the appropriate intermediate temperature range, the atoms will have sufficient energy to move to the proper position on the surface and be incorporated into the growing crystal. The growth mechanism of MBE is shown schematically in Figure 1.15.

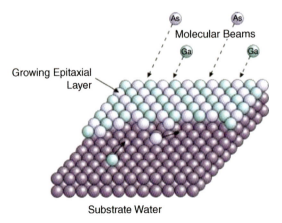

Figure 1.15 The molecular beam epitaxy growth mechanism.

During the MBE process, a range of structural and analytical probes can be used to monitor film growth *in situ*, in real time, on a sub-nanometer scale:

- Reflection high-energy electron diffraction (RHEED), using forward scattering at the grazing angle; this shows a maximum when there is a completed monolayer, and a minimum when there is a partial layer, which produces more scattering.
- Low-energy electron diffraction (LEED) takes place in backscattering geometry, and can be used to study surface morphology, but not during growth.
- Auger electron spectroscopy (AES), records the type of atoms present.
- Modulated beam mass spectrometry (MBMS) allows the chemical species and reaction kinetics to be studied.
- Reflectance difference spectroscopy (RDS).
- Scanning tunneling microscopy (STM) and atomic force microscopy (AFM).

1.3.2.3 Sputter Deposition

Sputtering is one of the most important PVD methods, as it involves the physical vaporization of atoms from a surface by momentum transfer from bombarding, energetic, atomic-sized particles. Sputter deposition permits a better control of the composition of multi-element films, and a greater flexibility in the types of materials that may be deposited.

Although first reported by Wright in 1877, the sputter deposition of films became feasible only because a relatively poor vacuum is needed for its operation. Despite the fact that Edison patented a sputter deposition process for depositing silver onto wax photograph cylinders in 1904, the process was not used widely in industry until the advent of magnetron sputtering in 1974. The application of sputter deposition led to an acceleration in the development of reproducible, stable long-lived vaporization sources for production purposes. Following the use of a magnetic field that would confine the motion of the secondary electrons close to the target surface, planar magnetron sputtering has become the most widely used sputtering configuration, having been derived originally from the development of the microwave klystron tube in World War II, from the investigations of Kesaev and Pashkova (in 1959) on confining arcs, and of Chapin (in 1974) on developing the planar magnetron sputtering source [86–89]. The operating principles of both direct current (DC) and radio-frequency (RF) sputtering systems are illustrated schematically in Figure 1.16 [71].

Effective sputter deposition can be achieved in:

- a good vacuum ($<10^{-5}$ Torr) using ion beams;
- a low-pressure gas environment, where sputtered particles are transported from the target to the substrate without gas-phase collisions (i.e., a pressure less than about 5 mTorr), using a plasma as the ion source of ions; and
- a higher-pressure gas, where gas phase collisions and "thermalization" of the ejected particles occurs but the pressure is low enough that gas-phase nucleation is not important (i.e., a pressure greater than about 5 mTorr but less than about 50 mTorr).

Currently, plasma-based sputtering is the most common form of sputtering, in which a plasma is present and positive ions are accelerated to the target which is at

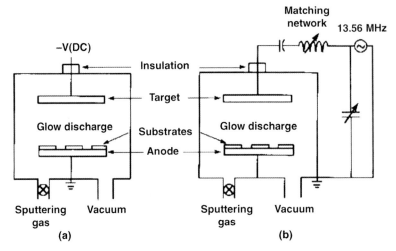

Figure 1.16 Schematic diagram of the principles of (a) direct current (DC) and (b) radiofrequency (RF) sputtering systems.

a negative potential with respect to the plasma. At higher pressures, the ions suffer physical collisions and charge-exchange collisions, so that there is a spectrum of energies of the ions and neutrals bombarding the target surface. At low pressures, the ions reach the target surface with an energy which is given by the potential drop between the surface and the point in the electric field where the ion is formed. In vacuum-based sputtering, however, an ion or plasma beam is formed in a separate ionization source, accelerated, and then extracted into a processing chamber which is maintained under good vacuum conditions. In this process, the mean bombarding energy is generally higher than in the plasma-based bombardment, and the reflected high-energy neutrals are more energetic.

Sputter deposition could be used to deposit films of elemental materials, and also to deposit alloy films and maintain the composition of the target material. This is possible by virtue of the fact that the material is removed from the target in a layer-by-layer fashion, which is one of the main advantages of the process. This allows the deposition of some rather complex alloys such as W : Ti for semiconductor metal-lization [90], Al : Si : Cu for semiconductor metallization [91], and Metal–Cr–Al–Y alloys for aircraft turbine blade coatings.

The deposition of films of compound materials by sputtering can be achieved either by sputtering from a compound target, or by sputtering from an elemental target in a partial pressure of a reactive gas (i.e., "reactive sputter deposition"). In most cases, the sputter deposition of a compound material from a compound target results in a loss of some of the more volatile material (e.g., oxygen from SiO_2); however, this loss is often made up by deposition in an ambient containing a partial pressure of the reactive gas – a process known as "quasi-reactive sputter deposition." In the latter case, the partial pressure of reactive gas that is needed is less than that used for reactive sputter deposition.

The advantages of sputter deposition include:

- Any material can be sputtered and deposited, including elements, alloys, or compounds.
- The sputtering target provides a stable, long-lived vaporization source.
- Vaporization is from a solid surface and can occur up, down, or sideways.
- In some configurations, the sputtering target can provide a large-area vaporization source.
- In some configurations, the sputtering target can provide specific vaporization geometries, for example, a line source from a planar magnetron sputtering source.
- The sputtering target can be made conformal to a substrate surface, such as a cone or sphere.
- Sputtering conditions can easily be reproduced from run to-run.
- There is little radiant heating in the system compared to vacuum evaporation.
- In a reactive deposition, the reactive species can be activated in a plasma.
- When using chemical vapor precursors, the molecules can be either fully or partially dissociated in the plasma.
- The utilization of sputtered material can be high.
- *In situ* surface preparation is easily incorporated into the processing.

1.3.3
Chemical Vapor Deposition (CVD)

Chemical vapor deposition (CVD) is a method of forming a thin solid film on a substrate by the reaction of vapor-phase chemicals which contain the required constituents. The decomposition of source gases is induced by various energy forms such as chemical, thermal, plasma or photon, and reacted on and/or above the temperature-controlled surface to form the thin film. *Thermal CVD* is the deposition of atoms or molecules by the high-temperature (range from 300 to 900 °C) reduction or decomposition of chemical vapor precursor species which contain the material to be deposited [92–94]. Normally, the reduction is accomplished by hydrogen at an elevated temperature, while the decomposition is accomplished by thermal activation. The deposited material may react with other gaseous species in the system to produce compounds (e.g., oxides, nitrides). In general, CVD processing is accompanied by volatile reaction byproducts and unused precursor species. The CVD process has been studied extensively and is very well documented [95–97], largely due to the close association with solid-state microelectronics.

In CVD the source materials are brought in a gas phase flow into the vicinity of the substrate, where they decompose and react to deposit the film onto the substrate. Any gaseous byproducts are then pumped away, as shown schematically in Figure 1.17.

The CVD process can be generalized in a sequence of steps:

- Reactants are introduced into reactor;
- The gas species are activated and/or dissociated by mixing, heat, plasma or other means.

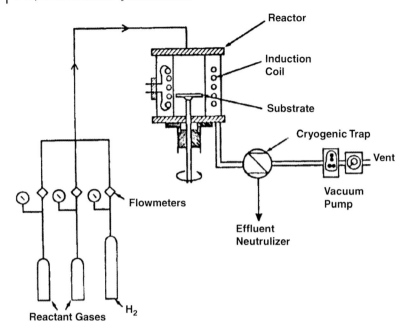

Figure 1.17 The chemical vapor deposition (CVD) process. The source materials are brought in gas phase flow into the vicinity of the substrate, where they decompose and react to deposit film on the substrate. Both, gas-phase transport and surface chemical reactions are important for film deposition.

- The reactive species are adsorbed on the substrate surface.
- The adsorbed species undergo chemical reaction or react with other incoming species to form a solid film.
- The reaction byproducts are desorbed from the substrate surface.
- The reaction byproduct is removed from the reactor.

Due to the versatile nature of CVD, the number of potential chemistries leading to the commonly used films is huge; details of those chemistries that have been, and still are, widely used are listed in Table 1.2. The gas-phase (homogeneous) reactions and surface (heterogeneous) reactions are intricately mixed, but with increasing temperature and partial pressure of the reactants the gas-phase reactions will become progressively more important. Extremely high concentrations of the reactants will cause the gas-phase reactions to become predominant, resulting in homogeneous nucleation. The wide variety of chemical reactions involved can be grouped into: pyrolysis; reduction; oxidation; compound formation; disproportionation; and reversible transfer, depending on the precursors used and the deposition conditions applied.

1.3.3.1 Reaction Kinetics

CVD is a nonequilibrium process that is controlled by chemical kinetics and transport phenomena, with the reaction rates obeying Arrhenius behavior. In case

Table 1.2 Reactions used in chemical vapor deposition.

Reaction	Equation
Pyrolysis	SiH_4 (g) → Si (s) + 2 H_2 (g)
Reduction	$SiCl_4$ (g) + 2 H_2 (g) → Si (s) + 4 HCl (g)
Hydrolysis	$SiCl_4$ (g) + 2 H_2 (g) + O_2 (g) → SiO_2 (s) + 4 HCl (g)
Compound formation	$SiCl_4$ (g) + CH_4 (g) → SiC(s) + 4HCl(g)
	$TiCl_4$ (g) + CH_4 (g) → TiC(s) + 4HCl(g)
Disproportionation	2 GeI_2(g) → Ge(s) + $^\bullet GeI_4$(g) at 300 °C
Reversible transfer	As_4(g) + As_2(g) + 6GaCl(g) + 3H_2(g) → 6GaAs(s) + 6HCl(g)

of the deposition rate determined at several temperatures, the activation energy E_a can be extracted from the Arrhenius formula. The magnitude of the activation energy gives hints to possible reaction mechanisms.

For most CVD reactions, two temperature regimes can be found (Figure 1.18). Here, when the temperature is low the surface reaction rate is low, and there is an overabundance of reactants; the reaction is then in the *surface reaction-limited regime*. The rate of silicon nitride deposition from SiH_2Cl_2 at 770 °C is approximately 3.3 nm min^{-1}, but this is compensated by the fact that the deposition can take place simultaneously on up to 100 wafers.

As the temperature increases, the reaction rate on the surface is increased exponentially such that, above a certain temperature, all of the source gas molecules will react at the surface. The reaction is then in the *mass transport-limited regime*, because the rate is dependent on the supply of a new species to the surface. The fluid dynamics of the reactor then plays a major role in both deposition uniformity and the reaction rate.

1.3.3.2 Variants of CVD Methods [98]
The conventional CVD process, which is based on thermally activated CVD, uses inorganic precursor sources, with the deposition process being initiated by thermal

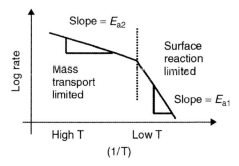

Figure 1.18 Surface reaction-limited versus mass transfer-limited CVD reactions.

energy and occurs at atmospheric pressure, low pressure, or ultrahigh vacuum. The deposition often requires relatively high temperatures (typically 500–1400 °C), depending on the type of inorganic precursor used (e.g., halides, hydrides). According to the forms of energy introduced to the system in order to activate the chemical reactions desired to deposit solid films onto substrates, a variety of CVD methods and CVD reactors have been developed, including PECVD and photo-assisted CVD (PACVD) which use plasma and light, respectively, to activate the chemical reactions. Atomic layer epitaxy (ALE) represents a special mode of CVD where a "monatomic layer" can be grown in sequence by employing sequential saturating surface reactions, while metal–organic CVD (MOCVD) uses a metal–organic precursor rather than an inorganic precursor as used in conventional CVD methods.

These CVD variants are useful when there is a need to control the growth of epitaxial films, and to fabricate tailored molecular structures. Other CVD variants, such as pulsed-injection MOCVD and aerosol-assisted CVD use special precursor generation and delivery systems, unlike conventional CVD; for example, flame-assisted vapor deposition (FAVD) uses a flame source to initiate the chemical reaction and/or heat the substrate. Electrochemical vapor deposition (EVD) represents another variant of CVD that has been tailored to deposit dense films onto porous substrates. In addition, chemical vapor infiltration (CVI) is a form of CVD that has been adapted for the deposition of a dense ceramic matrix during the fabrication of ceramic fiber-reinforced ceramic matrix composites.

Currently emerging low-cost, non-vacuum CVD-based techniques (e.g., aerosol-assisted and flame-assisted CVD) have the potential to be scaled up for large area or mass production. Although most of these variants can also be carried out at either atmospheric or reduced pressure, PACVD must be conducted at low pressure (typically 1.3 to 1333 Pa) in order to generate the plasma.

1.3.3.3 Advantages of CVD

Although CVD is a complex chemical system, it has its distinctive advantages. Notably, the process is gas phase in nature; hence, given a uniform temperature within the coating retort and uniform concentrations of the depositing species, then the rate of deposition will be similar on all surfaces. Consequently, variable shaped surfaces such as screw threads, blind holes and channels or recesses, if provided with reasonable access to the coating powders or gases, can be coated evenly without any build-up on the edges.

In some cases, it is possible to form ductile CVD layers, (e.g., chromizing of low-carbon mild steel). (*Note*: "Chromizing" refers to a type of coating process developed for coinage production, in which chromium is deposited onto mild steel blanks by CVD and diffused into the surface to generate a layer that is, effectively, a ferritic stainless steel.) Given that the processing temperature will normally anneal any hilly ferrous substrate onto which the CVD layer is deposited, it would then become practicable to form, press or bend these components successfully after coating. This is in direct contrast with stainless steel components, which become significantly work-hardened during any forming or pressing, and may cause the rapid wearing of any tooling used in the process.

The high temperatures used during CVD results in a considerable amount of diffusion of the coating into the substrate; consequently, if the thermal expansion coefficients are compatible between the coating and substrate, then the adhesion will be excellent. In many cases the substrate can be heat-treated after CVD coating, with no distress to the coating.

1.3.4
Atomic Layer Deposition (ALD)

Atomic layer deposition (ALD), a unique thin film-deposition technique, is based on the sequential use of a gas-phase chemical process with atomic-scale precision, and differs significantly from other thin film-deposition methods. By keeping the precursors separate throughout the coating process, the thickness of the film grown can be controlled down to the atomic/molecular scale per monolayer [99, 100]. Some excellent reviews have been produced by Ritala and Leskela [101, 102] on the subject of ALD which, in the literature, is also referred to as ALE, atomic layer growth (ALG), atomic-layer CVD (ALCVD), and molecular layer epitaxy (MLE). In comparison with other thin film-deposition techniques, ALD is relatively new and was first used to grow ZnS films [103]. Additional details on ALD were reported during the early 1980s [104–106]. ALD can be considered as a special modification of CVD, or even as a combination of vapor-phase self-assembly and surface reaction. It is similar in terms of its chemistry to CVD, except that in ALD the CVD reaction is broken into two half-reactions; this allows the precursor materials to be kept separate during the reaction, so that they can react with a surface one-at-a-time, in sequential manner.

ALD was developed during the late 1970s, and subsequently introduced worldwide as ALE [107]. The ALD deposition method was mainly developed in response to the need for thin-film electroluminescent (TFEL) flat-panel displays, as these require high-quality dielectric and luminescent films on large-area substrates. Subsequently, interest in ALD increased stepwise during the mid-1990s and 2000s, with interest focused on silicon-based microelectronics. In this respect, reviews produced by Ritala [108] and Kim [109] represent recent key references. Today, both the equipment required for ALD, and the processes, have moved through two generations and are approaching a third generation to be hall-marked by its higher productivity, reliability, and other enhancements. Currently, ALD is considered to be the deposition method with the greatest potential for producing very thin, conformal films and, in particular, an ability to control the thickness and composition of the films at the atomic level. One major driving force in this area has been the recent interest in using ALD to scale down microelectronic devices. In fact, the recently demonstrated ability of ALD to produce outstanding dielectric layers and attracts for the semiconductor industry for use in high-K dielectric materials has led to an acceleration of ALD development. A typical atomic layer deposition system is illustrated schematically in Figure 1.19.

1.3.4.1 ALD Process
The growth of material layers by ALD consists of repeating the following characteristic four steps:

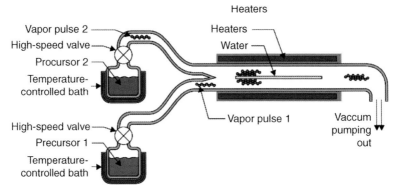

Figure 1.19 Schematic image of a typical atomic layer deposition system.

- Exposure of the first precursor.
- Purging or evacuation of the reaction chamber to remove the nonreacted pre-cursors and the gaseous reaction byproducts.
- Exposure of the second precursor, or another treatment to activate the surface again for the reaction of the first precursor.
- Purging or evacuation of the reaction chamber.

1.3.4.2 Types of ALD Reaction

Today, ALD may be carried out by either thermal reactions or by plasma-assisted processes (which are also partially thermally activated). Almost of all these reactions comprise a two-step ALD process, with single unbalanced heuristic chemical reactions being used unless the reaction chemistry is unclear without an explicit two-step description. Some of the reactions selected from important examples of films used in the development of ALD technology and applications are detailed in the following sections.

Thermal ALD

1) Depositing Compounds

In this class of reactions, metal halides are reacted with hydrides, such as H_2O or NH_3. Although $TiCl_4$ and WF_6 are well-known halide sources with good vapor pressures, many other metallic halides may often exist as solids and may sublime at convenient source temperatures, but have low vapor pressures. A thermal ALD reaction of note using metal halides is the $HfCl_4$ chemistry:

$$HfCl_4 + 2H_2O \rightarrow HfO_2 + 4HCl.$$

Recently, HfO_2 has emerged as a promising high-K dielectric because of its chemical stability with silicon relative to ZrO_2. A basic $HfCl_4/H_2O$ process has been demonstrated [110]. Other metal oxides with known halide reactions include: ZrO_2 [111], Ta_2O_5 [112], Al_2O_3 [113], and TiO_2 [114, 115].

The use of metal–organic (MO) chemistry reactions represents another means of forming compounds. Indeed, although the early ALD processes were often developed with halide/hydride chemistry, the use of trimethyl aluminum (TMA) for aluminum-bearing films was an important exception.

Moving from halide sources to MO sources eliminates trace Cl or F, but introduces the presence of trace C or N, but this is a necessary trade-off as organic chemistry provides a wide diversity of materials. Among other precursor characteristics, it may be desirable to develop liquid precursors with a higher pressure and, concurrently, with a greater thermal stability.

Although the ALD process for Al_2O_3, using the TMA/H_2O chemistry [116], was the "standard" process for many years, semiconductor device leakage characteristics were subsequently found to be better with TMA/O_3 chemistry [117].

$$Al(CH_3)_3 + HOH \rightarrow Al_2O_3 + CH_4.$$

$$Al(CH_3)_3 + O_3 \rightarrow Al_2O_3 + H, C, O \text{ containing by products.}$$

2) Depositing Elemental Films

Reactions forming elemental films using halide–hydride chemistry have been developed, in which alternating pulses of a silicon halide and silicon hydride can lead to the formation of elemental silicon [118].

An early demonstration of the ALD formation of elemental W films was using metal halides with silane reduction chemistry [119]:

$$WF_6 + SiH_4 \rightarrow W + SiF_xH_y + SiF_4 + H_2.$$

As the strong bonding energy of the SiF_x byproduct compound essentially leaves no Si to react with the metal, WSi_x is not formed. This chemistry is similar to that known for CVD W processes. Other refractive metals can be formed using silane or other hydride-based reduction reactions.

3) Depositing Noble Metals with O_2 Chemistry

This type of chemical reaction [120] may run counter to initial intuition, as oxygen "combustion" is used to create an elemental material. However, RuO is an intermediate, and once RuO_x forms on the substrate surface it is further reduced by Ru $(Cp)_2$ to form an elemental material:

$$RuO_x + RI(Cp)_2 \rightarrow Ru Ru(Cp) + CO_2 + H_2O$$

$$Ru (Cp) + O_2 \rightarrow RuO_x + CO_2 + H_2O$$

where $(Cp)_2 = (C_5 H_5)_2$. After each of the O_2 half-reactions, the surface is terminated in RuO_x; however, after each pair of half-reactions an additional layer of Ru is added to the bulk film. The concentration of the O may have to be controlled in order to avoid oxidation of the underlying layers.

Plasma-Assisted ALD

1) Depositing Elemental Films

An early Si elemental ALD thermal process which used SiH_2, Cl_2/H_2 [121] was demonstrated by using metal or silicon halides with atomic H; however, the reaction proceeded only above $800\,°C$, which was too high for many applications. Thus, ALD saturation and elemental Si (or Ge) were achieved by using atomic H for reduction at approximately $540\,°C$ [122]. Still later, others utilized the same reaction principle to deposit non-Group IV elements, and produced elemental Ti and Ta [122].

$$SiCl_4 + {}^*H \rightarrow Si\text{-}H + HCl$$

$$TiCl_4 + {}^*H \rightarrow Ti\text{-}H + HCl$$

where * indicates a radical or plasma environment. Hence, plasma-assisted ALD may occur by direct plasma, remote apparatus configurations, or combinations thereof.

2) Depositing Metal Compounds

Plasma-assisted metal precursors use metal halides or MO compounds to make metal nitrides:

$$TiCl_4 + {}^*NH_3 \rightarrow TiN\text{-}H\ CO_2 + HCl$$

The reaction takes place at approximately $100\,°C$ lower than its thermal counterpart. Metal nitrides or oxides may be formed using halide precursors and plasma containing either oxidants (O_3, H_2O) or nitridants (NH_3) [123], as well as otherwise nonreactive gases such as O_2 and N_2/H_2.

1.3.4.3 Advantages and Disadvantages

When using ALD, the film thickness will depend only on the number of reaction cycles, which in turn makes the thickness control accurate and simple. Unlike CVD, there is less need for reactant flux homogeneity, which gives a large area (large batch and easy scale-up) capability, excellent conformality and reproducibility, and also simplifies the use of solid precursors. The growth of different multilayer structures is also straightforward. Taken together, these advantages make the ALD method highly attractive for microelectronics, and notably for the manufacture of future-generation integrated circuits. The other advantages of ALD include the wide range of film materials that is available, as well as the high density and low impurity level. A lower deposition temperature may also be used in order not to affect sensitive substrates.

1) Advantages
   - Stoichiometric films with large area uniformity and 3-D conformality.
   - Precise thickness control.
   - Low-temperature deposition possible.
   - Gentle deposition process for sensitive substrates.

1) Disadvantages
    - Deposition rate slower than CVD.
    - The number of different material that can be deposited is fair compared to MBE.

1.4
Pattern Transfer

In the manufacture of nanostructures via top-down fabrication methods, one vital step is that of pattern transfer, where the pattern is defined through two steps: (i) lithographic resist patterning; and (ii) subsequent etching of the underlying material. Etching and lift-off represent the two ways of developing the transfer the pattern onto the substrates. As shown in Figure 1.20, the transfer can be either additive (lift-off) or subtractive (etch), although in practice the subtractive processes are preferred as they have a greater reliability and so a higher yield. Subtractive processing involves either etching or the removal of material; this can be achieved either by using suitable wet

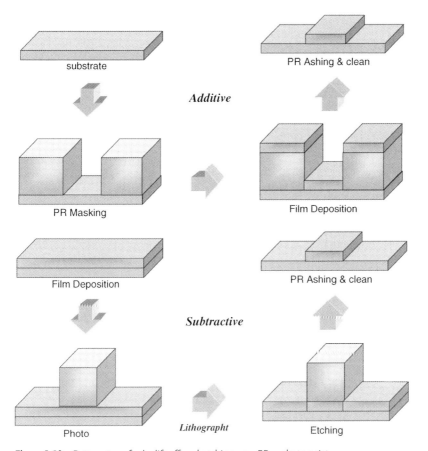

Figure 1.20 Pattern transfer by lift-off and etching way. PR = photoresist.

chemicals, or by dry etching in a vacuum system with the assistance of ions formed by an electrical discharge in a gas. Although the resist pattern can always be removed if found to be faulty on inspection, once the pattern has been transferred onto a solid material by etching, then any reworking is much more difficult, and often impossible.

1.4.1
Etch

Etching is the process of removing regions of the underlying material that are no longer protected by photoresist after development. There are two major types of etching: wet etching and dry etching.

1.4.1.1 Wet Etching
In wet etching, liquid chemicals or etchants are used to remove materials from the wafer, during which time the substrates are immersed in a reactive solution (etchant). As the layer to be removed is "etched away" by chemical reaction or by dissolution, the reaction products must be soluble so that they can be carried away by the etchant solution.

A basic wet etching process may be broken down into three basic steps: (i) diffusion of the etchant to the surface for removal; (ii) reaction between the etchant and the material being removed; and (iii) diffusion of the reaction byproducts from the reacted surface. The mechanisms fall into two major categories:

- metal etching (electron transfer):

$$M\,(s) \rightarrow M^{n+}\,(aq) + ne^-$$

- insulator etching (acid–base reaction):

$$SiO_2 + 6HF \rightarrow H_2SiOF_6\,(aq) + 2H_2O$$

Wet etching has found widespread use because of its special advantages of: (i) low cost; (ii) high reliability; (iii) high throughput; (iv) excellent selectivity in most cases with respect to both mask and substrate materials; (v) greater ease of use; (vi) higher reproducibility; and (vii) better efficiency in the use of etchants. Many of the materials used in microelectronics can be etched using wet etching methods.

Silicon Dioxide Etch HF-based etchants are widely used for etching silicon dioxide; hence, for pure HF-etching the overall reaction could be described as [124, 125]:

$$SiO_2 + 6\,HF \rightarrow H_2 + SiF_6 + 2H_2O.$$

Here, a 5 : 1 buffered hydrofluoric acid (BHF) solution (also known as buffered oxide etch, BOE) is a commonly used SiO_2 etchant formulation, and the reaction involved in the process is:

$$SiO_2 + 4HF + 2NH_4F \rightarrow (NH_4)_2SiF_6 + 2H_2O$$

$$SiO_2 + 3HF_2^- + H^+ \rightarrow SiF_6^{2-} + 2H_2O.$$

Here, "5:1" refers to five parts by weight of 40 wt% ammonium fluoride (the "buffer") to one part by weight of 49 wt% HF; this results in a total of about 33% NH_4F and 8.3% HF by weight [126], and the pH-value is about 3. HF is a weak acid, and except when present in very small concentrations it does not completely dissociate into H^+ and F^- ions in water [127]. Judge [128] and Deckert [129] have each shown the etch rate of both silicon dioxide and silicon nitride to increase linearly with the concentrations of both HF and HF_2^-. However, for concentrations below 10 M, whilst being independent of the concentration of F^- ions alone, the HF_2^- complex attacks oxides much faster than HF. Thus, the etch rate increases more than linearly with respect to the HF concentration.

Poly-Silicon Etch   Silicon is usually wet-etched using a mixture of nitric acid (HNO_3) and HF [2, 24, 25], which may be masked by the photoresist.

A simplified description of the reaction is that the HNO_3 in the solution oxidizes the silicon, followed by the oxidized compound being etched by the HF (formed from the fluoride ions in this acidic solution). Many metal-etches also remove material in a two-step manner, the overall reaction being [125, 130]:

$$3Si + 4HNO_3 + 18HF \rightarrow 3H_2SiF_6 + 4NO(g) + 8H_2O$$

Although the etching of silicon with HNO_3 and HF is an isotropic approach, on occasion it does not meet the requirements for microelectronics. Orientation-dependent silicon wet etchants have also been developed. For example, KOH is used for the orientation-dependent etching (ODE) of single-crystal silicon. ODEs attack {111}-type planes, which have a high bond density, much more slowly than other planes [124, 131]. Occasionally, isopropyl alcohol may be added to the KOH solutions; this decreases the etch rate but improves uniformity, thus reducing the requirement for stirring [132]. In this case the gross reaction is:

$$Si + 2OH^- \rightarrow SiO_2(OH)_2^{2-} + 2H_2(g)$$

Metal Wet Etch   The wet etching of aluminum and aluminum alloy layers may be achieved using slightly heated (35–45 °C) solutions of phosphoric acid, acetic acid, nitric acid, and water. This is a multistep etch process, which could also be masked by a photoresist. The aluminum is first oxidized by the nitric acid, while the phosphoric acid and water simultaneously etch the resulting oxide [133].

A solution with a constituent of H_2O_2 (30%; i.e., hydrogen peroxide, 30% by weight) is used to wet-etch tungsten and its alloys (where HF is the active ingredient in the etchant) and also etched oxides. Raising the proportion of HF in the solution causes an increase in the etch rate. In this etching, a film of tungsten oxide is formed that is dissolved in the hydrogen peroxide [134]. This etchant can also be used to etch tungsten–titanium alloys, but not pure titanium.

A wet process is also used for the cleaning of wafers before use. For example, Piranha – a hot solution of H_2SO_4 and H_2O_2 mixed in any ratio – has been used for decades for wafer cleaning [135–137]. With a lower ratio of H_2SO_4 to H_2O_2, as for other acidic hydrogen peroxide solutions, Piranha will first strip off the photoresist and any other organics by oxidizing them, and then remove any metals by forming complexes that remain in solution [138, 139]. This does not adversely affect the silicon dioxide and silicon nitride, and has only a minor effect on the bare silicon of forming a thin layer of hydrous silicon oxide. However, after the Piranha clean and rinse the silicon oxide can easily be removed with quick (10 s) dip into 10 : 1 or 25 : 1 HF. Other materials on the wafer may be wet-etched by using the appropriate etching solutions.

As with any process, wet etching has its own certain disadvantages. Typically, wet etching is isotropic in nature, and the etched feature will have curved walls and its width will differ from that of the opening in the resist. If the aspect ratio (the ratio of depth to width) of the desired feature is small, then the isotopic nature of the etching is often not important; however, in the closely packed structures found in very large-scale integration (VLSI) integrated circuits it is not acceptable. An additional problem is that, after wet chemical etching, disposal of the partly used reagent may raise environmental issues. A further problem is that monolayer-thick layers of hydro-carbons can inhibit wet etching, such that the *in situ* control of etch depth is made difficult.

Silicon of $\langle 110 \rangle$ orientation offers an interesting possibility for the anisotropic wet etching of perfectly vertical walls when the mask is aligned so that slow-etching (111) planes form the sidewalls. The side walls and bottom surfaces shown in Figure 1.21b contain a large number of facets when etched at 70 °C in KOH–water without the addition of 2-propanol; however, the microchannel sidewalls are clearly still vertical. In contrast, Figure 1.21a shows a less-pronounced surface structure with a definite slope in the side walls when etched in a solution containing 2-propanol [140].

1.4.1.2 Dry Etching

Unlike wet etching processes, dry etching does not utilize any liquid chemicals or etchants to remove materials from the wafer; rather, the substrates are immersed in a reactive gas (plasma), and in the process only volatile byproducts are generated. As with wet etching, dry etching also follows the resist mask patterns on the wafer; that

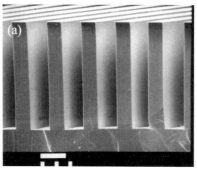
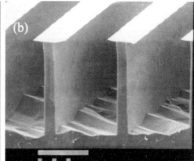
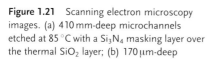

Figure 1.21 Scanning electron microscopy images. (a) 410 mm-deep microchannels etched at 85 °C with a Si₃N₄ masking layer over the thermal SiO₂ layer; (b) 170 μm-deep microchannels etched at 70 °C with a 1 mm-thick SiO₂ masking layer, showing side hanging of the masking layer over the microchannels.

is, it only etches away materials that are not covered by mask material (and are therefore exposed to its etching species), while leaving areas covered by the masks almost (but not perfectly) intact. These masks were previously deposited on the wafer using a wafer fabrication step known as "lithography."

Dry etching may be accomplished by any of the following: (i) through chemical reactions that consume the material, using chemically reactive gases or plasma; (ii) by physical removal of the material, usually by momentum transfer; or (iii) by a combination of both physical removal and chemical reactions.

In a plasma discharge, a number of different mechanisms for gas-phase reactions are operative. Discharge generates both ions and excited neutrals, and both are important for etching.

$$\text{Ionization}: \text{e}^- + \text{Ar} \rightarrow 2\text{e}^- + \text{Ar}^+$$

$$\text{Excitation}: \text{e}^- + \text{O}_2 \rightarrow \text{e}^- + \text{O}_2{}^*$$

$$\text{Dissociation}: \text{e}^- + \text{SF}_6 \rightarrow \text{e}^- + \text{SF}_5{}^* + \text{F}^*$$

Silicon Dioxide Etch Fluorocarbon–Plasma (CF_4 + CHF_3 + He) is used for silicon dioxide dry etching. In this case, it appears that the CF_x ($x \leq 3$) radicals are chemisorbed onto the SiO_2 and become dissociated; the radicals then supply carbon to form CO, CO_2, and COF_2 gases from the oxygen in the film. They also supply fluorine to form SiF_4 gas [141]. The overall reactions that occur are as followings [124]:

$$3SiO_2 + 4CF_3 \rightarrow 2CO + CO_2 + 3SiF_4$$

$$SiO_2 + 2CHF_2 \rightarrow 2CO + H_2 + SiF_4$$

Plasma HF-vapor is another method using for the dry etching of silicon dioxide. As with liquid-based HF etches, the HF vapor etches silicon dioxide and has been used to remove native oxide from silicon before the growth of epitaxial silicon and other processes, such as the XeF_2 etching of silicon. In the process, the HF/H_2O vapor condenses into droplets on the surfaces of the oxide samples during a 1-minute etch, such that a faster etching is caused where the droplets had formed. The related reaction in this process is [142]:

$$SiO_2 + 4HF \rightarrow SiF_4 + H_2O.$$

Silicon Etch Fluorine-, chlorine-, and bromine-based processes represent standards for silicon etching, and result in reaction products of SiF_4, $SiCl_4$ and $SiBr_4$, respectively. Fluorine-based processes are safer to use, but are seldom fully aniso-tropic, while chlorine-based processes result in vertical sidewalls inherently (the same applies to bromine-based processes). Importantly, both chlorine and bromine are highly toxic, and it is essential that the equipment used for Cl_2 or HBr etching must be equipped with a loadlock.

First synthesized in 1962 [143], XeF_2 has the unusual capability to etch silicon at a significant rate, without requiring a plasma to generate reactive species, and has been used for silicon etching [143, 144]. Notably, XeF_2 has one major advantage over wet silicon etchants in that will gently etch without the application of any forces. In addition, it has the advantage over plasma etching of being extremely selective over almost all of the traditional masking layers, including silicon dioxide, some silicon nitrides, and photoresists. XeF_2 has also been used to micromachine free-standing structures made from aluminum and polysilicon protected by a layer of oxide [145].

During the etch process, the XeF_2 molecules are physisorbed onto the silicon surface and dissociate to release volatile xenon atoms, while the fluorine atoms remain to react with the silicon to form volatile SiF_4. The overall reaction is:

$$Si + 2XeF_2 \rightarrow SiF_4 + 2Xe.$$

The etching of silicon with plasma represents an anisotropic approach, normally using Cl_2 + He, HBr + Cl_2, as the plasma source. When Cl_2 + He is applied to etch silicon, a previous SF_6 step is typically used to break through the native oxide. In this case, the chlorine atoms are chemisorbed one at a time onto the silicon surface, eventually forming volatile $SiCl_4$ [146]. This method has been used to etch 80 pm-deep trenches with fairly vertical sidewalls [147]; the overall reaction is:

$$4Cl + Si \rightarrow SiCl_4.$$

HBr + Cl_2 plasma represents yet another anisotropic silicon plasma etch source, but this has a better selectivity of silicon over oxide, whereby the bromine atoms most likely react with silicon in a manner similar to chlorine (as described above).

The chlorine etching of undoped silicon occurs very slowly in the absence of ion bombardment [147]. Unlike F-atom silicon etches, Cl- and Br-based etches tend to be vertical [148].

Silicon Nitride Etches   Fluorine-Atom-Plasma (SF_6 + He or CF_4 + CHF_3 + He) is used to plasma-etch silicon nitride, and this can be masked with a photoresist. The etch is anisotropic and results in fairly vertical sidewalls. In this case, the fluorine atoms are adsorbed onto the surface one at a time, in a surface reaction, and volatile products are formed. The overall reaction is [124]:

$$12FCl + Si_3N_4 \rightarrow SiF_4 + 2N_2.$$

Plasma Metal Etches Cl_2 + BCl_3 + $CHCl_3$ + N_2 is used to dry etch aluminum, which is an anisotropic etch due to the side-wall inhibitor formed from the $CHCl_3$ [149]. Due to poor selectivity, when etching the thick layers of Al, a thicker photoresist, a plasma-hardened photoresist, or a more durable masking layer must be used. Usually, a higher temperature is used to keep the etch product volatile so that it leaves the wafer [124] and does not coat the chamber or exhaust the plumbing. Cl_2 rather than Cl appears to be the main etchant [149], and the etch product becomes $AlCl_3$ at higher temperatures [149, 150]. The dominant overall reaction below 200 °C is:

$$12Al + 3Cl_2 \rightarrow Al_2Cl_3$$

SF_6 is used for tungsten plasma etching, with the etch process function being fairly isotropic. CF_4 is often added to the feed gas, and increases the anisotropy as side-wall polymers form, although the etch rate will be slowed down. In this case, the chuck can be heated to enhance the etch rate. The overall reaction is:

$$6F + W \rightarrow WF_6$$

Shown in Figure 1.22 are the SEM images of surface structures of silicon that have been etched with SF_6/O_2 plasma in an RIE etching manner. The clearly visible difference between these figures relates to the fact that the substrate in Figure 1.22a was pretreated with BHF and acetone, whereas that in Figure 1.22b was pretreated only with BHF. The width of the needles is almost 200 nm. The morphology of the silicon surfaces etched in Figure 1.22b was found to be uniform, and the formation of columnar nanostructures with diameters <100 nm and depths >300 nm were possible [151].

The dry etching method has the following advantages:

- The elimination of handling dangerous acids and solvents.
- The use of only small amounts of chemicals.
- The production of isotropic or anisotropic etch profiles.
- Directional etching can be achieved, without using the crystal orientation of Si.
- Lithographically defined photoresist patterns are faithfully transferred into the underlying layers
- High resolution and cleanliness.
- Less undercutting.
- No unintentional prolongation of etching.
- Better process control.
- Ease of automation (e.g., cassette loading).

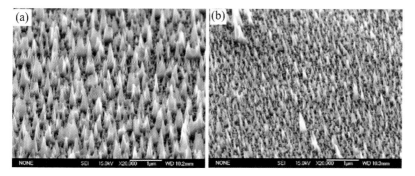

Figure 1.22 Scanning electron microscopy images of needle-like nanostructures of the silicon surface by using RIE in a parallel-plate plasma system. (a) Pretreatment with BHF and acetone; (b) Pretreatment only with BHF.

1.4.1.3 A Comparison of Wet and Plasma Etching

Wet etching is usually isotropic (which is desirable in some cases), it may provide a selectivity that is dependent on the crystallographic direction, and it can be very selective over the masking and underlying layers. In contrast, plasma etching uses fresh chemicals for each etch (this results in a less chemical-related etch-rate variability) and it can be vertically anisotropic (as well as isotropic), thus allowing the patterning of narrow lines. One drawback of wet etching is that, when removing a sacrificial layer in micromachining, there will be a capillary-force pull down of any free-standing structures [152]. However, this can be overcome by using a supercritical-liquid drying process [153] or by switching to a dry-etched sacrificial layer [154, 155].

In many applications, the choice of wet versus plasma etching is a question of convenience – whether certain equipment or an etch bath is available, or a suitable masking material is at hand. However, when sloped etch profiles are required, or when under-cutting is needed, then isotropic etching must be used. One particular benefit is that the isotropic wet etching of silicon can be achieved at fairly high rates, at microns or even tens of microns per minute.

1.4.2
Lift-Off Processes

The pattern-transfer technique – *lift-off*– refers to the process of creating patterns on the wafer surface through an additive process, as opposed to the more familiar patterning techniques that involve subtractive processes, such as etching. Lift-off is most commonly employed in patterning metal films for interconnections.

The steps of the technique are shown schematically in Figure 1.20. The resist is first exposed to radiation via the pattern-carrying mask, and the exposed areas of the resist are then developed (as shown in Figure 1.20). A film is then deposited over the resist and substrate. Prior to film deposition – and particularly for sputtering or evaporation processes – a "post-develop bake" is recommended, which will drive off any excess solvent so that there will be less out-gassing during the film deposition. The film thickness must be smaller than that of the resist. By using an appropriate solvent (such as acetone), the remaining parts of the resist and the deposited film atop these parts of the resist can be lifted off (see Figure 1.20). The lift-off technique is capable of high resolution, and often used for the fabrication of discrete devices.

Depending on the type of lift-off process used, patterns can be defined with extremely high fidelity and for very fine geometries. Lift-off, for example, is the process of choice for patterning electron-beam-written metal lines, because the film remains only where the photoresist has been cleared. The defect modes are the opposite what might be expected for etching films, as the defects may occur in the underlaying photoresist layer; for example, particles that underlay the photoresist may lead to open or other unwanted shapes on the substrate, whereas in case of metal lift-off the scratches may lead to unwanted areas of the metal layer remaining on the wafer.

Any deposited film can be lifted-off, provided that:

- During film deposition, the substrate does not reach temperatures that are high enough to burn the photoresist.
- The film quality is not absolutely critical; a photoresist will outgas very slightly in vacuum systems, which may adversely affect the quality of the deposited film.
- The adhesion of the deposited film on the substrate is very good.
- The film can be easily wetted by the solvent.
- The film is thin enough and/or grainy enough to allow solvent to seep underneath; the thickness of the film being lifted off should be preferably kept at less than one-third of the total photoresist thickness.
- The film is not elastic, and is thin and/or brittle enough to be torn along the adhesion lines.

References

1 Thompson, L.F. (1983) *Introduction to Microlithography* (eds L.F. Thompson, C.G. Willson, and M.J. Bowden), The American Chemical Society, Washington, DC, p. 1.

2 Moreau, W.M. (1988) *Semiconductor Lithography: Principles and Materials*, Plenum, New York.

3 Suzuki, K., Matsui, S., and Ochiai, Y. (2000) *Sub-Half-Micron Lithography for ULSIs*, Cambridge University Press, Cambridge.

4 Gentili, M., Giovannella, C., and Selci, S. (1993) *Nanolithography: A Borderland between STM, EB, IS, and X-Ray Lithographies*, Kluwer, Dordrecht, The Netherlands.

5 Brambley, D., Martin, B., and Prewett, F.D. (1994) *Adv. Mater: Opt. Electron.*, **4**, 55.

6 Bernard, F. (2002) *Microelectron. Eng.*, **61–62**, 11.

7 Moore, G.E. (1995) *Proc. SPIE*, **2440**, 2–17.

8 Mack, C. (1996) *Opt. Photo. News*, **April**, 29–33.

9 Dammel, R. (1993) *Diazonaphth-oquinone-Based Resists*, vol. **TT11**, SPIE Optical Engineering Press.

10 Kumar, A., Abbot, N.A., Kim, E., Biebuyck, H.A., and Whitesides, G.M. (1995) *Acc. Chem. Res.*, **28**, 219.

11 Ulman, A. (1991) *An Introduction to Ultrathin Organic Films: From Langmuir-Blodgett to Self-Assembly*, Academic Press, San Diego, CA.

12 Huang, J., Dahlgren, D.A., and Hemminger, J.C. (1994) *Langmuir*, **10**, 626.

13 Chan, K.C., Kim, T., Schoer, J.K., and Crooks, R.M. (1995) *J. Am. Chem. Soc.*, **117**, 5875.

14 Bruning, J.H. (1997) *Proc. SPIE*, **3051**, 14.

15 Levinson, H.J. and Arnold, W.H. (1997) Optical lithography, *Handbook of Microlithography and Microfabrication*, vol. **1** (ed. P. Rai-Choudhury), SPIE, Bellingham, WA.

16 Sheats, J.R. and Smith, B.W.(eds) (1998) *Microlithography: Science and Technology*, Marcel Dekker, New York.

17 Bruning, J.H. (1980) *J. Vac. Sci. Technol.*, **17**, 1147.

18 Smith, B.W. (2002) *J. Microlith. Microfab. Microsyst.*, **1**, 95.

19 Levenson, M.D., Viswanathan, N.S., and Simpson, R.A. (1982) *IEEE Trans. Electron Devices*, **ED29**, 1812.

20 Shibuya, M. (1987) Projection master for transmitted illuminated. Japanese Patent Gazette No. 62-50811

21 Smith, H.I., Anderson, E.H., and Schattenburg, M.L. (1989) Lithography mask with a p phase shifting attenuator, U.S. Patent 4,890,309

22 Flanders, D.C. and Smith, H.I. (1982) Spatial period division exposing. U.S. Patent 4,360,586

23 Tananka, T., Uchino, S., Hasegawa, N., Yamanaka, T., Terasawa, T., and Okazaki, S. (1991) *Jpn. J. Appl. Phys. Part I*, **30**, 1131.

24 Rogers, J.A., Paul, K.E., Jackman, R.J., and Whitesides, G.W. (1998) *J. Vac. Sci. Technol. B*, **16**, 59.

25 Aizenberg, J., Rogers, J.A., Paul, K.E., and Whitesides, G.M. (1998) *Appl. Opt.*, **37**, 2145.

26 Aizenberg, J.J., Rogers, A., Paul, K.E., and Whitesides, G.M. (1997) *Appl. Phys. Lett.*, **71**, 3773.

27 Terazawa, T., Hasegawa, N., Fukuda, H., and Katagiri, S. (1991) *Jpn. J. Appl. Phys.*, **30**, 2991.

28 Tritchkov, A., Jeong, S., and Kenyon, C. (2005) *Proc. SPIE*, **215**, 5754.

29 Perlitz, S., Buttgereit, U., Scherubl, T., Seidel, D., Lee, K.M., and Tavassoli, M. (2007) *Proc. SPIE*, **6607**, 66070Z.

30 Luo, Y. and Misra, V. (2006) *Nanotechnology*, **17**, 4909.

31 McCord, M.A. and Rooks, M.J. (2000) *Handbook of Microlithography, Micromachining and Microfabrication*, (ed. P. Rai-Coudhury), vol. 2, SPIE, Washington.

32 Brewer, G.R. (1980) *Electron-Beam Technology in Microelectronic Fabrication*, Academic Press, New York.

33 Chen, W. and Ahmed, H. (1993) *Appl. Phys. Lett.*, **62**, 1499.

34 Craighead, H.G., Howard, R.E., Jackel, L.D., and Mankievich, P.M. (1983) *Appl. Phys. Lett.*, **42**, 38.

35 Chou, S.Y. (1997) *Proc. IEEE*, **85**, 652.

36 Vieu, C., Carcenac, F., Pepin, A., Chen, Y., Mejias, M., Lebib, A., Manin-Ferlazzo, L., Couraud, L., and Lunois, H. (2000) *Appl. Surf. Sci.*, **164**, 111.

37 Yesin, S., Hasko, D.G., and Ahmed, H. (2001) *Appl. Phys. Lett.*, **78**, 2760.

38 Rosenfield, M.G., Thomson, M.G.R., Coane, P.J., Kwietniak, K.T., Keller, J., Klaus, D.P., Volant, R.P., Blair, C.R., Tremaine, K.S., Newman, T.H., and Hohn, F.J. (1993) *J. Vac. Sci. Technol. B*, **11**, 2615.

39 Rishton, S.A., Schmid, H., Kern, D.P., Luhn, H.E., Chang, T.H.P., Sai-Halasz, G.A., Wordeman, M.R., Ganin, E., and Polcari, M. (1988) *J. Vac. Sci. Technol. B*, **6**, 140.

40 Fujita, J., Ohnishi, Y., Ochinai, Y., Nomura, E., and Matsui F S. (1996) *J. Vac. Sci. Technol. B* **14**, 4272.

41 Thompson, L.F. and Bowden, M.J. (1983) *Introduction to Microlithography* (eds L.F. Thompson, C.G. Willson, and M.J. Bowden), The American Chemical Society, Washington, DC, p. 15.

42 Spears, D.L. and Smith, H.I. (1972) *Solid State Technol.*, **15**, 21.

43 Smith, H.I. (1996) *Phys. Scr.*, **T61**, 2631.

44 Perlman, M.L., Rowe, E.M., and Watson, R.E. (1974) *Phys. Today*, **27**, 30.

45 Kunz, C. (1976) *Physik Bl.*, **32**, 55.

46 Dagneaux, P., Depautcx, C., Dhez, P., Durup, J., Farge, Y., Fourme, R., Guyon, P.M., Jaegle, P., Leach, S., Lopez-Delgado, R., Morel, G., Pinchaux, R., Thiry, P., Vermeil, C., and Wuilleumier, F. (1975) *Ann. Phys. (Paris)*, **9**, 9.

47 Kunz, C. (1974) *Vacuum Ultraviolet Radiation Physics* (eds E.E. Koch, R. Haensel, and C. Kunz), Vieweg, Braunschweig, p. 753.

48 Kitayama, T., Itoga, K., Watanabe, Y., and Uzawa, S. (2000) *J. Vac. Sci. Technol. B*, **18**, 2950.

49 Smith, H.I., Spears, D.L., and Bemacki, S.E. (1973) *J. Vac. Sci. Technol.*, **10**, 913.

50 Bemacki, S.E. and Smith, H.I. (1974) *Proceedings 6th International Conference Electron and Ion Beam Science and Technology, 1974, San Francisco, CA* (ed. R. Bakish), The Electrochemical Society, Princeton, NJ.

51 Bemacki, S.E. and Smith, H.I. (1975) *IEEE Trans. Elec. Dev.*, **ED22**, 421.

52 Chou, S.Y., Smith, H.I., and Antoniadis, D.A. (1985) *J. Vac. Sci. Technol. B.*, **3**, 1587.

53 Shahidi, G.G., Antoniadis, D.A., and Smith, H.I. (1988) *IEEE Elect. Dev Lett.*, **EDG9**, 94.

54 Ismail, K., Bagwell, P.F., Orlando, T.P., Antoniadis, D.A., and Smith, H.I. (1991) *Proc. IEEE*, **79**, 1106.

55 Scott-Thomas, J.H.F., Field, S.B., Kastner, M.A., Smith, H.I., and Antoniadis, D.A. (1989) *Phys. Rev. Lett.*, **62**, 583.

56 Simon, G., Haghiri-Gosnet, A.M., Bourneix, J., Decanini, D., Chen, Y., Rousseaux, F., Launios, H., and Vidal, B. (1997) *J. Vac. Sci. Technol. B*, **15**, 2489.

57 Gerlach, R. and Utlaut, M. (2001) *Proc. SPIE, Charged Particle Detection, Diagnostics, and Imaging*, **4510**, 96.

58 Prewett, P.D. and Mair, G.L.R.(eds) (1991) *Focused Ion Beams from Liquid Metal Ion Sources*, John Wiley & Sons, New York.

59 Hall, T.M., Wagner, A., and Thompson, L.F. (1979) *J. Vac. Sci. Technol.*, **16**, 1889.

60 Seliger, R.L., Kubena, R.L., Olney, R.D., Ward, J.W., and Wang, V. (1979) *J. Vac. Sci. Technol.*, **16**, 1610.

61 Gierak, I., Septierl, A., and Vieu, C. (1999) *Nucl. Instrum. Methods Phys. Res. Sect. A*, **A421**, 91.

62 Matsui, S. and Ochiai, Y. (1996) *Nanotechnology*, **7**, 247.

63 Gamo, K. (1996) *Microelectron. Eng.*, **32**, 159.

64 Morimoto, H., Sasaki, Y., Saitoh, K., Watakabe, Y., and Kato, T. (1986) *Microelectron. Eng.*, **4**, 163.

65 Melngailis, J. (1987) *J. Vac. Sci. Technol.*, **B5**, 469.

66 Zachariasse, J. and Walker J. (1997) *Microelectron. Eng.*, **35**, 63.

67 Adesida, I. (1983) *Nucl. Instrum. Methods*, **209–210**, 79.

68 Harthey, M., Shaver, D., Shepard, M., Melngailis, J., Medvedev, V., and Robinson, W. (1991) *J. Vac. Sci. Technol.*, **B9**, 3432.

69 Herbert, P., Braddell, J., MacKenzie, S., Woodham, R., and Cleaver, J. (1994) *Microelectron. Eng.*, **23**, 263.

70 Kuwano, H. (1984) *J. Appl. Phys.*, **55**, 1149.

71 Ohring, M. (1992) *The Materials Science of Thin Films*, Academic Press, San Diego, CA.

72 Vossen, J.L. and Kern, W.(eds) (1991) *Thin Film Processes II*, Academic Press, San Diego, CA.

73 Nalwa, H.S.(ed.) (2002) *Handbook of thin Film Materials, Vol. I: Deposition and Processing of Thin Films*, Academic Press, San Diego, CA.

74 Chambers Scott A. (2000) *Surf. Sci. Rep*, **39**, 105.

75 Faraday, M. (1857) *Philos. Trans.*, **147**, 145.

76 Holland, L. (1957) *Vacuum Deposition of Thin Films*, Chapman & Hall, London.

77 Deshpandey, C.V. and Bunshah, R.F. (1991) *Thin Film Processes II* (eds J.L. Vossenand W. Kern), Academic Press, San Diego, CA.

78 Glang, R. (1970) *Vacuum Evaporation, Handbook of Thin Film Technology* (eds L.I. Maisseland R. Glang), McGraw-Hill, pp. 1–26.

79 Pulker, H.K. (1984) Chapter 6, Film Formation Methods: Coatings on Glass, in *Thin Films: Science and Technology Series*, No. 6, Ch. 6 Elsevier.

80 Koleshko, V.M. (1987) *Vacuum*, **36**, 689.

81 Perry, A.J. (1981) *Wear*, **67**, 381.

82 Buckley, D.H. (1981) *Surface Effects in Adhesion, Friction, Wear, and Lubrication, Tribology Series 5*, Elsevier, p. 613.

83 Herman, M.A. and Sitter, H. (1989) *Molecular Beam Epitaxy-Fundamentals and Current Status*, Springer-Verlag, Berlin.

84 Kasper, E. and Bean, J.C.(eds) (1988) *Silicon-Molecular Beam Epitaxy I and II*, CRC Press, Boca Raton, FL.

85 Parker, E.H.C.(ed.) (1985) *The Technology and Physics of Molecular Beam Epitaxy*, Plenum Press, New York.

86 Wehner, G.K. (1955) *Adv. Electron. Electron Physics*, **7**, 239.

87 Kay, E. (1962) *Adv. Electron. Electron Physics*, **17**, 245.

88 Maissel, L.I. (1966) The deposition of thin films by cathode sputtering, *Physics of Thin Films*, vol. 3 (eds G. Hassand R.E. Thun), Academic Press, p. 61.

89 Holland, L. (1961) Cathodic sputtering, in *Vacuum Deposition of Thin Films*, Ch. 14, Chapman & Hall.

90 Nowicki, R.S. (1982) *Solid State Technol.*, **21**, 127.

91 Gadepally, K.V. and Hawk, R.M. (1989) *Proc. Arkansas Acad. Sci.*, **43**, 29.

92 Morosanu, C.E. (1990) *Thin Films by Chemical Vapor Deposition*, Elsevier, Amsterdam.

93 Cooke, M.J. (1985) *Vacuum*, **35**, 67.

94 Pierson, H.O. (1992) *Handbook of Chemical Vapor Deposition: Principles, Technology and Applications*, Noyes Publications.

95 Jensen, K.F. and Kern, W. (1991) *Thin Film Processes II* (eds J.L. Vossenand W. Kern), Academic Press, San Diego, CA.

96 Hitchman, M.L. and Jensen, K.F.(eds) (1993) *CVD Principles and Applications*, Academic Press, San Diego.

97 Ser, P., Kalck, P., and Feurer, R. (2002) *Chem. Rev.*, **102**, 3085.

98 Choy, K.L. (2003) *Prog. Mater. Sci.*, **48**, 57.

99 Herrmann, C.F., DelRio, F.W., George, S.M., and Bright, V.M. (2005) Micromachining and Microfabrication Process Technology, (eds M.-A. Maherand H.D. Stewart), *Proceedings SPIE*, vol. 5715, SPIE, Bellingham, WA. Available at: http://ald.colorado.edu/J_Phys_Chem_100.pdf.

100 Wikipedia: The Free Encyclopedia (2006) Atomic Layer Deposition. Wikimedia Foundation, 24 April 2006.

101 Ritala, M. and Leskela, M. (2002) *Handbook of Thin Film Materials, 61.1: Deposition and Processing of Thin Films* (ed. H.S. Nalwa), Academic Press, San Diego, CA, p. 103.

102 Ritala, M. and Leskela, M. (1999) *Nanotechnology*, **10**, 19.

103 Suntola, T. and Simpson, M. (1990) *Atomic Layer Epitaxy* (eds T. Suntolaand M. Simpson), Blackie, New York, pp. 3–5.

104 Ahonen, M. and Pessa, M. (1980) *Thin Solid Films*, **65**, 301.

105 Pessa, M., Makela, R., and Suntola, T. (1981) *Appl. Phys. Lett.*, **38**, 131.

106 Suntola, T. and Hyvarinen, J. (1985) *Annu. Rev. Muter. Sci.*, **15**, 177.

107 Suntola, T. and Antson, J. (1977) Methods for producing compound thin films. U.S. Patent No. 4058430

108 Ritala, M. and Leskela, M. (2002) Deposition and processing of thin films, in *Handbook of Thin Film Materials*, vol. 1 (ed. H. Nalwa), Academic Press, San Diego, p. 103.

109 Kim, H. (2003) *J. Vac. Sci. Technol. B*, **26**, 2231.

110 Ott, A.W., Klaus, J.W., Johnson, J.M., and George, S.M. (1997) *Thin Solid Films*, **292**, 135.

111 Aarik, J., Aidla, A., Mändar, H., Uustare, T., Kukli, K., and Schuisky, M. (2001) *Appl. Surf. Sci.*, **173**, 15.

112 Ritala, M. and Leskelä, M. (1994) *Appl. Surf. Sci.*, **75**, 330.

113 Zang, H., Solanki, R., Roberds, B., Bai, G., and Banerjee, I. (2000) *J. Appl. Phys.*, **87**, 1921.

114 Yun, S.-J., Kang, J.S., Paek, M.C., and Nam, K.S. (1998) *J. Korean Phys. Soc.*, **33**, S170.

115 Aarik, J., Aidla, A., Uustare, T., and Sammelselg, V. (1995) *J. Cryst. Growth.*, **148**, 268.

116 Sammelselg, V., Rosental, A., Tarre, A., Niinisto, L., Heiskanen, K., Ilmonen, K., Johansson, L.-S., and Uustare, T. (1998) *Appl. Surf. Sci.*, **134**, 78.

117 Kim, Y.K., Lee, S.H., Choi, S.J., Park, H.B., See, Y.D., and Chin, K.H. (2000) *IEDM Tech. Dig.*, 369, (IEEE Cat No: 00CH38138).

118 Yokoyama, S., Ohba, K., and Nakajima, A. (2001) *Appl. Phys. Lett.*, **79**, 617.

119 Klaus, J.W., Ferro, S.J., and George, S.M. (2000) *Thin Solid Films*, **360**, 145.

120 Aaltonen, T., Alen, P., Ritala, M., and Leskela, M. (2003) *Chem. Vap. Deposition*, **9**, 45.

121 Nishizawa, J., Aoki, K., Suzuki, S., and Kikuchi, K. (1990) *J. Cryst. Growth*, **99**, 502.

122 Rossnagel, S., Sherman, A., and Turner, F. (2000) *J. Vac. Sci. Technol.*, **B18**, 2016.

123 Londergan, A. (2002) *Rapid Thermal and Other Short Time Processes III, Proceedings, Vol. 2002–11*, The Electrochemical Society, Inc.

124 Runyan, W.R. and Bean, K.E. (1990) *Semiconductor Integrated Circuit Processing Technology*, Addison-Wesley, Reading, MA.

125 Ghandi, S.K. (1983) Silicon and gallium arsenide, *VLSI Fabrication Principles*, John Wiley & Sons, New York.

126 J.T. Baker, Inc . (1993) Product Specifications for Product No. 5192, Buffered Oxide Etch, 5:1, J.T. Baker, Inc., Phillipsburg, NJ, Tech. support, 7 June 1995.

127 Kikyuama, H., Miki, N., Saka, K., Takano, J., Kawanabe, I., Miyashita, M., and Ohmi T. (1991) *IEEE Trans. Semicond. Manuf.*, **4**, 26.

128 Judge, J.S. (1971) *J. Electrochem. Soc.*, **118**, 1772.

129 Deckert, C.A. (1978) *J. Electrochem. Soc.*, **125**, 320.

130 Turner, D.R. (1960) *J. Electrochem. Soc.*, **107**, 810.

131 Kendall, D.L. (1990) *J. Vac. Sci. Technol. A*, **8**, 3598.

132 Amulya, K.N. and Goldemberg, J. (1990) *J. Electrochem. Soc.*, **137**, 3612.

133 Elliot, D.J. (1989) *Integrated Circuit Fabrication Technology*, 2nd edn, McGraw-Hill, New York, p. 355.

134 van den Meerakker, J.E.A.M., Scholten, M., and van Oekel, J.J. (1992) *Thin Solid Films*, **208**, 237.

135 Wolf, S. and Tauber, R.N. (1986) *Silicon Processing for the VLSI Era*, vol. 1, Lattice, Sunset Beach, CA.

136 Yang, M.G. and Koliwad, K.M. (1975) *J. Electrochem. Soc.*, **122**, 675.

137 Pintchovski, F., Price, J.B., Tobin, P.J., Peavey, J., and Kobold, K. (1979) *J. Electrochem. Soc.*, **126**, 1428.

138 Kem, W. and Puotinen, D.A. (1970) *RCA Review*, **30**, 187.

139 Amick, J.A. (1976) *Solid State Technol.*, **19**, 47.

140 Dwivedi, V.K., and Ahmad, R.G.S. (2000) *Microelectron. J.*, **31**, 405.

141 Dwivedi, V.K., Gopal, R., and Ahmad, S. (2000) *Microelectron. J.*, **31**, 405.

142 Kuiper, A.E.T. and Lathouwers, E.G.C. (1992) *J. Electrochem. Soc.*, **139** (9), 2594–2599.

143 Oxtoby, D.W. and Nachtrieh, N.H. (1986) *Principles of Chemistry*, Saunders College Pub., Philadelphia, p. 728.

144 Winters, H.F. and Cobum, J.W. (1979) *Appl. Phys. Lett.*, **34**, 70.

145 Hoffman, E., Warneke, B., Kruglick, E., Weigold, J., and Pister, K.S.J. (1995) 3D structures with piezoresistive sensors in standard CMOS, Proceedings, IEEE Micro Electro-Mechanical Systems 1995, Amsterdam, The Netherlands, January-February, vol. 1, p. 288.

146 Manos, D.M. and Flamm, D.L.(eds) (1989) *Plasma Etching: An Introduction*, Academic, Boston.

147 Keller, C.G. and Howe, R.T. (1995) Nickel-filled thermally actuated hexsil tweezers, Technical Digest, 8th International Conference on Solid-state Sensors and Actuators (Transducers '95), Stockholm, Sweden, p. 376.

148 Rossnagel, S.M., Cnomo, J.J., and Westwood, W.D.(eds) (1990) *Handbook of Plasma Processing Technology*, Noyes, Park Ridge, NJ.

149 Lieberman, M.A. and Lichtenherg, A.J. (1994) *Principles of Plasma Discharges and Materials Processing*, John Wiley & Sons, New York.

150 Kem, W. and Deckert, C.A. (1978) Chemical etching, *Thin Film Processes*, (eds J.L. Vossenand W. Kem), Ch. V-1, Academic, New York, p. 413.

151 Jung, S., Kim, K., Park, D., Sohn, B.H., Jung, J.C., Zin, W.C., Hwang, S., Dhungel, S.K., Yoo, J., and Yi, J. (2007) *Mater. Sci. Eng. C*, **27**, 1452.

152 Mastrangelo, C.H. and Hsu, C.H. (1993) *IEEE J. Microelectromech. Syst.*, **2**, 44.

153 Mulhem, G.T., Soane, D.S., and Howe, R.T. (1993) Supercritical carbon dioxide drying of microstructures, Technical Digest, 7th International Conference on Solid- State Sensors and Actuators (Transducers '93), Yokahama, Japan, June.

154 Sampsell, J.B. (1993) The digital micromirror device and its application to projection displays, Technical Digest, 7th International Conference on Solid-State Sensors and Actuators (Transducers '93), Yokahama, Japan, June 1993, p. 24.

155 Storment, C.W., Borkholder, D.A., Westerlind, V., Suh, J.W., Maluf, N.I., and Kovacs, G.T.A. Flexible, dry-released process for aluminium electrostatic actuators (1994) *IEEE J. Microelectromech. Syst.*, **3** (3), 296–299.

2
Scanning Probe Microscopy as a Tool for the Fabrication of Structured Surfaces

Claudia Haensch, Nicole Herzer, Stephanie Hoeppener, and Ulrich S. Schubert

2.1
Introduction

The invention of scanning probe microscopy (SPM) by Binnig and Rohrer [1, 2] during the 1980s represented an important milestone in the field of surface sciences. Soon after its invention, the capability of the SPM technique (and its variations) to manipulate matter by means of the scanning tip inspired the development of new approaches for nanofabrication. The desire to generate ever-smaller structures that cannot easily be fabricated using conventional structuring tools, as well as very large-scale integration and complementary metal-oxide-semiconductor approaches, fuelled a major interest in using SPM methods to create structures with nanometer resolution. Although not the primary example of manipulating surfaces by means of SPM, the studies of Dagata *et al.* should be mentioned as being an important step in this development. Thus, it was shown that by applying voltage pulses, first via scanning tunneling microscopy (STM) [3] and later via an atomic force microscopy (AFM) tips [4], oxide structures could be formed with nanometer resolution. Subsequently, Day *et al.* were the first to investigate site-selective oxidation on silicon [4], when they used two different silicon substrates for patterning, namely silicon with a thermally grown 10 nm-thick layer of silicon oxide and silicon with native oxide; the inscribed features were then analyzed using AFM technique. As a result, patterning structures were obtained with a height of 2.8 nm, and which were recessed about 3.8 nm after etching with hydrofluoric acid (HF). Notably, these results indicated not only the formation of silicon dioxide but also consumption of the silicon substrate during oxide formation, since the hole structures had been created after the etching process. Although the obtained line widths were only 85 nm, this could be further improved by using sharper tips. Shortly afterwards, Yasutake and coworkers described the patterning of Si(100) and hydrogen-terminated Si surfaces by the application of a negative voltage between an Au-coated Si_3N_4 tip and the Si [5]. Subsequent AFM and Auger electron spectroscopy investigations were carried out to investigate the height and chemical composition of the obtained features. A schematic representation of the local anodic oxidation (LAO) process is shown in Figure 2.1.

Nanotechnology, Volume 8: Nanostructured Surfaces. Edited by Lifeng Chi
Copyright © 2010 WILEY-VCH Verlag GmbH & Co. KGaA, Weinheim
ISBN: 978-3-527-31739-4

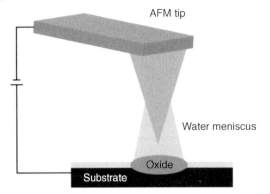

Figure 2.1 Schematic representation of the local anodic oxidation process.

In this case, the AFM tip serves as the cathode whilst the substrate acts as the anode. As this method is dependent on an electrical current, both the AFM tip and substrate must be conductive [6]. The water meniscus which is formed between the tip and the surface can be seen as a nanometer-sized electrical cell [7], and also provides the electrolytes for the LAO, which is essential for the patterning. The applied voltage induces an electric field with a value of $10^9 \, \text{V} \, \text{m}^{-1}$ as the threshold for the LAO process [8]. In fact, this electrical field is responsible for ionizing the water molecules to form reactive ionic species necessary for the LAO process [6]. In this way, the tip was used to create a nanometric electrochemical cell that consisted of the substrate, the tip itself, and the water meniscus (which is present under atmospheric conditions). At the anode – that is, the sample surface – an oxidation reaction takes place as described by Garcia *et al.* [7, 9], whilst at the cathode (in this case, the SFM tip) hydrogen is generated:

$$Si + 2H^+ + 2OH^- \rightarrow Si(OH)_2 \rightarrow SiO_2 + 2H^+ + 2e^-$$

$$(M + nH_2O \rightarrow MO_n + 2nH^+ + 2ne^-)$$

$$2H^+_{aq} + 2e^- \rightarrow H_2.$$

Investigations of the oxidized structures are carried out by taking measurements of the obtained height, since the silicon oxide features reveal an increase in height after the LAO [8]. This might be explained by the molecular volume of the oxides, which is normally larger than that of the substrate, and therefore the raised features would be formed during the LAO reaction [10]. In this situation, the hydrolysis of water from the water meniscus plays an essential role, and emphasizes the importance of the reliable formation of a water meniscus between the tip and the sample. The typical size of the water meniscus at different ambient conditions can be investigated using environmental scanning electron microscopy (ESAM), as depicted in Figure 2.2.

Whereas, the majority of LAOs were performed in a water meniscus, some examples have been reported where organic solvents were used as the reaction media for the inscription of nanometer-sized structures. Garcia and coworkers

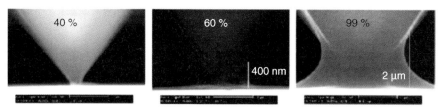

Figure 2.2 Environmental scanning electron microscopy investigation of the typical size of the water menisci at different relative humidities. Reproduced with permission from Ref. [11].

described a comparison of the LAO process in water and ethanol [12] where the LAO was found to be increased in time, supposedly as the result of a reduction in the trapped charges within the growing oxide. These ethanol menisci were later used for the fabrication of nanometer-sized carbide structures [13], whereby the inscribed nanowires were written with a 70 nm distance between each other and with diameters less than 45 nm, demonstrating the high accuracy of the LAO. Additional studies included the use of octane and 1-octene as organic liquids in the meniscus for the LAO of sub-10 nm-sized structures [14]. Further reports have described the LAO in hexadecane [15], in hydrocarbon solvents (e.g., n-octane, toluene, dioxane) [16] and in HF/ethanol [17]. The LAO has been reported for a wide variety of different substrates, including semiconductors, metals, and self-assembled monolayers (SAMs). Whereas, the LAO on silicon [18–29] was subject of the primary experiments, other semiconductors such as gallium arsenide [30–36], germanium [37–39] and silicon nitride [40–45] have been shown to be of interest for the fabrication of electronic devices. In addition to semiconductors, many different metals have been investigated for the LAO, including titanium [46–51], ferromagnetic metals [52–55], niobium [56, 57], molybdenum [58–60], aluminum [61, 62], and zirconium [63]. Furthermore, patterning was also achieved on both diamond [64–66] and graphene [67, 68] substrates. Since the first experiments related to LAO, several research groups have conducted investigations into the mechanism and reaction kinetics of this process [69–85]. Notably, such studies have addressed the dependence of the LAO process on various parameters, including the relative humidity, tip geometry, tip–substrate distance, applied voltage, and the oxidation time. Various explanations for the LAO behavior have been proposed by different models, including the Cabrera–Mott model, the power-law model, the direct-log kinetic model, and the space charge model [10]. Moreover, several groups have described a linear relationship between the thickness of the oxide layer and the applied voltage [6, 69]. When Avouris and coworkers discussed the rate of the LAO process, they proposed that this would decrease rapidly while the oxide layer was increasing, and that this effect could be explained by a self-limiting influence of the decreasing strength of the applied field and a build-up of stress [71]. These findings were subsequently supported by Sugimura and Nakagiri [9]; moreover, the resolution of the oxidized patterns could be controlled by the shape of the tip [70]. In addition to the commercially available conductive SPM tips that have in the past generally been used for LAOs, several groups have demonstrated the use of carbon nanotube (CNT) probes to improve the resolution of the oxidized features [86–89]. This effect could be explained by a decrease in the water meniscus between the tip and the substrate. Kuramochi and coworkers, for example, demonstrated the fabrication of a lattice structure with line widths of 15 nm and a spacing of 35 nm, as well as concentric circles with 25 nm line widths and 25 nm spacing with multiwalled CNTs used as probes [90]. The size of the oxide features depend on the field strength applied between the tip and the substrate [79]. In subsequent studies, Kuramochi and coworkers quantified the role of the relative humidity compared to the size of the oxide structures [82] and showed that, whilst operating under constant humidity, the size would increase in line with the applied voltage and exposure time, but decrease in line with the speed of the tip. However, if the humidity was to be increased, the size of the features would increase if the applied voltage and exposure time were kept constant.

This electro-oxidation of the surfaces inspired a number of research projects that focused on investigating the nature and formation process of these structures. By using secondary ion mass spectroscopy (SIMS), it could be shown that the formed structures consisted of silicon oxide [91], and this was confirmed using X-ray photoelectron spectroscopy (XPS) [30]. This fact is of particular importance since the processing of silicon oxide is performed routinely via wet-etching processes, as implemented in microelectronics. Indeed, it was shown that the formed silicon oxide structures could be used in a similar way and could be developed into topographic features, for example by applying HF etching [4], anisotropic wet-etching (e.g., with hydrazine or aqueous solutions of potassium hydroxide) [92, 93], or dry-etching procedures [94]. This compatibility with standard structuring techniques would allow the rational and efficient design of functional devices, such that the SPM could be used to generate sophisticated, small features that cannot easily be produced using conventional methods. This led to the application of LAO lithography not only for the fabrication of etched masks [40] and high-density read-only storage devices [49], but also in the fabrication of device structures that have since achieved a remarkable level of sophistication.

The major drawbacks of this patterning technique are the slow acquisition of the image, the exposure rate, and the obtainable size of the LAO structures [94]. The area of the features is limited by the size of the piezoelectric scanner [95], which in turn limits the industrial application of the system. Consequently, several attempts have been made to produce centimeter-sized areas by using a parallel lithography method. As an example, Minne *et al.* demonstrated a reliable electro-oxidation process that employed an array of two cantilevers, although unfortunately an array of five cantilevers showed different qualities of the electro-oxidation patterns for every individual tip [94]. However, this problem could be overcome by the use of a 2×1 array of individually controlled cantilevers [96]. While using a modular micromachined parallel AFM tip array combined with large displacement scanners, the electro-oxidation of centimeter-sized areas is possible, and also in high resolution [97]. Another interesting approach towards upscaling the LAO process would be the use of metalized stamps [95, 98–100]. For this, e.g., a metalized digital video disc (DVD) polymeric support with multiple protrusions was used as cathode, so as to generate a large amount of features with line widths down to 100 nm [95].

And, only three years later the same group introduced an instrument that could perform anodic oxidation in parallel fashion [101], opening the possibility of fabricating silicon oxide patterns over square-centimeter regions in an operation time of less than one minute.

Villarroya *et al.* reported the fabrication of a new cantilever-based sensor system for biochemical detections to be operated within liquid environments, and which employed conventional micro-electro-mechanical system (MEMS) technology and AFM-based lithography. The key feature of the sensor layout here was the implementation of electrical elements for the deflection detection of the cantilever. This was realized by measuring the change in electrochemical current between the mobile cantilever of the sensor and another electrode that was fixed at the free extreme of the cantilever. In this way, a finger-like array of electrodes with high spring constants could be fabricated on the microfabricated sensor cantilever. As a result of the cantilever deflection the relative positions of the electrodes would be altered, and this would result in a change in the electrochemical current to be measured. Hence, advantage could be taken of the heavy dependence of the electrochemical potential on the effective facing cross-sections of both electrodes. In order to ensure a sufficient sensitivity of this detection principle, it was necessary that the distance between the electrodes was less than 100 nm, and that they were patterned by using the AFM electro-oxidation of aluminum oxide on the microfabricated cantilever itself. This led to an increase in the thickness of the aluminum oxide, which subsequently was removed to generate the finger-electrodes.

Minne *et al.* demonstrated the fabrication of 0.1 μm metal oxide semiconductor field effect transistors (MOSFETs) on amorphous silicon (α: Si) films [102]. The probe-induced oxide pattern was first transferred onto α: Si by plasma dry etching, after which the gate contact pad was masked by the photoresist and the gate masked by oxide, leaving the α: Si in these regions intact. The authors reported later on a parallel lithography approach in which the direct electro-oxidation process was coupled with arrays of cantilevers (maximum 50) [96, 97, 102]. Wilder and Quate introduced a cantilever within an integrated MOSFET as a current source for the on-chip control of the exposure current.

Moreover, electro-oxidation of the substrate allows the direct manipulation of the electronic properties of the substrate, with nanometer precision. Campbell *et al.* used the electro-oxidation of Ti films to fabricate metal-oxide-metal devices [103], by scanning a biased tip across a predefined area to define a wire structure which restricted the current flow. The tip was subsequently repositioned on the nonoxidized side of the wire and scanned towards the wire. Due to the constriction of the electro-oxidation process, the electrical resistance was increased as the tip was moved towards the oxide wire. The measurement of the device's resistance during the electro-oxidation process allowed a precise control of the width and the resistance of the junctions and, as a result, structures with dimensions of less than 10 nm and precisely tailored electrical properties could be obtained.

Ishii *et al.* used a AlGaAs/GaAs heterostructure containing a two-dimensional (2-D) electron gas as substrate for electro-oxidation [104]. The group observed that the electro-oxidation of the GaAs cap layer resulted in an increase of the resistance within the 2-D electron gas. Later, Ensslin *et al.* showed that the 2-D electron gas was depleted by a local oxidation of the cap layer [105] if the electron gas was less than 50 nm beneath the surface, and used this process to produce a large variety of sophisticated devices. It appears that a depletion of the electron gas results from the fact that, during the electro-oxidation process, the surface/electron gas distance is reduced and thus the number of surface states is slightly increased. The majority of the donor electrons from the doping layer is then used to fill up these surface states, whilst only a small number of electrons move into the electron gas. The change in the internal electric field is regarded as the reason for the depletion of the electron gas, and one-dimensional (1-D) simulations using a Poisson–Schrödinger solver were used to confirm this mechanism. In this case, the line structures typically showed a width of 100 nm and a height of 8–10 nm. Moreover, it was found that an increase occurred in the resistance in the 2-D electron gas below the oxidized area, and the introduction of additional top and gate layers allowed efficient tuning of the device's characteristics. Similar to the electro-oxidation of the GaAs cap layer, this approach could also be used to pattern the thin Ti gate electrodes to create, for example, quantum point contacts [106]. Consequently, a wide variety of different structures was fabricated to study not only the conductance but also conductance fluctuations in quantum wires [105], four-terminal quantum dots (QDs) and a double quantum dot system with integrated charge readout [107]. Coulomb blockade oscillations in in-plane gate singe-electron transistors [108], the conductance in single-electron transistors and quantum point contacts [109], as well as quantum rings [110], magnetotransport in antidot arrays [111], Aharonov–Bohm oscillations in quantum ring structures [112] and Coulomb blockade resonances in single-electron transistors [113] are all examples demonstrating the impressive capabilities of this patterning approach.

These examples stress some of the advantages of SPM-based structuring techniques. In particular, the wide variety of structuring modes that can be used to modify the surface itself as well as its properties are very versatile. Besides the electro-oxidative modification schemes introduced here, many other interactions can be used to inscribe features onto a surface. Notably, mechanical, thermal, electrostatic and chemical interactions (or combinations of these) have been used to structure surfaces at the nanoscale by means of SPM-based approaches [114] and, as a result, the versatility and variety of materials and structures that can be produced has fuelled extensive interest in SPM-based lithography. The reported surfaces and materials that can be patterned include semiconducting materials such as silicon, metals and rare-earth metal oxide blends, and also molecularly functionalized surfaces including thiols, silanes, DNA, proteins, biomolecules, and nanoparticles [115, 116]. One other important advantage of SPM-based structuring methods is an ability to visualize the inscribed features at high resolution, directly after the patterning process [117, 118]. From a technical point of view, SPM-based techniques are simpler and do not require the expensive fabrication of masks (as do other nanostructuring methods), and consequently the technique is much cheaper, especially for prototyping purposes. With regards to instrumental requirements the technique is very cost-effective, as only a relatively cheap AFM/STM set-up is required [117]. Furthermore, the method offers a complete freedom of pattern choice, a very high spatial precision, and produces structures with a resolution of <10 nm (a value that requires significant know-how if it is to be achieved using conventional structuring methods) [119–122]. A molecular precision of the measured objects can be achieved (and even improved) by using an ultrasharp tip [119]. Likewise, from a practical aspect it is possible to use the same tip to pattern the substrate and to image the inscribed structure *in-situ* after the writing process, thus implementing a direct control of the fabrication step. Whereas, STM-based lithography is mainly performed in ultra-high vacuum, structuring methods based on AFM can be carried out in an ambient environment and under liquid conditions [119, 122]; thus, AFM-based lithography shows great promise for the structuring of biomaterials *in-vitro,* and also for imaging under physiological conditions. Of interest to chemists is the possibility to investigate nanometer-sized features, such as molecular-scale chemical syntheses [115]. Systematic studies of the size-dependent properties of the inscribed nanostructures can be performed directly using AFM, based on an ability to make *in situ* changes to the nanometer-sized features. Another important aspect of these nanometer-sized structures is the possible investigation of molecular recognition processes, the electronic behavior of small clusters of molecules, and the manipulation and organization of biomaterials [115]. Moreover, additional studies may provide information on tip–surface interactions, structures and properties on a nanometer level [119].

Unfortunately, however, SPM-based lithography has certain well-known limitations when implementing fabrication applications. Notably, the fabrication of nanostructures is serial in nature and therefore rather slow [115, 119]; consequently, until now SPM-based patterning techniques have been the subject of research mainly at the academic level. Although the use of SPM-based lithography as a manufacturing tool for high-throughput applications still presents a major challenge, much effort has been made during the past decade to increase the writing speed with a single tip, and to pattern simultaneously with multiple tips [120, 123–132]. For example, Cruchon-Dupeyrat *et al.* introduced an automated vector-scanning scanning probe lithography (SPL) instrument, which could be programmed or linked to computer-assisted design software [120]. However, due to drift and creep of the piezo scanner, and to electronics and/or cantilever artifacts, the inscribed text files and filled structures fidelity of the process have not yet been perfected. Never the less, many of these problems could be solved by using a closed-looped feedback sensor, or by choosing a cantilever with the correct spring constant. More recently, centimeter-scale imaging and lithography with tip arrays of up to 50 cantilevers were reported by Minne *et al.* [97]. In this case, a modular micromachined parallel AFM array was combined with a large displacement scanner and used to produce nanometer-sized features over a large area. Likewise, Wouters and coworkers reported details of the large-scale constructive nanolithography of *n*-octadecyltrichlorosilane (OTS) monolayers via two different methods [127]. The first method used automated AFM where, with a single tip, approximately 1000 structures could be transferred onto the substrate, whilst in a second approach a four-cantilever array was used to inscribe different patterns. Both methods produced structures of high resolution that could be further modified by, for example, the self-assembly of nanomaterials. A cantilever array of five probes for the parallel SPL of *n*-octadecyltrimethoxysilane monolayers was successfully demonstrated by Kakushima *et al.* [128]. In addition, the fabrication of an AFM array with a single-electron transistor has been reported, which can be combined with ultraviolet (UV) lithography for application in quantum devices. Mirkin and coworkers reported the fabrication of a nanoplotter with an array of microfabricated probes for application in parallel dip-pen nanolithography (DPN) [123]. During these investigations, two types of tip array were developed. The first type consisted of 32 silicon nitride cantilevers, separated by 100 μm; although this provided straightforward writing and imaging of the structures, the sharpness of the tips that could be produced was greatly limited by the conformal blanket deposition of the silicon nitride thin film. The second type of probe array, which consisted of eight boron-doped silicon tips separated by 310 μm, provided structures with line widths down to 60 nm and increased imaging capabilities, but the probe density was diminished. One of the first probes to have a large number of tip arrays (created by IBM) incorporated a 2-D array of 32×32 (1024) AFM cantilevers [125]. The information densities of the array were in the order of 650 to 1300 Gb cm^{-2}, and the unit showed great promise for nanostructuring due to its high-speed/large-scale imaging properties. Recently, a 2-D cantilever array consisting of 55 000 tips was reported by Mirkin *et al.* [130]. One other major disadvantage of SPM-based lithography is the limited layer thickness that can be patterned at high resolution. When compared to patterning techniques that use electron beams (when relatively thick layers of resist material can be created), SPL methods are unable to produce thick layers without a significant decrease in resolution. This leads to their applications being limited to selective etching processes, as the thin resist layers are often unable to withstand the extreme conditions of the etching method.

Possible resist layers can be based on SAMs. These are parts of two main categories of which have been used basically in recent research: (i) silane-based monolayers, which react with silicon, glass and activated metal surfaces such as Al; and (ii) thiol monolayers, which react on gold or silver substrates. Thiol-based monolayers were first utilized in 1983 by Nuzzo *et al.* [133], whereas silane-based monolayers were introduced slightly earlier, in 1980, by Sagiv [134]. Until now, the thiol/gold combination has received the most attention, mainly due its easy preparation. Overviews of thiol-based monolayers and their applications have been provided by Ulman *et al.* [135, 136], Everhart [137], Whitesides *et al.* [138], Woodruff [139], and Mutzutami [140].

Nevertheless, silane-based monolayers demonstrate certain advantages over thiols, notably the high stability of the monolayer which results from a covalent network formation, consisting of three bonds, between the surface and the silane molecules. In particular, silane-based SAMs are stable and closely packed, which allows them to serve as a good resist layer for chemical transformation, and also to provide insulating layers. Such high stability also allows further modification steps to be carried out, without affecting the monolayer, in particular at higher temperatures. Moreover, silane-based monolayers are also compatible with silicon technology; notably, the electronic properties of silicon can be influenced by the presence of SAMs, as reported by Peor *et al.* [141], whereby alkyl-, benzyl-, chloro-methylbenzyl-, chlorobenzyl-, bromobenzyl- and iodobenzyltrichlorosilanes were each self-assembled and studied using Kelvin probe techniques. The two main parameters required to tune the electronic properties were coverage of the substrate and the molecular dipole moment of the molecules [141]. Subsequently, Rittner *et al.* investigated the electrical properties of SAMs on hydroxylated silicon surfaces by utilizing C_{18} alkyl chains bearing methyl, thiol, thiophene, phenoxy, and biphenyl end groups. Of particular interest here were the insulating properties of the monolayers and the breakdown voltage. For example, the fact that iodine doping led to an increase in conductivity suggested that it might be possible to build a nanomolecular transistor by using the functional end group as an active layer for the deposition of a conductive layer on the SAM dielectric layer [142]. In further studies, Li *et al.* self-assembled ferrocene-containing monolayers onto silicon and investigated both their capacity and conductance. Interestingly, because they are reversibly chargeable, such monolayers might not only find potential applications in memory devices [143] but also permit the use of optical techniques (e.g., fluorescence spectroscopy) in their investigation. For example, Lee *et al.* described the preparation of spot arrays for protein synthesis by patterning through a photoresist, followed by perfluorination and finally amination with various silane monolayers. In order to achieve this, Fmoc (9-fluorenylmethyl chloroformate) amine acid was first coupled onto the glass surface, followed by fluorescent labeling that allowed the reaction to be monitored via fluorescence imaging. This allowed the creation of a model library of amino acids, with the α-chymotrypsin subsite specificities being replicated by coupling Cy5–streptavidin to the remaining biotin, following enzymatic digestion [144].

These monolayers, and their effective implementation into structuring and nanofabricaton schemes, achieved significance when it was first realized that SAMs and their surface reactions could prove valuable in SPM-based lithography for tuning the surface properties towards specific applications. In particular, based on their inherent hydrophobicity, monolayers showed a potential to improve the resolution of electro-oxidative nanolithography methods, and it soon became clear that the nature of the terminal end groups played an important role in reducing the dimensions of the water meniscus required for the electro-oxidation process. The SAM/ceramic bilayer coatings have also been shown to play important roles in the protection of silicon devices or other electronic applications. For example, Salami *et al.* have described a series of phosphonato-based triethoxysilanes used to manipulate the growth of zirconium oxide [145].

The thermal stability of silane-based SAMs renders them compatible with chemical transformations at higher temperatures, and also allows a wide variety of chemical surface reactions to be conducted, including surface-initiated atom transfer radical polymerization (ATRP) at 100 °C [146], surface initiated reversible addition fragmentation chain transfer (RAFT) radical polymerizations, which were carried out at up to 90 °C [147], and/or the formation of an imide bond between an amine acid salt bilayer at temperatures up to 210 °C [60]. These examples indicate the versatility of functional or reactive SPM-modified substrates to tune the surface's properties, to render its functionality, or simply to attach objects to that surface. Thus, the implementation of such substrates into nanometric frameworks represents a promising approach to the creation of nanometer-sized functional structures by means of SAM-based lithographic techniques.

This brief overview of SPM-based lithography, and its possible combination with SAMs, is indicative of the high potential of this method; hence, extensive investigations have been conducted in this area during the past decade.

During the past decade, the integration of SAMs into SPM lithographic approaches has fuelled sustained research activities, such that a variety of modification schemes has been developed. In the following sections, a brief overview will be provided, highlighting (with selected examples) the potential that derives from the implementation of monolayers in nanofabrication processes. In the past, although mechanical, thermal, electrostatic and chemical interactions have each been used for the inscription of structures, the following relates to two main approaches. The first approach is focused on the patterning methods relating to structuring with SAMs, with the DPN method being used as an example. Next, SPM lithographic methods will be discussed, by which patterned features can be obtained on SAMs on different materials. In addition to nanografting and nanoshaving, the mechanical fabrication routes used to develop nanometer-sized features – notably electro-oxidative nano-lithography and the chemical activation of SAMs by means of tip-induced surface reactions – will each be discussed in greater detail. Following a description of the details of the ready-made silane-based monolayers and surface reactions of SAMs that can be implemented into the nanofabrication route. Discussion will be centered on the combination of patterning and surface chemistry of SAMs towards multi-functional surfaces.

2.2
Structuring with Self-Assembled Monolayers

2.2.1
Dip-Pen Nanolithography

Since its development in 1999, the fabrication of nanometer-sized features by DPN has attracted significant attention in the field of nanotechnology [114, 148–155]. This technique, which was introduced by Mirkin *et al.*, uses an AFM tip to directly transfer an ink onto a substrate via capillary transport, so as to create patterned surfaces [156]. Such transport is possible due to the formation of a water meniscus between the AFM tip and the substrate, while the driving force behind the transfer of the ink to the surface is the chemisorption between the ink molecules and the surface [148]. The chemisorption of these molecules leads to the fabrication of stable surface structures. A schematic representation of the DPN technique is illustrated in Figure 2.3.

Although Mirkin and coworkers were the first to introduce the concept of DPN, the initial experiments for depositing ink from an AFM tip were described by Jaschke and Butt back in 1995 [157], with the deposition of 1-octadecanethiol (ODT) onto mica via an AFM tip. In this case, two main results were noted in terms of the ODT depositions. In some experiments, transfer of the ODT onto the surface occurred

AFM tip

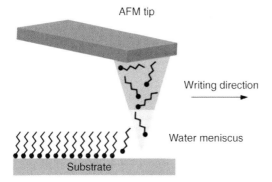

Writing direction

Water meniscus

Substrate

Figure 2.3 Schematic representation of the dip-pen nanolithography (DPN) technique.

immediately after contact of the tip with the mica; however, in other cases a slow growth of small and randomly placed structures was observed, although the inscribed structures were homogeneous in terms of their height and also stable. Four years later, Mirkin and colleagues carried out a further series of experiments on the deposition of thiols onto Au with ODT as the ink [156], in which case the formation of stable surface structures was achieved by the covalent linkage of −SH moieties to the Au surface. After having dipped an AFM tip into a solution of ODT in acetonitrile for 1 min, lateral force microscopy (LFM) measurements were carried out to investigate, in direct manner, the successful deposition of the transferred ink to the surface (Figure 2.4). This was verified by a lower frictional contrast of the inscribed features compared to the bare gold substrate, as illustrated in Figure 2.4a. The lattice-resolved LFM image (Figure 2.4b) confirmed the formation of a highly ordered, densely packed monolayer of thiol molecules.

In further experiments, ODT and 16-mercaptohexadecanoic acid (MHA) were combined as an ink for the fabrication of multicomponent nanostructures by a stepwise writing process [158]. In this way, two differently coated AFM tips were applied for the fabrication of parallel lines consisting of ODT and MHA, while subsequent LFM investigations revealed the precise inscription of six parallel lines of the two inks. These results showed that it was possible not only to create accurate nanostructures with multiple inks, but also to align them with a precision better than 5 nm. In a further experiment, where a pattern of MHA was "overwritten" with ODT, the previously inscribed structures were not influenced by any subsequent writing process, due to the fact that the ink had become linked exclusively to the surface areas, where it had a chemical affinity.

The method of DPN depends on several different aspects, each of which must be taken into account. The resolution of the patterns relies on various parameters, including the grain size of the substrate, the chemical affinity of the ink molecules to the substrate, the contact time between the tip and the substrate, the tip radius and the material of the tip, the writing speed, and the relative humidity [156]. Whereas, a grainy surface leads to interrupted lines, smooth substrates are suitable for the writing of long lines with nanometer-sized widths and high quality. As the formation of stable structures relies mainly on the chemisorption of the ink molecules to the

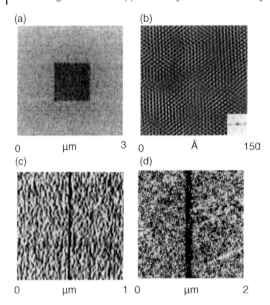

Figure 2.4 (a) Lateral force microscopy image of a square of 1-octadecanethiol inscribed on Au (1 μm × 1 μm); (b) Lattice-resolved, lateral force microscopy image of an 1-octadecanethiol self-assembled monolayer on Au(111)/mica; (c) Lateral force microscopy image of a 30 nm- wide line by dip-pen nanolithography (DPN); (d) Lateral force microscopy image of a 100 nm line by DPN. The darker regions correspond to areas of relatively lower friction. Reproduced with permission from Ref. [156].

substrate, the choice of ink is an important parameter for the fabrication of well-ordered features. In general, it is possible to use different types of ink on various substrates. Notably, the relative humidity controls the size of the water meniscus formed between the tip and the substrate, and this, in turn, offers the possibility to control the ink transport rate, the feature size, and therefore also the line widths [158]. Recently, some critical questions arose regarding the role of the water meniscus, which was proposed to mediate the transport of ink to the surface [159]. However, the question remained as to how water-insoluble inks could be transferred to the surface. In an attempt to resolve this problem, Sheehan and Whitman conducted a study regarding the role of the relative humidity and thiol diffusion on DPN [160], and showed that such ink deposition could be observed after 24 h, even under dry air or in a N_2 atmosphere. These results suggested that the water meniscus was not necessary for the transfer process. In a later study, Schwartz also reported on the molecular transport from the AFM tip [159], where the patterning was investigated under various parameters including temperature, relative humidity, and an ethanol vapor, while the patterning was carried out using different tip coatings. The study results indicated that the writing process was not necessarily dependent on the water meniscus, since both ODT and MHA could also be patterned under 0% humidity. However, the resolution of the inscribed features was seen to depend on the relative humidity during the structuring process. A higher resolution of the inscribed patterns could also be obtained by using sharper tips. The amount of material transferred to the surface was also seen to be a crucial parameter for the writing time and the number of features which can be inscribed, as well as for the size of the inscribed structures. Consequently, several different methods have been reported to increase the amount of ink that is adsorbed on the AFM tip [149, 161, 162]. The use of tips that are made from, or are coated with, polydimethylsiloxane (PDMS), represents one possibility of enhancing the amount of ink molecules deposited [152, 163, 164]. Other favorable characteristics of PDMS include the wide variety of inks that can be coated onto the tip, the reduced evaporation of the adsorbed ink, and the utilization for the patterning of rough surfaces due to its elastic properties [165]. The modification of the tip with a layer of, for example, 1-dodecylamine, alters the surface property to hydrophilic, and this leads to an improved quality of the LFM measurements due to a reduction in the capillary force and a higher resolution of soft-inked materials [166]. The transport of the ink to the surface, which in turn influences the quality of the patterns, is a complex process that is influenced by different parameters [151, 152, 167], notably the purity of the ink and the surface, the shape of the tip, and also the material, the relative humidity, the temperature during the writing process, and so on.

2.2.1.1 Thermal Dip-Pen Nanolithography

In an attempt to expand the number of usable inks for patterning, a variation of the normal DPN approach was developed, termed thermal dip-pen nanolithography (tDPN) [167–170]. In this process, the tip is first coated with a material that is solid at room temperature, and then brought into contact with the surface, such that the ink is transferred to the substrate when the cantilever is heated. Not only can tDPN be used to control the rate of deposition onto a localized area, but the writing can also be switched on and off. Furthermore, when compared to the normal DPN process, tDPN excludes any contamination of the inscribed structures during the imaging step, due to the on/off deposition of the ink. Reported materials that have been inscribed via tDPN range from organic molecules (e.g., octadecylphosphonic acid), metals (e.g., indium) and the polymers poly(N-isopropylacrylamide) (PNIPAAM) and poly(3-dodecylthiophene). In seeking a system that did not require a thermal cantilever, Mirkin and coworkers described a DPN technique that used high-melting temperature molecules, but did not need tDPN [171]. On investigating the patterning of various inks with melting points between 99 and 231 °C, Mirkin's group showed that if the conditions of the writing process were carefully optimized, then no heatable tips would be required for the inscription. However, for any inks that were poorly water-soluble, tDPN represented an important improvement compared to "normal" DPN.

In comparison to other nanofabrication techniques, DPN demonstrates several clear advantages. One important characteristic of the DPN method is its ability to use a wide range of different substrates, including metals, insulating, and semiconducting surfaces [149], as well as a wide variety of inks (including diverse chemical moieties) that may lead to functional surface patterns. Examples of these substrates include alkanethiols [156, 158, 172], silanes [173, 174], polymers [175–177], metal ions [178], and biomolecules [179–181] such as DNA [182–185], proteins [186–192], and peptides [193]. The wide variety of materials that can be used as inks allows the possibility of investigating a number of different processes, such as biorecognition, the control of single virus particles on a surface, virus–cell infectivity processes, cell–cell adhesion and the mechanism of cell migration, as well as studies related to nanoscale phenomena and the monitoring of molecular processes *in-situ*, such as monolayer nucleation and growth [149, 194, 195]. In particular, the inscription process is not limited to one ink; in fact, it is possible to write with several different inks on the same substrate. The preparation of pristine multiple ink nanostructures can be used in the study of molecule-based electronics, catalysis and molecular diagnostics [158]. Compared to other nanofabrication techniques, DPN requires only small amounts of material to create nanometric features [156], and neither does it depend on the use of harsh conditions such as electron-beam, UV-light and/or development steps [149] to fabricate nanometer-sized features, and this helps to prevent contamination and destruction of the substrate. The resolution of the inscribed structures is less than 50 nm, which in turn leads to line widths in the range of 15 nm being achieved, and an alignment resolution of approximately 5 nm [150, 196]. Compared to other patterning techniques, DPN is a direct-write technique [151], with no need for any preparation of resist layers, stamps (as in micro-contact printing) or masks, nor the use of commercially non-available equipment [150, 154, 156, 158]. On a practical point, as the inscription process can be operated under either ambient or inert conditions, no ultrahigh-vacuum techniques are required [150]. Moreover, the fact that both the writing and imaging of the obtained features can be carried out with a single tip represents an important point for efficient writing and scanning processes [148]. Notably, the tips most frequently used for DPN are commercially available, while conductive tips are not required at all.

Two important disadvantages of DPN when used to fabricate large patterns are the speed of the writing process, and the size of the obtained features [154]. When implementing into high-throughput systems, the technique must be expanded from a serial to a parallel set-up, and various attempts have been made to overcome this limitation. Two strategies are available to achieve this: (i) the fabrication of a passive-pen array, where each tip duplicates the desirable structure [197]; and (ii) the use of an active array with individually addressable tips. Of these two methods, the passive array is the most applicable because the ink transfer appears to be force-independent, while the implementation of a nanoplotter with an array of probes for applications in parallel DPN has been introduced and further improved [123, 198, 199]. Others have reported the writing of large structures with three different probe arrays (with the number of tips ranging from 26 to 250) and a deposition speed of $0.935 \, \text{cm min}^{-1}$. Currently, for DPN the largest number of tips used in an array has been 55 000 [130, 200]; when in 2-D format, such an array can be used for patterning over an area of several square centimeters, and with a resolution of less than 100 nm. As an example, when the successful writing of the image of Thomas Jefferson from a US five cent coin was achieved by the patterning of ODT on gold, 55 000 duplicates of the cover of the coin were written with high precision. The patterning of phospholipids has also been demonstrated using this array, with each tip writing the letter combination "INT" three times within only 12 s, over an area of $1 \, \text{cm}^2$.

The second strategy involves the addressability of the individual tips. Actuation of the tip can be achieved in different ways, including thermal [132, 201, 202], piezoelectric, or electrostatic [203]. The *thermal actuation* of a tip array has been used most frequently, due to the easy fabrication process, the use of simple materials, and the large displacement of the tip array and performance at low voltages [201]. The main disadvantage of this method is the thermal crosstalk that occurs between neighboring tips, due to heat transfer between the probes; the technique is also unsuitable for use with temperature-sensitive materials [203]. Mirkin *et al.* demonstrated a thermally actuated array of 10 tips for the inscription of ODT on Au with sub-50 nm line widths [132, 201, 202]. An alternative approach to actuate the individual tips, *electrostatic actuation*, occurs due to the generation of electrostatic attraction forces [201] and is produced by the presence of two oppositely charged electrodes. In contrast to thermal actuation, the electrostatic method depends on a complex fabrication process, as the probes are not heated during the patterning process it is possible to inscribe temperature-sensitive materials [203]. The actuator crosstalk is also reduced in the case of electrostatic actuation. Recently, Bullen and Liu described the successful patterning of ODT using electrostatic-actuated tips with line widths down to 25 nm, which was comparable to the commercially available silicon nitride cantilevers that are used for ink transfer.

Since its introduction, the use of DPN has been reported using a wide variety of different inks and substrates. A selection of experiments and interesting examples from various research areas are outlined in the following sections.

2.2.1.2 DPN with Biomolecules

The construction of protein arrays represents an important area in the field of proteomics, cell research and diagnostics, among others [186]. For example, Mirkin and coworkers described the fabrication of arrays of MHA features on a background of passivating 11-mercaptoundecyl-tri(ethylene glycol). When the substrates were subsequently immersed in solutions of different proteins to test their adsorption behavior, the proteins assembled selectively on the MHA features, but no nonspecific adsorption occurred on the background layer. Most importantly, the proteins demonstrated biological activity after the adsorption process. Subsequently, cell-adhesion tests were carried out on patterns of Retronectin, adsorbed onto MHA, where the cells were attached selectively only onto the patterned areas. A direct approach for writing patterns of proteins was reported later by the same group [204]. When both rabbit immunoglobulin G (IgG) and anti-rabbit IgG nanostructures were inscribed on negatively charged and aldehyde-terminated substrates, fluorescence imaging was used to reveal the chemical identity of the fluorophore-labeled anti-rabbit IgG protein. Additional studies were carried out on the high throughput production of large protein patterns [205], in which features of *N*-hydroxysuccinimide (NHS) were inscribed on gold for selective reactions with a variety of proteins; the proteins were later labeled with Alexa Fluor 594 to investigate the biological activity of the antibodies when located on the protein structures (Figure 2.5). The tapping mode height and fluorescence images confirmed the antibody adsorption onto the protein-array templates.

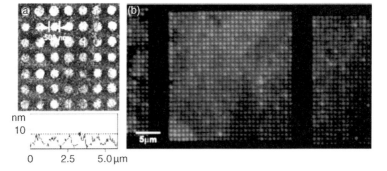

Figure 2.5 (a) Tapping mode height image and height profile of fluorescein isothiocyanate Alexa Fluor 594-labeled human immunoglobulin G (IgG) nanoarrays immobilized onto protein A/G templates; (b) Fluorescence microscopy image of Alexa Fluor 594-labeled antibody nanoarray patterns. Reproduced with permission from Ref. [205].

Further studies in the field of biomolecules were conducted by Li *et al.*, who reported the fabrication of nanopatterns on individual, stretched DNA molecules [206]. Nanostructures of gold, created by using DPN, can be used to assemble thiol-terminated DNA molecules [207], after which the DNA structures can further react with complementary DNA, or with particles modified with complementary DNA. This process was used also by Chung and coworkers to assemble single DNA-functionalized nanoparticles into the gap regions of single-electrode junctions [185]. The method described might be useful for the development of biosensors and to investigate electrical transport through such features. Other experiments related to the fabrication of functional electrical gaps for the detection of DNA have been recently reported by Li *et al.* [208]. In this case, DPN was used to pattern chip DNAs into micrometer-sized electrical gap structures, after which the DNA assemblies were reacted with target single-stranded DNA and DNA-functionalized nanoparticles to form structures capable of conducting an electrical current. The patterning of enzymes onto DNA-terminated monolayers leads to the possibility of performing nanoscale enzymology [209]. Hyun *et al.* demonstrated the writing of DNase 1 onto oligonucleotide SAMs, with a subsequent treatment of the surface with Mg^{2+} ions so as to create hole structures, caused by digestion of the surface-bound substrate by the enzyme.

2.2.1.3 **DPN with Polymers**
The patterning of polymers represents an interesting area of research, based on the possibility of using these structures to fabricate sensors, in catalysis, and for optical devices. In particular, the patterning of conductive polymers has attracted significant attention, as they might be used for the fabrication of nanodevices and nanosensors. Lim *et al.* described the deposition of nanometer-sized structures of self-doped sulfonated polyaniline and doped polypyrrole onto positively and negatively charged surfaces via electrostatic interactions [210], with the obtained features being characterized by LFM and electrochemical measurements. The writing of polythiophene

nanowires on semiconducting and insulating substrates was demonstrated by Maynor and coworkers [211], who used a variation of the normal DPN process, the so-called "electrochemical DPN." For this, the monomer units were polymerized at the tip–substrate interface, which led to the creation of conducting polymeric nanowires with a resolution of more than 100 nm. Other examples included the combination of DPN and ring-opening metathesis polymerization (ROMP) to create combinatorial libraries of functional polymer features [212], the guided pattern formation in spin-coated polymer blend films from DPN-inscribed surface templates [177], and the creation of nanostructures in poly(4-vinylpyridine) by local protonation with a pH 4 buffer solution used as ink [213].

2.2.1.4 DPN with Fluorescent Dyes

Patterned areas of fluorescent dyes have the potential for application in high-density optical information storage, optoelectronic devices, and biological staining [214, 215]. When Su and Dravid demonstrated the inscription of different organic dyes on both bare and modified silicon substrates [214], characterization of the structures by fluorescence microscopy showed the emission of, for example, eight parallel lines of rhodamine 6G (R6G) on negatively charged silicon. Notably, the line widths could be controlled by changing the scanning speed of the tip. Other examples included the fabrication of luminescent patterns of R6G and their characterization, using scanning confocal microscopy, down to the single-molecule level [215], the placement of fluorescent-labeled silazanes [216], and the deposition of fluorescent adamantyl-functionalized molecules on β-cyclodextrin monolayers [217].

2.2.1.5 DPN in the Field of Electrolytes

The fabrication of polyelectrolyte structures via layer-by-layer formation might be incorporated into applications such as nanoelectronics, and also in the study of cell-adhesion characteristics. Yu and coworkers described the fabrication of polyelectrolyte structures on different surfaces [218], whereby poly(diallyldimethylammonium) chloride (PDDA) and poly(styrenesulfonate) (PSS) were used as inks to obtain positively and negatively charged nanofeatures. The method demonstrated a potential for implementation into other surface-engineering applications, such as directed cell growth and surface-mediated molecular assemblies. Lee *et al.* created polyelectrolyte multilayers of PDDA and PSS on structured MHA patterns on gold [219], after which the background was filled with different molecules, such as ODT or poly(ethylene glycol) (PEG), to prevent any nonspecific adsorption of the polyelectrolytes. Fabrication of the multilayer was achieved by alternating the assembly of PDDA and PSS onto the MHA structures. The features were then characterized using fluorescence microscopy, after having labeled the multilayers with a fluorescein solution to reveal uniform fluorescein structures on the surface.

2.2.1.6 DPN with Nanomaterials

The use of nanomaterials in the process of DPN offers the possibility to guide, for example, the assembly of individual particles on a surface to study quantum phenomena or particle–particle and particle–substrate interactions; moreover, nanoelectronic structures and devices could be designed by the patterning of metallic materials. The reported examples of different nanomaterials used in DPN range from gold [220–222], platinum [223] and magnetic nanoparticles [224–227], cadmium selenide nanostructures [228] and SnO_2 [229], positively charged modified polystyrene spheres [230], nanowires [231, 232] to single-wall carbon nanotubes (SWCNTs) [233]. The first report of the formation of metallic nanostructures by an electroless metal deposition process was reported by Maynor *et al.* [222]. In these studies, the water meniscus between the AFM tip and the surface acted as a reactor vessel, causing the metal ions to be reduced to metal atoms with subsequent deposition of the nanofeatures. The structures showed a high stability against several washing steps, as well as thermal stability up to 300 °C. Porter and coworkers also demonstrated the writing of gold and palladium lines via electroless deposition [234], obtaining line widths of 30 nm with a height of 10 nm. The generation of arrays of magnetic particles was demonstrated by Liu [224], where a pattern of MHA and ODT, fabricated by DPN, served as a template for the selective assembly of pre-prepared magnetic Fe particles. Further experiments of the fabrication of "hard" magnetic nanostructures were performed with barium hexaferrite [225], in which the writing of an ink containing iron nitrate and barium carbonate yielded BaFe particles with sub-100 nm diameters. The magnetic properties of the inscribed features were characterized by magnetic force microscopy (MFM), which revealed the magnetic nature of the particles. Basner and coworkers described an interesting approach for the generation of metallic nanowires [232] in which enzymes modified with Au nanoparticles were used as biocatalytic inks for the inscription of lines of different metals. This method proved to be useful for the generation of complex nanocircuitry.

2.2.1.7 Chemical DPN

Finally, DPN has been used in the field of chemical surface reactions, with Degenhart and coworkers reporting the fabrication of robust micrometer- and nanometer-sized reaction areas on surfaces [235]. For this purpose, NHS-terminated monolayers on gold were used for patterning with $-NH_2$-functionalized polyamidoamine dendrimers, which then underwent a chemical surface reaction (amide linkage formation), with the formation of covalently attached structures. As these structures are highly stable, they could be used in a variety of applications, including chemical sensors. Additional nanometric surface reactions were demonstrated by Chi and Choi [236], in which an interchain carboxylic anhydride (ICA)-terminated monolayer was used for patterning with alkylamines to form stable surface structures via amide bond formation. The ICA-terminated SAM was prepared by the treatment of a carboxylic acid-functionalized SAM on Au with trifluoroacetic anhydride and triethylamine. Subsequent characterization of the inscribed features, using LFM, revealed a lower friction of the structures compared to the background. Long and coworkers demonstrated the localized click chemistry by using DPN [237], where acetylene-terminated silicon substrates served as surface templates for the patterning of azide-modified dendrimers. The $-C\equiv CH$ end groups were obtained via a two-step synthesis, starting from an amino-terminated SAM, which was treated with an acetylene-functionalized carboxylic acid under peptide bond formation conditions. Coupling of the azide dendrimer was achieved via a Cu(I)-catalyzed cycloaddition, while LFM was carried out to detect any changes in composition after the DPN process.

These selected examples of nanostructures that can be obtained by using DPN demonstrate the versatility of the method. Due to the fact that a wide range of materials can be patterned on different substrates, the procedure has many potential applications, including the fabrication of sensors, as electronic devices, and in studies of biorecognition processes. Moreover, its implementation in high-throughput experimentation has demonstrated the possibility of patterning large surface areas and large amounts of structures, with high quality.

2.3
Structuring of Self-Assembled Monolayers

Compared to the above-described DPN approach, the following structuring methods employ SAMs that have been self-assembled on various substrates and subsequently patterned. The main advantages of using SAMs are the thermal, chemical and physical stability of the system and the densely packed nature of the monolayers. Structuring with an AFM tip by employing mechanical forces (e.g., nanoshaving and nanografting) and by applying a bias voltage between the substrate and the tip – that is, with LAO and a constructive nanolithography approach – are detailed in the following sections.

2.3.1
Nanoshaving

The first stages of fabricating the nanometer-sized features of SAMs by mechanical forces with the aid of an AFM tip were reported by Liu *et al.* in 1994 [238]. Here, the structure and stability of $CH_3(CH_2)_9SH$ ($C_{10}SH$) and ODT, self-assembled on Au (111), were investigated by using AFM. Under sufficiently high loads of the AFM tip, the molecules could be removed from the surface; moreover, the process was seen to be reversible and, by applying a decreased load, the thiol molecules were able to diffuse back to the surface. This area of research was extended in 1995 with studies of alkylsilanes on mica [239], examining the displacement of monolayers of octadecyl-triethoxysilane on mica and characterizing their stability by means of AFM. A comparison with their thiol analogues showed that a much greater force was needed to displace the silane-based SAMs. When compared to thiols on gold, the process was seen to be irreversible, due to a reduced diffusion and mechanical strength.

This effect is used in the so-called "nanoshaving" approach to create negative structures by the displacement of a SAM with an AFM tip under a high local pressure [115, 119, 153, 240]. This process can be divided into three steps: (i) characterization of the surface, using AFM operated at low forces; (ii) removal of the SAM to inscribe the nanofeatures (this causes the AFM tip to be scanned at a high local pressure over the surface, resulting in a high shear force on the contact areas and subsequent displacement of the SAM) and (iii) imaging and visualization of the

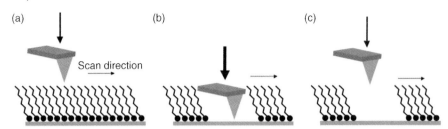

Figure 2.6 Schematic representation of the nanoshaving process. (a) Imaging of the surface; (b) Patterning of the self-assembled monolayer (SAM) under high local pressure; (c) Imaging of the surface.

inscribed structures, again under reduced loads. The manipulation via nanoshaving is shown schematically in Figure 2.6.

This process is highly dependent on the force applied to the surface [119, 240]. Whilst a very high force of the AFM tip can lead to plastic deformation or displacement of the substrate, low forces will result in an incomplete removal of the SAM; therefore, it is required that each system is investigated carefully and independently. The fabrication of high-resolution patterns depends on different parameters, including a molecule-by-molecule displacement, an immediate removal of the SAM, and a slow readsorption rate in order to prevent any backfilling of the structures with the self-assembled molecules that have been removed. Readsorption of the adsorbates depends on the environment of the fabrication route [119]. During the patterning of thiols on gold in air or water, the readsorption rate is higher than in the case of, for example, ethanol or 2-butanol; hence, the solubility of the thiols in the solvent used has a clear influence on the readsorption rate. Whilst thiols are not (or are only poorly) soluble in water, the removed adsorbates will remain weakly bound to the gold surface, and consequently a reversible displacement of the thiols will lead to low-resolution patterns. As the solubility of thiols is greater for ethanol and 2-butanol, however, the readsorption will be decreased and sharp patterns are obtained. The structuring of siloxane monolayers on mica can be achieved under different conditions. Due to the presence of only a few covalent bonds between the mica substrate and the siloxanes, the system has no long-range order. Furthermore, the siloxane molecules are connected via Si−O−Si bonds, which are responsible for the formation of a stable network. Following the nanoshaving process, the siloxane molecules that have been removed will show a low reactivity towards the mica substrate, and it is for this reason that the displacement of the molecules is irreversible and the structures obtained will have sharp features with a high resolution. Several examples have been reported where nanoshaving has been used not only to create structures with a high resolution, but also on a variety of substrates to demonstrate the potential of the technique in the fabrication of nanoelectronics. The production of functional semiconducting wires from sexithiophene, using an AFM tip, was described by Chwang *et al.* [241], who created wires between 300 and 70 nm wide via this approach. In order to investigate the electrical properties of these products, both photoconductivity and temperature-dependent transport measurements were carried out to compare them with single grains of sexithiophene. This study also demonstrated the possibility of using other organic semiconductors to create nanometer-sized structures for applications in nanoelectronics. Liu and coworkers described the precise positioning of gold nanoparticles, surrounded by a shell of alkanethiol and alkanedithiol molecules [242]. In this case, an alkylthiol monolayer was used as a background for the nanostructuring by a sharp AFM tip. The nanoparticles adsorbed only onto the inscribed structures, such that the alkenedithiols served as anchoring groups for attachment to the surface. The construction of three-dimensional (3-D) protein–DNA features on gold substrates was demonstrated by Zhou *et al.* [243], whereby a thiolated DNA as monolayer was used as the base for patterning to obtain hole structures of $400 \times 400 \, nm^2$. As this background layer proved to be resistant to the nonspecific adsorption of DNA–streptavidin assemblies, 3-D structures of DNA and streptavidin could be created via a step-by-step growing procedure. Zauscher *et al.* described the fabrication of stimuli-responsive nanopatterned polymer brushes of PNIPAAM onto gold surfaces [244, 245]. Here, a monolayer of ODT was formed as a resist layer onto Au, to serve as a template for the structuring by nanoshaving. Subsequent backfilling of the nanometer-sized features was achieved using a thiol-terminated initiator for the polymerization of NIPAAM. These findings might be important for the fabrication of silicon-based devices, where nanometer-sized polymer brushes could serve as barriers to different wet chemical etchants. The patterning of 1-alkenes, self-assembled onto hydrogen-passivated silicon surfaces, was described by Berrie and coworkers [246]. These authors showed that, depending on the applied load and the number of etching scans under high loads, the depths of the structures in the alkyl monolayer could be varied between 2 and 15 nm. Furthermore, these results were compared to the patterning of alkyl siloxane monolayers on silicon and mica. The reversible, templated nanostructure electrodeposition on a Au(111) surface by means of a "write, read and erase" nanolithographic approach was demonstrated by Borguet *et al.* [247], where a monolayer of ODT on gold was used for the inscription of nanometer-sized patterns of Ag. Deposition of the Ag structures was achieved by using electrochemistry, and was also reversible, depending on the applied voltage. Thus, this process would be suitable for the *in situ* deposition of metal structures for the fabrication of complex nanostructures. Cremer and coworkers reported on the fabrication of supported phospholipid bilayers with a resolution of less than 100 nm [248]. In this case, a bovine serum albumin (BSA) monolayer was patterned by an ultrasharp AFM tip under an applied force of approximately 300 nN. The inscribed structures were then backfilled with a vesicle solution which consisted of 1-palmitoyl-2-oleoyl-*sn*-glycero-3-phosphocholine and a dye-labeled lipid. After washing with a phosphate-buffered saline solution, investigations using fluorescence microscopy revealed a uniform fluorescence from the 55 nm-wide lines.

To summarize, nanoshaving represents a simple method for the fabrication of nanometric features via the mechanical removal of SAMs with an AFM tip. Under ambient conditions, nanoshaving enables patterning with high resolution, as well as an immediate characterization of the structures obtained. Various reports have outlined the possible use of this approach to fabricate complex 3-D biomolecular structures, to create organic semi-conductor nanowires for transport studies, or in the "grafting from" technique of functional monomers. Nevertheless, the writing process must be carefully optimized to ensure not only that no damage of the underlying substrate occurs, but also that there is a complete removal of the SAM. either without or with less readsorption of the molecules onto the surface.

2.3.2
Nanografting

Nanografting represents an alternative patterning method, where thiol chemistry on gold is combined with AFM to create nanometer-sized features [249]. This technique is similar to nanoshaving, but includes an additional step. The procedure begins with the imaging of a SAM on the surface, under low pressure, in a liquid medium containing a second reactive adsorbate [115, 119, 240]. The AFM tip is then scanned with higher forces over the surface so as locally to remove any self-assembled molecules, which are then transported into the liquid. In the meantime, the second adsorbate molecules are adsorbed onto the freshly created structures, after which the nanostructures may be imaged under low force with the AFM tip to investigate the inscribed structures. A schematic overview of the fabrication of nanostructures in this way is shown in Figure 2.7.

Both, nanografting and nanoshaving, are heavily influenced by the applied force of the AFM tip onto the surface [119, 240]. As noted above, an excessively high load of the tip can results in a plastic deformation or displacement of the underlying substrate. although if the force is too low the SAM cannot be completely removed.

The term "nanografting" was first coined in 1997 by Xu and Liu [250], who used a $C_{10}SH$ monolayer on gold as a resist for patterning the surface with the AFM tip. In this case, ODT was chosen as the reactive second thiol compound for backfilling of the nanometer-sized features. The subsequent characterization using AFM revealed a height difference of 8.8 Å, which could be correlated to a crystalline-phase SAM (Figure 2.8); furthermore, no exchange between the ODT and $C_{10}S$–Au was observed in the remaining background layer. In addition, the ability to obtain multiple nanostructures by altering the thiol compound before each fabrication step opened

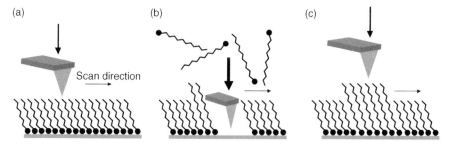

Figure 2.7 Schematic representation of the nanografting process. (a) Imaging of the surface; (b) Patterning of the self-assembled monolayer (SAM) under high local pressure with simultaneous adsorption of a second adsorbate molecule; (c) Imaging of the surface.

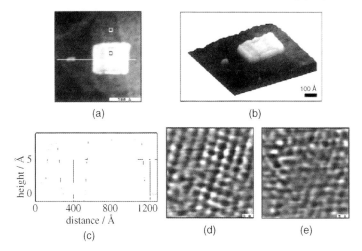

Figure 2.8 (a, b) Topographic images of the created square structures of the $CH_3(CH_2)_9SH$–Au resist (bright square = 1-octadecanethiol–Au; dark area = $CH_3(CH_2)_9SH$–Au); (c) Height profile of the 1-octadecanethiol–Au square; (d, e) Molecular-resolution images of the $CH_3(CH_2)_9SH$–Au and 1-octadecanethiol–Au areas. Reproduced with permission from Ref. [250].

the possibility of using the technique to fabricate, for example, nanoelectronic devices.

Further studies of the nanografting technique were performed and expanded by the group of Liu [251–259]; notably, investigations were also conducted into the kinetics of the self-assembly process of thiols on bare gold surfaces, compared to a spatially confined area [251]. In this way, an acceleration of the kinetics was observed for the nanometer-sized features, due to the generation of a transient reaction environment. Additional studies have been related to using an inscribed structure, backfilled with chemically active thiols, for the selective immobilization of proteins via electrostatic interactions or covalent binding [253]. Moreover, 3-D nanostructures could be obtained via selective surface reactions [255]. Depending on the resist layer on gold (such as ODT or 11-mercapto-1-undecanol), either positive or negative nanopatterns could be created, with the obtained features being backfilled with either an alkylthiol or an −OH-terminated thiol compound. In a third fabrication step, the −OH functionalities were reacted with OTS to construct structures in the third dimension.

Biorelated research in the field of nanografting – for example, concerning the fabrication of protein or enzyme patterns – has been conducted by several groups [256, 258, 260–268]. One such example included the incorporation of parallel, three-helix bundle metalloproteins on a gold surface via nanografting [260], while another described a double-cysteine-terminated maltose-binding protein that could be immobilized onto Au substrates at well-defined locations, with subsequent investigations being carried out using *in situ* AFM friction measurements to characterize the bioactivity of the protein products [262, 263]. Further investigations were conducted, using AFM force–compression measurements, to probe the ligand-induced changes in the mechanical properties of the maltose-binding proteins. In this case, both positive and negative patterns were created containing –OH functionalities on gold. These hydroxyl groups would react with trichlorosilanes to build bilayer systems. Thiolated, single-stranded DNA could also be patterned in this way to provide biostructures with nanometer resolution, that might potentially be of interest for fabricating DNA biosensors and biochips [256, 258]. Further studies addressing the construction of 3-D protein nanostructures were detailed by Abell *et al.* [269], whereby an alkanethiol, terminated with a hexa(ethyleneglycol) group and self-assembled onto Au, was used as a base for the nanopatterning of three differently charged thiol compounds in the construction of multifunctional, nanometer-sized features. For this, various proteins were immobilized onto the surface to investigate the pH-dependency of protein adsorption. DeYoreo and coworkers reported on the structuring of virus particles on gold surfaces [270] which could be modified either genetically or chemically and attached onto the SAM. Additional studies were carried out on the covalent linkage of oligonucleotides on nanometer patterns for the formation of Pd crystals. In the field of nanochemistry, further investigations were conducted by using nanografting to fabricate the nanometer-sized features of maleimide [271]. Such nanoscale structures could then be coupled via a Michael addition with *p*-xylylenediamine to obtain free amine functionalities, which would further react with 11,11′-dimaleimidoundecyldisulfide. This step-by-step surface chemistry led to the build-up of 3-D features. A modified variant of nanografting – the so-called "nano-pen reader and writer process" – which was developed by Liu and coworkers [272] combined nanografting on a thiol-terminated gold surface with DPN. The tip to be used for patterning of the SAM was precoated with another thiol compound to create structures with multiple components. The construction of large patterned areas was also described by the groups of both Liu and Garno, using an automated nanografting approach [120, 273]. Notably, the group of Liu described computer-assisted design and automated vector SPL, while Garno's group focused their attention on the mechanics of automated nanografting, and demonstrated results for the different writing strategies.

The technique of nanografting is not limited to thiols on gold surfaces, but can also be applied to silicon substrates and self-assembled silane monolayers [274, 275]. Linford *et al.* described the successful patterning of monolayers of octadecyl- and octyldimethylmonochlorosilane on thin and thick silicon substrates, using an AFM tip, with the inscribed structures being backfilled with perfluorinated silanes and aminosilanes. The $-NH_2$ functionalities introduced were then used for the attachment of DNA strands and Pd cations, which could in turn be applied to testing of the electrical properties of nanoscale objects.

To summarize, nanografting represents a powerful technique for the fabrication of nanometer-sized features, with high spatial resolution. One advantage of nanografting in comparison to nanoshaving is the *in situ* backfilling of the created structures with chemically active self-assembling molecules. Consequently, this approach can be used for biorecognition and protein immobilization approaches, as well as for the investigation of reaction kinetics and mechanisms of surface reactions. Moreover, the technique has the potential to create a variety of different structured monolayers with various functional elements. Yet, the disadvantages of nanografting are similar to those of nanoshaving, as it is equally necessary carefully to adjust the force applied to remove the SAMs, so as to prevent destruction of the substrate and of any remaining material. It is also important that the molecules being used to backfill the structures show a higher adsorption rate than the removed molecules, in order to prevent the formation of mixed monolayers, or the adsorption of the initial SAM molecules.

2.3.3
Electro-Oxidative Lithography

In electro-oxidative lithography processes, a bias voltage is applied between a substrate and the AFM tip, and this results in the creation of a localized electric field. This field can lead to physical and/or chemical modifications of the substrate or the SAM (as outlined in the introduction), which can be used to structure surfaces in the nanometer range. Thus, electro-oxidation has been defined as two discrete areas: (i) LAO, which, as described above, provides the possibility of generating oxide patterns on different substrates; and (ii) electro-oxidation, which focuses on the chemical modification of terminal end groups on a SAM.

2.3.3.1 Local Anodic Oxidation
At this point, electro-oxidative patterning will be reviewed with special emphasis on the possibility to structure and/or locally modify SAMs. Next to the anodic oxidation of semiconductors and metals, the method can also be applied to pattern molecularly functionalized surfaces. This area of LAO includes SAMs on silicon and gold, Langmuir–Blodgett (LB), and polymeric thin films. The use and patterning of these functionalized surfaces permits the introduction of various chemical functionalities in the patterned areas, so as to fabricate multifunctional surfaces. A brief overview of LAO on various modified substrates is provided in the following subsections.

LAO on SAMs on Silicon   One of the first reports on the oxidation of organosilane-terminated monolayers was provided by Sugimura [276, 277], where a trimethylsilyl (TMS) SAM on Si was used to fabricate silicon oxide patterns. These oxide features were later etched in a mixture of $NH_4F/H_2O_2/H_2O$, which resulted in the formation of nanometer-sized grooves. The patterning was carried out with a conductive AFM tip with positive as well as negative bias voltages. Further studies were performed to investigate the effect of humidity, bias voltage, and probe scan rate on the degradation of the TMS monolayer. Further oxidation experiments included the use of octadecyldimethylmethoxysilane [278, 279], octadecyltrimethoxysilane [280], 1-dodecene [281, 282], 1-octadecene [283] and OTS [284, 285] monolayers to investigate the growth of silicon oxide features on various SAMs. Besides the oxidation of these $-CH_3$-terminated monolayers, which are chemically inert, other monolayers with functional end groups were also applied to LAO. For example, Zheng and coworkers reported on the anodic oxidation of thiol-terminated monolayers on Si [286]; this involved the use of Au nanoparticles being attached to the −SH functionalities, as a lithographic mask, and preventing oxidation of the covered areas. This approach offered the possibility of controlling the size of the inscribed feature, simply by changing the size of the nanoparticles. Later, the group of Fréchet demonstrated the high-resolution anodic oxidation of SAMs of dendrimers on silicon and titanium [287, 288]. The dendrimers were modified either with a chlorosilane group or with a triethoxysilane group to enable self-assembly onto the substrates, and this allowed features with dimensions less than 60 nm to be fabricated on silicon. TiO$_2$ patterns were also created with line widths of 25 nm, heights of 12 nm, and spacing between individual lines of 50 nm; these monolayers could be used as both positive and negative tone resists in SPL. Other examples have demonstrated the oxidation of ester-terminated SAMs, for example, with methyl 10-undecenoate [283], amine-functionalized monolayers [289–291] and bromine-modified SAMs (C. Haensch *et al.*, unpublished results). Together, these examples not only demonstrate the variety of surface moieties that can be patterned, but also represent interesting candidates for the fabrication of bifunctional and multifunctional surfaces. Shortly after the first anodization of SAMs on silicon, some interesting post-modifications of the inscribed structures were reported which demonstrated the potential of this technique for the fabrication of molecular assemblies. As an example, Sugimura *et al.* demonstrated the combination of LAO with the self-assembly of organosilane molecules [292]. In this case, following the oxidation of a TMS monolayer, the created patterns were modified with a layer of (3-aminopropyl)triethoxysilane (APTES) to introduce chemical functionalities. These amino moieties were labeled with aldehyde-modified fluorescent latex nanoparticles, and investigated using fluorescence optical microscopy to reveal the selective attachment of particles on the −NH$_2$ groups. Sugimura and coworkers also described the fabrication of a coplanar nanostructure which consisted of a surface pattern of octadecyltrimethoxy-silane and fluoroalkylsilane [293]. These structured features were characterized using Kelvin probe force microscopy to investigate their surface potential properties. When the fabrication of positive and negative patterns was demonstrated by Graaf *et al.* [294], a pattern of dodecyl and silicon oxide features was used for the self-assembly of different molecules and nanomaterials, namely R6G molecules and CdSe/ZnS nanocrystals. The R6G was selectively self-assembled on the oxide structures due to electrostatic interactions, whereas the nanoparticles (which were surrounded by a hydrophobic shell) self-assemble only on the alkyl-terminated layer. The nanoscale deposition of manganese single-molecule magnets on silicon oxide features was presented by Martínez and coworkers [291]. Here, the magnets were deposited site-selectively onto the SiO$_2$ features due to the positive charges of the magnets, and no self-assembly onto the −NH$_2$ structures was observed. The site-selective self-assembly of gold nanoparticles on the pattern of OTS and amine-terminated oxide features was described by Li and coworkers [285], while an interesting method for detecting metal ions by using LAO was provided by Kim and coworkers [295]. A pattern of (3-mercaptopropyl)trimethoxysilane (MPTMS) and APTES was used for the self-assembly of Au nanoparticles, which self-assembled only on the −SH functionalities. This part of the surface served as the fixed electrode, whereas the amine groups were used for the self-assembly of other metal ions (i.e., Cu^{2+}). Notably, the conductance of the resultant structures depended on the concentration of the metal ions. When He *et al.* reported on the site-specific growth of SWCNTs on Si [290], the iron nanoparticles were selectively assembled onto oxide features due to electrostatic interactions, whereas the amine-terminated background layer was modified with sodium dodecyl sulfate to prevent any unspecific self-assembly of the Fe particles onto the $-NH_2$ groups. These particles subsequently acted as a catalyst for the growth of SWCNTs via chemical vapor deposition (CVD). These findings might be important for the development of SWCNT-based electronic devices. Other interesting research studies have focused on the alignment and stretching of λ-DNA wires into parallel patterns of OTS and $-NH_2$ functionalities [296, 297]. For this, the DNA wires were self-assembled selectively onto the inscribed features, due to coulombic interactions between the amine groups of the substrate and the phosphate backbone of the DNA. Other biorelated examples were demonstrated by Yoshinobu and coworkers [289], who utilized the anodic oxidation of OTS and APTES monolayers for the selective patterning of proteins in the fabrication of positive- and negative-tone structures. Lee *et al.* employed the oxidation of a monolayer of octadecyldimethylmethoxysilane fabricating nanopatterns for the modification with polymer brushes [298]. In this case, a ruthenium-based metathesis catalyst was assembled onto the silicon oxide features to serve as an initiator for the surface-initiated ROMP. Two different monomer units were tested for the site-selective growth of polymer brushes, and the obtained features were characterized using electric force microscopy.

Further interesting non-organosilane molecules used in the anodization process have included metal phosphate monolayers, fabricated via a two-step procedure [279, 299, 300]. This involved the reaction of an –OH-terminated silicon substrate with $POCl_3$ and subsequent reaction with, for example, Zr^{4+}, Hf^{4+}, Ca^{2+}, and Mg^{2+} ions. Such reaction with tetravalent metal ions led to the fabrication of positively charged phosphate monolayers, whereas with divalent metal ions the surface appeared to be neutral. A comparison of the two surfaces revealed a need for a lower threshold voltage for oxidation of the positively charged surfaces than for the neutral substrates.

The group of Lee investigated the anodization of SAMs of 1,12-diaminododecane·dihydrochloride (DAD × 2HCl) and *n*-tridecylamine·hydrochloride (TDA × 2 HCl) [122, 279, 301–304] and, in particular, the influence of the surface functionalities on the anodization process. When mixed monolayers of DAD × 2HCl and TDA × HCl were tested for this purpose, the DAD × 2HCl monolayer led to a positively charged surface due to the presence of the ammonium chloride moieties, whereas the TDA × HCl SAM was uncharged, because of the terminal $-CH_3$ groups. The terminal end group of DAD × 2HCl was found to lead to an enhancement of the oxidation [301]. Moreover, the positively charged surface of the DAD × 2HCl SAM was responsible for an increase in the line widths and the heights of the inscribed structures, an effect which could be explained by an enlargement of the water meniscus between the AFM tip and the substrate, due to surface charges [122, 303].

LAO on SAMs on Gold   Jang and coworkers described the characterization of the desorption and oxidation of thiol-terminated gold substrates [305], having first prepared the gold surface by depositing a layer of Au onto silicon. Depending on the monolayer, two processes can occur and result in the formation of two different patterns: (i) removal of the SAM with the formation of recessed structures; and (ii) the formation of silicon oxide structures.   Jang *et al.* investigated eleven different monolayers on Au, including $-CH_3$-, $-COOH$-, $-PO_3H_2$-, $-OH$-, $-NH_2$-, $-CF_3$-, and $-(OCH_2CH_2)_3OH$-terminated SAMs. The parameters that controlled the mode of patterning were the SAM chain length, the functional end group, the bias voltage, the local pH value, and the hydroxide anion accessibility.

LAO on LB Films   Investigations conducted by Bourgoin and coworkers highlighted the potential to oxidize not only SAMs on Si or Au, but also organic films prepared by the LB technique [306]; indeed, phthalocyanine LB films could be patterned with line widths down to 50 nm. Further investigations were carried out on LB films of palmitic acid to study the bias dependence of the LAO process [307] and, by changing the applied voltage, it was possible to create both positive and negative patterns. Mixed LB films of hexadecylamine and palmitic acid were also studied to analyze the mixing and charge effects on the anodization, and to investigate the mechanism of the patterning process [81, 308].

LAO on Polymeric Films   The anodic oxidation of polymeric films offers the possibility to construct patterns that can be used for the site-selective self-assembly of protein molecules. This was shown by Yam *et al.*, who oxidized oligo(ethylene glycol)-terminated films on silicon to test the specific adsorption of fibrinogen, avidin and BSA onto silicon oxide patterns [309]. Choi and coworkers described the *in situ* observation of biomolecules [310], whereby a methoxy-PEG-terminated monolayer was oxidized and served as a passivation background, whilst the patterns were used for the site-selective immobilization of streptavidin, labeled with Au particles, and pure streptavidin. The nonlabeled streptavidin patterns were further investigated for the detection of biotinylated materials. These findings demonstrated the potential of polymeric films for applications in biosensing devices.

The anodic oxidation process represents an interesting method for the construction of nanometer-sized features on a large variety of different substrates. In addition to the widely investigated silicon substrates, other semiconductors and metals formed the focus of these studies. In order to introduce chemical functionalities, LAO was applied to organic layers of various materials on silicon surfaces, which in turn opened the possibility of functionalizing the surface with multiple chemically active groups. Potential applications of these patterns may be found in the fabrication of metal-oxide-semiconductor transistors and biosensor devices, and also for investigating chemical processes at the nanometer scale. One disadvantage of this patterning technique, however, is the possible destruction of the underlying substrate, and the process must be very carefully tuned. The technique is also rather slow, such that its use in high-throughput strategies would not easily be realized.

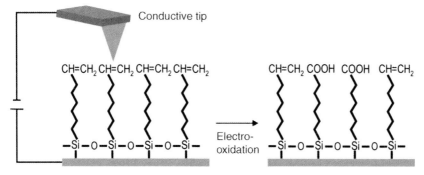

Figure 2.9 Schematic representation of the electro-oxidation on self-assembled monolayers of 18-nonadecenyltrichlorosilane on silicon.

2.3.3.2 Chemical Activation of Self-Assembled Monolayers

In 1999, Sagiv introduced another electro-oxidation process of SAMs, namely "constructive lithography" or the electro-oxidation process [311]. In contrast to the above-described anodization process, the monolayer will not be degraded while the features are inscribed, but the terminal end groups will be chemically activated. In the first of these experiments, which was carried out with a monolayer of 18-nonade-cenyltrichlorosilane (NTS), a conductive AFM tip was used to pattern the SAM, and the terminal $-CH=CH_2$ groups were converted to carboxylic acid functionalities (Figure 2.9). A bilayer of OTS was then self-assembled onto the $-COOH$ groups to create multilayer structures. Depending on the voltage applied, the patterning process would induce an electro-chemical surface transformation of the terminal end group of the monolayer, although the overall structure of the monolayer would, ideally, not be influenced.

This process was later applied also to OTS monolayers on silicon [312], where the terminal $-CH_3$ groups were converted to $-COOH$ moieties. Transformation to the carboxylic acid functionalities was followed by AFM and Fourier transform infrared (FT-IR) spectroscopy. Subsequent contact-mode AFM measurements allowed characterization of both the topographic and (especially) the frictional changes of the oxidized monolayers. FT-IR spectroscopy on a macroscale structured surface showed the $-CH_2$ vibrations to be preserved, but the terminal $-CH_3$ vibration to be greatly reduced. A further indication of carboxylic acids formation was the appearance of an absorption peak for $-C=O$ at $1713 \, \text{cm}^{-1}$. As an additional surface-sensitive technique for investigating chemical transformations, time-of-flight secondary ion mass spectrometry (TOF-SIMS) represents an interesting alternative [313]. For this, Pignataro and coworkers used patterns of a 1-octadecene monolayer, self-assembled on hydrogen terminated silicon, to analyze the transformation process [314], and obtained both elemental and molecular information concerning the chemical features after modification. The modified areas showed the presence of C_xH_yO- and C_xH_yN-type peaks, both of which increased with in line with higher bias voltages and were related to the formation of organic polar moieties. In contrast, a reduction in the SiC_xH_y signal was observed. The characterization of micrometer-sized features can also be addressed by using XPS to analyze the chemical structure. For example, Andruzzi *et al.* used a micrometer pattern of OTS and PEG for their XPS analysis [315].

Nonetheless, the characterization of nanometer-sized structures is, in general, a difficult process, and very few techniques allow investigations to be made of the chemical state of the features. Furthermore, the sensitivity and resolution of the different techniques are frequently insufficient. Consequently, the most frequently used technique for the indirect characterization of nanometric features is that of AFM, which demonstrates mainly the changes in frictional and topographic properties following the oxidation process. When Wouters *et al.* used AFM to investigate the influence of applied voltage and pulse duration on the electro-oxidation process of OTS on silicon [316], the formation of silicon oxide structures resulted in an increase of the topographic image. Moreover, the carboxylic acid-terminated structures showed a change in height, depending on the direction of the scan (this was in fact correlated to a crosscoupling of the friction and the height signal). The change in height was used as an indication for the formation of −COOH moieties, whilst degradation of the monolayer under harsher conditions was associated with a detectable positive change in the height images, independent of the scan direction. The dependence of oxidation time versus the bias voltage is shown in Figure 2.10, where a small window for the oxidation of OTS was observed. Above a certain threshold – that is, at high pulse duration and bias – the monolayer was degraded and silicone oxide formed, but below the threshold line no oxidation had occurred, due to short pulses and low bias voltages.

Hoeppener *et al.* described a series of AFM studies to investigate surface properties during the oxidation process, and at the transition state of monolayer oxidation and degradation [318]. In general, the writing process itself was seen to depend heavily on

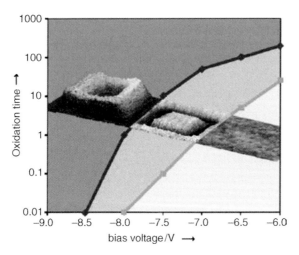

Figure 2.10 Dependence of oxidation time on bias voltage. Reproduced with permission from Ref. [317].

a number of parameters, while the choice of conducting AFM tip and its geometry had a critical influence on the required oxidation voltages and times, and also affected the size of the inscribed structures. In order to reduce the size of the patterned areas, the tip diameter could be reduced by using highly doped and/or noncoated tips. The humidity of the environment during the writing process was identified as another important issue; whilst a low humidity resulted in longer writing times and incomplete pattern formation, a too-high humidity resulted in wider line widths.

One limiting factor when implementing electro-oxidation into high-throughput strategies is that the actual process is rather slow, though this might be overcome by using an automated writing process with a software-driven AFM set-up. The use of such a system with conductive parallel cantilever arrays was demonstrated by Wouters *et al.* for fabricating large areas of oxidized surface patterns [127]. By using an automated oxidation set-up, 1000 circles could be inscribed onto an OTS monolayer on silicon. Following the *in situ* imaging of the features, it was clear that the conductive coating of the tip had not been degraded during the patterning, as indicated by a constant line width and the intensities of the friction signals measured on the circles. Moreover, these structures could be used for the self-assembly of nanoparticles, which occurred exclusively onto the oxidized areas, rather than on the OTS background. Another way to increase the patterning speed would be to use an array of four cantilevers for the oxidation process; in this way, a successful oxidation of square structures was demonstrated on OTS, with the subsequent self-assembly of CdSe/ZnS particles. Following this, Cai and coworkers introduced an alternative method of reducing the writing and fabrication times of nanometer-sized patterns [319], when they described the process of electro-pen nanolithography (EPN). This was a combination of electro-oxidation with an AFM tip and DPN, in which an ink-coated conducting AFM tip was used to oxidize an OTS monolayer. In this way, patterns of $-COOH$ could be created, with the ink being transferred directly onto the patterned features due to the higher surface energy of the OTS_{ox} areas. The structures obtained revealed line widths of approximately 50 nm, and were inscribed at a writing speed of 10 μm s^{-1}. In addition, different inks could be used to introduce chemical functionalities onto the patterns, and in particular trialkoxysilanes and quaternary ammonium salts. The self-assembly of MPTMS molecules resulted in an availability of $-SH$ moieties, and to prove a successful transfer of the thiol molecules, functionalized gold nanoparticles were self-assembled onto the surface. Subsequent AFM investigations revealed the self-assembly of particles only on the nanopatterns, as well as an increase in height of 2 nm, which was in good agreement with the diameter of the Au particles. This process might have a future role in the fabrication of 3-D structures and, depending on the ink used, also for the direct writing of biological patterns. In order to obtain areas in the range of square micrometers, the AFM tip could be exchanged with a conductive metal stamp, which enabled the pattern of the grid to be transferred onto the SAM [320]. Hoeppener and coworkers later described an oxidation process which employed a metal stamp, composed of a Cu transmission electron microscopy (TEM) grid, onto SAMs of OTS on silicon. Following its exposure to a saturated water vapor atmosphere, the copper grid was pressed against the monolayer-terminated surface. Compared to the oxidation process using an AFM tip, the inscription with a TEM grid required longer oxidations times of approximately 30 s, and a higher voltage of 30–35 V. The need for longer patterning times and higher voltages might be due to the larger distance between the TEM grid and the surface, and also to the presence of a thicker water layer. An alternative approach towards patterning SAMs utilized a patterned monolayer on silicon; this could first be pressed onto another SAM, after which a bias voltage would be applied to transfer the structures onto the unmodified surface [321].

The inscribed structures could, furthermore, be used after the electro-oxidation process for a large variety of different post-modification steps, including the self-assembly of different nanomaterials (e.g., nanoparticles, nanowires), the formation of multilayers, and also for the application of nanometric surface chemistry. An overview of the different possibilities for post-modification of the inscribed features is shown in Figure 2.11, where different driving forces have been used to add nanomaterials or functional molecules to the structures.

Self-Assembly of Additional Silane Molecules onto the Nanopatterns In 2000, Sagiv and colleagues had already suggested many different possible post-modification reactions of the oxidized areas, via a variety of chemical transformations based on pattern functionalization [312]. The $-COOH$ functionalities, created during the oxidation process, are suitable for the self-assembly of a second layer of reactive trichlorosilanes, due to the reaction of $-SiCl_3$ groups with carboxylic acid moieties. Examples of this include the self-assembly of NTS [312], 11-bromoundecyltrichlorosilane (BTS) [322], 11-undecyltrichlorosilane (UTS) [325], and others. Wouters and coworkers also demonstrated the self-assembly of quaternary ammonium salts (e.g., trimethyloctadecylammonium bromide) onto the acid structures [325]. The formation of a bilayer can lead to the introduction of different chemical active functionalities. Moreover, these moieties can be used for other modification sequences, such as nanometer-sized surface chemistry and the site-selective self-assembly of nanomaterials (e.g., nanoparticles). Some interesting examples of this are described in the following subsections.

Surface Chemistry on the Nanopatterns One important application of the oxidized areas is their use in surface chemistry, when it is necessary to utilize surface reactions that have high yields and can be carried out under mild reaction conditions, with readily available starting materials. Examples include the reaction of the terminal end groups of NTS monolayers (ethylenic functionalities) with H_2S and $BH_3 \times THF$ (tetrahydrofuran), which leads to $-SH$ moieties, whereas oxidation of the ethylenic groups with $KMnO_4$ and KIO_4 creates $-COOH$ end groups [312, 327]. The formation of $-NH_2$ functionalities can be obtained by a photoreaction with formamide; this results in the creation of amide moieties, while a subsequent reduction with $BH_3 \times THF$ leads to amine functionalities [328]. One concept that fulfils the criteria for surface reactions is the so-called "click chemistry" approach, as introduced by Sharpless in 2001 [329]. Until now, one of the most important click

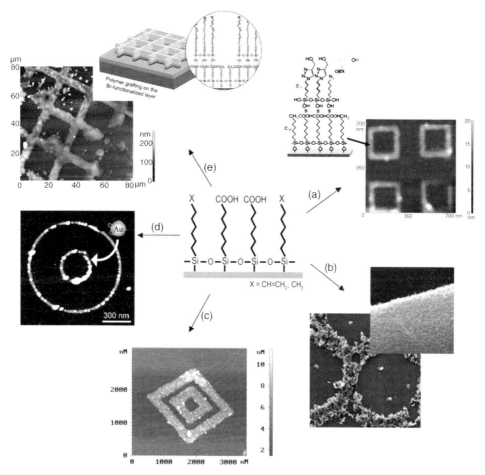

Figure 2.11 Examples of the post-modification of oxidized nanometer-sized structures on SAMs on silicon. (a) Clicking on the nanometer-scale (reproduced with permission from Ref. [322])); (b) Patterned growth of carbon nanofibers [323]; (c) Site-selective assembly of Fe(II) salt (reproduced with permission from Ref. [324]); (d) Self-assembly of Au nanoparticles onto the nanostructures (reproduced with permission from Ref. [325]); (e) Polymer brushes (reproduced with permission from Ref. [326]).

reactions is the 1,3-dipolar cycloaddition of terminal acetylenes and organic azides, which results in the regioselective formation of 1,4-disubstituted triazoles [330]. Haensch et al. reported the details of a 1,3 dipolar cycloaddition of nanometer-sized azide structures with propargyl alcohol with line widths of 50 nm on a background layer of OTS [322]. A subsequent characterization of the obtained features was carried out using AFM, and the results were confirmed on nonstructured functional substrates using FT-IR spectroscopy and XPS. The major advantage of this reaction scheme is the wide diversity of clickable moieties, including phosphorescent iridium complexes [331], gold nanoparticles [332], CNTs [333], dendritic systems [334], and others [335]. Willner and coworkers used the tip-mediated oxidation of monolayers of OTS, and activated the surface templates via a secondary enzymatic reaction for further purpose [336]. The −COOH functionalities formed during the oxidation process were reacted with tyramine, which itself can be oxidized biocatalytically (with the enzyme, tyrosinase) to catechol moieties that control the self-assembly of magnetic nanoparticles and boronic acid-terminated gold nanoparticles. This approach permits the possible fabrication of nanobiosensors and/or nanocircuitry. Andruzzi *et al.* combined the electro-oxidation of OTS with a conductive stamp with NHS chemistry to obtain bioselective patterns of PEG and OTS [315]. Here, carbodiimide NHS chemistry was used to react NHS-terminated micrometer-sized patterns with an amino-terminated PEG, and the PEG/OTS patterns were later applied to protein adsorption studies with fluorescently labeled BSA. The characterization of the features, using fluorescence microscopy, showed a reduced adsorption on the chemically modified lines. Furthermore, although a significant inhibition of cell adhesion onto the PEG patterns was noted, cell growth was maintained on the functionalized areas. Wouters *et al.* reported successive functionalization reactions on patterns of OTS with 40 nm resolution [325], where UTS was used for bilayer formation on the structures, so as to fabricate a pattern for the radical polymerization of styrene. Yet, only a partial increase in pattern height was observed, this being related to the UTS structure possibly undergoing horizontal polymerization. The results presented by these authors might lead potentially to applications in electronics, or perhaps for DNA and protein sensors. The fabrication of polymer brushes on micrometer-sized surface areas was demonstrated by Becer *et al.*, who attached BTS as a chemically active molecule onto the patterns [326]. In this way, the bromine functionality could be used as an initiator for the ATRP of, for example, styrene. This "grafting-from" approach led to the creation of polymer brushes of various heights, depending on the reaction time. Notably, the height of the polymer brush was seen to increase linearly with the polymerization time, and was indicative of a controlled polymerization process. In an additional test to determine whether the polymer terminated with bromine end groups, a second ATRP polymerization with *tert*-butyl acrylate was performed, and this revealed an increase in polymer brush height of about 20–40 nm. Clearly, the functionalization of patterned substrates with defined polymer block systems promises much with regards to biomedical applications, and/or for the creation of responsive brush systems.

Self-Assembly of Different Nanomaterials onto Nanopatterns The self-assembly of nanomaterials onto the structured features can be achieved via two different strategies. For the first strategy, carboxylic acid functionalities were used directly for the attachment of nanoparticles. For example, Hoeppener *et al.* demonstrated the site-selective binding of magnetic Fe_3O_4 particles onto predefined surface areas of −COOH moieties [337]. In this case, the particles self-assembled onto the −COOH features due to hydrophilic interactions of the acid functionalities with the ligand shell. Subsequent treatment of the surface with conventional adhesion tape led to the removal of unspecifically bonded material, but without destroying the created structures. The same method was also used to create nanostructures of Fe particles by the subsequent reduction of Fe(II) ions assembled onto the oxidized areas [324]; here, the typical particle size was 6–7 nm, with a high degree of uniformity. Following this, magnetic force microscopy (MFM) measurements were conducted to investigate the magnetic properties of the nanoparticles, thus revealing their magnetic origin. The fabrication of such nanosystems permits the possible creation of magnetic structures with decreasing device dimensions. For example, Wouters and colleagues described the self-assembly of positively charged gold nanoparticles onto −COOH patterns [325], after which tapping mode AFM studies revealed an increase in height of 18–20 nm, in good agreement with the diameter of the Au particles. The subsequent successful self-assembly of two differently sized gold nanoparticles onto oxidized nanopatterns was demonstrated by the same group [338], when they investigated the sequential oxidation steps performed on the OTS and the subsequent self-assembly of various nanoparticles. The Au particles, which were self-assembled in an initial step, had to be stabilized (e.g., by thermal annealing at 90 °C for 6 h) to prevent their exchange during a second self-assembly step. Druzhinina and coworkers described the growth of carbon nanofibers and nanotube patterns on OTS/-COOH structures [323]; in this case, iron acetate was assembled onto the acid moieties and subsequently reduced to metallic Fe particles that acted as a catalyst for carbon nanofiber growth under microwave irradiation. Today, applications of these structures can be found in electronic devices.

The second strategy involved the self-assembly of a second layer on top of the −COOH features, before the selective self-assembly process can be performed Previously, examples of surface chemistry conducted on nanopatterns were given to demonstrate the potential of chemical modification schemes for introducing a wide variety of chemical functionalities. Such chemical end groups are suitable for the selective self-assembly of different nanomaterials; for example, thiol and carboxylic acid groups can be used to deposit various materials such as gold, silver, or cadmium selenide and $[Au]_{55}$ clusters [312, 327, 339]. Hoeppener *et al.* demonstrated the self-assembly of Cd^{2+} ions on functionalized −SH nanopatterns [339], where cadmium cations were self-assembled onto thiol groups and were then reacted with H_2S to create CdS particles. The latter particles could then be metalized by treatment with an aqueous solution of $HAuCl_4$, with the formation of Au structures being confirmed by subsequent silver deposition from a silver enhancer solution on the gold patterns. The same authors also demonstrated the creation of millimeter-sized silver electrodes via a monolayer photodesorption with gallium onto OTS monolayers, creating molecularly sharp boundaries in the process. Surface chemistry was then used to functionalize fabricated surface structures also with thiol moieties, so as to assemble silver onto the oxidized structures. Liu *et al.* demonstrated the site-selective deposition of $[Au_{55}(Ph_2PC_6H_4SO_3Na)_{12}Cl_6]$ clusters onto −SH nanopatterns [327]; these features were stable against thermal treatment and structurally robust (e.g., cleaning with "Scotch tape" did not disturb the structures, but any unspecifically bound material was removed). Liu *et al.* reported on the hierarchical self-assembly of colloidal gold particles on silicon [328], where nanopatterns of −NH_2 functionalities could be created via the chemical reaction of ethylenic groups with formamide and $BH_3 \times THF$. Protonation of the amine moieties led to positively charged surface features that were suitable for the attachment of negatively charged particles via electrostatic interactions [340–344]. The latter interactions were responsible for the spontaneous self-assembly of [Au-citrate] particles (which were negatively charged) onto the nanostructures. Such defined molecular templates could be used to fine-tune the distances between nanomaterials which are anchored to the surface, and might also be used in the advancement of 3-D nanofabrication techniques. The construction of hydride metal–organic surface nanostructures was demonstrated by Maoz *et al.* [345], when a monolayer of a thiol-functionalized silane was loaded with silver ions and used to create nanometer-sized structures on specific surface areas via either a chemical or a tip-induced reduction of the Ag ions to metallic nanoparticles. Hoeppener *et al.* demonstrated the preparation of amine-terminated nanostructures for the selective binding of CNTs [346]; in this case, the $-NH_2$ moieties were obtained by a vapor-phase self-assembly process of 3-aminopropyltrimethoxysilane (APTMS) onto the electro-oxidized surface areas, while the CNTs selectively self-assembled onto the amine features. These investigations might have important implications for the future, notably in the field of nanoelectronics.

Wetting-Driven Self-Assembly Concept   Another versatile approach to the template-guided fabrication of metal nanopatterns is that of wetting-driven self-assembly, as recently introduced by Sagiv and coworkers [347]. This process utilizes the selective adhesion of nanosized volumes of wetting liquids to the lyophilic surface structures of a lyophilic/lyophobic substrate, where the lyophilic/lyophobic surface consists of a pattern of $-COOH$ areas versus OTS. The patterns were fabricated by retraction of the COOH/OTS surface from the melt of three different compounds, namely eicosene, ODT, and dodecanoic acid. This method has allowed the introduction of various chemical functionalities by the use of readily available and cheap functional alkanes. Post-modification of the obtained terminal surface groups led to templates for the site-specific self-assembly of metallic gold and silver. Checco *et al.* used the strong hydrophilic/hydrophobic contrast between oxidized structures and the OTS monolayer to study the wetting behavior of ethanol and octane on patterned line features [348, 349]. This allowed the precise control and stabilization of liquid objects in desired confinements, enabled studies of the wetting phenomenon to be conducted, and allowed the determination of liquid profile shapes with sub-100 nm resolution. Cai *et al.* studied the liquid-behavior at the nanometer level on iodine patterns which had been inscribed by the electro-oxidation process [350]. As iodine serves as a good tracing and visualizing agent in this type of study, such investigations may provide an understanding of the evaporation dynamics of liquid solvents on nanometer-sized structures. Depending on the deposition method used, the nanometer-sized structures can be either gel-like (solution–deposition method) or dendritic, snowflake-shaped polycrystalline iodine sheets (vapor-phase–condensation method).

These examples stress the versatility of the structuring approach, and are potentially compatible with other surface-chemistry schemes.

2.3.4
Catalytic Lithography

The fabrication of nanometer-sized structures is possible not only via the electro-
oxidation or anodization of SAMs, but also by catalyzing a surface reaction with an
AFM tip [351]. As the reaction takes only place in those areas where the tip is in
contact with the surface, this approach will lead to a selective functionalization of the
terminal end groups, without applying an electrical current and without destroying
the underlying monolayer [352]. Hence, this technique is not limited to the use of
conducting substrates; rather, a wide variety of different substrates can be used.
Despite the fact that the technique represents a promising approach to performing
nanometric surface chemistry, very few examples have been reported to date. Müller
et al. were among the first to describe the use of an AFM tip coated with a catalyst to
perform nanochemistry [353], and to modify the surface functionalities of spatially
defined areas on a silicon substrate. In this case, the hydrogenation of an azide-
terminated silicon surface with a platinum-coated AFM tip was investigated as a
model reaction; the reaction scheme is depicted in Figure 2.12, where the terminal
$-N_3$ groups were converted to amine functionalities that could be used for further
modification sequences to yield more complex structures. Fluorescence labeling with
fluorescein-labeled, aldehyde-modified latex beads or 3-(2-furoyl)quinoline-2-carbox-
aldehyde (ATTO-TAG) was chosen as post-modification reaction. When investigations of the modified areas were performed using confocal scanning laser microscopy, the measurements revealed brightly fluorescent squares that represented the
reacted surface areas, but imaging of the azide-terminated surface, after derivatiza-
tion with the fluorescent compounds, showed no signal. These studies led to the
development of a general approach that used AFM coated tips to perform nanometric
catalytic surface chemistry.

The catalysis of chemical surface reactions by a palladium-coated AFM tip for the
fabrication of nanometer-sized features was demonstrated by Blackledge *et al.* [352].

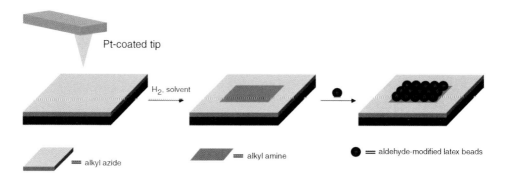

Figure 2.12 A Pt-coated AFM tip is scanned
over an azide-terminated substrate in the
presence of H_2, resulting in the formation of
$-NH_2$ groups. The obtained amine
functionalities were modified with fluorescein-
labeled latex beads or ATTO-TAG to yield a site-
selective self-assembly of fluorescent dyes on
specific surface areas.

Two example reactions included the hydrogenation of azide groups and *N*-benzyloxy-carbonyl-protected amines to $-NH_2$ functionalities, while a third reaction scheme showed the addition of aminobutyldimethylsilane (ASiH) to terminal carbon–carbon double bonds. The inscribed amine end groups were subsequently labeled with 5- and 6-carboxytetramethylrhodamine succinimidyl esters in order to conduct fluorescence measurements on the obtained structures. The reaction mechanism described proposed the formation of a reactive palladium–organosiloxane intermediate that could only be formed if the monolayers were to be deformed during the structuring process. The Langmuir–Hinshelwood mechanism, which was suggested as a possible reaction model, includes chemisorption of the terminal end group of the monolayer and H_2 or ASiH on the Pd-coated tip, and a subsequent reaction. Davis and colleagues described surface-confined Suzuki and Heck carbon–carbon coupling reactions under Pd catalysis [354, 355]; the schematic outline of the surface reactions is depicted in Figure 2.13a and b. In this case, 4-bromo-*N*-(3-(methylthio)-propyl)-4-vinylbenzamides and a styrene (*N*-3(methylthio)-propyl)-4-vinylbenzamide, self-assembled on gold, were used as functional monolayers for the spatially controlled surface modification sequences. The Suzuki reaction was performed with a poly-vinylpyrollidone (PVP)-Pd nanoparticle-functionalized AFM tip at a pressure of 15 to 25 nN, and in a reaction solution of methanol, sodium acetate and 3-aminophenyl-boronic acid or phenylboronic acid. The Heck reaction was performed in a solution of dimethylformamide (DMF) with sodium hydrogen carbonate and 4-iodobenzoic acid under a pressure of 25 to 40 nN, which led to line widths of 12 to 15 nm being achieved. The successful reaction sequences were proven by a combination of fluorescence tagging, frictional imaging, and labeling with appropriate nanoparticles. The fluorescence image of a Suzuki-catalyzed square functionalized with NHS–fluorescein revealed a brightly fluorescent rectangle (see Figure 2.14a), while the AFM height image of a Suzuki-catalyzed square functionalized with aldehyde-terminated nanospheres that were attached only to the inscribed structures, is shown in Figure 2.14b.

The reduction of a monolayer of imines, using an AFM tip coated with a reducing agent, was investigated by Blasdel *et al.* (Figure 2.13c) [356]. For this, sodium triacetoxyborohydride ($Na(OAc)_3BH_4$) was used as reducing agent to form the corresponding secondary amines, the generation of which was confirmed using a chloranil test. The colorless amine was then reacted with acetaldehyde and tetra-chloro-*p*-benzoquinone to yield a bright blue tertiary amine. Visualization of the inscribed structures was achieved using inverted optical microscopy under bright-field illumination.

Bis(ω-*tert*-butyldimethyl-siloxyundecyl)disulfide (TBDMS) monolayers on gold could be hydrolyzed in the contact areas of an acidic tip to create nanopatterns of hydrolyzed TBDMS SAMs [357]. In this case, 2-mercapto-5-benzimidazole sulfonic acid was attached to the Au tips as the catalytic species, such that inscribed features with a line width of approximately 25 nm were obtained. Cleavage of the bulky terminal end group led to the formation of spaces between the residual monolayer that could be refilled with dendritic wedges. The corresponding AFM height images revealed an increase in height of 1.3 nm, indicating a successful filling with the

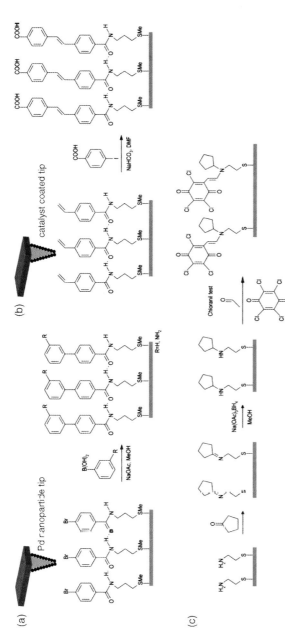

Figure 2.13 (a) Suzuki reaction between an aryl bromide monolayer and phenylboronic acid/3-aminophenylboronic acid in methanol and sodium acetate with a Pd nanoparticle-coated AFM tip; (b) Heck reaction between an aryl styrene monolayer and an aryl halide in DMF and sodium hydrogen carbonate with a catalyst-coated AFM tip; (c) An amine-terminated monolayer was reacted with cyclopentanone to yield an intermediate imine, which was scanned in methanol and Na(OAc)₃BH₄ with an AFM tip to react to secondary amines; the chloranil test revealed the formation of bright-blue tertiary amine functionalities.

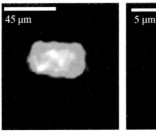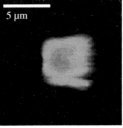

Figure 2.14 (a) Fluorescence image of a Suzuki-catalyzed square functionalized with NHS-fluorescein; (b) AFM height image of a Suzuki-catalyzed square functionalized with aldehyde-terminated nanospheres. (Reproduced with permission from Ref. [354]).

dendritic ligands. Zorbas and coworkers described the photochemical reaction of a dye layer with a chemically modified AFM tip [358]; here, the dye used was a commercially available Procion Red MX-5B that was oxidized under UV-mediated photocatalysis, while the catalytic species were TiO_2 particles attached to an AFM probe. Subsequent AFM, optical microscopy and mid-FT-IR investigations revealed the photocatalytic degradation of the dye molecules. The fabrication of nanometer-sized features by applying a Diels–Alder reaction onto silicon was shown by Matsubara *et al.* [359]. For this, a monolayer terminated with alkene functionalities was reacted with an AFM tip that had been coated with a solution of 2-(13-hydroxy-2-oxatridecanyl)furan. As a consequence, a force of 32 nN and a writing speed of $0.2\,\mu m\,s^{-1}$ were sufficient to successfully couple the furan molecules onto the terminal surface groups. Wang and coworkers demonstrated the tip-assisted hydrolysis of a monolayer of dithiobis(succinimidoundecanoate) on gold [360], where the base hydrolysis of the ester-terminated surface was accelerated after contact mode imaging, due to the implementation of a disorder into the structure. It appears that hydroxide ions have an easier access to the acyl carbon atoms of the monolayer, and this resulted in an accelerated hydrolysis. A localized click chemistry was reported by Long *et al.* [361], who used an acetylene-terminated surface as the template for a nanometer-scale cycloaddition reaction. This was achieved by using an AFM tip immersed in a solution of an azide reagent and the Cu catalyst. Later, a new and versatile patterning approach – the so-called thermochemical nanolithography (TCNL) – was introduced by Szoszkiewicz *et al.* [362]. In this case, a heatable AFM tip was used to inscribe features onto polymeric substrates with line widths in the region of 12 nm. The deprotection of an ester moiety to acid functionalities was tested as a possible model reaction, while the change in hydrophilicity was investigated using LFM. The parallelization of individually addressable tips was also demonstrated for the preparation of large-scale patterning.

The combination of catalytic chemistry with the application of bias voltages has led to some interesting methods for creating nanometer-sized surface patterns. As an example, Fresco and coworkers demonstrated the chemical activation of protected amine and thiol surfaces by applying a bias voltage between the substrate and the AFM tip [363, 364]. In this case, the α,α-dimethyl-3,5-dimethoxybenzyloxycarbonyl

(DZZ) group was selected as a protective moiety, due to the mechanism of cleavage of this functionality via an ionic intermediate, with 3,5-dimethoxy-α-styrene and carbon dioxide being released and primary amine and thiol functionalities being obtained. The inscribed amino groups were used in further modification steps for the reaction with a dendrimer and a dendronized polymer. The AFM images revealed increases in height of 1 nm and 4 nm, respectively, while the line widths of the structures were broadened due to the flexibility of the polymer chain. Furthermore, exposure of the thiol functionalities to a solution of gold nanoparticles resulted in the selective self-assembly of the particles onto the $-SH$ groups. Consequently, the placement of single particles could be achieved by a programmed application of electrical pulses to the surface. The electro-oxidation of thiol-terminated monolayers on both nonstructured and nanometer-sized surfaces, by applying a positive voltage to the surface, was reported by Pavlovic *et al.* [365, 366]. This activation resulted in the formation of thiolsulfinates and thiolsulfonates, which could be used for the covalent immobilization of biomolecules; release of the biomolecules was detected by treating the surface with a disulfide-cleaving reagent. Sugimura and coworkers introduced the reversible nanochemical conversion of amino-terminated monolayers with an AFM tip [367, 368] when, by applying a positive bias voltage to the surface, the terminal $-NH_2$ groups could be converted to $-NO$ functionalities. The nitroso-terminated SAM could then be reduced to $-NH_2$ moieties by changing the voltage to negative values, and surface potential measurements confirmed the chemical surface reaction. The fabrication of metallic structures on the nanometer scale via an AFM tip was achieved by Li *et al.* [223]. For this, a positive bias voltage was applied to a tip, which had been coated with H_2PtCl_6; the latter then dissolved in the water meniscus, such that the platinum(IV) was reduced to metallic Pt. This protocol demonstrated an interesting approach to using the water meniscus as a reaction vessel for a wide range of different surface reactions.

To summarize, these examples have demonstrated the potential of catalytic lithography for the chemical functionalization of nanometer-sized features. Moreover, a range of surface reactions can be applied to yield a wide variety of terminal end groups, while the modified functionalities can be used for fluorescent labeling, for the self-assembly of nanoparticles, and for the preparation of metallic nanostructures. Moreover, this approach enables a preservation of the underlying substrate and also of the monolayer, which is not in contact with the AFM tip.

2.4
Surface Chemical Reactions for Structured Surfaces

The key feature of the previously introduced patterning is the combination of surface structures with functional moieties. Clearly, the use of SAMs represents a versatile method for implementing a wide variety of chemical functions that provide access to surface reactions conducted on the nanometer scale. Moreover, a whole range of chemical interactions, including electrostatic and covalent binding, hydrogen bonding, hydrophilic/hydrophobic interactions and complex formation, are available to attach and stabilize nanomaterials to the structures. Additional possibilities for expanding the capabilities of a combination of lithography and functional SAMs has emerged from the field of surface chemistry, which allows the implementation of many reaction schemes to obtain different surface functionalizations. To date, a wide range of synthetic routes that uses different precursor molecules to form dense monolayers have been described, and some examples are provided in the following sections. These reactions have been conducted on nonpatterned surfaces and on both micrometer and nanometer scales, in combination with alternative structuring approaches or by using techniques discussed earlier in the chapter. Nonetheless, each of the described reactions is suitable for implementation in a range of lithographic techniques. Due to the greater stability of silane-based monolayers compared to thiol monolayers on gold, attention will be focused at this point on the surface chemistry performed on SAMs on silicon-based substrates.

2.4.1
Molecular Overlayers – Functionalization – Precursors

The formation of SAMs on silicon surfaces can be carried out using either silane-based precursor molecules that self-assemble on oxidized silicon-based surfaces (such as glass or silicon [134]), or via activation by $SiCl_4$ and $HNEt_2$, followed by the addition of hydroxyl-functionalized molecules [369, 370]. Yet, a conceptually different approach for the formation of SAMs on silicon substrates is the hydrogenation of the silicon substrate and reaction with alkene-functionalized molecules [371].

Silane-based precursor molecules are mainly functionalized with a trichlorosilane, trimethoxysilane or triethoxysilane group that reacts with the surface to form a covalent network. In this respect, trichlorosilane is the most reactive precursor, and trimethoxysilane and triethoxysilane are less reactive. Although, a wide variety of functional moieties can be implemented into the silane-based monolayers by utilizing the terminal groups of the silane precursors, these functional groups must be compatible with certain criteria. For example, the introduced functional group should not interact with the surface, and/or should not react with the silane group in order to avoid the formation of multilayers, or destruction of the silane group. The spacer, which usually is an alkyl chain, also plays an important role, with longer alkyl chains resulting in the formation of more stable and densely packed SAMs [134]. Most patterning approaches concentrate on the use of commercially available silane-based molecules such as OTS, BTS, 1H, 1H, 2H, 2H-perfluorodecyltri-chlorosilane (PFDTS), N-[3-(trimethoxysilyl)propyl]ethylenediamine (EDATMS), APTMS, APTES, N-(6-aminohexyl)-3-aminopropyltrimethoxysilane (AHAPS), MPTMS, and PEG silanes.

In general, OTS and PFDTS are used as passivation layers, due to the hydrophobic and chemically relative inert properties of the formed layers. BTS is applied mostly for surface reactions such as substitution reactions, or it may act as an initiator for polymerization reactions. Amino-terminated SAMs are used for the binding of negatively charged nano-objects as well as for surface reactions, such as Schiff base reactions or esterifications. MPTMS is used for the binding of nano-objects, while

PEG silanes have been extensively studied as bio-repellent materials that demonstrate their importance in biorelated systems and find applications in cell and protein micropatterning. These systems are also of significant importance in research related to the development of biosensors, lab-on-a-chip devices, tissue engineering, fundamental cell biology studies, drug screening, or medical diagnostics. Some examples of these precursor molecules in their fields of application are provided in the following subsections.

Typically, these materials are applied for purposes that include protein and cell-adhesion studies. Notably, OTS and PFDTS can each be self-assembled so as to obtain mixed monolayers that demonstrate varying protein-adsorption behaviors. For example, protein adsorption can be suppressed compared to the pure monolayer, with adsorption occurring preferentially on PFDTS [372]. When Hoffman *et al.* investigated the protein-repellent properties of mixed PEG silane-based monolayers and alkyl silane-based monolayers, the pure PEG silane monolayer was shown to be fully protein repellent, whereas on the mixed monolayer no protein absorption was observed above a PEG silane content of 90% [373]. Yap *et al.* created a micro pattern with topographical features for selective cell adhesion by modifying a silicon substrate with a PEG silane to create a nonfouling background. The PEG-modified surface was then patterned by photolithography, using a photoresist layer placed on top of the SAM, such that the free positions were subsequently functionalized with [3-(2-aminoethylamino)propyl]trimethoxysilane. When the polystyrene latex beads were later self-assembled on an amine-functionalized surface, HT-29 cancer cells were shown to adhere preferentially to the hydrophilic substrate areas, with the increasing distance between the adhesive sites promoting cell adhesion [374]. When gas-phase soft lithography was used to pattern APTMS and MPTMS, a PDMS could be applied to a master such that its shape became adapted. After curing, the PDMS mold was peeled off and placed in a reaction chamber with APTMS or MPTMS. The PDMS mold was then pressed onto the silicon substrate, and the ink was transferred by diffusion to react with the surface. The presence of amine groups was demonstrated by the adsorption of an oligonucleotide by the negatively charged phosphate groups [375], while the precursor molecules could be used to guide nano-objects onto certain positions. The fabrication of a gold nanoparticle array was achieved by first creating an OTS and an APTMS patterned surface; in this way, an OTS monolayer was self-assembled and patterned by AFM anodization (as described earlier). The oxidized areas were then used to self-assemble the APTMS, and this bifunctional template was subsequently used to self-assemble the gold nanoparticle array [285]. Guidance of the gold nanoparticle assembly into nanometer arrays could also be achieved with a hexadecene monolayer attached to a hydrogenated silicon surface. For this, the monolayer could be patterned by LAO and used to self-assemble APTMS that could, in turn, be used to guide the gold nanoparticles [376]. Moreover, APTMS can be used to self-assemble well-dispersed CNTs on the oxidized silicon surface [377]. Pang *et al.* demonstrated the improved patternability and adhesion of poly(3,4-ethylenedioxythiophene) (PEDOT) by the microcontact printing of OTS and subsequent filling of the nonfunctionalized areas with amine-functionalized SAMs. Following this, $FeCl_3$ could be selectively spincoated onto the amine-functionalized areas, and PEDOT films were grown selectively on the amine-functionalized surface by vapor-phase polymerization. The amine-functionalized monolayer and FeCl$_3$ resulted in an improved adhesion of the PEDOT film [378].

SAMs are also frequently used to tune the surface properties, with the hydrophobic coatings playing an important role in the fluid–surface interactions of microfluids. Thus, Feng *et al.* investigated the influence of OTS on the fluid dynamics of chemically modified silicon dioxide and glass microchannels [379].

Whilst these few examples highlight the wide variety of applications able to benefit from surface modifications with commercially available precursor molecules, significant interest remains in widening the availability of the precursor molecules. Hence, two quite different strategies can be used to generate functionalized monolayers. The first strategy relates to the synthesis of new precursor molecules that provide tailor-made functional groups, while the second strategy involves the implementation of new functionalities and focuses on the chemical modification of conventional precursor layers.

Notably, three alternative approaches have been proposed that describe the route to synthesize trichlorosilane precursor molecules; this is illustrated schematically in Figure 2.15.

The first synthesis of a silane-based monolayer was described by Netzer *et al.*, who initially converted the hydroxyl group of a 10-undecenyl alcohol into a chloride group that was then activated by Mg; tetrachlorosilane was subsequently added to form the trichlorosilane group. An extension of the alkyl chain length can be achieved by adding oxirane or oxetane to introduce either two or three methylene groups to the Mg-activated molecule [380]. Other possible approaches to the synthesis of silane-based molecules include the synthesis of alkene-functionalized molecules, which can be converted by adding HSiCl$_3$ and H$_2$PtCl$_6$ as a catalyst, or by the use of bromine-functionalized molecules, which can be converted to silane molecules by adding Mg, followed by the addition of SiCl$_4$ (as in the above-described approach). Maoz *et al.* described the synthesis of *trans*-13-docosenyltrichlorosilane [381], while Wasserman reported the synthesis of methyl 11-(trichlorosilyl)decanoate via a platinum-catalyzed method and the synthesis of 16-hepatdecenyltrichlorosilane and 10-uncecenyltrichlorosilane via a magnesium-activated approach [382].

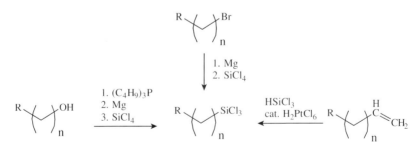

Figure 2.15 An overview of the synthesis routes to obtain trichlorosilane-based functional molecules.

Based on these general strategies, several functional precursor molecules have been synthesized, demonstrating the versatility of this approach. The synthesis of cyano-, bromo-, thiocyanato-, and thioaceto-terminated C_{16} trichlorosilanes was introduced by Balachander *et al.*, using the platinum catalyst-mediated process [383]. Additionally, the synthesis of iodo-, chloroacetate-, iodoacetate-, benzyl bromide-, and benzyl iodide-terminated C_{16} trichlorosilanes has been established using the same method [384]. Phthalocyanine molecules, which may have potential applications in display technology, as chemical sensors or as photoconducting devices [385], have been functionalized with an alkyltrichlorosilane group via the platinum catalyst pathway, and can be self-assembled on silicon. For this purpose, an 11-(3-thienyl) undecenyltrichlorosilane could be synthesized via a platinum catalyst method and then used for the self-assembly onto surfaces. These SAMs were proposed for use in thiophene polymerizations, to form conductive layers [386]. A maleiimido-terminated alkyl trichlorosilane molecule has also been synthesized using the platinum catalyst method. In this case, the maleiimido group can be utilized for the covalent binding of nucleophilic heterocycles, alkylthiols or amines, thus making the attachment of a wide class of molecules to the surface possible [387]. The synthesis of C_{10-12} alkyl chains terminated with a functional hydroxyl group and a PPh_2 group was reported for the self-assembly on silicon surfaces via activation of the surface by $SiCl_4$ and diethylamine, and the attachment of hydroxyalkylphosphine. Here, the PPh_2 end group could act as a ligand for Rh catalysts on the surface, or reaction of the Rh could be performed prior to the self-assembly process. The covalently attached Rh catalyst was tested for the hydrogenation of tolan [388]. When Zhang *et al.* demonstrated the formation of a PEG silane by the reaction of PEG with tetrachlorosilane, an effective depression of plasma protein adsorption and cell attachment was noted on these surfaces [389]. Subsequently, Sharma *et al.* described the development of ultrathin, uniform, stable *in-vivo*-like environments and conformal PEG films for silicon-based microdevices. For this, the surface-reactive PEG molecule was prepared by dissolving PEG in anhydrous toluene, followed by successive triethylamine addition. A tetrachlorosilane was then added so as to form a trichlorosilane group on the hydroxyl group. Different reactions, including the functionalization of PEG hydroxyl groups, as well as a reaction of tetrachlorosilane with several PEG chains up to cycle formation, might occur during this process. Nonetheless, the PEG silane was shown to form uniform films on silicon surfaces with a degree of roughness less than 1 nm by optimization of the self-assembly conditions [390]. Chi *et al.* synthesized an imidazolium chloride-functionalized triethoxy silane by the reaction of methylimidazole with a triethoxysilane-functionalized alkyl chloride. These authors investigated the use of such SAMs for controlling the wettability of silicon substrates by anion exchange, and showed that the water contact angle could be varied from 28 to 42° simply by exchanging the counterion, from choride to PF_6^- [391]. Each of these examples underlines the major impact of silane-based molecules on adding chemical functionality to SAMs, and the possibility of expanding the availability of tailor-made functional groups to bind and/or stabilize nano-objects, or for subsequent chemical modification schemes.

2.4.2
Surface Chemistry

Besides the (sometimes difficult to control) synthesis of functional silane precursor molecules – due to the high reactivity and water-sensitivity of the reactants – an alternative route has been proposed to acquire functional SAMs. This approach employs chemical reactions that are performed on SAMs that consist of silanes and which are known to form monolayers of reliable quality. The advantage of this technique is seen in the better quality of the starting monolayer, the possibility of avoiding undesired interactions between the silane and the functional group, and no need to optimize the self-assembly process for each individual precursor molecule. However, the subsequently performed surface reaction should be highly efficient in order to maximize the availability of the desired surface functionalities. Sagiv *et al.* reported the first chemical reaction on a covalently attached SAM, by demonstrating the conversion of a double bond to a hydroxyl function by treatment with B_2H_6 and successive reaction with $H_2O_2/NaOH$ solution; the newly formed alcohol end groups were then used for the formation of multilayer systems [380]. Based on these initial studies, a substantial research activity on surface chemistry in the field of functional silane-based monolayers has subsequently emerged.

As a result, substitution, esterification, Schiff base reactions, the formation of thiourea and ureas, click chemistry, photochemistry, oxidation, and the growth of polymer brushes – among others – have each been introduced and are discussed with respect to their applications in surface chemistry in the following subsections. A schematic overview of these reaction schemes is provided in Figure 2.16.

2.4.2.1 **Substitution**
Substitution reactions utilize the displacement of one functional group by another, such as the displacement of bromide by a thiocyanate or an azide (Figure 2.16). The substitution is mainly divided into *nucleophilic substitution*, whereby an anion attacks the functional group, or an *electrophilic substitution*, where a cation replaces the functional group. For surface reactions, BTS monolayers are mainly used for nucleophilic substitution reactions. In particular, Balachander *et al.* self-assembled a BTS monolayer and demonstrated replacement of the bromine group by substitution with azide or thiocyanate [383]. Furthermore, bromine- or chlorine-terminated SAMs can be substituted with iodine, as demonstrated by Lee; the function can subsequently be replaced with decanethiol, *n*-decylamine, *p*-nitrothiolphenol, glutathione and lamini fragment peptides [384]. Additionally, Fryxell *et al.* demonstrated the substitution of a bromine SAM with molecules such as cysteine and amines [392]. Shuye *et al.* enlarged the available functional groups by conducting a nucleophilic substitution of a bromine-functionalized SAM with thioacetate, sulfonate, and nitrile [393], while Haensch *et al.* self-assembled BTS monolayers and showed the substitution of bromine with primary amines such as propargylamine and 5-(2,2:6,2″-terpyridin-4yloxy)pentylamine; here, the terpyridine moiety was further used for complexation with $PEG_{70}–RuCl_3$ [394]. Another possible means of introducing terpyridine moieties is via reaction with an acetylene-modified Fe(II) complex;

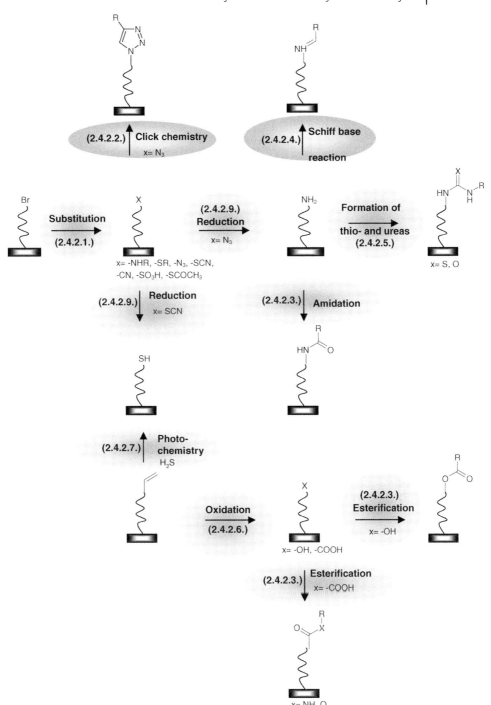

Figure 2.16   A schematic overview of possible modification schemes that can be implemented by surface reactions.

this can be initiated by treatment with HCl, with the free terpyridine moieties which can subsequently being closed with other metal ions such as Ir(III) or Zn(II) [395].

The nucleophilic substitution reaction scheme can be also used for structured surfaces. For example, Herzer *et al.* prepared chemical nanostructures by utilizing a high-resolution lithographic technique to form replaceable barrier nanostructures of triangular shape. For this purpose, an OTS monolayer was self-assembled onto a glass substrate patterned with the gold barrier structures. Then, after removal of the barrier structure, a BTS monolayer was self-assembled selectively onto the former positions of the barrier structures. The BTS monolayer was converted first, via substitution, into a thiocyanate monolayer, and subsequently to a thiol by reduction. Site-selective binding of gold nanoparticles could be demonstrated with high sensitivity on the thiol functional group [396]. Haensch *et al.* demonstrated the patterning of a BTS monolayer via a selective degradation of the BTS monolayer by LAO, with PFDTS being self-assembled in site-selective fashion as a passivation layer onto the oxidized areas. The BTS monolayer was subsequently substituted with azide and successively converted into an amine group by reduction, which could site-selectively bind silicon nanoparticles [397] (also C. Haensch *et al.*, unpublished results).

The substitution reaction represents a powerful tool for creating a large variety of versatile functionalized surfaces, and thus introducing a wide diversity of surface properties, such as charges or biofunctionalities. These properties can be utilized in a variety of applications, such as biosensors, for the growth or deposition of inorganic materials, in microfluidics, for the microengineering of smart surfaces for bioseparation or data storage, as sensors, or in the microfabrication of controlled-release devices.

2.4.2.2 Click Chemistry

The now widely used click chemistry was introduced in 2001 by Sharpless [329]. The main characteristics of a click reaction include its modularity, the wide scope, the high yield, and the lack of formation of any byproducts (or, at least, of byproducts that can be removed using nonchromatographic methods, such as crystallization or distillation). Furthermore, the reaction must be stereospecific, the reaction conditions mild, and the starting materials and reactants readily available. Furthermore, no solvents or easily removable solvent should form any part of the reaction, and the products should show a good stability under physiological conditions. The most commonly used click reaction on surfaces is the 1,3 dipolar cycloaddition of azide-functionalized surfaces with acetylene-functionalized molecules (see Figure 2.16). The first example of click chemistry to be conducted on a silica surface was described by Lummerstorfer *et al.* in 2004 [398], when BTS was self-assembled on a silicon wafer and the bromine functions were subsequently converted into azide groups via a substitution reaction. The azide functions were later used for the Huisgen 1,3-dipolar cycloaddition reaction [330] with three differently substituted acetylenes, for example, $R-C\equiv C-R'$ ($R,R' = C_6H_{13}$, H; $COOCH_3$, H; $COOC_2H_5$, $COOC_2H_5$). In this case, only ester-functionalized acetylenes showed a quantitative conversion, whilst for hexyl-substituted acetylene no reaction was observed (this was explained by the influence of electron-withdrawing ester groups). Rohde *et al.* described the activation of a hydrogenated surface by chlorination to bind sodium acetylene. Here, the acetylene functionality was used to click the electroactive benzoquinone which, when covalently attached, was reduced to a primary amine group by the application of a voltage that was used to covalently bind a ferrocene complex via an amide linkage [399]. The covalently attached electro-active ferrocene molecules might find potential applications in charge–storage molecular devices. Ciampi *et al.* described the covalent immobilization of commercially available diacetylene compounds on hydrogenated silicon surfaces via a hydrosilylation procedure; after which the alkyne end group was used to click various azide compounds [400]. The clicking of molecules such as polymers [401] and dyes [402] has also been demonstrated.

Click reactions have also been demonstrated on structured surfaces. For example, an *n*-octyldimethylchlorosilane monolayer was gradually modified following exposure to UV light to generate ozone to form acid groups. The acid groups were then used to bind acetylene-terminated molecules, which were further used to click peptides via the 1,3-dipolar cycloaddition, via the formation of a triazole ring [403]. Click chemistry based on microcontact printing has also been demonstrated by Rozkiewicz *et al.* to obtain structured surfaces. These authors self-assembled BTS and substituted the bromine with azide, after which a PDMS stamp was inked with the acetylene-terminated molecules and pressed onto the azide-terminated surface [404]. Ravoo *et al.* demonstrated, moreover, the preparation of carbohydrate microarrays by using microcontact click chemistry. For this purpose, BTS was self-assembled on glass or silicon surfaces, and subsequently converted to an azide moiety by substitution. Previously, alkyne-functionalized carbohydrates have been synthesized and clicked onto the azide-functionalized surface by pressing the PDMS stamp, inked with the carbohydrates, $CuSO_4$ and ascorbic acid, onto the substrate. Lines with dimensions of down to 5 µm could be created in this way [405]. Click chemistry, directed using scanning electrochemical microscopy, was first introduced for the self-assembly of a BTS monolayer onto a glass slide, with subsequent conversion into an azide group by a substitution reaction. In this way, a gold microelectrode could be used to transfer the acetylene-functionalized fluorescent dye and to create Cu(I) ions locally between the tip and the substrate, to catalyze the click reaction. By using this method, features of about 500 µm were created [406]. Oxidative nanolithography has been also combined with the click chemistry approach, when an OTS monolayer was oxidized with a biased AFM tip and BTS was site-selectively self-assembled onto the activated region. The bromine end group was replaced with azide and used to click propargyl alcohol; in this way, surface reactions on feature sizes down to 50 nm could be performed [448].

These few examples of click reactions highlight the versatility of the process, with both biomolecules and electroactive molecules being introduced onto the surfaces to demonstrate potential future applications in areas such as electronics, sensors, or glycomics.

2.4.2.3 Esterification/Amidation

Another possible means for binding functional molecules onto a surface is that of esterification or amidation, which utilizes the reaction of an acid or ester group with a hydroxyl or with an amine group, as depicted in Figure 2.16. In this way, either carboxylic acid- or ester-functionalized molecules can be introduced onto the surface; alternatively, amine- or hydroxyl-functionalized molecules can be used. Esterification and amidation reactions are important for biological applications, as they may be used to attach biomolecules such as DNA or biotin. These types of functionalized patterns are also important for the placement of cells, and to study cellular interactions.

Fryxell *et al.* demonstrated the formation of amide bonds, by the reaction of a trifluoroethylester SAM with primary amines [392], thus providing a possible means of covalently attaching amine molecules to the surface. Maoz *et al.* described the microwave-induced reaction of an acid-salt-terminated SAM and an amine-functionalized alkyl chain, which permitted amine-functionalized molecules to be bound onto the surface [407]. Flink *et al.* demonstrated the chemical functionalization of APTES with acid chloride-, thionylchloride- and carboxylic acid-functionalized molecules [408], thus opening the possibility to covalently attach carboxylic acid-functionalized molecules.

These reactions were also used to create functionalized patterns, and some representative processes are highlighted here. For example, Zhang *et al.* patterned a self-assembled PFDTS monolayer by using electron beam lithography (EBL), with APTMS subsequently being self-assembled on the irradiated spots and further functionalized with biotin by reaction of the amine group with an activated acid group attached to the biotin so as to form an amide bond. By using this method, nanostructures down to 250 nm could be created [409]. Normally, the direct attachment of amine-functionalized molecules to carboxylic acid-functionalized surfaces leads to salt formation, rather than to the creation of the desired amide bond. Hence, the attachment of an amine to carboxylic acid-functionalized surfaces must be carried out by activation with NHS (Figure 2.17).

In this reaction, NHS reacts with the carboxylic acid groups under the formation of a succinate ester, which presents a good leaving group and can subsequently be reacted with the desired amine molecules, forming of an amide bond. Previously, this method has been used by Fabre *et al.*, who self-assembled an ethyl undecylenate and a 1-decene monolayer on a hydrogenated silicon surface. The ethyl undecylenate SAM

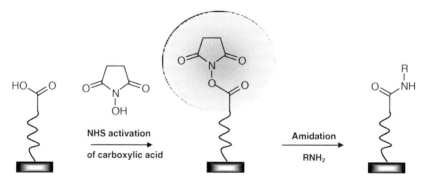

Figure 2.17 NHS activation of carboxylic acid for the binding of amine-functionalized molecules.

was activated with NHS by immersing the substrate into a solution of 1-(3-dimethyl-aminopropyl-3-ethylcarbodiimide) and NHS. A 2- aminoethylferrocenylmethylether was then covalently attached to the NHS-activated ethyl undecylate SAM, with formation of the amide bond [410]. The intact amine was used to bind DNA by first reacting with succinimidyl-4-[maleimidophenyl]butyrate to form an ester bond, after which the thiol-functionalized DNA was covalently attached [411]. An improved method for the reduction of nonspecific protein adsorption was introduced via the self-assembly of 7-octenyltrimethoxysilane and successive EBL, during which the irradiated areas were used for the self-assembly of APTES and the vinyl groups of the 7-octenyltrimethoxysilane were converted to hydroxyl groups. The binding of pro-teins onto amine groups was suitable to create patterns with a resolution down to 250 nm [412]. Crivillers *et al.* demonstrated the amidation of EDATMS by reaction with a carboxylic acid-terminated radical; in this case, the radical functionalized surface could be reversibly oxidized and showed different absorption spectra in the oxidized and reduced states. This approach proved to be highly attractive, as it provided a chemical redox-switchable surface that led to changes in the optical and magnetic responses of the system. It was also proposed that patterns of these radical molecules could be created by micro-contact printing, and this was subsequently demonstrated by inking the PDMS stamp with the radicals and pressing the stamp onto an amine-functionalized surface [413]. Duan *et al.* described the bifunctional chemical patterning of APTMS and PFDTS by micro-contact printing, whereby the APTMS was functionalized with a fluorescent dye by esterification, thus opening the possibility for further modification processes [414].

2.4.2.4 Schiff Base Reactions

Amine-terminated surfaces can be functionalized with aldehyde molecules via Schiff base reactions to form an imine bond, or vice versa (Figure 2.16). La *et al.* demon-strated the nanopatterning of SAMs via a selective chemical transformation induced by soft X-ray irradiation. For this purpose, (3-aminopropyl)diethoxymethylsilane was self-assembled on a silicon surface and functionalized with 4-nitrobenzaldehyde or 4-nitrocinnamaldehyde, under the formation of an imine bond. A nitrosubstituted phenyl-imine SAM was then converted into a secondary amine monolayer by selective X-ray irradiation, and the nonirradiated areas were later hydrolyzed to amines. Moreover, the amines could be converted with a Cy3-tagged oligonucleotide, with selective conversion of the amine by the Cy3-tagged oligonucleotide being confirmed by fluorescence imaging [415]. The Cy3-tagged oligonucleotides may also be attached covalently to the amine by using an esterification reaction, as previously introduced and described by Chen *et al.* [411]. Rozkiewicz also demonstrated the Schiff base reaction of an amine-functionalized monolayer, such that the EDATMS was self-assembled on silicon surfaces and the amine functionality was converted to an imine bond by reaction with different aldehydes. The imine bond can also be formed by microcontact printing of the aldehyde onto an amine-functionalized surface, as demonstrated by microcontact printing of the fluorescent dye Lucifer Yellow on amine-functionalized glass [416]. Schiff base reactions have also been shown capable of successfully immobilizing cytophilic proteins by microcontact printing, utilizing a similar approach to that described above. The amine monolayers were first self-assembled and reacted with terephthalaldehyde; the proteins were then contact-printed onto these aldehydes with feature sizes down to 100 μm, and the remaining areas were filled with amine-functionalized PEG [417]. Moreover, a mixed aldehyde/alkyl organic monolayer that had been self-assembled on a hydrogenated silicon surface was selectively functionalized on the aldehyde group by amine-functionalized biomolecules, such as the lysine groups of proteins [418].

To summarize, Schiff base reactions have been applied in particular for the binding of biomolecules, providing the reaction scheme with possible future applications in bioassays and other cell-related studies.

2.4.2.5 Formation of Thioureas and Ureas

The formation of thioureas and ureas has also been used to introduce functional moieties into SAMs (see Figure 2.16). Flink *et al.* demonstrated the chemical functionalization of APTES with isothiocyanate- and isocyanate-functionalized molecules to form thiourea or urea groups on the SAM [408].

This chemical reaction can be shown as being compatible with patterning methods, with a self-assembled EDATMS monolayer being patterned using nanoimprint lithography, for example. In this case, the amine function was used in the reaction with 1,4-diphenylene diisothiocyanate, and then successively reacted with cyclodextrin-functionalized gold or silicon nanoparticles. The same template was further utilized to monitor host–guest interactions with suitable molecules, as well as for two types of layer-by-layer assembly [419]. Maury *et al.* used nanoimprint lithography to create nanopatterns of His-tagged proteins, and thus prepared EDATMS–PEG or –PFDTS patterns. Using these structures, protein adsorption experiments were conducted via electrostatic and supramolecular interactions. The amine was also reacted with a 1,4-phenylene diisothiocyanate, and *N*-nitrilotriacetic acid subsequently attached; a protein was then attached to the nitrilotriacetic acid after treatment with a Ni(II) solution. Such protein interactions have been shown to be reversible by exchanging the Ni(II) with a strong competing ligand [420].

The formation of thioureas and ureas represents a highly compatible reaction scheme that can be integrated into several different patterning approaches, notably in the efficient binding of biomolecules that could be employed for biological applications.

2.4.2.6 Oxidation

Oxidation has been used to introduce hydroxyl- or acid-functionalized moieties onto SAMs, which can in turn be used for the esterification reactions described above to introduce other molecules (as shown in Figure 2.16). Netzer *et al.* described the oxidation of alkene end-functionalized trichlorosilane SAMs with different alkyl chain lengths to hydroxyl groups by treatment with B_2H_6 and subsequent treatment with a mixture of H_2O_2 and NaOH; hence, hydroxyl-functionalized SAMs were used for the formation of multilayers [380, 421]. Maoz *et al.* also demonstrated the oxidation of unsaturated alkyl trichlorosilane SAMs by crown ether-solubilized $KMnO_4$ to cleave the alkene bond, under the formation of a covalently attached alkyl silane-acid salt and an alkyl acid salt, that is removed from the surface. The length of the alkyl chain was seen to depend on the length and position of the starting unsaturated trichlorosilane [422]. Wasserman *et al*. demonstrated the oxidation of alkene or methyl functional groups of SAMs to carboxylic acid groups by $KMnO_4$, $NaIO_4$, and K_2CO_3 [382], while Shyue *et al*. reported the oxidation of nitrile-functionalized SAMs to carboxylic acid by stirring the substrates in a solution of sodium bicarbonate [393].

Oxidation can also be carried out on structured surfaces, and some examples of this are provided at this point. Maoz *et al*. described the oxidation of a methyl-terminated alkyl chain with an AFM tip (for details of this reaction, see Chapter 2.3.3.2), and also demonstrated the possibility of forming multilayer systems on the nanometer scale [311]. Miyaki *et al*. reported the details of the high-resolution EBL of octenyl-trimethoxysilane, where the vinyl groups were converted into hydroxyl groups by treatment with $BH_3 \times THF$ and a mixture of H_2O_2 and NaOH, following the previously introduced approach [380, 421]. Feature sizes down to 18 nm could be achieved using this method [423].

Oxidation reactions allow, in particular, the formation of multilayer systems, which in turn might allow the introduction of both ready-made and synthesized silane-based molecules, in addition to their combination with esterification reactions. Such a scheme would permit a wide variety of possible applications, depending on the nature of the introduced molecules as well as the formation of 3-D structures.

2.4.2.7 Photochemistry

Photochemical reactions represent an additional powerful means of functionalizing SAMs. Previously, Frydman described the photochemical conversion of a NTS SAM to a thiol-functionalized monolayer by treatment with H_2S and UV-irradiation at 254 nm (see Figure 2.16) [424], with the formed disulfide bonds being cleaved by treatment with either $NaBH_4$ [339] or $BH_3 \times THF$ [327]. A similar photochemical conversion into thiol-functionalized SAMs was also implemented into surface-structuring techniques, whereby the electro-oxidation of an OTS monolayer was applied and the NTS self-assembled onto locally formed acid groups. The double bond was subsequently utilized for the formation of thiol-functionalized groups, where both Ag and CdSe nanoparticles could be assembled [312] to form macrosopic electrodes on the surfaces. Such a modification scheme would be compatible with constructive electro-oxidation lithography, and might represent a technique for the creation of conductive metallic wires, with nanometer resolution [339].

Photochemistry can also be applied to photoisomerization reactions, with azo-silanes being synthesized and self-assembled on silicon oxide substrates. Following irradiation with UV light (360 nm), a *trans–cis* photoisomerization was observed, whereas UV-light irradiation at 450 nm triggered a *cis-trans* molecular isomerization. These changes in molecular photoisomerization were investigated using surface plasmon resonance spectroscopy (SPRS), a technique that allows the detection of very small changes in the thickness of these ultrathin layers [425]. These reversible transitions within the monolayers represent an example of the light-triggered reversible switching of the layer thickness.

Hozumi *et al.* described the photochemical conversion of an aldehyde-functionalized SAM to carboxylic acid-functionalized SAMs by irradiation using 172 nm vacuum UV light [426].

Brandow *et al.* reported on the self-assembly of *p*-chlorophenyltrichlorosilane which could be patterned through a photomask by irradiation with UV light (193 nm). In this way, the chlorine groups on the irradiated region were converted into aldehyde groups, which in turn were further converted to amines by treatment with NH_4OAc and $NaBH_3CN$. Subsequently, the amine moieties were used for the self-assembly of a Pd(II) catalyst, which catalyzed the electroless deposition of nickel [427]. Hong *et al.* demonstrated the photoreactivity of *n*-octadecyltrimethoxysilane by irradiation (through a photomask) with vacuum UV light of 172 nm, and observed the formation of carboxylic acid groups whilst the alkyl chain was degraded. The carboxylic acid moieties were further used for the binding of fluoro-functionalized silane molecules or of (*p*-chloromethyl)phenyltrimethoxysilane [428]. Chen *et al.* demonstrated the patterning by UV-light irradiation at 193 nm through a photomask of (aminoethyl-aminoethyl)phenylsiloxane (PEDA) SAMs. In this case, the benzylic C−N bond was cleaved on the irradiated regions, followed by the formation of an aldehyde. The intact amine was used to bind DNA by first reacting it with succinimidyl-4-[maleimido-phenyl]butyrate to form an ester bond, after which the thiol-functionalized DNA became attached covalently [411].

Photochemistry represents a powerful tool for the creation of functional patterns in a one-step procedure, notably because of its similarity to the patterning of resist materials, and hence its compatibility with standard photolithography. In particular, the functional groups can be used for further chemical reactions, not only to introduce functional moieties but also for the preparation of light-induced switches.

2.4.2.8 Polymer Brushes

Polymers can be used to "tune" the properties of a surface, a procedure that is highly desirable in many areas of research, and especially in biotechnology and advanced microelectronics. Although, the primary method for attaching polymeric brushes to a surface is via the adsorption of block copolymers [429–431], it is the noncovalent nature of this procedure that becomes its major weakness. Yet, such limitations can be relatively easily overcome by providing a *covalent* attachment of the polymers onto the surface, and for this two different strategies are favored: (i) a "grafting- from" approach; and (ii) a "grafting-to" approach. Whilst both methods permit the surfaces to be functionalized with polymer chains, the "grafting-from" method involves a polymer being grown from the surface, whereas the "grafting-to" method involves the attachment of pre-synthesized polymeric chains.

In 1996, Chang *et al.* were the first to demonstrate different ways of constructing SAMs of poly(γ-benzyl-L-glutamate) on silicon substrates, using both "grafting-from" and "grafting-to" methods. In the first of these methods, the preformed polymer is "grafted-to" the surface via a chloroformat group, whereas in the second method poly(γ-benzyl-L-glutamate) is first functionalized with a triethoxysilane head group and then attached to the silicon surface, using the triethoxysilane groups. As an alternative, the polymerization could be initiated by attaching APTES to the surface. It was concluded by these authors that "grafting-to" was more promising than "grafting-from," mainly because of the low degree of polymerization observed for the surface-initiated polymerization [432]. Based on these results, an extensive search was undertaken in the field of surface-initiated polymerizations, and a schematic overview of the various polymerization methods used on different surfaces is shown in Figure 2.18. The polymerization techniques are explained in detail, and representative examples discussed, in the following subsections.

"Grafting-From" Approach   In the past, a number of different polymerization techniques have been used to produce the polymeric building blocks needed to carry out a "grafting-from" approach. The most notable of these were controlled radical polymerization techniques, including atom transfer radical polymerization (ATRP), reversible addition-fragmentation chain transfer (RAFT) polymerization and nitroxide-mediated polymerization (NMP). All three methods have been shown to provide well-defined polymer materials for surface-initiated polymerizations. Husseman *et al.* were the first to discuss the possible synthesis of a silane-based initiator for NMP and ATRP, whereby monosilane or trichlorosilane groups could be introduced to allow attachment of the initiators to the surface. Subsequently, the successful growth of different homo-, random, and block copolymers using these initiators was demonstrated [433]. Matyjaszewski *et al.* also described the ATRP of styrene and methyl acrylate from an initiator that had been attached covalently to the silicon surface. The initiator was first synthesized via an esterification of 10-undecen-1-ol and 2-bromoisobutyl bromide, respectively, and this reaction was followed by hydrosilylation, which led to a highly reactive trichlorosilane group that could be used to form a covalent bond to the substrate. The living character of the polymerization was demonstrated by a linear increase in layer thickness with increasing polymerization time; and the possibility of growing block copolymers was also demonstrated [146]. Rowe-Konopacki *et al.* demonstrated the surface-initiated RAFT polymerization of diblock copolymers, using the same trichlorosilane molecules as described by Matyjaszewski, and converted them with a dithiobenzoyl disulfide to obtain a RAFT initiator on the surface [147].

   Each of these methods has also been shown as suitable for the generation of patterned polymer brushes. For example, Piech *et al.* described the surface-initiated ATRP polymerization of spirobenzopyran-*co*-methylmethacrylate from quartz slides, onto the surfaces of which an ATRP initiator was self-assembled and, subsequently, ATRP polymerization performed. The polymer film produced was selectively irradiated by a focused 366 or 780 nm pulsed laser beam, so as to pattern the polymer film by inducing a ring-opening isomerization of the spirobenzopyran to a zwitterionic merocyanine isomer. This reaction was demonstrated to be reversible by, for example, heating or irradiation with light at 585 nm, with a color change from light yellow to purple/red on the irradiated areas indicating successful conversion. Following treatment of the spirobenzopyran-*co*-methylmethacrylate copolymer, the modified colloids self-assembled preferentially onto the irradiated regions [434]. Becer *et al.* carried out the patterning of an OTS monolayer on silicon by using

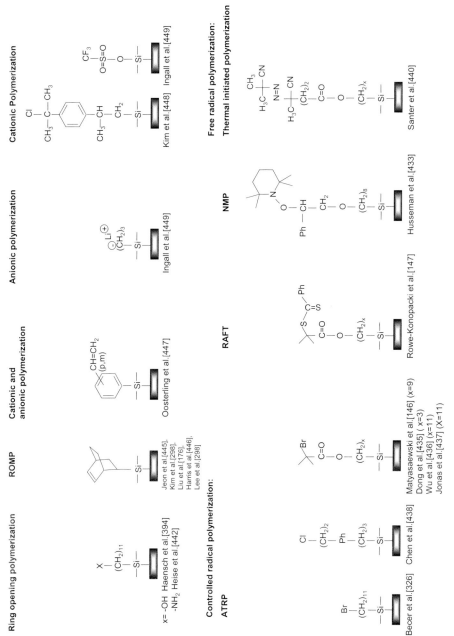

Figure 2.18 A schematic representation of surface-initiated polymerizations.

constructive electro-oxidative nanolithography, starting from a BTS monolayer which was self-assembled on the surface and utilized for the ATRP polymerization not only of styrene but also of block-copolymers. Polymer brushes with a line width of 70 nm could be obtained in this way [326, 397]. Later, Dong *et al.* showed that PEG/ polyacrylic acid patterns obtained by photolithography could be used to obtain structured polymer brush surfaces. As an example, PEG trichlorosilane was self-assembled on a silicon wafer and coated with a photoresist that had been patterned through a photo mask; the PEG was later removed from the non-covered areas by O_2 plasma. An ATRP initiator with a surface-reactive chlorosilane group was then self-assembled onto the now free areas, and the polymerization of acrylic acid was carried out. In an attempt to attach proteins to the polyacrylic acid, the acid groups were activated by *N*-(3-dimethylaminopropyl)*N'*-ethylcarbodiimide, NHS, and 4-morpho-line-ethanesulfonic acid, after which the amine-terminated proteins were attached covalently to the polymeric chains [435]. Wu *et al.* prepared a mixed OTS/polyacrylic acid pattern in which the base OTS monolayer was formed using a vapor diffusion technique, while the unmasked regions were used for the subsequent self-assembly of the ATRP initiator that was used to perform the polymerization of the acrylic acid [436]. Alternatively, patterning using either nanoimprint lithography or EBL was used to create nanometer-sized patterns of an ARTP initiator and PEG. After having first deposited a 100 nm-thick poly(methylmethacrylate) (PMMA) film on a silicon wafer, and creating a nanopattern, the ATRP initiator was self-assembled onto the exposed areas; following removal of the PMMA layer, the PEG monochlorosilane was self-assembled and the 2-(2-methoxyethoxy)ethyl methacrylate finally polymerized. In this way, polymer brush features with a lateral resolution down to 35 nm could be created [437]. Chen *et al.* described the formation of various polymer brush patterns prepared by the treatment of the hydroxylated silica surface, utilizing hexamethyldi-silazane self-assembly and the subsequent activation of the Si–CH$_3$ groups by O_2-plasma and/or EBL. The locally formed, higher reactive Si–O species could be used to bind the ATRP initiator (4-chloromethyl)phenyltrichlorosilane. These surface-bond-ed initiators were used to polymerize the methylacrylate, such that features down to 5 μm in size could be obtained [438]. Brinks *et al.* also highlighted the possible use of NMP for surface structuring; in this case, the NMP-polymerized brushes were used on patterns formed by LB structuring, after which LB lithography was carried out utilizing L-α-dipalmitoyl-phosphatidylcholine (DPPC) and the triethoxysilane-func-tionalized NMP initiator; this resulted in a surface that was patterned with uniform DPPC lines. Ultimately, when the initiator was attached covalently and the DPPC removed from the substrate, monomers such as styrene and acrylate became polymerized [439].

Another possible method of implementing surface-initiated polymerization is that of free radical polymerization [440] (which is also compatible with several structuring techniques), or an electrochemical polymerization approach that permits the poly-merization of monomers such as thiophene, which has an important role in electronic devices. Inaoka *et al.* demonstrated the electrochemical polymerization of different thiophene derivatives from a self-assembled oligothiophene-substituted alkylsilane [441].

Ring-opening polymerization (ROP) has also been used as a "grafting-from" technique. For example, Heise *et al.* prepared a mixed monolayer of BTS and 1-trichlorosilylundecane, whereby the bromine functional group was converted via an azide substitution and reduction to an amine functional group. The amine group was then used for the polymerization of benzyl γ-benzyl-L-glutamate N-carboxyanhydride [442]. Choi *et al.* demonstrated the surface-initiated ROP of ε-caprolactone from a N-(2-aminoethyl)-3-aminopropyltrimethoxy SAM [443], while Yoon *et al.* reported the ROP of poly(p-dioxanone). The same authors self-assembled (N-triethoxysilylpropyl)-O-poly(ethylene oxide)urethane on a silicon surface, and utilized the hydroxyl functional group for the $Sn(Oct)_2$-catalyzed ROP [444]. The possibility of introducing this polymerization approach to patterned substrates was shown by Haensch *et al.*, when the electro-oxidation of an OTS monolayer, the self-assembly of a BTS, and subsequent substitution to an azide was used to link propargyl alcohol to the surface structures, using the 1,3-dipolar cycloaddition. The propargyl alcohol was subsequently used to perform the ROP of L-lactide.

The ROMP technique was also used on silicon and patterned surfaces, with Jeon *et al.* demonstrating the patterning of OTS via micro-contact printing and a ROMP catalyst. In this case, the OTS was transferred via a PDMS stamp onto the substrate, and the non-covered areas were later filled with norbonyl trichlorosilane. The latter was activated with a ruthenium catalyst to surface-initiate the polymerization of derivatives of norbornene; use of this method led to smallest feature sizes of 2 μm being obtained [445]. Liu *et al.* described a combination of DPN and ROMP, and in particular demonstrated the successful transfer of 5-(bicycloheptenyl)trichlorosilane onto a Si substrate via an AFM tip, a subsequent activation of the structures with the first-generation Grubbs catalyst, and the subsequent polymerization of norbornene derivatives [176]. The photolithographic patterning of a ROMP catalyst was introduced as another method to obtain structured linear and crosslinked polymer brushes, and for this the inactivation of an Ru catalyst by exposure to UV-light was utilized. Consequently, the silicon wafer was functionalized with the initiator, which was in turn activated in a second step by a Ru catalyst. The substrates were illuminated through a mask that had been placed onto the substrate. Finally, the patterned catalyst layer was immersed in a solution containing the norbomyl monomer, and the polymer observed to grow only on the nonilluminated areas of the substrate. Features with a resolution of 4.3 μm could be created in this way [446]. Lee *et al.* used AFM anodization lithography to obtain nanometer-sized features of polymer brushes, with octadecylmethyldiethoxysilane being used as a resist layer. With a biased AFM tip the monolayer was locally removed, and SiO_2 was grown. Onto these features the 5-(bicycloheptenyl)triethoxysilane was self-assembled and, after activation, the polymers were grown. By using this method, feature sizes down to 75 nm could be prepared [298].

Other possible ways of performing surface-initiated polymerizations are anionic and cationic in nature. Oosterling *et al.* demonstrated the possibility of anionic polymerization from silicon surfaces by self-assembling p(m)-vinylbenzyltrichlorosilane on the surface, and then polymerizing monomers such as MMA [447]. Kim *et al.* prepared chlorosilyl-functionalized initiators and carried out a surface-initiated living cationic polymerization of isobutylene [448]. Both, cationic and anionic, surface-initiated polymerization techniques have been shown suitable for the patterning, for example, by Ingall *et al.* These authors carried out the patterning of a phenylsilane monolayer by irradiation through a mask with 193 nm UV light. The nonirradiated areas were first functionalized by treating the monolayer with trifluoric acid to replace the phenyl ring, after which the triflat was substituted by nucleophils or monomers – that is, $-C \equiv CH$, $-OCH_2CF_3$, $-O(CH_2)_6NH_2$. The triflat function could be used for the cationic polymerization of MMA to form polymer films of PMMA or poly(propylene oxide) (PPO). The anionic polymerization of acrylonitrile has been performed from a bromine-functionalized silane monolayer, which could be activated using lithium-*tert*-butylphenyl [449].

In summary, almost all standard polymerization techniques have been applied to the fabrication of polymer brushes via the "grafting-from" method, and these examples highlight the versatility of this approach, whereby uniform brushes with various properties can be obtained. Nevertheless, characterization of the polymer brushes – in particular on the nanometer scale – is difficult, as the growth kinetics might be influenced by the surface and/or the dense organization of the individual polymer chains. The "grafting-to" method (see below) has the advantage that the polymeric material can be characterized prior to the polymers being attached to the substrate. Moreover, the polymer systems can be synthesized under optimal conditions, while conventional characterization and purification tools can be used to prepare well-defined polymer systems that subsequently will be linked to the surface.

"Grafting-To" Approach   Among the "grafting-to" approaches used to covalently bind polymers onto silicon surfaces, the most obvious has been a functionalization of the polymer chain with surface-active silanes. Park *et al.* demonstrated the "grafting-to" of a rod–coil diblock copolymer to a silicon surface via immersion, casting, or contact printing. The rod–coil diblock copolymer consisted of a polystyrene part and a 3-(triethoxysilyl)-propylisocyanate, where the triethoxysilyl group could be attached covalently to the silicon surface. In this way, micropatterns of the polymer with 7.5 μm line width could be fabricated [450]. In particular, the grafting of PEG onto surfaces was of special interest, on the basis of its repellent properties towards proteins and cells. A PEG alkyltrichlorosilane pattern was fabricated by using a five-step procedure where first, a PMMA film was structured by EBL to selectively remove the PMMA from the silicon. The alkyltrichlorosilane was then self-assembled from the gas phase on the irradiated areas, the PMMA mask was removed, and the PEG trimethoxysilane was grafted onto the remaining silicon surface. These substrates were utilized so as to selectively adsorb collagen onto the hydrophobic alkyl tracks, which had a line width of between 30 and 90 nm [451]. Alternatively, a PEG silane could be self-assembled and spin-coated. As an example, Brough *et al.* used an eight-arm amine-terminated PEG to crosslink PEG by EBL in solution, after which biotin was immobilized on the amine-terminated PEG spots by the formation of an amide bond. The biotin was then used successively to immobilize streptavidin, and this was suitable to initiate the polymerization of actin [452]. Gaubert *et al.* demonstrated the preparation of biologically active, large-scale nanopatterns by utilizing nanoimprint lithography as a patterning technique, such that a gold silicon pattern was obtained. In particular, the self-assembly of a commercially available PEG silane onto the silicon oxide regions was used, and passivation of the noncovered gold areas with hexadecanthiol was subsequently performed. Cell-adhesion experiments demonstrated PEG's cell-adhesive/cell-repellent properties, with patterns down to 60 nm being created on a polyethylene background [453]. Dekeyser *et al.* investigated the "grafting-to" of PEG-trimethoxysilanes and trichlorosilanes with different chain lengths under different conditions, in order to develop procedures for the preparation of nanostructured surfaces for biomaterial applications using EBL. For this, although the layer thickness was about 1–2 nm, no significant difference was identified for the use of hexane or toluene as solvent; however, the grafted silane was not stable under standard incubation conditions (37 °C, 24 h, phosphate-buffered saline). As a consequence, the grafted PEG could not be used as a repellent polymer for proteins, though this problem was not observed at room temperature [454]. Whilst the bulk of the investigations was based on the self-assembly of silane-based PEG, the reaction of poly(ethyleneglycol methylether) with a hydrogenated surface has also been reported [455]. An additional method that can be used for the "grafting-to" approach is that of click chemistry (see above). As an example, Ostaci *et al.* demonstrated the self-assembly of ethynylenedimethylchlorosilane onto silicon substrates fabricated by the 1,3-dipolar cycloaddition of different polymers such as PEG-N_3 or PMMA-N_3 [401]. LeMieux and coworkers described the "grafting-to" of carboxylic-terminated polystyrene and poly(butyl acrylate) on epoxysilane SAMs on silicon, where the total layer thickness was 1–3 nm. However, by varying the concentration of each polymer and the molar mass, very finely defined structured surfaces could be obtained with approximately 10 nm phase domains and less than 0.5 nm roughness. Due to the immiscibility of the two polymers, switching of the surface nanomechanical properties could be observed. The surface wettability was also shown to be affected by hydrolysis of the poly(butyl acrylate) to the corresponding acid [456].

In conclusion, the possible use of "grafting-from" and "grafting-to" methods to create polymer brushes on surfaces was achieved by using different strategies that enabled the properties of surfaces to be engineered; this represents an important step in the development of "smart" materials. It also provides access to a large number of potential applications in coatings, microfluidics devices, and other systems. Clearly, polymerization techniques that include controlled living radical polymerization, ROMP and cationic and anionic polymerization, have been shown suitable for the creation of nanopatterned polymer brushes.

2.4.2.9 Others

The wide variety of chemical modification schemes used to introduce functionality to monolayers and to tune the surface properties, highlights the versatility of using functional SAMs. In addition to the examples discussed in this chapter, a number of other chemical reactions have been used to modify surfaces. These include the Sonogashira coupling, as performed by Qu, where the authors self-assembled a 1-(allyoxy)-4-iodobenzene on a hydrogenated silicon surface, after which the iodine functional group was coupled to an 1-ethynyl-4-fluorobenzene or 1-chloro-4-ethy-nylbenzene by a palladium-catalyzed Sonogashia reaction [457]. Shuye *et al.* demonstrated the hydrolysis of a thioester-functionalized SAM into a thiol by immersion in hydrochloric acid solution [393], while Balachander *et al.* described the formation of amino-terminated substrates, by the reduction of either azide- or nitrile-functionalized SAMs. Thiol-terminated substrates may be obtained via the reduction of thiocyanate- or thioester-functionalized SAMs (see Figure 2.16) [383]. Wasserman *et al.* introduced the bromination of alkene-functionalized SAMs by reaction with elemental bromine [382], whereby a mixed SAM of 1-octadecene and 11,11′-oxybis-1-undecene was prepared on a hydrogenated silicon substrate. The alkene functional groups of 11,11′-oxybis-1-undecene were successfully reacted with a first-generation Grubbs catalyst and different substituted alkenes [458].

It has been shown that most of these reactions may also be carried out on structured surfaces, so as to create tailor-made surface properties and binding sites in confined surface areas. Yet, surprisingly few reports are available concerning any structuring approaches that permit the introduction of more than two functional groups. Although, without doubt, these investigations have had a major impact on many fields of research, and also on a wide variety of applications (e.g., as sensor devices and in diagnostics), the issue of preparing such multifunctional structures will place additional demands on the fabrication process, a point which is discussed in the following subsections.

2.4.3
Multifunctionality

Today, the preparation of patterned multifunctional surfaces remains a challenge because compatible functionalization approaches must be used. In this respect, it will become necessary to identify surface reactions and structuring methods that are not exclusive of one another, nor do they destroy the integrity of the individual functional groups. To date, very few research groups have succeeded in preparing such multifunctional surfaces. Indeed, the methods applied have used either photochemical reactions, whereby irradiation is performed through a mask, or the selective deposition of molecules onto a certain spot, whether by pipetting, micro-contact printing, or DPN.

Two research groups in particular have reported the fabrication of multifunctional surface by using chemical photolithography, such that different molecules were self-assembled which provided photocleavable groups required different wavelengths for their cleavage. When irradiation of the first wavelength was applied through a photomask, the first photolabile group was cleaved; after moving the photomask to a different area of the surface, a second wavelength was applied that cleaved the second photolabile group. Ryan *et al.* prepared photosensitive thiol chains that contained two different photocleavable bonds: an *ortho*-nitrobenzyl amine-protecting group that cleaved at 365 nm; and a thiolate bond that cleaved at 220 nm. These thiols were self-assembled onto a gold surface and the substrate was illuminated through a photomask that permitted illumination only at specific wavelengths, and in specific areas. By using this method, it was possible to introduce three different functional groups onto one substrate [459].

The second method, as introduced by del Campo *et al.*, employed photosensitive triethoxysilanes that had been self-assembled onto quartz or silicon substrates. In a first step, only those molecules with one photocleavable group were assembled; illumination of the substrates through a photomask at a certain wavelength was sufficient to cleave the photosensitive group resulting in the formation of a bifunctional substrate. Moreover, if two different photo-cleavable molecules were introduced, this approach proved to be viable for creating patterns with four different functional regions [460].

Two other groups have reported an ability to prepare multifunctional surfaces by applying micro-contact printing. Renault and coworkers described the formation of patterns with several binding sites for proteins on a surface, by using affinity contact printing, and proceeded to functionalize a PDMS stamp with a protein that acted as antigen when the stamp was immersed in a solution containing different antibodies. The result was that each antigen was bound specifically to a complementary antibody such that, when the stamp was brought into contact with a substrate, the antibodies would be transferred to the surface, creating a microarray of printed proteins [461]. An alternative approach, reported by Geissler *et al.*, involved edge-spreading lithography. This concept was based on the fact that alkanethiol molecules are delivered from a PDMS stamp onto a coinage-metal substrate by a relief structure. From a practical standpoint, silicon beads were used as guides and a PDMS stamp inked with an alkanethiol was pressed onto the gold surface covered with the silicon beads. The ink was transferred to the contact areas of the stamp and the silica beads, and formed a ring around the silica beads on the gold surface. In a further step, a second thiol was delivered by a PDMS stamp onto the gold substrate and formed another circle that nucleated at the edges of the first monolayer. By using this method, concentric rings consisting of different monolayers could be obtained [462].

Multifunctional surfaces were investigated for different biological assays as shown by, for example, Zammatteo *et al.* These authors investigated the coupling of DNA onto glass for creating DNA microarrays by comparing amino-, acid- and aldehyde-functionalized surfaces, and coupling the DNA via either acid- or amine-functional groups. In this way, DNA spots of 400 μm diameter were created on the amino-functionalized surfaces [463]. Beyer *et al.* described the preparation of multifunctional PEG-based arrays, whereby 7-octenyl trichlorosilane and OTS were self-assembled on a glass slide and activated by UV-ozone; subsequently, a UV-induced graft polymerization of PEGMA was performed. On the amine-terminated PEGMA functionalized glass slides, different peptides could be coupled by placing spots of 200 μm diameter, with the spot arrays being utilized as immunoassays [464]. Kim *et al.* prepared spot arrays on glass surfaces to measure the coupling competition of Fmoc amino acids; after optimization, the synthesis of model libraries of biotin-Gly-Ala-P_1-Gly (P_1: one of 19 amino acids) could be performed. These spot arrays were prepared by patterning with a photoresist and perfluorination, after which the photoresist was washed off and amination performed on the free areas, using various silanes and polymers [144].

2.5
Summary and Outlook

In this chapter, an overview has been presented with regards to the fabrication schemes used to create structured surfaces. The aim was to introduce SPM-based structuring techniques that are especially powerful when combined with self-assembly techniques, as well as functional molecular layers that can be further modified in a chemical sense. The wide diversity of applications that might profit from this concept highlights the importance of further developments in this field. Notably, the special demands of this research requires a strong interaction of different disciplines; indeed, only a combination of different fields of science can provide solutions to the major problems that presently prevent these techniques from being implemented into "real" fabrication processes. Whilst engineering will, to some degree, support the development of instrumental implementations, chemists and materials scientists alike must contribute towards significant improvements of the modification schemes, as highlighted in this chapter. Although, to date, many developments have been made, only selected examples have been included here; however, the wide diversity of chemical reactions and molecular building blocks should enable the incorporation of chemical surface reactions into new fabrication concepts. Furthermore, the availability of a plethora of assembly schemes, confined locally by different structuring techniques and combined with the rules of chemical interactions, may be seen as the major strengths of this nanofabrication strategy.

Overall, the combination of chemically addressable surface templates that can be formed via lithographic techniques, together with reliable modification routines, holds great promise for the realization of a wide variety of structural features that can be implemented to create functional device structures, microfluidic devices, sensors, and diagnostic arrays in the future.

References

1 (a) Binnig, G. and Rohrer, H. (1984) European patent 27517-B1; (b) Binnig, G. and Rohrer, H. (1984) European patent 27517-A1, (c) Binnig, G. and Rohrer, H. (1984) Swiss patent 643397-A5; (d) Binnig, G. and Rohrer, H. (1984) European patent 27517-A; (e) Binnig, G. and Rohrer, H. (1984) US patent 4343993-A; (f) Binnig, G. and Rohrer, H. (1984) European patent 27517-B; (g) Binnig, G. and Rohrer, H. (1984) German patent 3066598-G; (h) Binnig, G. and Rohrer, H. (1984) Swiss patent 643397-A.

2 Binnig, G., Quate, C.F., and Gerber, C. (1986) *Phys. Rev. Lett.*, **56**, 930–933.

3 Dagata, J., Schneir, J., Harary, H.H., Evans, C.J., Postek, M.T., and Bennett, J. (1990) *Appl. Phys. Lett.*, **56**, 2001–2003.

4 Day, H.C. and Allee, D.R. (1993) *Appl. Phys. Lett.*, **62**, 2691–2693.

5 Yasutake, M., Ejiri, Y., and Hattori, T. (1993) *Jpn. J. Appl. Phys.*, **32**, L1021–L1023.

6 Tseng, A.A., Notargiacomo, A., and Chen, T.P. (2005) *J. Vac. Sci. Technol. B*, **23**, 877–894.

7 Garcia, R., Martinez, R.V., and Martinez, J. (2006) *Chem. Soc. Rev.*, **35**, 29–38.

8 Stiévenard, D. and Legrand, B. (2006) *Prog. Surf. Sci.*, **81**, 112–140.

9 Sugimura, H. and Nakagiri, N. (1995) *Jpn. J. Appl. Phys.*, **34**, 3406–3411.

10 Xie, X.N., Chung, H.J., Sow, C.H., and Wee, A.T.S. (2006) *Mater. Sci. Eng. R-Rep.*, **54**, 1–48.

11 Weeks, B.L., Vaughn, M.W., and DeYoreo, J.J. (2005) *Langmuir*, **21**, 8096-2098.

12 Tello, M. and Garcia, R. (2003) *Appl. Phys. Lett.*, **83**, 2339–2341.

13 Tello, M., Garcia, R., Martin-Gago, J.A., Martinez, N.F., Martin-González, M.S., Aballe, L., Baranov, A., and Gregoratti, L. (2005) *Adv. Mater.*, **17**, 1480–1483.

14 Martinez, R.V. and Garcia, R. (2005) *Nano Lett.*, **5**, 1161–1164.

15 Kinser, C.R., Schmitz, M.J., and Hersam, M.C. (2005) *Nano Lett.*, **5**, 91–95.

16 Suez, I., Backer, S.A., and Fréchet, J.M. (2005) *Nano Lett.*, **5**, 312–324.

17 Kim, Y., Kang, S.K., Choi, I., Lee, J., and Yi, J. (2005) *J. Am. Chem. Soc.*, **127**, 9380–9381.

18 Wang, D., Tsau, L., and Wang, K.L. (1994) *Appl. Phys. Lett.*, **65**, 1415–1417.

19 Snow, E.S., Juan, W.H., Pang, S.W., and Campbell, P.M. (1995) *Appl. Phys. Lett.*, **66**, 1729–1731.

20 Snow, E.S., Campbell, P.M., Twigg, M., and Perkins, F.K. (2001) *Appl. Phys. Lett.*, **79**, 1109–1111.

21 Chien, F.S.-S., Hsieh, W.-F., Gwo, S., Vladar, A.E., and Dagata, J.A. (2002) *J. Appl. Phys.*, **91**, 10044–10050.

22 Garcia, R., Calleja, M., and Pérez-Murano, F. (1998) *Appl. Phys. Lett.*, **72**, 2295–2297.

23 Garcia, R. and Calleja, M. (2000) *Appl. Phys. Lett.*, **76**, 3427–3429.

24 Pérez-Murano, F., Abadal, G., Barniol, N., Aymerich, X., Servat, J., Gorostiza, P., and Sanz, F. (1995) *J. Appl. Phys.*, **78**, 6797–6801.

25 Clément, N., Tonneau, D., Dallaporta, H., Bouchiat, V., Fraboulet, D., Mariole, D., Gautier, J., and Safarov, V. (2002) *Physica E*, **13**, 999–1002.

26 Losilla, N.S., Oxtoby, N.S., Martinez, J., Garcia, F., Garcia, R., Mas-Torrent, M., Veciana, J., and Rovira, C. (2008) *Nanotechnology*, **19**, 455308/1–455308/6.

27 Ma, Y.-R., Yu, C., Yao, Y.-D., Liou, Y., and Lee, S.-F. (2001) *Phys. Rev. B*, **64**, 195324/1–195324/5.

28 Vijaykumar, T., Raina, G., Heun, S., and Kulkarni, G.U. (2008) *J. Phys. Chem. C*, **112**, 13311–13316.

29 Mo, Y., Wang, Y., and Bai, M. (2008) *Physica E*, **41**, 146–149.

30 Mori, G., Layyarino, D., Ercolani, L., Sorba, L., Heuen, S., and Locatelli, A. (2005) *J. Appl. Phys.*, **97**, 114324/1–114324/8.

31 Martin-Sánchez, J., Gonzáles, Y., Gonzáles, L., Tello, M., Garcia, R., Ranados, D., Garcia, J.M., and Briones, F. (2005) *J. Cryst. Growth*, **284**, 313–318.

32 Cambel, V. and Soltys, J. (2007) *J. Appl. Phys.*, **102**, 74315/1–74315/7.

33 Lazzarino, M., Padovani, M., Mori, G., Sorba, L., Fanetti, M., and Sancrotti, M. (2005) *Chem. Phys. Lett.*, **402**, 155–159.

34 Okada, Y., Iuchi, Y., Kawabe, M., and Harris, J.S.Jr (2000) *J. Appl. Phys.*, **88**, 1336-1140.

35 Tsai, C.-H., Jian, S.-R., and Wen, H.-C. (2007) *Appl. Surf. Sci.*, **254**, 1357–1362.

36 Jian, S.-R., Fang, T.-H., and Chuu, D.-S. (2005) *J. Phys. D*, **38**, 2424–2432.

37 Lu, Y.F., Mai, Z.H., Qui, G., and Chim, W.K. (1999) *Appl. Phys. Lett.*, **75**, 2359–2361.

38 Hanke, M., Boeck, T., and Gerlitzke, A.-K. (2006) *Appl. Phys. Lett.*, **88**, 173106/1–173106/6.

39 Bo, X.-Z., Rokhinson, L.P., Yin, H., Tsui, D.C., and Strum, J.C. (2002) *Appl. Phys. Lett.*, **81**, 3263–3265.

40 Gwo, S. (2001) *J. Phys. Chem. Solids*, **62**, 1673–1687.

41 Chien, F.S.-S., Chan, J.-W., Lin, S.-W., Chou, Y.-C., Chen, T.T., Gwo, S., Chao, T.-S., and Hsieh, W.-F. (2000) *Appl. Phys. Lett.*, **76**, 360–362.

42 Chien, F.S.-S., Chou, Y.-C., Chen, T.T., Hsieh, W.-F., Chao, T.-S., and Gwo, S. (2001) *J. Appl. Phys.*, **89**, 2465–2472.

43 Fernandez-Cuesta, I., Borrisé, X., and Pérez-Murano, F. (2006) *J. Vac. Sci. Technol. B*, **24**, 2988–2992.

44 Hsu, H.-F. and Lee, C.-W. (2008) *Ultramicroscopy*, **108**, 1076–1080.

45 Choi, I., Yang, Y.I., Kim, Y.-J., Kim, Y., Hahn, J.-S., Choi, K., and Yi, J. (2008) *Langmuir*, **24**, 2597–2602.

46 Unal, K., Aronsson, B.-O., Mugnier, Y., and Descouts, P. (2002) *Surf. Interface Anal.*, **34**, 490–493.

47 Kim, T.Y., Di Zitti, E., Ricci, D., and Cincotti, S. (2008) *Physica E*, **40**, 1941–1943.

48 Kim, T.Y., Di Zitti, E., Ricci, D., and Cincotti, S. (2004) *J. Phys. D*, **37**, 1357–1361.

49 Cooper, E.B., Manalis, S.R., Fang, H., Dai, H., Matsumoto, K., Minne, S.C., Hunt, T., and Quate, C.F. (1999) *Appl. Phys. Lett.*, **75**, 3566–3568.

50 Matsumoto, K., Gotoh, Y., Maeda, T., Dagata, J.A., and Harris, J.S. (2000) *Appl. Phys. Lett.*, **76**, 239–241.

51 Kim, J., Kim, J., Song, K.-B., Lee, S.-Q., Kim, E.-K., and Park, K.-H. (2003) *Jpn. J. Appl. Phys.*, **42**, 7635–7639.

52 Takemura, Y., Kidaka, S., Watanabe, K., Nasu, Y., Yamada, T., and Shrakashi, J.-I. (2003) *J. Appl. Phys.*, **93**, 7346–7348.

53 Lin, H.-N., Chang, Y.-H., Yen, J.-H., Hsu, J.-H., Leu, I.-C., and Hon, M.-H. (2004) *Chem. Phys. Lett.*, **399**, 422–425.

54 Hsu, J.-H., La, H.-W., Lin, H.-N., Chuang, C.-C., and Huang, J.-H. (2003) *J. Vac. Sci. Technol. B*, **21**, 2599–2601.

55 Takemura, Y., Hayashi, S., Okazaki, F., Yamada, T., and Shirakashi, J.-I. (2005) *Jpn. J. Appl. Phys.*, **44**, L285–L287.

56 Bouchiat, V., Faucher, M., Thirion, C., Wernsdorfer, W., Fournier, T., and Panncticr, B. (2001) *Appl. Phys. Lett.*, **79**, 123–125.

57 Snow, E.S., Campbell, P.M., Rendell, R.W., Buot, F.A., Park, D., Marrian, C.R.K., and Magno, R. (1998) *Appl. Phys. Lett.*, **72**, 3071–3073.

58 Amato, J.C. (2004) *Appl. Phys. Lett.*, **85**, 103–105.

59 Archanjo, B.S., Silveira, G.V., Gocalves, A.-M.B., Alves, D.C.B., Ferlauto, A.S., Lacerda, R.G., and Neves, B.R.A. (2009) *Langmuir*, **25**, 602–605.

60 Rolandi, M., Quate, C.F., and Dai, H. (2002) *Adv. Mater.*, **14**, 191–194.

61 Davis, Z.F., Abadal, G., Hansen, O., Borisé, X., Barniol, N., Pérez-Murano, F., and Boisen, A. (2003) *Ultramicroscopy*, **97**, 467–472.

62 Snow, E.S., Park, D., and Campbell, P.M. (1996) *Appl. Phys. Lett.*, **69**, 269–271.

63 Farkas, N., Zhang, G., Evans, E.A., Ramsier, R.D., and Dagata, J.A. (2003) *J. Vac. Sci. Technol. A*, **21**, 1188–1193.

64 Tachiki, M., Fukuda, T., Sugata, K., Seo, H., Umezawa, H., and Kawarada, H. (2000) *Appl. Surf. Sci.*, **159–160**, 578–582.

65 Tachiki, M., Seo, H., Banno, T., Sumikawa, Y., Umezawa, H., and Kawarada, H. (2002) *Appl. Phys. Lett.*, **81**, 2854–2856.

66 Loh, K.P., Xie, X.N., Lim, Y.H., Teo, E.J., Zheng, J.C., and Ando, T. (2002) *Surf. Sci.*, **505**, 93–114.

67 Masubuchi, S., Ono, M., Yoshida, K., Hirakawa, K., and Machida, T. (2008) *Cond. Matter.*, arXiv:0812.0048v1.

68 Weng, L., Zhang, L., Chen, Y.P., and Rokhinson, L.P. (2008) *Appl. Phys. Lett.*, **93**, 93207/1–93207/3.

69 Gordon, A.E., Fayfield, R.T., Litfin, D.D., and Higman, T.K. (1995) *J. Vac. Sci. Technol. B*, **13**, 2805–2808.

70 Stiévenard, D., Fontaine, P.A., and Duboirs, E. (1997) *Appl. Phys. Lett.*, **70**, 3272–3274.

71 Avouris, P., Hertel, T., and Martel, R. (1997) *Appl. Phys. Lett.*, **71**, 285–287.

72 Dagata, J.A., Inoue, T., Itoh, J., and Yokoyama, H. (1998) *Appl. Phys. Lett.*, **73**, 271–273.

73 Dagata, J.A., Inoue, T., Itoh, J., Matsumoto, K., and Yokoyama, H. (1998) *J. Appl. Phys.*, **84**, 6891–6899.

74 Marchi, F., Bouchiat, V., Dallaporta, H., Safarov, V., Tonneau, D., and Doppelt, P. (1998) *J. Vac. Sci. Technol. B*, **16**, 2952–2956.

75 Garcia, R., Calleja, M., and Rohrer, H. (1999) *J. Appl. Phys.*, **86**, 1898–1902.

76 Dagata, J.A., Perez-Murano, F., Abadal, G., Morimoto, K., Inoue, T., Itoh, J., and Yokoyama, H. (2000) *Appl. Phys. Lett.*, **76**, 2710–2712.

77 Dubois, E. and Bubendorff, J.-L. (2000) *J. Appl. Phys.*, **87**, 8148–8154.

78 Snow, E.S., Jernigan, G.G., and Campbell, P.M. (2000) *Appl. Phys. Lett.*, **76**, 1782–1784.

79 Jungblut, H., Wille, D., and Lewerenz, H.J. (2001) *Appl. Phys. Lett.*, **78**, 168–170.

80 Tello, M. and Garcia, R. (2001) *Appl. Phys. Lett.*, **79**, 424–426.

81 Ahn, S.J., Jang, Y.K., Lee, H., and Lee, H. (2002) *Appl. Phys. Lett.*, **80**, 2592–2594.

82 Kuramochi, H., Ando, K., and Yokoyama, H. (2003) *Surf. Sci.*, **542**, 56–63.

83 Dagata, J.A., Perez-Murano, F., Martin, C., Kuramochi, H., and Yokoyama, H. (2004) *J. Appl. Phys.*, **96**, 2386–2392.

84 Dagata, J.A., Perez-Murano, F., Martin, C., Kuramochi, H., and Yokoyama, H. (2004) *J. Appl. Phys.*, **96**, 2393–2399.

85 Lee, S., Pyo, E.K., Kim, J.O., Noh, J., Lee, H., and Ahn, J. (2007) *J. Appl. Phys.*, **101**, 44905/1–44905/5.

86 Daia, H., Frankin, N., and Han, J. (1998) *Appl. Phys. Lett.*, **73**, 1508–1510.

87 Kuramochi, H., Tokizaki, T., Yokoyama, H., and Dagata, J.A. (2007) *Nanotechnology*, **18**, 135703/1–135703/6.

88 Kuramochi, H., Tokizaki, T., Ando, K., Yokoyama, H., and Dagata, J.A. (2007) *Nanotechnology*, **18**, 135704/1–135704/7.

89 Choi, J.S., Bae, S., Ahn, S.J., Kim, D.H., Jung, K.Y., Han, C., Chung, C.C., and Lee, H. (2007) *Ultramicroscopy*, **107**, 1091–1094.

90 Kuramochi, H., Ando, K., Shikakura, Y., Yasutake, M., Tokizaki, T.K., and Yokoyama, H. (2004) *Nanotechnology*, **15**, 1126–1130.

91 Sugimura, H., Uchida, T., Kitamura, N., and Masuhara, H. (1993) *Jpn. J. Appl. Phys.*, **32**, L553.

92 Campbell, P.M. and Snow, E.S. (1998) *Mater. Sci. Eng. B*, **51**, 173–177.

93 Zhang, Y.Y., Zhang, J., Luo, G., Zhou, X., Xie, G.Y., Zhu, T., and Liu, Z.F. (2005) *Nanotechnology*, **16**, 422–428.

94 Minne, S.C., Flueckiger, P., Soh, H.T., and Quate, C.F. (1995) *J. Vac. Sci. Technol. B*, **13**, 1380–1385.

95 Cavallini, M., Mei, P., Biscarini, F., and Garcia, R. (2003) *Appl. Phys. Lett.*, **83**, 5286–5288.

96 Minne, S.C., Manalis, S.R., Atalar, A., and Quate, C.F. (1996) *J. Vac. Sci. Technol. B*, **14**, 2456–2461.

97 Minne, S.C., Adams, J.D., Yaralioglu, G., Manalis, S.R., Atalar, A., and Quate, C.F. (1998) *Appl. Phys. Lett.*, **73**, 1742–1744.

98 Albonetti, C., Martinez, J., Losilla, N.S., Greco, P., Cavallini, M., Borgatti, F., Montecchi, M., Pasquali, L., Garcia, R., and Biscarini, F. (2008) *Nanotechnology*, **19**, 435303/1–435303/9.

99 Farkas, N., Comer, J.R., Zhang, G., Evans, E.A., Ramsier, R.D., Wight, S., and Dagata, J.A. (2004) *Appl. Phys. Lett.*, **85**, 5691–5693.

100 Martinez, R.V., Losilla, N.S., Martinez, J., Tello, M., and Garcia, R. (2008) *Nanotechnology*, **18**, 84021/1–84021/6.

101 Martinez, J., Losilla, N.S., Biscarini, F., Schmidt, G., Borzenko, T., Molenkamp, L.W., and Garcia, R. (2006) *Rev. Sci. Instrum.*, **77**, 86106/1–86106/3.

102 Minne, S.C., Soh, H.T., Flueckiger, P., and Quate, C.F. (1995) *Appl. Phys. Lett.*, **66**, 703–705.

103 Snow, E.S. and Campbell, P.M. (1995) *Science*, **270**, 1639–1641.

104 Ishii, M. and Matsumoto, K. (1995) *Jpn. J. Appl. Phys.*, **34**, 1329–1331.

105 Heinzel, T., Held, R., Lüscher, S., Ensslin, K., Wegschneider, W., and Bichler, M. (2001) *Physica E*, **9**, 84–93.

106 Lüscher, S., Held, R., Fuhrer, A., Heinzel, T., Ensslin, K., Bichler, M., and Wegschneider, W. (2001) *Mater. Sci. Eng. C*, **15**, 153–157.

107 Sigrist, M., Fuhrer, A., Ihn, T., Ensslin, K., Driscol, D.C., and Gossard, A.C. (2004) *Appl. Phys. Lett.*, **85**, 3558–3560.

108 Lüscher, S., Fuhrer, A., Held, R., Heinzel, T., and Ensslin, K. (1999) *Appl. Phys. Lett.*, **75**, 2452–2454.

109 Lüscher, S., Fuhrer, A., Held, R., Heinzel, T., Ensslin, K., Bichler, M., and Wegschneider, W. (2002) *Microelectron. J.*, **33**, 319–321.

110 Fuhrer, A., Lüscher, S., Ihn, T., Heinzel, T., Ensslin, K., Wegschneider, W., and Bichler, M. (2002) *Microelectron. Eng.*, **63**, 47–52.

111 Dorna, A., Sigrist, M., Fuhrer, A., Ihn, T., Heinzel, T., Ensslin, K., Wegschneider, W., and Bichler, M. (2002) *Physica E*, **13**, 719–722.

112 Grbic, B., Leturcq, R., Ihn, T., Ensslin, K., Reuter, D., and Wieck, A.D. (2008) *Physica E*, **40**, 1273–1275.

113 Grbic, B., Letrucq, R., Ensslin, K., Reuter, D., and Wieck, A.-D. (2005) *Appl. Phys. Lett.*, **87**, 232108/1–232108/3.

114 Wouters, D. and Schubert, U.S. (2004) *Angew. Chem., Int. Ed.*, **43**, 2480–2495.

115 Krämer, S., Fuierer, R.R., and Gorman, C.B. (2003) *Chem. Rev.*, **103**, 4367–4418.

116 Rolandi, M., Suez, I., Scholl, A., and Fréchet, J.M.J. (2007) *Angew. Chem., Int. Ed.*, **46**, 7477–7480.

117 Zauscher, S. (2004) Polymeric and biomolecular nanostructures: fabrication by scanning probe lithography, in *Dekker Encyclopedia of Nanoscience and Nanotechnology* (eds J.A. Schwarz, I. Contescu, and K. Putyera), Marcel Dekker, New York.

118 Tang, Q., Shi, S.-Q., and Zhou, L. (2004) *J. Nanosci. Nanotechnol.*, **4**, 948–963.

119 Liu, G.-Y., Xu, S., and Qian, Y. (2000) *Acc. Chem. Res.*, **33**, 457–466.

120 Cruchon-Dupeyrat, S., Porthun, S., and Liu, G.-Y. (2001) *Appl. Surf. Sci.*, **175–176**, 636–642.

121 Wu, C.-H., Sheu, J.-T., Chen, C.H., and Chao, T.-S. (2007) *Jpn. J. Appl. Phys.*, **46**, 6272–6276.

122 Lee, S., Kim, J., Lee, W.S.K., Shin, H.-J., Koo, S., and Lee, H. (2004) *Mater. Sci. Eng.*, **C24**, 3–9.

123 Zhang, M., Bullen, D., Chung, S.-W., Hong, S., Ryu, K.S., Fan, Z., Mirkin, C.A., and Liu, C. (2002) *Nanotechnology*, **13**, 212–217.

124 Wilder, K., Soh, H.T., Atalar, A., and Quate, C.F. (1999) *Rev. Sci. Instrum.*, **70**, 2822–2827.

125 Vettiger, P., Despont, M., Drechsler, U., Dürig, U., Häberle, W., Lutwyche, M.I., Rothuizen, H.E., Stutz, R., Widmer, R., and Binnig, G.K. (2000) *IBM J. Res. Develop.*, **44**, 323–340.

126 Minne, S.C., Adams, J.D., Yaralioglu, G., Manalis, S.R., Atalar, A., and Quate, C.F. (1998) *Appl. Phys. Lett.*, **73**, 1742–1744.

127 Wouters, D. and Schubert, U.S. (2007) *Nanotechnology*, **18**, 485306/1–485306/7.

128 Kakushima, K., Watanabe, T., Shimamoto, K., Gouda, T., Ataka, M., Mamura, H., Isono, Y., Hashiguchi, G., Mihara, Y., and Fujita, H. (2004) *Jpn. J. Appl. Phys.*, **43**, 4041–4144.

129 Watanabe, F., Arita, M., Motooka, T., Okano, K., and Yamada, T. (1998) *Jpn. J. Appl. Phys.*, **37**, L562–L564.

130 Lenhert, S., Sun, P., Wang, Y., Fuchs, H., and Mirkin, C.A. (2007) *Small*, **3**, 71–75.

131 Bullen, D., Wang, X., Zou, J., Chung, S.-W., Mirkin, C.A., and Liu, C. (2004) *Micromech. Syst.*, **13**, 594–602.

132 Bullen, D., Chung, S.-W., Wang, X., Zou, J., Mirkin, C.A., and Liu, C. (2004) *Appl. Phys. Lett.*, **84**, 788–791.

133 Nuzzo, R.G. and Allara, D.L. (1983) *J. Am. Chem. Soc.*, **105**, 4481–4483.

134 Sagiv, J. (1980) *J. Am. Chem. Soc.*, **102**, 92–98.

135 Ulman, A. (1996) *Chem. Rev.*, **96**, 1533–1554.

136 Ulman, A., Kang, J.F., Shnidman, Y., Liao, S., Jordan, R., Choi, G.-Y., Zaccaro, J., Myerson, A.S., Rafailovich, M., Sokolov, J., and Fleischer, C. (2000) *Rev. Mol. Biotechnol.*, **74**, 175–188.

137 Everhart, D.S. (2002) Self-assembling monolayers: alkaline thiols on gold, in *Handbook of Applied Surface and Colloid Chemistry*, vol. 2 (ed. K. Holmberg), Wiley, pp. 99–116.

138 Love, J.C., Estroff, L.A., Kriebel, J.K., Nuzzo, R.G., and Whitesides, G.M. (2005) *Chem. Rev.*, **105**, 1103–1169.

139 Woodruff, D.P. (2007) *Appl. Surf. Sci.*, **254**, 76–81.

140 Mizutani, F. (2008) *Sens. Actuators, B*, **130**, 14–20.

141 Peor, N., Sfez, R., and Yitzchaik, S. (2008) *J. Am. Chem. Soc.*, **130**, 4158–4165.

142 Rittner, M., Martin-Gonzalez, M.S., Flores, A., Schweizer, H., Effenberger, F., and Pilkuhn, M.H. (2005) *J. Appl. Phys.*, **98**, 54312/1–54312/7.

143 Li, Q., Mathur, G., Homsi, M., Surthi, S., Misra, V., Malinovskii, V., Schweikart, K.-H., Yu, L., Lindsey, J.S., Liu, Z., Dabke, R.B., Yasseri, A., Bocian, D.F., and Kuhr, W.G. (2002) *Appl. Phys. Lett.*, **81**, 1494–1496.

144 Kim, D.-H., Shin, D.-S., and Lee, Y.-S. (2007) *J. Pept. Sci.*, **13**, 625–633.

145 Salami, T.O., Yang, Q., Chitre, K., Zarembo, S., Cho, J., and Oliver, S.R.J. (2005) *J. Electron. Mater.*, **34**, 534–540.

146 Matyjaszewski, K., Miller, P.J., Shukla, N., Immaraporn, B., Gelman, A., Luokala, B.B., Siclovan, T.M., Kickelbick, G., Vallant, T., Hoffmann, H., and Pakula, T. (1999) *Macromolecules*, **32**, 8716–8724.

147 Rowe-Konopacki, M.D. and Boyes, S.G. (2007) *Macromolecules*, **40**, 879–888.

148 Mirkin, C.A., Hong, S., and Demers, L. (2001) *ChemPhysChem*, **2**, 37–39.

149 Salaita, K., Wang, Y., and Mirkin, C.A. (2007) *Nat. Nanotechnol.*, **2**, 145–155.

150 Mirkin, C.A. (2000) *Inorg. Chem.*, **39**, 2258–2272.

151 Ginger, D.S., Zhang, H., and Mirkin, C.A. (2004) *Angew. Chem., Int. Ed.*, **43**, 30–45.

152 Haaheim, J. and Nafday, O.A. (2008) *Scanning*, **30**, 137–150.

153 Leggett, G.J. (2005) *Analyst*, **130**, 259–264.

154 Huck, W.T.S. (2007) *Angew. Chem., Int. Ed.*, **46**, 2754–2757.

155 Li, X.-M., Huskens, J., and Reinhoudt, D.N. (2004) *J. Mater. Chem.*, **14**, 2954–2971.

156 Piner, R.D., Zhu, J., Xu, F., Hong, S., and Mirkin, C.A. (1999) *Science*, **283**, 661–663.

157 Jaschke, M. and Butt, H.-J. (1995) *Langmuir*, **11**, 1061–1064.

158 Hong, S., Zhu, J., and Mirkin, C.A. (1999) *Science*, **286**, 523–525.

159 Schwartz, P.V. (2002) *Langmuir*, **18**, 4041–4046.

160 Sheehan, P.E. and Whitman, L.J. (2002) *Phys. Rev. Lett.*, **88**, 156104/1–156104/4.

161 Kim, K.-H., Moldovan, N., and Espinosa, H.D. (2005) *Small*, **1**, 632–635.

162 Moldovan, N., Kim, K.-H., and Espinosa, H.D. (2006) *J. Microelectromech. Syst.*, **15**, 204–213.

163 Zhang, H., Elghanian, R., Disawal, N.A., Amro, S., and Eby, R. (2004) *Nano Lett.*, **4**, 1649–1655.

164 Zou, J., Wang, X., Bullen, D., Ryu, K., Liu, C., and Mirkin, C.A. (2004) *J. Micromech. Microeng.*, **14**, 204–211.

165 Wang, X., Ryu, K.S., Bullen, D.A., Zou, J., Zhang, H., and Mirkin, C.A. (2003) *Langmuir*, **19**, 895–8955.

166 Piner, R.D., Hong, S., and Mirkin, C.A. (1999) *Langmuir*, **15**, 5457–5460.

167 Nelson, B.A., King, W.P., Laracuente, A.R., Sheehan, P.E., and Whitman, L.J. (2006) *Appl. Phys. Lett.*, **88**, 33104/1–33104/3.

168 Sheehan, P.E., Whitman, L.J., King, W.P., and Nelson, B.A. (2004) *Appl. Phys. Lett.*, **85**, 1589–1591.

169 Lee, W.-K., Whitman, L.J., Lee, J., King, W.P., and Sheehan, P.E. (2008) *Soft Matter*, **4**, 1844–1847.

170 Yang, M., Sheehan, P.E., King, W.P., and Whitman, L.J. (2006) *J. Am. Chem. Soc.*, **128**, 6774–6775.

171 Hunag, L., Chang, Y.-H., Kakkassery, J.J., and Mirkin, C.A. (2006) *J. Phys. Chem. Lett. B*, **110**, 20756–20758.

172 Weinberger, D.A., Hong, S., Mirkin, C.A., Wessels, B.W., and Higgins, T.B. (2000) *Adv. Mater.*, **12**, 1600–1603.

173 Jung, H., Kulkarni, R., and Collier, C.P. (2003) *J. Am. Chem. Soc.*, **125**, 12096–12097.

174 Kooi, S.E., Baker, L.A., Sheehan, P.E., and Whitman, L.J. (2004) *Adv. Mater.*, **16**, 1012–1016.

175 Maynor, B.W., Filocamo, S.F., Grinstaff, M.W., and Liu, J. (2002) *J. Am. Chem. Soc.*, **124**, 522–523.

176 Liu, X., Guo, S., and Mirkin, C.A. (2003) *Angew. Chem., Int. Ed.*, **42**, 4785–4789.

177 Wei, J.H., Coffey, D.C., and Ginger, D.S. (2006) *J. Phys. Chem. B*, **110**, 24324–24330.

178 Basabe-Desmonts, L., Wu, C.-C., van der Werf, K.O., Peter, M., Bennink, M., Otto, C., Velders, A.H., Reinhout, D.N., Subramaniam, V., and Crego-Calama, M. (2008) *ChemPhysChem*, **9**, 1680–1687.

179 Willner, I., Baron, R., and Willner, B. (2007) *Biosens. Bioelectron.*, **22**, 1841–1852.

180 Zhang, H., Lee, K.-B., Li, Z., and Mirkin, C.A. (2003) *Nanotechnology*, **14**, 1113–1117.

181 Zhou, H., Li, Z., Wu, A., Wei, G., and Liu, Z. (2004) *Appl. Surf. Sci.*, **236**, 18–24.

182 Demmers, L.M., Ginger, D.S., Park, S.-J., Li, Z., Chung, S.-W., and Mirkin, C.A. (2002) *Science*, **296**, 1836–1838.

183 Nyamjav, D. and Ivanisevic, A. (2003) *Adv. Mater.*, **15**, 1805–1809.

184 Nyamjav, D. and Ivanisevic, A. (2005) *Biomaterials*, **26**, 2749–2757.

185 Cung, S.-W., Ginger, D.S., Morales, M.W., Zhang, Z., Chandrasekhar, V., Ratner, M.A., and Mirkin, C.A. (2005) *Small*, **1**, 64–69.

186 Lee, K.-B., Park, S.-J., Mirkin, C.A., Smith, J.C., and Mrksich, M. (2002) *Science*, **295**, 1702–1705.

187 Agarwal, G., Naik, R.R., and Stone, M.O. (2003) *J. Am. Chem. Soc.*, **125**, 7408–7412.

188 Lee, K.-B., Lim, J.-H., and Mirkin, C.A. (2003) *J. Am. Chem. Soc.*, **125**, 5588–5589.

189 Valiokas, R., Vaitekonis, S., Klenkar, G., Trinkunas, G., and Liedberg, B. (2006) *Langmuir*, **22**, 3456–3460.

190 Lee, M., Kang, D.-K., Yang, H.-K., Park, K.-H., Choe, S.Y., Kang, C., Chang, S.-I., Han, M.H., and Kang, I.-C. (2006) *Proteomics*, **6**, 1094–1103.

191 Kim, J.D., Ahn, D.-G., Oh, J.-W., Park, W., and Jung, H. (2008) *Adv. Mater.*, **20**, 3349–3353.

192 Lee, K.H., Kim, J.D., Kim, Y.J., Kang, S.H., Yung, S.Y., and Jung, H. (2008) *Small*, **4**, 1089–1094.

193 Jinag, H. and Stupp, S.I. (2005) *Langmuir*, **21**, 5242–5246.

194 Hong, S., Zhu, J., and Mirkin, C.A. (1999) *Langmuir*, **15**, 7897–7900.

195 Rosi, N.L. and Mirkin, C.A. (2005) *Chem. Rev.*, **105**, 1547–1562.

196 Zhang, Y., Salaita, K., Lim, J.-H., Lee, K.-B., and Mirkin, C.A. (2004) *Langmuir*, **20**, 962–968.

197 Mirkin, C.A. (2007) *ACS Nano*, **1**, 79–83.

198 Hong, S. and Mirkin, C.A. (2000) *Science*, **288**, 1808–1811.

199 Salaita, K., Lee, S.W., Wang, X., Huang, L., Dellinger, T.M., Liu, C., and Mirkin, C.A. (2005) *Small*, **1**, 940–945.

200 Salaita, K., Wang, X., Fragala, J., Vega, R.A., Liu, C., and Mirkin, C.A. (2006) *Angew. Chem., Int. Ed.*, **45**, 7220–7223.

201 Wang, X., Bullen, D.A., Zou, J., Liu, C., and Mirkin, C.A. (2004) *J. Vac. Sci. Technol. B*, **22**, 2563–2567.

202 Bullen, D., Wang, X., Zou, J., Chung, S.-W., Mirkin, C.A., and Liu, C. (2004) *J. Microelectromech. Syst.*, **13**, 594–601.

203 Bullen, D. and Liu, C. (2006) *Sens. Actuators A*, **125**, 504–511.

204 Lim, J.-H., Ginger, D.S., Lee, K.-B., Heo, J., Nam, J.-M., and Mirkin, C.A. (2003) *Angew. Chem., Int. Ed.*, **42**, 2309–2321.

205 Lee, S.-W., Oh, B.-K., Sanedrin, R.G., Salaita, K., Fujigaya, T., and Mirkin, C.A. (2006) *Adv. Mater.*, **18**, 1133–1136.

206 Li, B., Zhang, Y., Hu, J., and Li, M. (2005) *Ultramicroscopy*, **105**, 312–315.

207 Zhang, H., Li, Z., and Mirkin, C.A. (2002) *Adv. Mater.*, **14**, 1472–1474.

208 Li, S., Szegedi, S., Goluch, E., and Liu, C. (2008) *Anal. Chem.*, **80**, 5899–5904.

209 Hyun, J., Kim, J., Craig, S.L., and Chilkoti, A. (2004) *J. Am. Chem. Soc.*, **126**, 4770–4771.

210 Lim, J.-H. and Mirkin, C.A. (2002) *Adv. Mater.*, **14**, 1474–1476.

211 Maynor, B.W., Filocamo, S.F., Grinstaff, M.W., and Liu, J. (2002) *J. Am. Chem. Soc.*, **124**, 522–523.

212 Liu, X., Guo, S., and Mirkin, C.A. (2003) *Angew. Chem., Int. Ed.*, **42**, 4785–4789.

213 Maedler, C., Chada, S., Cui, X., Taylor, M., Yan, M., and LaRosa, A. (2008) *J. Appl. Phys.*, **104**, 14311/1–14311/4.

214 Su, M. and Dravid, V.P. (2002) *Appl. Phys. Lett.*, **80**, 4434–4436.

215 Noy, A., Miller, A.E., Klare, J.E., Weeks, B.L., Woods, B.W., and DeYoreo, J.J. (2002) *Nano Lett.*, **2**, 109–112.

216 Pena, D.J., Raphael, M.P., and Byers, J.M. (2003) *Langmuir*, **19**, 9028–9032.

217 Mulder, A., Onclin, S., Péter, M., Hoogenboom, J.P., Beijleveld, H.,

ter Maat, J., Garciá-Parajó, M.F., Ravoo, B.J., Huskens, J., van Hulst, N.F., and Reinhoudt, D.N. (2005) *Small*, **1**, 242–253.

218 Yu, M., Nyamjav, D., and Ivanisevic, A. (2005) *J. Mater. Chem.*, **15**, 649–652.

219 Lee, S.W., Sanedrin, R.G., Oh, B.-K., and Mirkin, C.A. (2005) *Adv. Mater.*, **17**, 2749–2753.

220 Zhang, H., Chung, S.-W., and Mirkin, C.A. (2003) *Nano Lett.*, **3**, 43–45.

221 Sheu, J.-T., Wu, C.-H., and Chao, T.-S. (2006) *Jpn. J. Appl. Phys.*, **45**, 3693–3698.

222 Maynor, B.W., Li, Y., and Liu, J. (2001) *Langmuir*, **17**, 2575–2578.

223 Li, Y., Maynor, B.W., and Liu, J. (2001) *J. Am. Chem. Soc.*, **123**, 2105–2106.

224 Liu, X., Fu, L., Hong, S., Dravid, V.P., and Mirkin, C.A. (2002) *Adv. Mater.*, **14**, 231–234.

225 Fu, L., Liu, X., Zhang, Y., Dravid, V.P., and Mirkin, C.A. (2003) *Nano Lett.*, **3**, 757–760.

226 Gundiah, G., John, N.S., Thomas, P.J., Kulkarni, G.U., Rao, C.N.R., and Heu, S. (2004) *Appl. Phys. Lett.*, **84**, 5341–5343.

227 Roy, D., Muny, M., Colombi, P., Bhattacharyya, S., Salvetat, J.-P., Cumpson, P.J., and Saboungi, M.-L. (2007) *Appl. Surf. Sci.*, **254**, 1394–1398.

228 Ding, L., Li, Y., Chu, H., Li, X., and Liu, J. (2005) *J. Phys. Chem. B*, **109**, 22337–22340.

229 Su, M., Liu, X., Li, S.-Y., Dravid, V.P., and Mirkin, C.A. (2002) *J. Am. Chem. Soc.*, **124**, 1560–1561.

230 Dimers, L.M. and Mirkin, C.A. (2001) *Angew. Chem., Int. Ed.*, **40**, 3069–3071.

231 Maynor, B.W., Li, J., Lu, C., and Mirkin, C.A. (2004) *J. Am. Chem. Soc.*, **126**, 6409–6413.

232 Basnar, B., Weizmann, Y., Cheglakov, Z., and Willner, I. (2006) *Adv. Mater.*, **18**, 713–718.

233 Zou, S., Maspoch, D., Wang, Y., Mirkin, C.A., and Schatz, G.C. (2007) *Nano Lett.*, **7**, 276–280.

234 Porter, L.A. Jr, Choi, H.C., Schmeltzer, J.M., Ribbe, A.E., Elliott, L.C.C., and Buriak, J.M. (2002) *Nano Lett.*, **2**, 1369–1372.

235 Degenhart, G.H., Dordi, B., Schönherr, H., and Vansco, G.J. (2004) *Langmuir*, **20**, 6216–6224.

236 Chi, Y.S. and Choi, I.S. (2006) *Adv. Funct. Mater.*, **16**, 1031–1036.

237 Long, D.A., Unal, K., Pratt, R.C., Malkoch, M., and Frommer, J. (2007) *Adv. Mater.*, **19**, 4471–4473.

238 Liu, G.-Y. and Salmeron, M.B. (1994) *Langmuir*, **10**, 367–370.

239 Xiao, X.D., Liu, G.-Y., Charych, D.H., and Salmeron, M.B. (1995) *Langmuir*, **11**, 1600–1604.

240 Liu, G.-Y. and Xu, S. (1999) *ACS Symp. Ser.*, **272**, 199–208.

241 Chwang, A.B., Granstrom, E.L., and Frisbie, C.D. (2000) *Adv. Mater.*, **12**, 285–288.

242 Garno, J.C., Yang, Y., Amro, N.A., Cruchon-Dupeyrat, S., Chen, S., and Liu, G.-Y. (2003) *Nano Lett.*, **3**, 389–395.

243 Zhou, D., Bruckbauer, A., Ying, L., Abell, C., and Klenerman, D. (2003) *Nano Lett.*, **3**, 1517–1520.

244 Kaholek, M., Lee, W.-K., LaMattina, B., Caster, K.C., and Zauscher, S. (2004) *Nano Lett.*, **4**, 373–376.

245 Kaholek, M., Lee, W.-K., Ahn, S.-J., Ma, H., Caster, K.C., Zauscher, B., and LaMattina, S. (2004) *Chem. Mater.*, **16**, 3688–3696.

246 Headerick, J.E., Armstrong, M., Cratty, J., Hammond, S., Sheriff, B.A., and Berrie, C.L. (2005) *Langmuir*, **21**, 4117–4122.

247 Seo, K. and Borguet, E. (2006) *Langmuir*, **22**, 1388–1391.

248 Shi, J. and Cremer, P.S. (2008) *J. Am. Chem. Soc.*, **130**, 2718–2719.

249 Liu, M., Amro, N.A., and Liu, G.-Y. (2008) *Annu. Rev. Phys. Chem.*, **59**, 367–386.

250 Xu, S. and Liu, G.Y. (1997) *Langmuir*, **13**, 127–129.

251 Xu, S., Laibinis, P.E., and Liu, G.Y. (1998) *Langmuir*, **14**, 9356–9361.

252 Xu, S., Miller, S., Laibinis, P.E., and Liu, G.Y. (1999) *Langmuir*, **15**, 7244–7251.

253 Wadu-Mesthridge, K., Xu, S., Amro, N.A., and Liu, G.-Y. (1999) *Langmuir*, **15**, 8580–8583.

254 Xu, S., Amro, N.A., and Liu, G.-Y. (2001) *Appl. Surf. Sci.*, **175–176**, 649–655.

255 Liu, J.-F., Cruchon-Dupeyrat, S., Garno, J.C., Frommer, J., and Liu, G.-Y. (2002) *Nano Lett.*, **2**, 937–940.

256 Liu, M., Amro, N.A., Chow, C.S., and Liu, G.-Y. (2002) *Nano Lett.*, **2**, 863–867.

257 Liu, G.Y. and Amro, N.A. (2002) *Proc. Natl Acad. Sci. USA*, **99**, 5165–5170.

258 Liu, G.-Y. (2005) *Langmuir*, **21**, 1972–1978.

259 Yu, J.J., Tan, Y.H., Li, X., Kuo, P.-K., and Liu, G.-Y. (2006) *J. Am. Chem. Soc.*, **128**, 11574–11581.

260 Case, M.A., McLendon, G.L., Hu, Y., Vanderlick, T.K., and Scoles, G. (2003) *Nano Lett.*, **3**, 425–429.

261 Hu, Y., Das, A., Hecht, M.H., and Scoles, G. (2005) *Langmuir*, **21**, 9103–9109.

262 Staii, C., Wood, D.W., and Scoles, G. (2008) *J. Am. Chem. Soc.*, **130**, 640–646.

263 Staii, C., Wood, D.W., and Scoles, G. (2008) *Nano Lett.*, **8**, 2503–2509.

264 Kenseth, J.R., Harnisch, J.A., Jones, V.W., and Porter, M.D. (2001) *Langmuir*, **17**, 4105–4112.

265 Jang, C.-H., Stevens, B.D., Carlier, P.R., Calter, M.A., and Ducker, W.A. (2002) *J. Am. Chem. Soc.*, **124**, 12114–12115.

266 Nuraje, N., Banerjee, I.A., MacCuspie, R.I., Yu, L., and Matsui, H. (2004) *J. Am. Chem. Soc.*, **126**, 8088–8089.

267 Wadu-Mesthrige, K., Amro, N.A., Garno, J.C., Xu, S., and Liu, G.-Y. (2001) *Biophys. J.*, **80**, 1891–1899.

268 Yu, J.-J., Nolting, B., Tan, Y.H., Li, X., Gervay-Hague, J., and Liu, G.-Y. (2006) *Nanobiotechnology*, **1**, 201–210.

269 Zhou, D., Wang, X.K., Birch, L., Rayment, T., and Abell, C. (2003) *Langmuir*, **19**, 10557–10562.

270 Chung, S.-W., Presley, A.D., Elhadj, S.K., Hok, S., Hah, S.S., Chernow, A.A., Francis, M.B., Eaton, B.E., Feldheim, D.L., and DeYoreo, J.J. (2008) *Scanning*, **30**, 159–171.

271 Wang, X., Zhou, D., Rayment, T., and Abell, C. (2003) *Chem. Commun.*, 474–475.

272 Amro, N.A., Xu, S., and Liu, G.-Y. (2000) *Langmuir*, **16**, 3006–3009.

273 Ngunjiri, J.N., Kelley, A.T., LeJeune, Z.M., Lewandowski, J.R.K., Li, B.R., Serem, W.K., Daniels, S.L., Lusker, K.L., and Garno, J.C. (2008) *Scanning*, **30**, 123–136.

274 Lee, M.V., Hoffman, M.T., Barnett, K., Geiss, J.M., and Smentkowski, V.S. (2006) *J. Nanosci. Nanotechnol.*, **6**, 1639–1643.

275 Lee, M.V., Nelson, K.A., Hutchins, L., Becerril, H.A., Cosby, S.T., Blood, J.C., Wheeler, D.R., Davis, R.C., Woolley, A.T., Harb, J.N., and Linford, M.R. (2007) *Chem. Mater.*, **19**, 5052–5054.

276 Sugimura, H., Okiguchi, K., and Nakagiri, N. (1996) *Jpn. J. Appl. Phys.*, **35**, 3749–3753.

277 Sugimura, H., Okiguchi, K., Nakagiri, N., and Mayashita, M. (1996) *J. Vac. Sci. Technol. B*, **14**, 4140–4143.

278 Kim, J., Oh, Y., Le, H., Shin, Y., and Park, S. (1998) *Jpn. J. Appl. Phys.*, **37**, 7148–7150.

279 Lee, H., Jan, Y.K., Bae, E.J., Lee, W., Kim, S.M., and Lee, S.H. (2002) *Curr. Appl. Phys.*, **2**, 85–90.

280 Sugimura, H., Takai, O., and Nakagiri, N. (1999) *J. Electroanal. Chem.*, **473**, 230–234.

281 Ara, M., Graaf, H., and Tada, H. (2002) *Appl. Phys. Lett.*, **80**, 2565–2567.

282 Graaf, H., Baumgärtel, T., Vieluf, M., and von Borczyskowski, C. (2008) *Superlattices Microstruct.*, **44**, 402–410.

283 Ara, M., Graaf, H., and Tada, H. (2002) *Jpn. J. Appl. Phys.*, **41**, 4894–4897.

284 Xie, X.N., Chung, H.J., Sow, C.H., and Wee, A.T.S. (2004) *Chem. Phys. Lett.*, **388**, 446–451.

285 Li, Q., Zheng, J., and Liu, Z. (2003) *Langmuir*, **19**, 166–171.

286 Zheng, J., Chen, Z., and Liu, Z. (2000) *Langmuir*, **16**, 9673–9676.

287 Tully, D.C., Wilder, K., Trimble, J.M., Fréchet, A.P., and Quate, C.F. (1999) *Adv. Mater.*, **11**, 314–318.

288 Rolandi, M., Suez, I., Dai, H., and Fréchet, J.M. (2004) *Nano Lett.*, **4**, 889–893.

289 Yoshinobu, T., Suzuki, J., Kurooka, H., Moon, W.C., and Iwasaki, H. (2003) *Electrochim. Acta*, **48**, 3131–3135.

290 He, M., Ling, X., Zhang, J., and Liu, Z. (2005) *J. Phys. Chem. B*, **109**, 10946–10951.

291 Martinez, R.V., Garcia, F., Garcia, R., Coronado, E., Forment-Aliaga, A., Romero, F.M., and Tatay, S. (2007) *Adv. Mater.*, **19**, 291–295.

292 Sugimura, H., and Nakagiri, N. (1997) *J. Am. Chem. Soc.*, **119**, 9226–9229.

293 Sugimura, H., Hanji, T., Hayashi, K., and Takai, O. (2002) *Adv. Mater.*, **14**, 524–526.

294 Graaf, H., Vieluf, M., and von Borczyskowski, C. (2007) *Nanotechnology*, **18**, 265306/1–265306/5.

295 Kim, Y., Kang, I., Choi, S.K., Choi, K., and Yi, J. (2005) *Microelectron. Eng.*, **81**, 341–348.

296 Shin, M., Kim, T., Kwon, C., Kim, S.K., Park, J.B., and Lee, H. (2006) *Jpn. J. Appl. Phys.*, **45**, 2076–2081.

297 Shin, M., Kwon, C., Kim, S.K., Kim, H.J., Roh, Y., Hong, B., Park, J.B., and Lee, H. (2006) *Nano Lett.*, **6**, 1334–1338.

298 Lee, W.-K., Caster, K.C., Kim, J., and Zauscher, S. (2006) *Small*, **2**, 848–853.

299 Kim, S.M., Ahn, S.J., Lee, H., Kim, E.R., and Lee, H. (2002) *Ultramicroscopy*, **91**, 165–169.

300 Kim, S.M. and Lee, H. (2003) *J. Vac. Sci. Technol. B*, **21**, 2398–2403.

301 Lee, H., Bae, E., and Lee, W. (2001) *Thin Solid Films*, **393**, 237–242.

302 Lee, W.B., Oh, Y., Kim, E.R., and Lee, H. (2001) *Synth. Met.*, **117**, 305–306.

303 Lee, W., Kim, E.R., and Lee, H. (2002) *Langmuir*, **18**, 8375–8380.

304 Lee, W., Lee, H., and Chun, M.S. (2005) *Langmuir*, **21**, 8839–8843.

305 Jang, J.-W., Sanedrin, R.G., Maspoch, D., Hwang, S., Fujigaya, T., Jeon, Y.-M., Vega, R.A., Chen, X., and Mirkin, C.A. (2008) *Nano Lett.*, **8**, 1451–1455.

306 Bourgoin, J.P., Sudiwala, R.V., and Palacin, S. (1996) *J. Vac. Sci. Technol. B*, **14**, 3381–3385.

307 Lee, H., Kim, S.A., Ahn, J., and Lee, H. (2002) *Appl. Phys. Lett.*, **81**, 138–140.

308 Ahn, S.J., Jang, Y.K., Kim, S.A., Lee, H., and Lee, H. (2002) *Ultramicroscopy*, **91**, 171–176.

309 Yam, C.M., Gu, J., Li, S., and Cai, C. (2005) *J. Colloid Interface. Sci.*, **285**, 711–718.

310 Choi, I., Kang, S.K., Lee, J., Kim, Y., and Yi, J. (2006) *Biomaterials*, **27**, 4655–4660.

311 Maoz, R., Cohen, S.R., and Sagiv, J. (1999) *Adv. Mater.*, **11**, 55–61.

312 Maoz, R., Frydman, E., Cohen, S.R., and Sagiv, J. (2000) *Adv. Mater.*, **12**, 725–731.

313 Pignataro, B., Panebianco, S., Consalvo, C., and Licciardello, A. (1999) *Surf. Interface Anal.*, **27**, 396–400.

314 Pignataro, B., Licciardello, A., Cataldo, S., and Marletta, G. (2003) *Mater. Sci. Eng. C*, **23**, 7–12.

315 Andruzzi, L., Nickel, B., Schwake, G., Rädler, J.O., Sohn, K.E., Mates, T.E., and Kramer, E.J. (2007) *Surf. Sci.*, **601**, 4984–4992.

316 Wouters, D., Willems, R., Hoeppener, S., Flipse, C.F.J., and Schubert, U.S. (2005) *Adv. Funct. Mater.*, **15**, 938–944.

317 Wouters, D., Hoeppener, S., and Schubert, U.S. (2009) *Angew. Chem., Int. Ed.*, **48**, 1732–1739.

318 Hoeppener, S., van Schaik, J.H.K., and Schubert, U.S. (2006) *Adv. Funct. Mater.*, **16**, 76–82.

319 Cai, Y. and Ocko, B.M. (2005) *J. Am. Chem. Soc.*, **127**, 16287–16291.

320 Hoeppener, S., Maoz, R., and Sagiv, J. (2003) *Nano Lett.*, **3**, 761–767.

321 Hoeppener, S., Maoz, R., and Sagiv, J. (2006) *Adv. Mater.*, **18**, 1286–1290.

322 Haensch, C., Hoeppener, S., and Schubert, U.S. (2009) *Nanotechnology*, **20**, 135302 (6pp).

323 Druzhinina, T., Weltjens, W., Hoeppener, S., and Schubert, U.S. (2009) *Adv. Funct. Mater.*, **19**, 1287–1292.

324 Hoeppener, S. and Schubert, U.S. (2005) *Small*, **1**, 628–632.

325 Wouters, D. and Schubert, U.S. (2003) *Langmuir*, **19**, 9033–9038.

326 Becer, C.R., Haensch, C., Hoeppener, S., and Schubert, U.S. (2007) *Small*, **3**, 220–225.

327 Liu, S., Maoz, R., Schmid, G., and Sagiv, J. (2002) *Nano Lett.*, **2**, 1055–1060.

328 Liu, S., Maoz, R., and Sagiv, J. (2004) *Nano Lett.*, **4**, 845–851.

329 Kolb, H.C., Finn, M.G., and Sharpless, K.B. (2001) *Angew. Chem., Int. Ed.*, **40**, 2004–2021.

330 Huisgen, R. (1984) in *1,3-Dipolar Cycloaddition Chemistry*, vol. 1 (ed. A. Padwa,), John Wiley & Sons, pp. 1–176.

331 Wang, X.-Y., Kimyonok, A., and Weck, M. (2006) *Chem. Commun.*, 3933–3935.

332 Flemming, D.A., Thode, C.F., and Williams, M.E. (2006) *Chem. Mater.*, **18**, 2327–2334.

333 Li, H., Cheng, F., Duft, A.M., and Adronov, A. (2005) *J. Am. Chem. Soc.*, **127**, 14518–14524.

334 Fernandez-Megia, E., Correa, J., and Riguera, R. (2006) *Biomacromolecules*, **7**, 3104–3111.

335 Moses, J.E. and Moorhouse, A.D. (2007) *Chem. Soc. Rev.*, **36**, 1249–1262.

336 Basner, B., Xu, J., Li, D., and Willner, I. (2007) *Langmuir*, **23**, 2293–2296.

337 Hoeppener, S., Susha, A.S., Rogach, A.L., Feldmann, J., and Schubert, U.S. (2006) *Curr. Nanosci.*, **2**, 135–141.

338 Wouters, D., and Schubert, U.S. (2005) *J. Mater. Chem.*, **15**, 2353–2355.

339 Hoeppener, S., Maoz, R., Cohen, S.R., Chi, L., Fuchs, H., and Sagiv, J. (2002) *Adv. Mater.*, **14**, 1036–1041.

340 Doron, A., Katz, E., and Willner, I. (1995) *Langmuir*, **11**, 1313–1317.

341 Zhu, T., Fu, X., Mu, T., Wang, J., and Liu, Z. (1999) *Langmuir*, **15**, 5197–5199.

342 Sato, T., Brown, D., and Johnon, B.F.G. (1997) *Chem. Commun.*, 1007–1008.

343 Yonezawa, T., Onoune, S.-Y., and Kunitake, T. (1998) *Adv. Mater.*, **10**, 414–416.

344 Liu, S., Zhu, T., Hu, R., and Liu, Z. (2002) *Phys. Chem. Chem. Phys.*, **4**, 6059–6062.

345 Maoz, R., Frydman, E., Cohen, S.R., and Sagiv, J. (2000) *Adv. Mater.*, **12**, 424–429.

346 Hoeppener, S., van Schaik, J.H.K., Wei, G., and Schubert, U.S. (2005) 13th International Conference on STM, 3–8 July, Sapporo, Japan, p. 234.

347 Chowdhury, D., Maoz, R., and Sagiv, J. (2007) *Nano Lett.*, **7**, 1770–1778.

348 Cheeco, A., Cai, Y., Gang, O., and Ocko, B.M. (2006) *Ultramicroscopy*, **106**, 703–708.

349 Cheeco, A., Gang, O., and Ocko, B.M. (2006) *Phys. Rev. Soc.*, **96**, 56104/1–56104/4.

350 Cai, Y. (2008) *Langmuir*, **24**, 337–343.

351 Woodsen, M. and Liu, J. (2007) *Phys. Chem. Chem. Phys.*, **9**, 207–225.

352 Blacklede, C., Engebretson, D.A., and McDonald, J.D. (2000) *Langmuir*, **16**, 8317–8323.

353 Müller, W.T., Klein, D.L., Lee, T., Clarke, J., McEuen, P.L., and Schultz, P.G. (1995) *Science*, **268**, 272–273.

354 Davis, J.J., Coleman, K.S., Bagshaw, K.L., and Busuttil, C.B. (2005) *J. Am. Chem. Soc.*, **127**, 13082–13083.

355 Davis, J.J., Bagshaw, C.B., Busuttil, K.L., Hanyu, Y., and Coleman, K.S. (2006) *J. Am. Chem. Soc.*, **128**, 14135–14141.

356 Blasdel, L.K., Banerjee, S., and Wang, S.S. (2008) *Langmuir*, **18**, 5055–5057.

357 Péter, M., Li, X.-M., Huskens, J., and Reinhoudt, D.N. (2004) *J. Am. Chem. Soc.*, **126**, 11684–11690.

358 Zorbas, V., Kanungo, M., Bains, S.A., Mao, Y., Hemraj-Benny, T., Misewich, J.A., and Wong, S.S. (2005) *Chem. Commun.*, 4598–4600.

359 Matsubara, S., Yamamoto, H., Oshima, K., Mouri, E., and Matsuoka, H. (2002) *Chem. Lett.*, 886–887.

360 Wang, J., Kenseth, J.R., Jones, V.W., Green, J.-B.D., McDermott, M.T., and Porter, M.D. (1997) *J. Am. Chem. Soc.*, **119**, 12796–12799.

361 Long, D.A., Unal, K., Pratt, R.C., Malkoch, M., and Frommer, J. (2007) *Adv. Mater.*, **19**, 4471–4473.

362 Szoszkiewicz, R., Okada, T., Jones, S.C., Li, T.-D., King, W.P., Marder, S.R., and Rieda, E. (2007) *Nano Lett.*, **7**, 1064–1069.

363 Fresco, Z.M., Suez, L., Backer, S.A., and Fréchet, J.M. (2004) *J. Am. Chem. Soc.*, **126**, 8374–8375,

364 Fresco, Z.M., and Fréchet, J.M. (2005) *J. Am. Chem. Soc.*, **127**, 8302–8303.

365 Pavlovic, E., Quist, A.P., Gelius, U., Nyholm, L., and Oscarsson, S. (2003) *Langmuir*, **19**, 4217–4221.

366 Pavlovic, E., Oscarsson, S., and Quist, A.P. (2003) *Nano Lett.*, **3**, 779–781.

367 Sugimura, H., Lee, S.-H., Saito, N., and Takai, O. (2004) *J. Vac. Sci. Technol. B*, **22**, L44–L46.

368 Saito, N., Lee, S.-H., Takahiro, I., Hieda, J., Sugimura, H., and Takai, O. (2005) *J. Phys. Chem. B*, **109**, 11602–11605.

369 Yam, C.M. and Kakkar, A.K. (1995) *J. Chem. Soc., Chem. Commun.*, 907–909.

370 Petrucci, M.G.L. and Kakkar, A.K. (1998) *Organometallics*, **17**, 1798–1811.

371 Linford, M.R., Fenter, P., Eisenberger, P.M., and Chidsey, C.E.D. (1995) *J. Am. Chem. Soc.*, **117**, 3145–3155.

372 Ge, S., Kojio, K., Takahara, A., and Kajiyama, T. (1998) *J. Biomater. Sci., Polym. Ed.*, **9**, 131–150.

373 Hoffmann, C. and Tovar, G.E.M. (2006) *J. Colloid Interface Sci.*, **295**, 427–435.

374 Yap, F.L. and Zhang, Y. (2007) *Biomaterials*, **28**, 2328–2338.

375 de la Rica, R., Baldi, A., Mendoza, E., Paulo, A.S., Llobera, A., and Fernandez-Sanchez, C. (2008) *Small*, **4**, 1076–1079.

376 Khatri, O.P., Han, J., Ichii, T., Murase, K., and Sugimura, H. (2008) *J. Phys. Chem. C*, **112**, 16182–16185.

377 Changa, L.-W., Yeha, Y.-C., and Lueb, J.-T. (2008) *Sensors & Transducers Journal*, **91**, 91–99.

378 Pang, I., Kim, S., and Lee, J. (2007) *Surf. Coat. Technol.*, **201**, 9426–9431.

379 Feng, Y., Zhou, Z., Ye, X., and Xiong, J. (2003) *Sens. Actuators A*, **108**, 138–143.

380 Netzer, L., Iscovici, R., and Sagiv, J. (1983) *Thin Solid Films*, **99**, 235–241.

381 Maoz, R., and Sagiv, J. (1987) *Langmuir*, **3**, 1045–1051.

382 Wasserman, S.R., Tao, Y.-T., and Whitesides, G.M. (1989) *Langmuir*, **5**, 1074–1087.

383 Natarajan Balachander, N. and Sukenik, C.N. (1990) *Langmuir*, **6**, 1621–1627.

384 Lee, Y.W., Reed-Mundell, J., Zull, J.E., and Sukenik, C.N. (1993) *Langmuir*, **9**, 3009–3014.

385 Cook, M.J., Hersans, R., McMurdo, J., and Russell, D.A. (1996) *J. Mater. Chem.*, **6**, 149–154.

386 Appelhans, D., Ferse, D., Adle, H.-J.P., Plieth, W., Fikus, A., Grundke, K., Schmitt, F.-J., Bayer, T., and Adolphi, B. (2000) *Colloids Surf. A*, **161**, 203–212.

387 Wang, Y., Cai, J., Rauscher, H., Behm, R.J., and Goedel, W.A. (2005) *Chem. Eur. J.*, **11**, 3968–3978.

388 Petrucci, M.G.L. and Kakkar, A.K. (1999) *Chem. Mater.*, **11**, 269–276.

389 Zhang, M., Desai, T. and Ferrari, M. (1998) *Biomaterials*, **19**, 953–960.

390 Sharma, S., Johnson, R.W., and Desai, T.A. (2003) *Appl. Surf. Sci.*, **206**, 218–229.

391 Chi, Y.S., Lee, J.K., Choi, S.-G., and Lee, I.S. (2004) *Langmuir*, **20**, 3024–3027.

392 Fryxell, G.E., Rieke, P.C., Wood, L.L., Engelhard, M.H., Williford, R.E., Graff, G.L., Campbell, A.A., Wiacek, R.J., Lee, L., and Halverson, A. (1996) *Langmuir*, **12**, 5064–5075.

393 Shyue, J.-J. and De Guire, M.R. (2004) *Langmuir*, **20**, 8693–8698.

394 Haensch, C., Ott, C., Hoeppener, S., and Schubert, U.S. (2008) *Langmuir*, **24**, 10222–10227.

395 Haensch, C., Chiper, M., Ulbricht, U., Winter, A., Hoeppener, S., and Schubert, U.S. (2008) *Langmuir*, **24**, 12981–12985.

396 Herzer, N., Hoeppener, S., Schubert, U.S., Fuchs, H., and Fischer, U.C. (2008) *Adv. Mater.*, **20**, 346–351.

397 Hoeppener, S. and Schubert, U.S. (2009) Electro-oxidative lithography and self-assembly concepts for bottom-up nanofabrication, in *Applied Scanning Probe Methods XIII* (eds B. Bhushan and H. Fuchs), ch. 20, Springer, pp. 45–67.

398 Lummerstorfer, T. and Hoffmann, H. (2004) *J. Phys. Chem. B*, **108**, 3963–3966.

399 Rohde, R.D., Agnew, H.D., Yeo, W.-S., Bailey, R.C., and Heath, J.R. (2006) *J. Am. Chem. Soc.*, **128**, 9518–9525.

400 Ciampi, S., Boecking, T., Kilian, K.A., James, M., Harper, J.B., and Gooding, J.J. (2007) *Langmuir*, **23**, 9320–9329.

401 Ostaci, R.-V., Damiron, D., Capponi, S., Vignaud, G., Leger, L., Grohens, Y., and Drockenmuller, E. (2008) *Langmuir*, **24**, 2732–3739.

402 Haensch, C., Hoeppener, S., and Schubert, U.S. (2008) *Nanotechnology*, **19**, 35703/1–35703/7.

403 Gallant, N.D., Lavery, K.A., Amis, E.J., and Becker, M.L. (2007) *Adv. Mater.*, **19**, 965–969.

404 Rozkiewicz, D.I., Janczewski, D., Verboom, W., Ravoo, B.J., and Reinhoudt, D.N. (2006) *Angew. Chem., Int. Ed.*, **45**, 5292–5296.

405 Michel, O. and Ravoo, B.J. (2008) *Langmuir*, **24**, 12116–12118.

406 Ku, S.-Y., Wong, K.-T., and Bard, A.J. (2008) *J. Am. Chem. Soc.*, **103**, 2392–2393.

407 Maoz, R., Cohen, H., and Sagiv, J. (1998) *Langmuir*, **14**, 5988–5993.

408 Flink, S., van Veggel, F.C.J.M., and Reinhoudt, D.N. (2001) *J. Phys. Org. Chem.*, **14**, 407–415.

409 Zhang, G.-J., Tanii, T., Zako, T., Hosaka, T., Miyake, T., Kanari, Y., Funatsu, T., and Ohdomari, I. (2005) *Small*, **1**, 833–837.

410 Fabre, B. and Hauquier, F. (2006) *J. Phys. Chem. B*, **110**, 6848–6855.

411 Chen, M.-S., Dulcey, C.S., Chrisey, L.A., and Dressick, W.J. (2006) *Adv. Funct. Mater.*, **16**, 774–783.

412 Miyake, T., Tanii, T., Kato, K., Zako, T., Funatsu, T., and Ohdomari, I. (2007) *Nanotechnology*, **18**, 305304/1–305304/6.

413 Crivillers, N., Mas-Torrent, M., Perruchas, S., Roques, N., Vidal-Gancedo, J., Veciana, J., Rovira, C., Basabe-Desmonts, L., Ravoo, B.J., Crego-Calama, M., and Reinhoudt, D.N. (2007) *Angew. Chem., Int. Ed.*, **46**, 2215–2219.

414 Duan, X., Sadhu, V.B., Perl, A., Peter, M., Reinhoudt, D.N., and Huskens, J. (2008) *Langmuir*, **24**, 3621–3627.

415 La, Y.-H., Jung, Y.J., Kim, H.J., Kang, T.-H., Ihm, K., Kim, K.-J., Kim, B., and Park, J.W. (2003) *Langmuir*, **19**, 4390–4395.

416 Rozkiewicz, D.I., Ravoo, B.J., and Reinhoudt, D.N. (2005) *Langmuir*, **21**, 6337–6343.

417 Rozkiewicz, D.I., Kraan, Y., Werten, M.W.T., de Wolf, F.A., Subramaniam, V., Ravoo, B.J., and Reinhoudt, D.N. (2006) *Chem. Eur. J.*, **12**, 6290–6297.

418 Rogero, C., Chaffey, B.T., Mateo-Marti, E., Sobrado, J.M., Horrocks, B.R., Houlton, A., Lakey, J.H., Briones, C., and Martin-Gago, J.A. (2008) *J. Phys. Chem. C*, **112**, 9308–9314.

419 Maury, P., Peter, M., Crespo-Biel, O., Ling, X.Y., Reinhoudt, D.N., and Huskens, J. (2007) *Nanotechnology*, **18**, 44007/1–44007/9.

420 Maury, P., Escalante, M., Peter, M., Reinhoudt, D.N., Subramaniam, V., and Huskens, J. (2007) *Small*, **3**, 1584–1592.

421 Netzer, L. and Sagiv, J. (1983) *J. Am. Chem. Soc.*, **105**, 674–676.

422 Maoz, R. and Sagiv, J. (1985) *Thin Solid Films*, **132**, 135–151.

423 Miyake, T., Tanii, T., Kato, K., Hosaka, T., Kanari, Y., Sonobe, H., and Ohdomari, I. (2006) *Chem. Phys. Lett.*, **426**, 361–364.

424 Frydman, E. (1999) Organic self-assembling monolayers as templates for deposition of inorganic materials, Ph.D. thesis, Weizmann Institute, Rehovot, Israel.

425 Sekkat, Z., Wood, J., Geerts, Y., and Knoll, W. (1996) *Langmuir*, **12**, 2976–2980.

426 Hozumi, A., Taoda, H., Saitoa, T., and Shirahatab, N. (2008) *Surf. Interface Anal.*, **40**, 408–411.

427 Brandow, S.L., Chen, M.-S., Aggarwal, R., Dulcey, C.S., Calvert, J.M., and Dressick, W.J. (1999) *Langmuir*, **15**, 5429–5432.

428 Hong, L., Sugimura, H., Furukawa, T., and Takai, O. (2003) *Langmuir*, **19**, 1966–1969.

429 Hadziioannou, G., Patel, S., Granick, S., and Tirrell, M. (1986) *J. Am. Chem. Soc.*, **108**, 2869–2876.

430 Dan, N. and Tirrell, M. (1993) *Macromolecules*, **26**, 4310–4315.

431 Belder, G.F., ten Brinke, G., and Hadziioannou, G. (1997) *Langmuir*, **13**, 4102–4105.

432 Chang, Y.-C. and Frank, C.W. (1996) *Langmuir*, **12**, 5824–5829.

433 Husseman, M., Malmstrom, E.E., McNamara, M., Mate, M.,

Mecerreyes, D., Benoit, D.G., Hedrick, J.L., Mansky, P., Huang, E., Russell, T.P., and Hawker, C.J. (1999) *Macromolecules*, **32**, 1424–1431.

434 Piech, M., George, M.C., Bell, N.S., and Braun, P.V. (2006) *Langmuir*, **22**, 1379–1382.

435 Dong, R., Krishnan, S., Baird, B.A., Lindau, M., and Ober, C.K. (2007) *Biomacromolecules*, **8**, 3082–3092.

436 Wu, T., Gong, P., Szleifer, I., Vlcek, P., Subr, V., and Genzer, J. (2007) *Macromolecules*, **40**, 8756–8764.

437 Jonas, A.M., Hu, Z., Glinel, K., and Huck, W.T.S. (2008) *Macromolecules*, **41**, 6859–6863.

438 Chen, J.-K., Hsieh, C.-Y., Huang, C.-F., Li, P.-M., Kuo, S.-W., and Chang, F.-C. (2008) *Macromolecules*, **41**, 8729–8736.

439 Brinks, M.K., Hirtz, M., Chi, L., Fuchs, H., and Studer, A. (2007) *Angew. Chem., Int. Ed.*, **46**, 5231–5233.

440 Santer, S., Kopyshev, A., Yang, H.-K., and Ruehe, J. (2006) *Macromolecules*, **39**, 3056–3064.

441 Inaoka, S. and Collard, D.M. (1999) *Langmuir*, **15**, 3752–3758.

442 Heise, A., Menzel, H., Yim, H., Foster, M.D., Wieringa, R.H., Schouten, A.J., Erb, V., and Stamm, M. (1997) *Langmuir*, **13**, 723–728.

443 Choi, I.S. and Langer, R. (2001) *Macromolecules*, **34**, 5361–5363.

444 Yoon, K.R., Chi, Y.S., Lee, K.-B., Lee, J.K., Kim, D.J., Koh, Y.-J., Joo, S.-W., Yund, W.S., and Choi, I.S. (2003) *J. Mater. Chem.*, **13**, 2910–2914.

445 Jeon, N.L., Choi, I.S., Whitesides, G.M., Kim, N.Y., Laibinis, P.E., Harada, Y.Y., Finnie, K.R., Girolami, G.S., and Nuzzo, R.G. (1999) *Appl. Phys. Lett.*, **75**, 4201–4203.

446 Harris, R.F., Ricci, M.J., Farrer, R.S., Praino, J., Miller, S.J., Saleh, B.E.A., Teich, M.C., and Fourkas, J.T. (2005) *Adv. Mater.*, **17**, 39–41.

447 Oosterling, M.L.C.M., Sei, A., and Schouten, A.J. (1992) *Polymer*, **33**, 4394–4400.

448 Kim, I.-J. and Faust, R. (2003) *J. Macromol. Sci. A*, **40**, 991–1008.

449 Ingall, M.D.K., Honeyman, C.H., Mercure, J.V., Bianconi, P.A., and

Kunz, R.R. (1999) *J. Am. Chem. Soc.*, **121**, 3607–3613.

450 Park, J.-W. and Thomas, E.L. (2002) *J. Am. Chem. Soc.*, **124**, 514–515.

451 Denis, F.A., Pallandre, A., Nysten, B., Jonas, A.M., and Dupont-Gaillain, C.C. (2005) *Small*, **1**, 984–991.

452 Brough, B., Christman, K.L., Wong, T.S., Kolodziej, C.M., Forbes, J.G., Wang, K., Maynard, H.D., and Ho, C.-M. (2007) *Soft Matter*, **3**, 541–546.

453 Gaubert, H.E. and Frey, W. (2007) *Nanotechnology*, **18**, 135101/1–135101/7.

454 Dekeyser, C.M., Buron, C.C., Mc Evoy, K., Dupont-Gaillain, C.C., Marchand-Brynaert, J., Jonas, A.M., and Rouxhet, P.G. (2008) *J. Colloid Interface Sci.*, **324**, 118–126.

455 Cecchet, F., De Meersman, B., Demoustier-Champagne, S., Nysten, B., and Jonas, A.M. (2006) *Langmuir*, **22**, 1173–1181.

456 LeMieux, M.C., Julthongpiput, D., Bergman, K.N., Cuong, P.D., Ahn, H.-S., Lin, Y.-H., and Tsukruk, V.V. (2004) *Langmuir*, **20**, 10046–10054.

457 Qu, M., Zhang, Y., He, J., Cao, X., and Zhang, J. (2008) *Appl. Surf. Sci.*, **255**, 2608–2612.

458 Dutta, S., Perring, M., Barrett, S., Mitchell, M., Kenis, P.J.A., and Bowden, N.B. (2006) *Langmuir*, **22**, 2146–2155.

459 Ryan, D., Parviz, B.A., Linder, V., Semetey, V., Sia, S.K., Su, J., Mrksich, M., and Whitesides, G.M. (2004) *Langmuir*, **20**, 9080–9088.

460 del Campo, A., Boos, D., Spiess, H.W., and Jonas, U. (2005) *Angew. Chem., Int. Ed.*, **44**, 4707–4712.

461 Renault, J.P., Bernard, A., Juncker, D., Michel, B., Bosshard, H.R., and Delamarche, E. (2002) *Angew. Chem., Int. Ed.*, **41**, 2320–2323.

462 Geissler, M., McLellan, J.M., Chen, J., and Xia, Y. (2005) *Angew. Chem., Int. Ed.*, **44**, 3596–3600.

463 Zammatteo, N., Jeanmart, L., Hamels, S., Courtois, S., Louette, P., Hevesi, L., and Remacle, J. (2000) *Anal. Biochem.*, **280**, 143–150.

464 Beyer, M., Felgenhauer, T., Bischoff, F.R., Breitling, F., and Stadler, V. (2006) *Biomaterials*, **27**, 3505–3514.

3
Physical, Chemical, and Biological Surface Patterning by Microcontact Printing

Jan Mehlich and Bart Jan Ravoo

3.1
Introduction

The technique of printing, which was invented by humankind many thousands of years ago, has through the years undergone steady improvements, notably due to the progress of technology [1–3]. Printing usually involves three components: an ink; an appropriate surface; and a stamp or a press.

Contact printing is an efficient method for pattern transfer, in which a conformal contact between the stamp and the surface of the substrate is the key to success. Printing has the advantage of simplicity and convenience: once a stamp has been made available, multiple copies of the pattern can be produced by repeated inking and printing. Printing is an additive process and, in comparison to lithography, the wastage of material is minimized. Printing can be used to pattern large areas. Furthermore, although contact printing is most suitable for two-dimensional (2-D) patterning, it can also be used to generate three-dimensional (3-D) structures through its combination with other processes.

Microcontact printing (µCP) was developed during the early 1990s by Whitesides and coworkers [4]. Just like conventional printing, µCP also involves an ink, a substrate and a stamp; however, in contrast to the dyes that are normally used for printing, the inks for µCP are printed in monomolecular layers and, instead of paper, clothing, stone or wood, the surfaces for µCP are usually ultraflat metal, silicon, or glass substrates. But, perhaps the most remarkable difference is that, instead of macroscopic patterns, the stamps for µCP carry features in the micrometer range [5], or even at the nanoscale [6, 7]. As a result, within less than two decades µCP has emerged as a straightforward and cheap bench-top method for the preparation of both microstructured and nanostructured surfaces.

In this chapter, the potential of µCP is reviewed with regards to the chemical, physical and biological patterning of surfaces by µCP. First, a general introduction to the method of µCP will be provided, including a short discussion of the main advantages and limitations of the process in the preparation of microstructured and nanostructured surfaces. The broad range of inks that can be printed in monolayers

Nanotechnology, Volume 8: Nanostructured Surfaces. Edited by Lifeng Chi
Copyright © 2010 WILEY-VCH Verlag GmbH & Co. KGaA, Weinheim
ISBN: 978-3-527-31739-4

by μCP, subject to a suitable modification of stamp and substrate, will then be described. In addition, an outline will be provided of the way in which μCP can provide physical surface structures by "soft lithography," and how μCP can be used to prepare biological microarrays. Exactly how μCP can be used to induce and direct chemical reactions on a surface will also be discussed. Finally, the major innovations that have been proposed to improve the resolution of μCP will be detailed, followed by a brief outlook of the situation.

At this point, it should be emphasized how quickly μCP has found widespread application throughout the scientific community. In fact, according to the ISI Web of Knowledge, almost 1000 articles involving μCP – including two recent reviews [8, 9] – have been produced to date. However, rather than simply provide an exhaustive review, the decision was taken to highlight the most important developments and applications of μCP for the preparation of microstructured and nanostructured surfaces.

3.2
What is Microcontact Printing?

In its most simple version, μCP is a nonphotolithographic method that readily provides patterned self-assembled monolayers (SAMs) with submicron lateral resolution. It offers remarkable experimental simplicity, and can be performed in almost any laboratory, without a need for "clean room" conditions. Moreover, as μCP is a cheap and straightforward process, it has rapidly found widespread applications in different areas of research since its invention during the early 1990s [4].

3.2.1
The "Master"

The initial step in each μCP experiment is the design and production of a "master" that can be designed with the help of simple computer software. The desired pattern is first transferred from the master to a surface of choice. When a master pattern has been established by common photolithographic methods on a flat substrate, such as a silicon wafer, it can easily be replicated by making elastomeric stamps with the negative image of the master. To achieve this, a liquid polymer precursor is poured onto the master, allowed to polymerize, and then released from the master such that the pattern is transferred as a microrelief structure at the surface of the hardened polymer. This stamp is then "inked" with the molecules that are to be printed, either by wetting the surface of the stamp with a solution of the ink molecules, by immersing the stamp in a solution of the ink, or simply by placing the stamp on an ink pad. In this situation, small, low-molecular-weight inks will be absorbed into the polymer network of the stamp, whereas large, high-molecular-weight inks, as well as nanoparticles (NPs) and colloids, will be coated onto the surface of the stamp. When the inked stamp is placed on a substrate, in those protruding areas where the stamp is in conformal contact with the substrate, the ink will be transferred. However, in the receding areas of the stamp there will be no contact with the substrate, and no ink will be transferred. The substrate may be a metal or metal oxide, a silicon wafer or glass, a polymer film, or a SAM, while the ink should possess functional groups that allow its chemisorption onto the surface. In the seminal studies conducted by Whitesides and coworkers, the stamp was prepared from polydimethylsiloxane (PDMS), the ink was *n*-octadecylthiol (ODT), and the substrate was a silicon wafer coated with a thin film of gold [4]. The entire procedure is illustrated schematically in Figure 3.1.

3.2.2
The Stamp

The stamp, which is key to the success of μCP as it is used to generate the pattern, is usually prepared from silicone polymers, among which PDMS (available commercially as Sylgard 184) is the most commonly used. Sylgard 184 is not only transparent but also has a low viscosity before being cured; both features are highly favorable when producing stamps for use in soft lithography. PDMS is also easy to handle and inexpensive (the typical cost of a stamp is much less than €1). Notably, PDMS has a very low resistance to most nonpolar solvents, and although it will not dissolve in such solvents it will undergo substantial deformation as a result of its swelling. Fortunately, however, the stamp will regain its original shape when the solvent has evaporated. Consequently, ink solutions should preferably be prepared in polar solvents such as ethanol, methanol, or water.

Sylgard 184 is a two-component heat-curing system; that is, it consists of a base and a curing agent mixed in a ratio of 10 : 1. The elastomer base is a PDMS with terminal ethylene groups, while the curing agent consists of much shorter PDMS chains, with many of the methyl groups substituted by hydrogen atoms. In the presence of Pt (in Sylgard 184, Pt is added to the base component) the polymerization follows the reaction shown in Scheme 3.1.

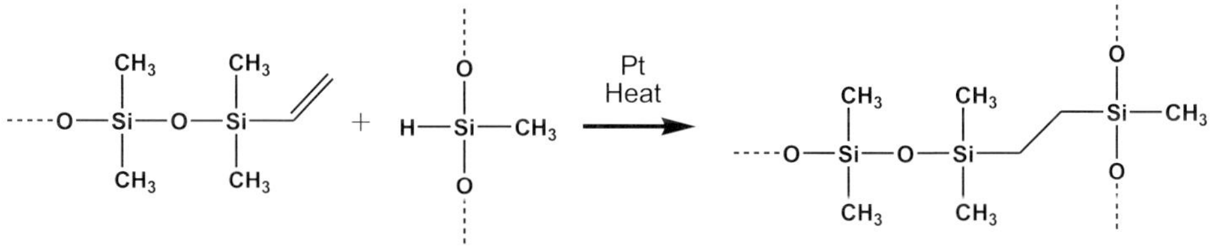

Scheme 3.1 Pt catalyzed cross linking of poly(dimethylsiloxane) (PDMS) with curing agent.

In the curing reaction of PDMS, the details of which have been elucidated [10], Pt(II) is initially coordinated by two terminal ethylene groups of the precursor polymer. In an oxidative addition – that is, when Pt(II) is oxidized to Pt(IV) – a hydrosiloxane unit of a curing agent molecule becomes coordinated to Pt. Then, after a migratory insertion of the hydrogen atom to one of the ethylene groups, the connection between the curing agent moiety and the PDMS polymer is made in a

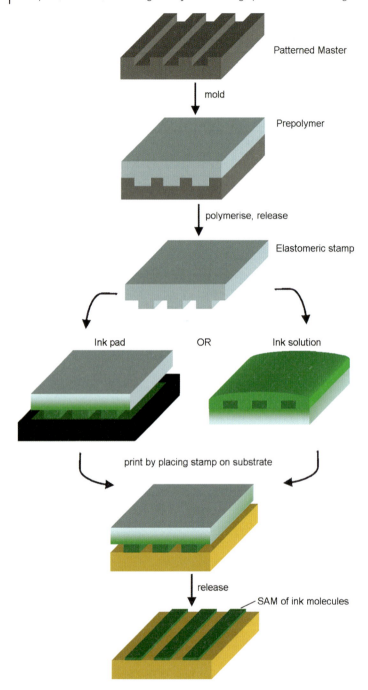

Figure 3.1 The principle of microcontact printing (μCP). The stages include: molding of a stamp; inking of a stamp; printing on a suitable substrate; and release of the stamp from the substrate. In the seminal studies of Whitesides and coworkers the stamp was produced from poly(dimethylsiloxane) (PDMS), the ink was *n*-octadecylthiol (ODT), and the substrate a silicon wafer coated with a thin film of gold [4].

reductive elimination – that is, Pt(IV) is reduced to Pt(II). Subsequently, another ethylene-terminated polymer can coordinate to Pt(II), and a further crosslink can be made such that the result is a more or less dense network of crosslinked polymer chains. Together, the curing time and temperature determine the extent of cross-linking, and hence the elasticity and the stiffness of the stamp. A significant shrinkage of the stamp must be taken into account when curing at high temperatures ($>100\,^{\circ}$C).

PDMS stamps are mainly characterized by the two opposing properties of stiffness and elasticity, which are expressed in the Young's modulus (which, for a PDMS stamp is typically about 1.5 MPa). On the one hand, a stamp should be mechanically stable or the pattern will be blurred upon contact with the substrate; this means that the stamp must be sufficiently stiff. On the other hand, as a conformal contact between the stamp and substrate is required, the elasticity of the stamp must be substantial. The stiffer the stamp, the greater will be the reduction in sagging and collapse of the stamp upon demolding. A stiffer stamp will also generally improve the accuracy of replication. Whilst the main disadvantage of a stiffer stamp is an increased brittleness, a greater elasticity will compensate for an uneven surface and ensure conformal contact also with uneven surfaces.

The principle of conformal contact is illustrated in Figure 3.2. Conformal contact comprises the macroscopic adaptation to the overall shape of the substrate, as well as the microscopic adaptation of a soft polymer layer to a rough surface, leading to an intimate contact without voids. The elastic adaption is caused by adhesion forces such that, even without the application of any external pressure, the stamp can sponta-neously compensate for some degree of substrate roughness, depending on the material's properties [11]. The elastomer (the light gray layer in Figure 3.2) com-pensates for local surface roughness amplitudes of up to 1 μm, whereas long-range warp (wavelengths >100 μm) is compensated by the flexibility of the backplane (the dark gray layer in Figure 3.2, which may be a metal, glass, or polymer). Conformal contact benefits from a low Young's modulus and a moderate (yet sufficient) work of adhesion.

The quality of the stamp also depends on the dimensions and depth of the pattern. The pattern dimensions can be characterized by the *aspect ratio* and the *fill ratio*. As illustrated in Figure 3.3, a microrelief stamp can be defined according to the width w of the protruding features, the height h of a protruding features, and the distance d between two protruding features (Figure 3.3a). The aspect ratio is the height h of features divided by their width, w, while the fill ratio is given by the width w of the features divided by their distance, d. Features of high aspect ratio ($h/w > 2$) exhibit

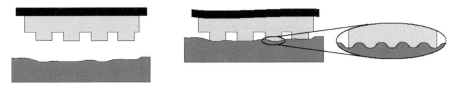

Figure 3.2 Conformal contact of an elastomer stamp (light gray) and a solid surface (dark gray).

(a)  (b) 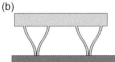 (c) (d)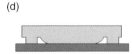

Figure 3.3 Effect of feature dimensions on the stability of an elastomer microrelief stamp. For details, see the text.

lateral instabilities (Figure 3.3b and c), where the structures collapse while peeling off the template or during the inking process due to capillary action (Figure 3.3b), or they collapse against the substrate such that a side of the feature comes into contact with the substrate (Figure 3.3c). On the other hand, voids in a stamp with a low fill ratio $(h/d < 0.2)$ are susceptible to sagging (Figure 3.3d) [11–13].

Typically, μCP is used for printing at the microscale – that is, with smallest features of about 0.5 μm. A number of factors determine the smallest features that can be printed, with the fundamental limits to printing being determined by three main constraints: (i) the minimum size of features in the stamp; (ii) the lateral dimensions and resolution of the ink; and (iii) the adhesion and spreading of the ink at the substrate surface. The smallest feature in the stamp depends on the size of features within the master, the fidelity of the molding process, and the ability of the elastomer mold to retain nanoscale features. Distortion of the stamp while in contact with the printed surface also limits the minimum size of the transferred feature. In the best case, composite stamps of PDMS can retain 100 nm features without collapse [14, 15]. Some strategies proposed to extend the resolution of μCP into the nanoscale are outlined in Section 3.7.

Inspired by the pioneering studies of Whitesides and colleagues, many research groups have since shown that the nature of the ink, the stamp, and the substrate can be widely modified, not only to improve the printing quality but also to exploit μCP for a broad range of applications. These achievements are described in detail in the following sections.

3.3
Inks and Stamps for Microcontact Printing

The role of μCP was first demonstrated for the preparation of patterned SAMs of *n*-alkylthiols on gold substrates [4, 16], and this remains today the most widely studied and best established use of the technique. Several points have been identified as being responsible for the success of this particular combination, namely:

- *n*-Alkylthiols are rapidly chemisorbed onto gold surfaces by the formation of a coordinative bond between gold and sulfur atoms.
- A dense and highly ordered monolayer of molecules is formed spontaneously, due to strong van der Waals interactions between the long alkyl chains.
- The self-limiting nature of the forming monolayer favors its confinement to the area of contact.

The basic process for forming patterned SAMs of *n*-alkylthiols on gold is conceptually simple. The stamp is first impregnated with a 1 mM solution of *n*-alkylthiol in ethanol, and then placed in contact with a clean gold surface; this causes the thiols to diffuse from the stamp onto the surface, where they assemble into an ordered monolayer. However, investigations into the details of this self-assembly phenomenon have suggested the process to be complex and to depend on a number of parameters, including the choice of the SAM-forming molecules, the concentration of molecules in the ink solution, the contact time, and the pressure applied to the stamp [17–19].

The mechanisms for the mass transport of thiols during μCP include (at least) the following:

- Diffusion from the bulk of the stamp to the interface between the stamp and the surface of the gold contacted by the stamp.
- Diffusion away from the edges of the stamp and across the surface of the gold substrate.
- Vapor transport through the gas phase (see Figure 3.1).

The first of these mechanisms is important for the formation of SAMs in regions where the stamp should be in contact with the surface; however, very little information is available regarding relevant parameters such as the rates of diffusion of *n*-alkylthiols (or other nonpolar molecules) in PDMS. The second and third mechanisms are important for understanding and controlling the lateral diffusion of SAMs into regions that are not contacted by the stamp. These are unwanted processes that lead to distortions of the lateral dimensions of the printed features and gradients of surface coverage at the edges of the printed structures. Whilst the relative contributions of each of these mechanisms in the formation of the SAMs in the area contacted by the stamp and in the noncontact area are not completely understood [19], much is known regarding the mechanisms of SAM formation, and the structure of *n*-alkylthiol SAMs on gold in particular. In general, these principles should be the same for μCP-mediated SAM formation in the contact areas between the stamp and the gold substrate. As with SAMs formed from solution, in μCP-controlled SAMs the monolayer not only contains perfect domains of slightly tilted aligned molecules but also invariably includes areas with less-ordered molecules, or even "collapsed" orientations with the molecules not standing upright but laying flat on the surface (Figure 3.4).

Patterned SAMs formed by μCP can be easily visualized using a range of techniques that include scanning electron microscopy (SEM), scanning probe microscopy (SPM), secondary ion mass spectrometry (SIMS), condensation figures observed in optical microscopy, and surface-enhanced Raman microscopy. In Figure 3.5 are shown the lateral force microscopy (LFM) images of patterned SAMs of *n*-hexadecanethiol (HDT) on gold [20]. In this case, the surface was patterned with HDT, after which the remaining regions were covered with 16-mercaptohexadecanoic acid (MUA) by immersing the patterned sample in an ethanolic solution of MUA. Relatively high frictional forces between the probe and the surface were detected in regions covered with a COOH-terminated SAM (light areas), while

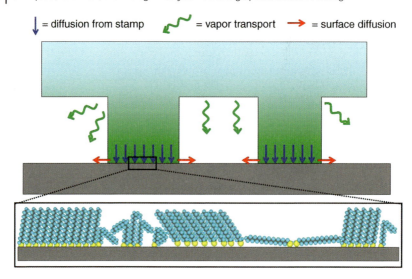

Figure 3.4 Ink transport in microcontact printing of *n*-alkylthiols and structure of *n*-alkylthiol SAMs on gold substrates.

relatively low frictional forces were measured in regions covered with a CH$_3$-terminated SAM (dark areas).

µCP is not limited to printing thiols on gold, however. Indeed, it has been shown that, subject to a suitable modification of stamp and substrate, other small molecules may also be printed. The µCP-mediated formation of patterned monolayers of *n*-alkylsilanes such as *n*-octadecyltrichlorosilane (OTS) adsorbed onto oxide surfaces such as glass, Al$_2$O$_3$, SiO$_2$, and ITO has been investigated in detail [21]. It has been found that the OTS chains can pack with densities approaching those found in bulk hydrocarbon crystals, but that even the highest-quality printed monolayers of *n*-alkylsilanes lack the long-range ordering found for *n*-alkylthiol SAMs on Au and Ag. It is generally believed that the adsorption of *n*-alkyltrichlorosilanes and other *n*-alkylsilanes with hydrolyzable bonds proceeds on hydrated surfaces via the formation of silanols as intermediates, which then react in turn laterally or with surface OH groups to form a network polymer which is covalently bound (to some degree) to the surface [22]. The resultant films have significant mechanical, thermal, and chemical stability, with infrared (IR) spectroscopy, ellipsometry, and contact angle measurements indicating a high degree of structural organization in such films. The largely all-*trans* alkyl chains are usually found to be tilted at ∼10° from the surface normal direction [23].

A PDMS stamp is quite hydrophobic and suitable for apolar ink molecules such as long-chain *n*-alkylthiols and *n*-alkylsilanes. However, polar and hydrophilic inks cannot be printed efficiently with PDMS stamps, and special surface treatments that enable the printing of such inks that otherwise would not adhere to PDMS due to its hydrophobic surface are required. When the PDMS surface is exposed to oxygen plasma or ozone, the surface becomes hydrophilic due to the formation of a thin and

COOH   CH₃

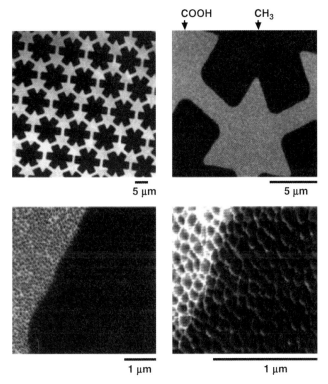

Figure 3.5 Lateral force microscopy at four different magnifications of a gold surface patterned with SAMs terminated in different head groups. Reproduced with permission from Ref. [20]; © 1995, American Chemical Society.

brittle silica-like layer that causes changes in the mechanical properties of PDMS. Owen and Smith [24] studied the formation of cracks in this silica-like layer, and showed that the cracks may allow the migration of low-molecular-weight PDMS fragments to the surface, leading to a recovery of the hydrophobic character of the PDMS surface. Hydrophobic recovery always occurs with time after exposure to oxygen plasma or ozone [25]. The chemical attachment of hydrophilic chlorosilanes and/or grafting of hydrophilic polymers on the oxidized PDMS surface to tune the surface energy of the PDMS stamp have been reported [26–28].

In view of the range of possible applications, there is today great interest in the patterning of bio(macro)molecules on surfaces. In particular, the mild conditions of µCP make it an attractive method for the patterning of biomolecules. For example, µCP can be used to transfer proteins onto a variety of substrate materials with-hydrophilic or hydrophobic surfaces, including bare and silanized glass, gold, silicon and silicon oxide, poly(styrene), poly(methylmethacrylate) (PMMA), and various monolayers on gold [29, 30]. One important advantage of µCP is that most proteins retain their biological activity after printing. When printing proteins on substrates, three types of immobilization can be distinguished, namely physisorption, chemisorptions, and attachment to protein-resistant surfaces. Similar to printing proteins, the μCP of DNA calls for carefully tailored surface properties of the PDMS stamps, since DNA is a highly negatively charged polyelectrolyte due to its phosphate backbone and electrostatic interactions may determine its adsorption and transfer properties [31]. Since μCP has today become a valuable tool in the preparation of biological microarrays, Section 3.5 of this chapter is focused on the μCP of biomolecules.

Supramolecular μCP

Supramolecular μCP is a variation of μCP where the interaction between ink and substrate is tuned by supramolecular (noncovalent) interactions. In a series of publications, Reinhoudt and Huskens and colleagues have shown that gold, glass and silicon surfaces functionalized with β-cyclodextrin host molecules form a suitable platform ("molecular printboard") to print guest molecules [32, 33]. The interaction between ink and substrate in supramolecular μCP is highly specific, and can be tuned via the multivalency of the ink – that is, the number of interactions with the substrate. Among others, these research groups have printed redox active dendrimers [34] and proteins [35] on such molecular printboards.

The terms "bottom-up" and "top-down" refer to two strategies in nanotechnology that are also evident in μCP with macromolecules. The term "printing polymers," for example, can be appreciated in two ways. In the top-down approach, a pattern of polymers is created by printing a polymer ink, such that a pattern of small features – usually just a monolayer on a substrate – is formed from a bulk polymer. In the bottom-up approach, either a monomer is patterned followed by polymerization on the substrate, or a "seed" for polymer growth is transferred in a patterned manner onto the substrate by μCP. Surface-initiated polymerization results in covalently bound, dense polymer brushes. The same principle applies to NPs and nanotubes (NTs), which can either be printed as such (e.g., with NP and NT inks) or synthesized on the substrate by printing a template. Since this is an important soft lithographic method underlining the importance of μCP for nanotechnology, this topic is described in more detail in Section 3.4; however, it should be noted that printing catalysts for the post-printing formation of much larger structures is possible. This illustrates the fact that μCP is not restricted to organic ink molecules (such as all inks discussed so far), but may also be applied to inorganic compounds.

Macromolecules are particularly useful as inks for μCP, as they tend to adhere strongly to the contact area and diffuse only slowly into noncontact areas. Simple polymers such as PMMA can be patterned using μCP, subject to some modification of the printing process [36]. As a stamp which is directly inked with a PMMA solution in chloroform will become deformed due to swelling, the stamp must be inked using the Langmuir–Schaefer film transfer technique. In this case, the inked stamp was brought into contact with a layer of PMMA on water, which resulted in a thin PMMA layer being deposited on the PDMS stamp. Printing the inked stamp on a silicon oxide substrate then led to the creation of patterned PMMA layers on the surface.

Silicon wafers were patterned with dendrimers of poly(amidoamine) (PAMAM) [6], resulting in 140 nm-wide lines of a single dendrimer layer. Patterns of amine-terminated PAMAM were used as stabilizers for the growth of photoluminescent CdS NPs, simultaneously functioning as adhesive layer between the particles and the silicon surface [37]. Amine-terminated PAMAM was also used to pattern reactive dendrimers on activated SAMs on gold [38]. The deposition of dendrimer multilayers on several substrates by μCP, and the effect of ink concentration, contact time and inking method have also been recently studied [39].

Unlike small apolar ink molecules such as *n*-alkylthiols, which are absorbed into the stamp and then transferred upon contact between the stamp and substrate, high-molecular-weight inks are not absorbed by the stamps but are merely adsorbed to the surface of the stamp. Hence, most of the ink is transferred in a single printing step, and re-inking is necessary after every print; however, this issue can be resolved by changing the composition and structure of the stamp. In this case, agarose has been exploited as a stamp material as it offers certain advantages, especially for printing large molecules such as biomolecules or even cells [40]. The high permeability of agarose for water makes it suitable for printing water-soluble biomacromolecules. In addition, the agarose stamp functions as an ink reservoir that releases the ink molecules slowly, which in turn enables multistep printing without re-inking.

More recently, an alternative method for microstructuring various polymer-based materials was developed, termed phase-separation micromolding (PSμM) [41, 42]. This versatile microfabrication technique can be used to structure a broad range of polymers, including block copolymers, and biodegradable and conductive polymers, without the need for clean room facilities. The method relies on the phase separation of a polymer solution while in contact with a structured mold. For this, a mixture of polymers is cast onto a patterned mold and then placed in a nonsolvent (e.g., water) where polymer chains of the soluble component leave the bulk-producing pores, which immediately become filled by the nonsolvent (Figure 3.6). By using such porous materials as stamps, high-molecular-weight polar inks such as poly(propylene imine) (PPI) dendrimer, HIgG-Fc protein, and functionalized silica NPs were successfully transferred from the stamps to the substrates [43]. The pores not only enable the attachment of such large molecules, but also serve as an ink reservoir for

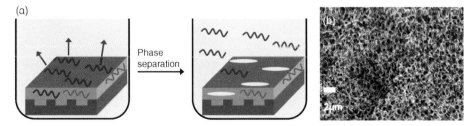

Figure 3.6 (a) The principle of phase separation micromolding: a polymer mixture on a mold is exposed to a nonsolvent; (b) Scanning electron microscopy image of a porous stamp. Reproduced with permission from Ref. [43]; © 2009, American Chemical Society.

repeated printing steps, without a need for re-inking and with no loss of printing quality. With these inks, the PDMS stamps can be used for only one printing step before showing a significant reduction in ink transfer.

Metals in the form of salts [44] and metal colloids [45] can also be patterned on appropriate substrates by using µCP. The µCP of colloids provides access to submicron metal structures, and is a flexible technique that allows patterning on a variety of substrates, including glass, (Si/SiO$_2$), and polymers. Moreover, both flat and curved surface substrates can be used without any loss of resolution. The µCP of colloids can also be used to produce free-standing metal structures and metal films with different thicknesses. For example, Hidber and coworkers used µCP to selectively seed substrates with palladium particles [45] by first coating a stamp with tetra-alkylammonium- or tetraoctadecylammonium-stabilized palladium NPs. The stamp was then contacted with a silanized substrate and the NPs were transferred, followed by electroless metallization with copper (Figure 3.7). The silane layer ensured bonding between the substrate and the NPs [45, 46]. Later, Kind and coworkers coated a stamp with a catalytic precursor ink [47], whereby the stamp was first brought into contact with a titanium-coated substrate, after which the Pd(II) in the ink and the titanium on the surface reacted chemically to form a Pd(0) catalytic pattern. Some additional applications of electroless deposition (ELD) are described in Section 3.4; these include the µCP of colloids for the preparation of surface-enhanced Raman scattering (SERS)-active substrates by attaching silver NPs to gold NP structures that have been patterned using µCP [48].

One final method should be mentioned that does not follow the typical principle of printing an ink onto a substrate but, without doubt, must be regarded as a variation of microcontact printing. Chen and coworkers recently reported the concept of "microcontact deprinting," which involved a microstructured poly(styrene) stamp placed on a monolayer of poly(styrene)-*block*-poly(2-vinylpyridine) micelles on a silicon wafer [49]. Lifting off the stamp caused the micelles in the contact area to be removed (Figure 3.8); these micelles served as initiators for the growth of NPs, such that a patterned bottom-up fabrication of NPs could be achieved.

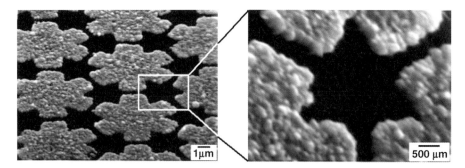

Figure 3.7 Scanning electron microscopy images of copper microstructures grown on poly (styrene) substrates patterned with palladium nanoparticles (NPs). Reproduced with permission from Ref. [46]; © 1996, American Chemical Society.

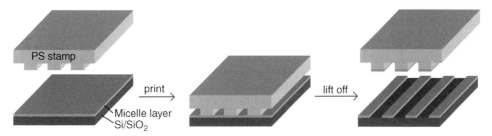

Figure 3.8 The principle of microcontact deprinting. A microstructured poly(styrene) stamp is placed on a monolayer of block copolymer micelles on silicon, and selectively removes the micelles in the contact area at lift-off.

In summary, although μCP was originally developed for the patterning of *n*-alkylthiol SAMs on gold substrates, it represents a straightforward method for the patterning of a wide variety of inks on all types of substrate, subject to an appropriate combination of ink, stamp, and substrate.

3.4
Microcontact Printing and Soft Lithography

Patterned SAMs on solid substrates are important for nanoscience and nanotechnology in two ways:

- They represent a nanostructured material that is easy to prepare and useful for the study of interfacial phenomena that are influenced by nanometer-scale topographies and composition.
- They serve as suitable templates for fabricating microstructures and nanostructures.

Some examples of interfacial phenomena studied with SAMs on thin films include wetting [50–52], corrosion [53, 54], adhesion [52, 55], tribology [56, 57], charge transfer through molecules [58, 59], nucleation and growth of crystals on surfaces [60], and model surfaces for biochemistry and cell biology [61, 62]. These studies depend primarily on the synthesis of SAMs with specific compositions, both in the plane of the surface and out of plane. However, some – such as electron-transfer processes – are extremely sensitive to the nanometer-scale thickness of the SAM. Other applications (such as resistance to etching and protein adsorption, modified electrodes for electrochemistry) rely on the ability of SAMs to prevent the diffusion of other molecules to the surface of the underlying substrate. The application of μCP, and its variations within the area of soft lithography, are detailed in the following subsections.

Hydrophobic SAMs of long-chain *n*-alkylthiols (16 carbons or more) can be used to protect metal films from aqueous wet etching [63]. Moreover, a combination of this ability with μCP makes it possible to fabricate microstructures and nanostructures composed of gold, silver, copper, palladium, platinum, and gold–palladium alloys.

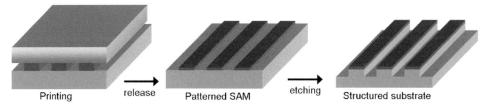

Figure 3.9 Lithography by μCP. A patterned SAM is used as an etch mask for the underlying metal substrate.

Indeed, this was the first application of μCP, and in fact was most likely the intention of its invention [64]. The principle is simple (see Figure 3.9): a substrate patterned by μCP with a SAM of an etch-resistant molecule is treated with an etching solution ("wet etching") or with an etching beam ("dry etching"). The SAM protects the underlying substrate areas from etching, so that the substrate material is removed only in the noncontact areas. This results in the creation of protruding features in the substrate that are similar to those of the stamp, and negative to those of the master that served as the mold for the stamp.

The parameters that determine the minimum dimensions and quality (as measured by the density of pinhole defects on etching and on the edge roughness) of the structures include the composition of the SAM, the density of defects in the SAM, the selectivity of the wet chemical etch, and the morphology of the thin film. A number of etching agents can selectively dissolve regions that are not derivatized with a SAM, and the compositions of these have been developed empirically. The addition of amphiphiles (e.g., *n*-octanol) or use of polymeric complexing agents (e.g., poly(ethyleneimine)) decreases the number of pits and pinholes produced in the surfaces of etched structures, controls the vertical profile of the edges of etched features, and also enables the use of SAMs as resists to pattern thick (>1 μm) electrodeposited films [65]. In the past, the density of pinholes in the SAM and the roughness of the edges of etched features have limited the use of μCP and selective wet etching for fabricating structures with lateral dimensions below 500 nm in gold [66, 67]. However, alternative substrates such as palladium or gold–palladium alloys ($Au_{60}Pd_{40}$) make it possible to generate etched structures that have smaller edge roughness and fewer pinholes than comparable structures in gold when SAMs are used as etch resists. An interphase of PdS that is formed between the bulk metal and the hydrophobic SAM enhances the contrast between the patterned and unpatterned regions [68]. An additional advantage of palladium and gold–palladium alloys as substrates is that they have small grain sizes (~15–30 nm); such morphology is better suited than that of gold (grain sizes ~35–75 nm) for fabricating metal lines with widths as small as 50 nm [69–71]. Unlike gold, palladium is compatible with complementary metal oxide semiconductor (CMOS) manufacturing processes [72]. μCP has also been used to etch Au/Ti layers on GaAs-based materials, and to this end layers of titanium and gold were first evaporated on top of GaAs/AlGaAs quantum well structures and then selectively etched away, using μCP-printed SAMs to protect particular areas of the surface [73]. Finally, the exposed GaAs could be etched away, transferring the pattern.

In conventional μCP followed by etching, the resultant topology is a positive replica of the stamp, and hence the negative of the master. However, in a newer variation of μCP the resultant topology is the negative of the stamp, and hence the positive of the master. This variation of μCP, which is termed "positive μCP" ((+)μCP) [74, 75], involves pattern replication by printing with a poorly etch-resistant ink, followed by immersion of the sample in a second, etch-resistant adsorbate solution that fills the available areas and acts as a resist in the etching step. An additional advantage of (+)μCP is that stamps with a high filling ratio can be used to replicate master features with a low filling ratio. Originally, pentaerythritol tetrakis(3-mercaptopropionate) (PTMP) was proposed as a positive ink, because it forms a stable SAM on gold and copper, is not replaced by etch-resistant thiols such as ODT, and does not provide significant etch resistance [74, 76, 77]. Whilst (+)μCP complements "standard" μCP, both techniques share similar attributes in terms of optimal contrast and resolution for patterning a metal substrate layer by printing and etching it selectively (Figure 3.10).

μCP can also be exploited to generate patterned metal structures or polymer brushes or nano-objects such as carbon nanotubes (CNTs) and NPs. As mentioned in Section 3.4, the patterned formation or growth of these structures by printing an initiator or a catalyst, followed by polymerization or nucleation reactions or selective deposition to build up the structures, represents an elegant "bottom-up" strategy to obtain nanostructured surfaces.

The ELD of metals onto patterned supporting metal features previously attached to substrates by μCP serves as a straightforward means of producing patterned metal structures on surfaces. The ability of printing to transfer chemical reagents from an elastomeric stamp to a substrate can be used to direct the ELD of copper [45–47]. Electroless deposition is a wet chemical metallization process that involves the reduction of a salt from solution onto a surface, using a reducing agent as the electron source. The presence of a catalyst on this surface is necessary to initiate ELD before the deposition can proceed in an autocatalytic manner (see Figure 3.11). The combination of printing with the ELD of a metal is of both scientific and technological interest.

A bottom-up approach is also followed when producing polymer brushes on substrates. These polymer brushes can, for example, increase the etch resistance of a monolayer on a gold substrate, with the initiator either being printed directly or being backfilled after printing another ink (Figure 3.12). Atom transfer radical polymerization (ATRP) can be used to grow polymer chains from an initiator template [78, 79], while $(BrC(CH_3)_2COO(CH_2)_{10}S)_2$ is often used as a polymerization initiator for the formation of polymer brushes of PMMA and various other poly(methacrylates) [78].

Following a similar patterning strategy, single-walled CNTs have been grown – using a chemical vapor deposition (CVD) technique – from methane and hydrogen on iron nitrate catalyst patterns, or on initiator polymer patterns prepared by μCP on suitable substrates (Figure 3.13) [80, 81]. It has also been shown that improved stamp production techniques can improve the quality of printing the catalyst necessary for NT growth [82]. Another approach enables the patterning of a substrate with isolated

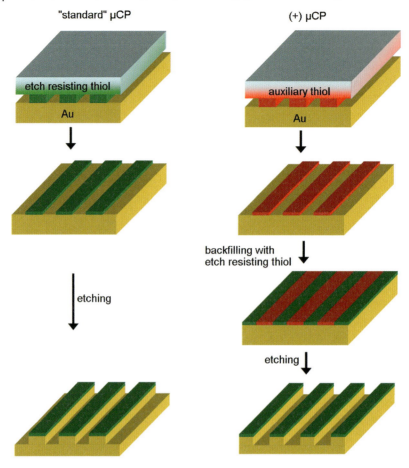

Figure 3.10 Lithography by $(+)\mu$CP compared to "standard" μCP. In standard μCP, a SAM is patterned by μCP, while the patterned SAM serves as an etch mask. Etching provides the positive of the stamp (and hence the negative of the master). In $(+)\mu$CP, a poorly etch-resistant SAM is patterned by μCP; the patterned SAM is then back-filled with a strongly etch-resistant SAM. Etching provides the negative of the stamp (and hence the positive of the master).

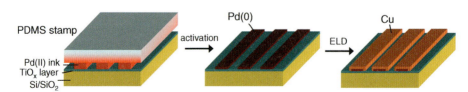

Figure 3.11 Metal structures by μCP. Left: Pd(II) salt is printed onto a TiO$_x$ layer on Si/SiO$_2$. Center: Pd(II) is reduced to Pd(0). Right: Pd(0) catalyzes the electroless deposition of copper.

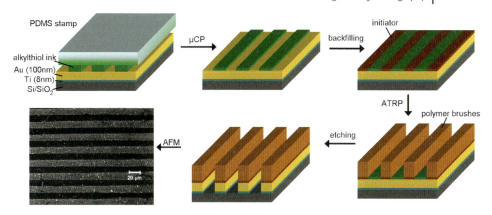

Figure 3.12 Formation of patterned polymer brushes by μCP and atomic force microscopy (AFM) image of patterned gold (dark areas, protected by PMMA) on glass (light areas). AFM image reproduced from Ref. [78]; © 2000, American Chemical Society.

CNTs by using a composite stamp, in this case, the growth of straight CNTs between the patterns was observed, and a method to promote the controlled growth of such isolated nano-objects considered conceivable [83].

Nanotransfer Printing

It is also possible to print a patterned thin film of metal by μCP. The process of transferring a solid nanofilm from a stamp with nanoscale patterned features to a substrate is referred to as "nanotransfer printing" [84–87], in which the stamp can be either a soft or a hard material such as PDMS or silicon. A typical procedure for this μCP technique, using a PDMS stamp, is illustrated in Figure 3.14. In this case, the stamp was coated with a continuous layer of gold (~20 nm thick), without an adhesion layer between the gold and the PDMS. The stamp was then brought into contact with a substrate coated with a dithiol (e.g., 1,8-octanedithiol) [85, 88], after

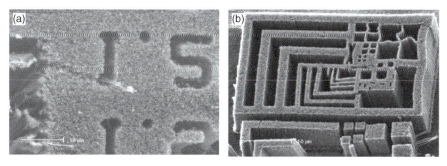

Figure 3.13 Growth of carbon nanotubes after patterning a substrate with iron catalyst with μCP. Image reproduced from Ref. [80]; © 2002, Elsevier.

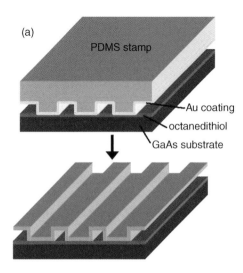
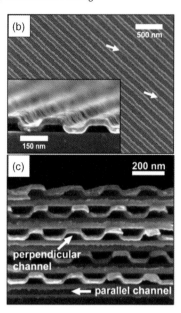

Figure 3.14 (a) The principle of nanotransfer printing (nTP); (b) SEM image of layer of gold on substrate; (c) SEM image of multiple layers after repeating the printing steps. Image reproduced from Ref. [91]; © 2003, American Chemical Society.

which the dithiol formed a SAM on the substrate (GaAs in this case) and the exposed thiol group was bound covalently to the gold layer in the regions of contact. Subsequent removal of the elastomeric stamp from the substrate left the gold layer bound to both the SAM and the underlying substrate. As an alternative, "cold welding" [89, 90] between two metal surfaces could be used to transfer the structured metal film, such that 3-D structures could be fabricated by repeating this procedure [91]. Notably, nanotransfer printing avoids any harsh processing conditions, allows the transfer of nanostructures to be achieved in one combined step [85, 92], and can also be used to pattern features with a lateral resolution of at least 70 nm and an edge roughness down to 10 nm [85, 93]. Another method for releasing the structured film relies on condensation reactions between surface-bound silanols (Si–OH) and/or titanols (Ti–OH) [85, 94]. Techniques that rely on noncovalent interactions between the metal film and the substrate have also been explored, with the minimum dimensions of transferred features currently in excess of 100 nm [95, 96].

As a contact printing technique, nanotransfer printing is well suited to transferring electrodes to fragile surfaces; in particular, it can be used to pattern parallel lines and circular dots as electrical contacts on SAMs [93], with such discontinuous structures adhering to the substrate under "Scotch tape" adhesive tests [92]. The components of devices fabricated directly on plastic substrates include complementary inverter circuits, organic thin-film transistors, capacitors, and electrostatic lenses. This nanotransfer patterning technique can also be used to transfer arrays of sacrificial etch masks and ferromagnetic stacks of cobalt. The morphology and continuity of the transferred metal structure is important in functional devices, with the uniformity of the metal film depending on the wetting and grain size of the metal on the stamp. Typically, a thin adhesion layer ($<2\,nm$ thick) will improve the uniformity of a gold layer on the PDMS stamp and in the transferred layer, although a metal film on an elastomeric stamp may crack due to thermal expansion during metal deposition. Such cracking can be prevented by the rapid deposition of metal and by cooling the stamp [88, 97]. The stress in the metal film from thermal expansion may also be avoided by depositing the metal onto a stamp with a higher thermal conductivity than PDMS (e.g., silicon or gallium arsenide), although the surfaces of these stamps must first be modified with a release layer. Mechanical stress during printing can also introduce cracks into the metal structure.

An alternative approach to printing structured materials is that of "decal transfer printing" [98, 99], whereby a structure (e.g., a PDMS membrane or isolated PDMS features) is transferred from one planar surface to another. In this case, the PDMS decals are made to adhere reversibly to the first substrate (a PDMS slab) [100, 101] while forming covalent bonds with the second substrate. The PDMS slab serves as a handle for patterning continuous or discontinuous features that are otherwise difficult to manipulate. Decal transfer printing can be used to transfer submicrometer features; however, extending the technique to nanoscale features will require further investigations of the interfacial adhesion between the PDMS (or other) substrate and the decal.

3.5
Microcontact Printing and Biological Arrays

During recent years, biological microarrays have rapidly developed into a essential tool for high-throughput genomic and proteomic analysis. Today, "DNA chips" are useful for large-scale parallel analyses of genome sequences and gene expression, for the detection of viruses and other pathogens, for monitoring mRNA expression, and for the classification and evaluation of tumors [102]. Similarly, "protein chips" are valuable for high-throughput diagnostics and drug discovery [103]. By comparison, "carbohydrate chips" have received much less attention to date [104].

Ideally, a biological microarray would have the following properties:

- A high and homogeneous probe density for optimal signal read-out.
- A submicron spot size and nanoscale spot resolution for high data density.
- Many thousands of different probes spotted identically and rapidly for large probe arrays.
- Simple, parallel manufacturing and analysis.

It is evident that state-of-the-art microarray technology falls short of this ideal, with inhomogeneous spots resulting when printing from pins or pipettes due to the evaporation of solvent. In particular, higher probe concentrations may remain at the edges (causing the "coffee-stain effect"), or the probe molecules may aggregate at only a few points within a spot. Hence, spot sizes are typically in the 50 μm range and are separated by at least 50 μm; moreover, significantly smaller spots can only be produced accurately by using time-consuming SPM-based serial processes. Although, admittedly, soft lithography methods such as μCP are not suitable for patterning multiple probes simultaneously, μCP has become a useful tool for the preparation of biological microarrays.

Biological microarrays can be provided in an "indirect" manner via conventional μCP, using molecular inks that provide a 2-D template for the selective adhesion of biomolecules, as well as of living cells. The earliest examples of this approach originate from the Whitesides group, who printed *n*-alkylthiol patterns on a gold-coated substrate and filled the noncontact area with an oligo(ethyleneglycol)-terminated thiol [105]. Subsequently, extracellular matrix (ECM) proteins (such as fibronectin, collagen and laminin) will be adsorbed onto the hydrophobic area, which in turn causes living cells of various types to adhere preferentially to the ECM-modified areas of the surface. In this way, μCP can be used to create microarrays of cells; moreover, as the cells are generally much larger than the resolution limit of μCP, the size and shape of the cell can be directed by its adhesion to a substrate patterned by μCP [106].

μCP can also be used to provide biological microarrays in a "direct" manner, since many biomolecules such as proteins, lipids or oligonucleotides may serve as suitable inks for μCP. Notably, the rather high molecular weight of biomolecules will enhance the formation of well-defined, high-contrast patterns as their diffusion is limited. The transfer of biomolecules from the stamp to the substrate by μCP depends on the surfaces properties of the stamp and substrate. Whilst the simplest μCP approach for patterning of biomolecules involves the direct transfer of ink molecules adsorbed onto the stamp to a target substrate by conformal contact, several important factors must be considered in this respect. Notably, the affinity of the biomolecule towards the stamp and substrate must be tailored such that it is higher for the latter than for the former. In addition, as μCP should not cause denaturation it is preferable that the use of hydrophobic stamps and substrates is avoided in the μCP of proteins. Finally, the biomolecule should, ideally, be printed in such a way that all of the active sites are exposed to the target molecules.

The first reports of the μCP of proteins were made in 1998 [29], when the process was deemed to be very straightforward, and involved: (i) the inking of a PDMS stamp with an aqueous protein solution; (ii) a period of incubation; (iii) air-drying of the stamp; and (iv) bringing the stamp into conformal contact with the substrate (Figure 3.15) [29, 107]. Tan and coworkers have demonstrated that both stamp and substrate wettability is crucial for biomolecule transfer [108]; indeed, a minimum wettability of the substrate was seen to be required for the successful μCP of proteins, but this would be lessened if the wettability of the stamp were to be reduced. Tan and coworkers also found the mechanism for the μCP of protein to differ from protein adsorption because: (i) those surfaces that are resistant to protein adsorption in an aqueous environment are susceptible to μCP under ambient conditions; and (ii) the amount of immobilized proteins and the wettability of the substrate varied gradually for adsorption, but displayed a threshold wettability for μCP.

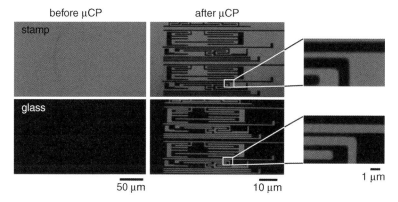

Figure 3.15 μCP of proteins. An IgG protein solution is incubated on the top of an elastomeric stamp. After drying, the stamp is brought into conformal contact with the glass substrate and transfer of proteins occurs only in the area of contact between the stamp and the substrate. Image reproduced from Ref. [29]; © 1998, American Chemical Society.

The patterning of proteins by μCP was demonstrated on different types of substrate, including glass, metal oxides, metals, and polymers. The concept of a direct μCP of protein onto a glass substrate was further extended to the fabrication of *single protein arrays* such as antibodies (e.g., immunoglobulin G; IgG) and green fluorescent proteins (GFPs) on glass [109]. ECM proteins such as laminins have also been patterned by μCP on silicon wafers to guide the growth of neurons for bioelectronic purposes [110]. It should be noted that, whilst many proteins are chemisorbed to gold substrates, the chemisorption often involves a reduction of the disulfides in the protein, leading in turn to denaturation. Gold-binding polypeptide (GBP) represents an interesting example of a protein that can be applied to direct μCP on gold surfaces [111]. Notably, GBP does not contain any cysteine residues that are known generally to form a covalent bond with gold; hence, the binding of GBP is independent of thiols, and offers a new means of interaction between the biomolecule and the surface. Likewise, a GBP–GFP–His$_6$ fusion protein could be printed directly onto a gold surface in a mixture of bovine serum albumin (BSA) and surfactant, such that the protein pattern could be applied as a template for the high-throughput assays of both protein–protein and DNA–DNA interactions [111]. Kwak and coworkers patterned cytochrome C onto gold surfaces using a nonmodified PDMS stamp [112]; in this case, the cytochrome C was used as an ink, while the protein arrays were transferred directly from the stamp to a SAM of mercaptohexanoic acid (MHA) on gold. Active enzymes were also successfully patterned using SAMs on gold surfaces [113]; for example, the metalloprotein azurin was printed on a glass substrate that had been modified with mercaptosilane and which allowed site-specific binding of the protein. The pattern obtained was investigated, using immunofluorescence, with anti-azurin serum [114].

Poly(lysine) was microcontact-printed onto a clean, nonmodified glass surface via an oxidized PDMS stamp by using electrostatic interactions between the positively charged polypeptide and the negatively charged glass surface [115]. Delamarche and coworkers proposed the use of hydrophilic PDMS stamps modified with poly (ethylene oxide) silanes [27, 116]. In this case, the modification was conducted by oxidation of the PDMS stamp and reaction with 3-aminopropyltriethoxysilane (APTES), followed by a reaction to conjugate the surface amino groups with poly (ethylene glycol) (PEG) chains. When PEG is grafted onto oxidized PDMS stamps it acts as a protein repellent layer, and this property was utilized to design a flat stamp with regions that could attract proteins (nonmodified PDMS) and regions modified with PEG that have protein-repellent properties [117]. The local modification of PDMS was conducted by oxidation in O_2-plasma with the application of metal mask (those areas covered by the mask were neither oxidized nor modified). When proteins are applied to such a stamp, they are directed towards its hydrophobic areas; hence, protein IgG was successfully transferred to the glass substrates and immobilized in a well-defined pattern with high accuracy and contrast. In a different approach, when the PEG-modified stamp (according to the procedure described above) was contacted with another flat, dry, nonmodified PDMS stamp (the "ink pad") that had been incubated in IgG buffer solution, a homogeneous layer of proteins was transferred to the PEG regions of the other stamp. The latter could then be contacted with a glass substrate and used to pattern IgG proteins.

Proteins may also be patterned on a flat stamp by using a microfluidic network [30], such that the patterned flat stamp can be contacted with glass or another substrate so as to transfer the pattern. Recently, this approach was extended to the high-resolution μCP of proteins, whereby a flat PDMS stamp was patterned with a nanoscale PEG pattern by using dip-pen nanolithography (DPN). The nanopattern could then be replicated as a protein nanopattern on a glass substrate [118].

Another means of overcoming the problems of PDMS stamps with regards to wettability and compatibility with aqueous solutions, would be to select alternative materials for fabrication of the stamp. One versatile approach here would be the use of agarose hydrogel stamps as a mold for transferring water-soluble biomolecules [40]. Since an agarose hydrogel stamp is highly permeable to water, it would also function as an ink reservoir; consequently, multiple stamping would be possible, without any need for intermediate re-inking of the stamp.

μCP of DNA

In the μCP of DNA, it is necessary to modify the stamp surface to ensure DNA–stamp attraction, and such modifications can be carried out by the addition of APTES, which confers a positive charge to the surface [31]. Perhaps the greatest benefit for the μCP of DNA is its ability to print multiple arrays from a single loaded stamp; indeed, this could ultimately result in both cost-saving and time-saving processes, especially for gene expression studies when it is the *ratio* of bound to labeled molecules that is important, and *not* the total amount of material present [31]. Subsequently, a much more efficient method of transferring the micropatterns of DNA and RNA to a surface was achieved by modifying the PDMS stamp with positively charged PPI dendrimers (creating the "dendri stamp") in a "layer-by-layer" arrangement (Figure 3.16) [119, 120]. The electrostatic interactions between dendrimers and

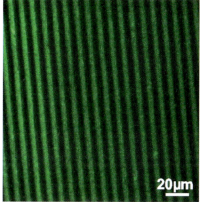
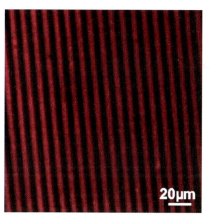

Figure 3.16 Transfer printing of DNA and RNA using "dendri-stamps." A PDMS stamp is oxidized and coated with a cationic PPI dendrimer. DNA and RNA bind to the dendrimer-coated stamp in a layer-by-layer arrangement. If the DNA (or RNA) is functionalized with an amine, it can be printed on an aldehyde-terminated self-assembled monolayer. The image shows a simultaneous fluorescence micrograph of DNA patterns after hybridization between a fluorescein-labeled probe that was obtained by μCP (left image) and its complementary Cy5-labeled target (right image). Image reproduced from Ref. [119]; © 2007, American Chemical Society.

oligonucleotides ensured a successful transfer of DNA or RNA to the target surface, while imine chemistry [119] or "click" chemistry [120] could be applied to bind the covalently modified DNA and RNA molecules to a chemically functionalized substrate (see Section 3.6). An alternative approach to patterning DNA molecules on the surface was proposed by Xu and coworkers [121], who prepared an "amphiphilic" DNA by attaching a hydrophobic alkyl chain to the 3' or 5' end, such that the hydrophobic tail enhanced the adsorption of DNA to the hydrophobic PDMS stamp. This in turn allowed for the efficient transfer and delivery of DNA to the surface.

It is also of interest to pattern phospholipids by μCP (Figure 3.17) [122]. Supported lipid bilayers are very fragile assemblies that are formed by lipids organized into two opposing leaflets on hydrophilic surfaces, such as glass or mica substrates, and can be patterned onto solid substrates. For phospholipid patterning, however, the μCP technique used differs slightly from that used with proteins or DNA. First, the bilayer must be formed on the oxidized PDMS stamp from the buffer solution by fusion of liposomes to the stamp surface. Second, the printing should be carried out in water, otherwise the bilayer will lose its structure. This method allows an efficient and reliable transfer of membrane patches to glass surfaces, which are of particular interest in investigations of biological membranes in general, and in the behavior of membrane proteins in particular. Alternatively, lipid bilayers can be patterned indirectly by μCP: in this case, either a template of proteins can be printed to which the lipid bilayer vesicles are fused, or a supported lipid bilayer is selectively removed in the contact areas by blotting through μCP with a bare stamp [123].

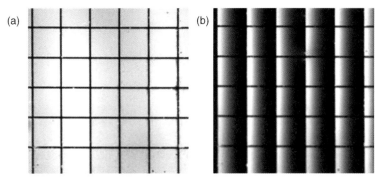

Figure 3.17 Patterning of phospholipids bilayers by μCP. (a) Fluorescence image of a patterned supported lipid bilayer that was printed onto a glass surface (egg phosphatidylcholine with 1 mol% Texas Red). The bright regions are fluorescence from the labeled lipids, and the dark grid pattern is the bare glass surface; (b) Fluorescence image taken after an electric field was briefly applied parallel to the bilayer plane, creating a steady-state gradient of the negatively charged labeled lipids and demonstrating long-range mobility. The dimensions of both images were 560 μm × 560 μm. Image reproduced from Ref. [122]; © 2001, American Chemical Society.

Affinity Contact Printing

Recently, an interesting concept for the simultaneous μCP of multiple probes has been proposed. "Affinity contact printing" (αCP) [124] relies on inking the surface of a PDMS stamp with antigens as "capture molecules" which allows the subsequent binding of selected antibodies from a solution containing mixtures of proteins (Figure 3.18). Affinity stamps were prepared by modification of the PDMS stamp with APTES and a crosslinker to produce an activated, hydrophilic surface. This activated stamp was then used to couple antigens to selected areas using: (i) microwells; (ii) microfluidic networks; and (iii) μCP. By repeating this procedure with a different type of antigen, the stamp could be functionalized with a pattern of various antigens, which would be valuable for microarray applications. When several types of antigen are immobilized on an activated stamp they can be exposed to a solution of different antibodies, so as to extract and immobilize a "matching partner." The captured antibodies can then be printed onto a glass substrate to form micro-arrays of antibodies.

An alternative form of affinity contact printing was demonstrated by Jang and coworkers [125], which relied on the modification of a PDMS stamp with amino-silanes and succinic anhydride to introduce carboxylic acid groups on the surface; this was followed by the immobilization of a monoclonal antibody (mAb) to the epidermal growth factor receptor (EGFR). The EGFR-antibody-modified stamp was then incubated with a solution of membrane proteins from cell membrane extracts and crude cell lysates. The stamp was contacted with a gold substrate that had been modified with an amino-terminated monolayer and, after μCP, the substrate was covered with a nematic liquid crystal (LC) film. The orientation of the LC film was

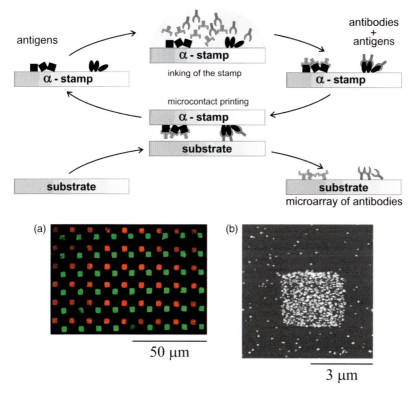

Figure 3.18 Upper panel: Affinity contact printing (αCP) relies on inking the surface of a PDMS stamp with antigens as "capture molecules"; this allows the subsequent binding of selected antibodies from a solution containing mixtures of proteins. Lower panel: (a) Fluorescence microscopy image showing the placement of the TRITC-anti-chicken and FITC-anti-goat antibodies from a stamp onto a glass substrate; (b) AFM image obtained on a spot of the array in which the printed anti-goat antibodies bound to Au-labeled goat antigens presented in solution. Detection of this binding was monitored by staining the Au labels with electroless-deposited silver particles of average diameter 80 nm. Images (a) and (b) reproduced from Ref. [124]; © 2002, Wiley-VCH.

found to be different on the amino-terminated surface and the regions of the surface presenting EGFR, thus providing a simple, label-free method for optically detecting the presence of EGFRs on the surface. In a similar manner, the group of Abbott used αCP to immobilize proteins that subsequently can be imaged with LCs [126]. This method relies on the covalent modification of PDMS stamp with a biotinylated BSA. In this case, the BSA-functionalized stamp was inked with anti-biotin IgG and brought into conformal contact with an amino-modified gold surface. After printing, the protein pattern was imaged by spreading an LC film onto the surface.

An interesting concept of pattern transfer of DNA using μCP was introduced by the groups of Crooks [127] and Stellaci [128]. These strategies relied on the fabrication of DNA arrays onto flat solid supports by immobilization via the 5′ end functionalized with, for example, amine linkers. The DNA array was further hybridized with complementary strands that possessed a capturing group at the 5′ end. These groups could be reacted with functionalized surfaces simply by bringing the surface into conformal contact with the DNA array. After reaction, the two surfaces could be separated and the pattern of single-stranded DNA transferred to the surface that was in contact with the patterned hybridized array. As a result, the strands would be mechanically separated and the new arrays of patterned DNA could be used for the next transfer of microarrays (Figure 3.19).

In conclusion, μCP has emerged as a versatile tool for the preparation of biological microarrays. Interesting methods for the simultaneous μCP of multiple inks have recently been reported. The highly selective molecular recognition of biomolecules may also be used in the replication of arrays by μCP.

3.6
Microcontact Printing and Surface Chemistry

One striking feature of μCP is the short contact time required to form a dense monolayer of ink on the substrate. Although, typically, the contact times are approximately 1 min, μCP has also been performed with millisecond contacts of the stamp and substrate [129]. In contrast, it takes several hours to prepare an *n*-alkylthiol or *n*-alkylsilane SAM from solution [130]. These observations indicate that μCP is a particularly effective method for preparing SAMs, even if this

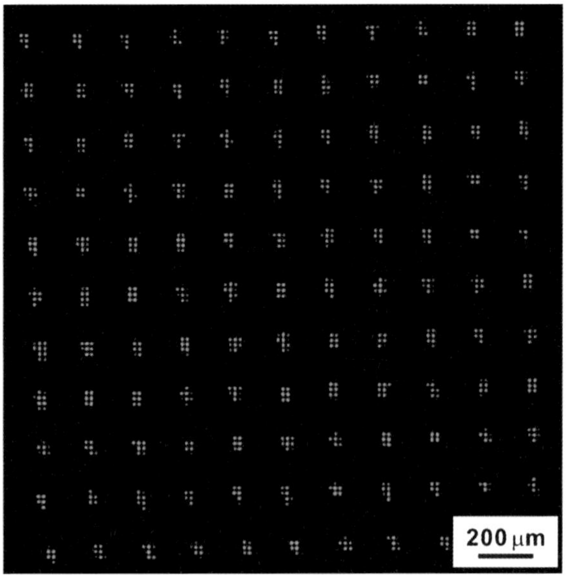

Figure 3.19 Fluorescence micrograph of an RNA microarray on a PDMS surface, which was fabricated using a master DNA array of 2500 spots (~70 μm in diameter). Image reproduced from Ref. [127]; © 2007, American Chemical Society.

involves a slow condensation reaction (as in the case of *n*-alkylsilane SAMs). This conclusion raises the interesting point of whether µCP could be used to accelerate surface reactions, for example by printing a molecular ink on top of a SAM [131]. It is known that reactions on SAMs are typically several orders of magnitude slower than reactions in solution [132]. It can be argued that the steric hindrance and conformational restraints encountered at the surface of a SAM (or any other surface) reduce the frequency of effective intermolecular collisions, and hence enhance the activation energy of reaction. Yet, it is likely that this kinetic barrier is more than compensated when a stamp saturated or densely covered with ink is brought into conformal contact with a SAM in which most of the reactive groups are exposed at the surface. In this case, a bimolecular reaction should benefit from the nanoscale confinement of highly concentrated reagents in the contact area between a stamp and a substrate.

Indeed, it has been demonstrated several times by Whitesides and colleagues that amides are formed when amines – small molecules as well as polymers – are printed on an anhydride-terminated or active ester-terminated SAM on gold [133]. However, it must be noted that this result is not surprising given the reactivity of amines towards anhydrides and active esters.

In 2004, Huck and coworkers described the formation of peptides by printing N-protected amino acids onto an amine-terminated SAM on gold (Figure 3.20) [133]. Of course, peptide bonds do not spontaneously form from carboxylic acids and amines under ambient conditions, and it was proposed by Huck that "...the nanoscale confinement of the ink at the interface between the stamp and the SAM, in combination with the pre-organization of the reactants in the SAM, facilitates the formation of covalent bonds" [134]. In a remarkable experiment, it was shown that the consecutive µCP of as many as 20 peptide nucleobases resulted in the formation of an oligopeptide nucleic acid that could selectively bind a complementary strand of DNA. These findings point to the fascinating potential of surface chemistry by µCP, that complex biomacromolecules could be synthesized simply by printing the monomers in the appropriate sequence!

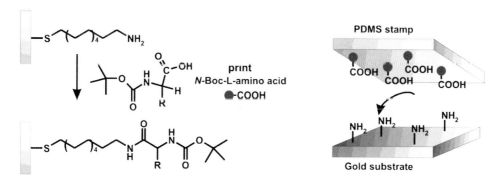

Figure 3.20 Peptide synthesis by µCP. An oxidized PDMS stamp is inked with an *N*-Boc-*L*-amino acid and pressed into a contact against an amino-functionalized gold substrate to yield a covalent peptide bond. Boc = *t*-butoxycarbonyl.

Subsequently, it was also shown that imines can be formed in a few minutes under ambient conditions by printing amines onto aldehyde-terminated SAMs [135]. The reaction of aldehydes and amines is an equilibrium reaction that is generally unfavorable unless water is removed from the reaction mixture. In addition, this reaction was applied to the preparation of biological microarrays: the μCP of RGD-containing proteins on aldehyde-terminated SAMs was used to direct the adhesion of cells in microarrays [136], while the μCP of amine-modified DNA on aldehyde-terminated SAMs provided DNA microarrays [119].

These reports point to a second advantage of surface chemistry by μCP, namely that biological arrays are generally prepared on transparent substrates (preferably glass) so that they can be read out with fluorescence; however, as biomolecules are not compatible with alkoxysilanes, an indirect immobilization and patterning method would be required for glass substrates. Microcontact chemistry on an intermediate SAM fulfills this requirement.

The Huisgen 1,3-dipolar cycloaddition of alkynes and azides can also be induced by μCP (Figure 3.21) [137]. The Cu(I)-catalyzed cycloaddition of alkynes and azides [138] is a prime example of "click chemistry" (i.e., a chemical reaction with near-quantitative yield, mild reaction conditions, and short reaction time) [139] that has found widespread use for the bio-orthogonal ligation of biomolecules to surfaces; moreover, its combination with μCP constitutes an attractive method for the preparation of microarrays. Triazoles are formed within minutes when an alkyne is printed on an azide-terminated SAM on a silicon wafer or glass, even in the absence of a Cu(I) catalyst that is normally used to accelerate this type of "click chemistry" [137]. It should be emphasized that the solution reaction in the absence of Cu(I) is slow unless electron-poor alkynes are used. The Huisgen cycloaddition induced by μCP was investigated in detail by printing a set of fluorescent alkynes on azide-terminated SAMs on glass substrates (J. Mehlich and B.J. Ravoo, unpublished results). When fluorescence microscopy was then used to monitor the extent

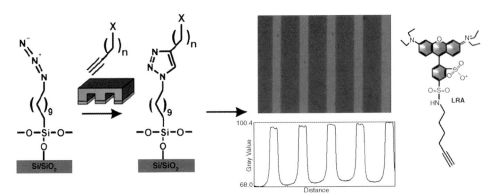

Figure 3.21 1,3-Dipolar cycloaddition reaction by μCP. Triazoles are formed within minutes when an alkyne is printed on an azide-terminated SAM on a silicon wafer or glass, even in the absence of a Cu(I) catalyst that is normally used to accelerate this type of "click chemistry."

of reaction on the glass surface, it was shown that the rate of cycloaddition depended on the reactivity of the alkyne and on the presence of Cu(I). Although the cycloaddition would be accelerated by Cu(I), it also proceeded readily in the absence of Cu(I).

"Click chemistry" by μCP was applied to print microarrays of alkyne-modified DNA [120] and alkyne-modified carbohydrates [140] on azide-terminated SAMs on Si wafers and glass. It was observed that, although DNA could be printed without a Cu(I) catalyst, the surface density of carbohydrates was low in the absence of a Cu(I) catalyst. In particular, for the preparation of biological microarrays it is advantageous to exclude the toxic Cu(I) catalyst.

μCP can also be used for the heterogeneous catalysis of chemical reactions in the contact area between stamp and substrate. In its most simple form, an oxidized PDMS stamp can be used as a heterogeneous acid catalyst to accelerate a hydrolysis reaction on a SAM. It has been shown that silylether-terminated SAMs are hydrolyzed to produce hydroxyl-terminated SAMs upon contact with an oxidized PDMS stamp for 5–10 min [141]. It was also shown that FMOC protecting groups can be removed from an amine-terminated SAM by contact with a piperidine-modified poly (urethane) stamp [142]. In this way, catalytic μCP can be used to replicate the microstructure of the stamp in the form of a chemical contrast on the substrate, without any ink transfer ("printing without ink"). In a more sophisticated approach to catalytic μCP, Toone and coworkers have shown that enzymes immobilized in a poly (acrylamide) stamp can induce the cleavage of surface-immobilized DNA in the area of contact between stamp and substrate [143].

Very recently, the heterogeneous catalysis of the Huisgen cycloaddition of alkynes and azides by μCP was reported. In this case, a microstructured PDMS stamp covered with a thin film of Cu (which had been air-oxidized to Cu_2O) was used to induce the cycloaddition of alkynes on an azide-terminated SAM on gold [144]. It was shown that the cycloaddition by μCP would proceed to completion (i.e., until all reactive sites on the surface were occupied) within a few hours if a Cu-coated stamp was used.

Finally, it must be emphasized that spatially controlled surface chemistry induced by μCP is not limited to reactions on SAMs on inorganic substrates. In particular, transparent polymer films represent attractive substrates for reactions induced by μCP. An early example of microcontact chemistry on polymer films was that described by Chilkoti and coworkers, who oxidized poly(olefin) and poly(ester) substrates, activated them with pentafluorophenyl esters, and subsequently patterned the polymer surface with amine-terminated biotin, using μCP [145]. In similar fashion, amine-modified proteins and DNA can be printed on N-hydroxysuccinimide-activated poly(methacrylate) films [146] (of course, these results should be expected, given the inherent reactivity of amines and active esters). Recently, the Cu (I)-catalyzed cycloaddition of alkynes and azides was also used to pattern the surface of a poly(alkyne) film by the μCP of azide-terminated biotin [147]. To this end, the Cu (I) catalyst was printed on a poly(alkyne) film covered with a thin layer of azide-terminated biotin. It is to be expected that less-reactive polymer films could also be functionalized with spatially patterned molecular monolayers.

Table 3.1 Surface chemical reactions induced by microcontact printing (μCP).

Substrate	Ink	Product	Catalyst	Reference(s)
Anhydride	Amine	Amide	—	[133]
Active ester	Amine	Amide	—	[145, 146]
Amine	Carboxylic acid	Amide	—	[134]
Aldehyde	Amine	Imine	—	[119, 135, 136]
Azide	Alkyne	Triazole	—	[120, 137]
Azide	Alkyne	Triazole	Cu(I)	[140]
Alkyne	Azide	Triazole	Cu(I)	[147]
Azide	Alkyne	Triazole	Cu stamp	[144]
Si-protected alcohol	—	Alcohol	Ox stamp	[141]
FMOC-protected amine	—	Amine	Pip stamp	[142]

In many respects, reactions induced by μCP follow the principles of click chemistry: near-quantitative yield (i.e., complete surface coverage); mild reaction conditions; and short reaction times [139]. Most interestingly, however, the scope of the reactions – including condensation, cycloaddition, nucleophilic substitution, and deprotection – continues to expand, and an overview of those induced by μCP to date is provided in Table 3.1.

Notably, reactions carried out using μCP can be combined with heterogeneous catalysis and applied to functionalize polymer films with molecular monolayers. The confinement of heterogeneous catalysts on a microstructured stamp also opens up the possibility to react highly volatile reagents with the substrate, which is not possible in conventional μCP. The limited resolution of μCP could possibly be overcome by using flat stamps with nanostructured heterogeneous catalysts (see Section 3.7). In summary, it can be foreseen that surface reactions induced by μCP will provide a straightforward and versatile method for surface chemistry in general, and for the fabrication of (bio)molecular microarrays and nanoarrays in particular.

3.7
From Micro to Nano: Increasing the Resolution of Microcontact Printing

As the name indicates, μCP is typically used for the structuring of surfaces at the microscale. A number of factors limit the resolution of conventional μCP to about 0.5 μm. The first major limitation is inherent to the flexible nature of the elastomer PDMS stamp. PDMS has a Young's modulus of about 1.5 MPa, which is soft enough to ensure a conformal contact with substrates so as to facilitate ink transfer. Unfortunately, however, a PDMS stamp can be easily deformed, and this imposes a limit on the aspect ratio (i.e., the height of a microstructure divided by its width) as well as the fill ratio (i.e., the width of a structure divided by the distance) of the stamp (see Figure 3.3). If the aspect ratio is too high (i.e., tall structures close together), then the microstructures will buckle and stick together. For conventional μCP with *n*-alkylthiol inks on gold, an aspect ratio of about 1 is considered optimal. However, if the fill ratio is too low (i.e., small structures far apart) then the stamp will sag and touch the substrate also in the noncontact area. A second major limitation to the resolution of μCP resides in the ink transfer from stamp to substrate: although, ideally, the ink should be transferred exclusively in the contact areas, the ink in fact tends to diffuse and spread to the noncontact areas during printing. In particular, when printing small features with low-molecular-weight inks, diffusion and spreading of the ink outside the contact area will adversely affect the edge resolution of μCP. The strategies proposed to extend the resolution of μCP into the nanoscale will be outlined in the following subsections.

One obvious approach would be to use "stiffer" stamps for μCP, so that deformations would occur less readily. For example, PDMS can be crosslinked more extensively, so that its Young's modulus would increase to about 10 MPa [11, 15]. Although such "hard" PDMS stamps would still be soft enough for conformal contact, their relief structure would less readily deform. Structures as small as 80 nm can be accurately replicated using hard PDMS stamps. Alternatively, stamps can be prepared from acryloxy perfluoropoly(ethers), which have a Young's modulus of about 10 MPa [148], or from poly(urethane acrylates), which have a modulus of about 20 MPa [149], or from poly(olefins), which can have a value of more than 40 MPa [18]. It has been shown that such "rigid" stamps can be used for the μCP of proteins in lines of 100 nm width with 3 μm periodicity (Figure 3.22) [150]. Deformation of the stamp can also be reduced by using a PDMS stamp on a rigid support [115, 151] that would prevent the stamp from sagging in the noncontact area, such that a substantially lower fill ratio would be possible. Another useful improvement is that of "submerged" μCP, where the μCP of *n*-alkylthiols is performed in water instead of

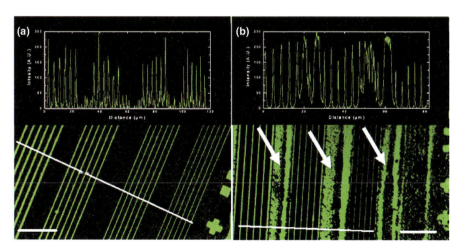

Figure 3.22 High-resolution μCP of proteins in lines of 100 nm width with 3 μm periodicity. μCP with poly(olefin) stamps (a) is clearly superior to μCP with conventional PDMS stamps (b). Image reproduced from Ref. [150]; © 2003, American Chemical Society.

air [152]. Here, the role of the water is to support the relief structure of the stamp, so that stamps with aspect ratios of 15 : 1 and higher can be used.

The diffusion and spreading of ink molecules into the noncontact areas can, of course, be limited by reducing the contact time of stamp and substrate. To this end, Wolf *et al.* have proposed "high-speed µCP" [129], which allows *n*-alkylthiol inks to be printed on gold substrates within 10 ms, while the resultant SAMs in the contact areas serve as effective etch resists, allowing the noncontact metal areas to be selectively etched. In fact, it has been shown that ultrafast µCP can be readily used for µCP at the submicron scale. As an alternative, the diffusion and spreading of ink into the noncontact area can be limited by inking the stamp through an ink pad, such that the stamp is inked only in the contact area [153].

Another obvious improvement would be to use inks that had a low diffusion coefficient and a low tendency to spread across the substrate. The diffusion rate of an ink correlates with its molecular weight; thus, a higher molecular weight will limit the diffusion of an ink into noncontact areas. To this end, the use of "heavy inks" has been proposed as an alternative to the simple *n*-alkylthiols, in particular for applications in high-resolution µCP for lithography. An early example of this so-called "nanocontact printing" was described by Huck *et al.*, who used a dendrimer ink and a submicron-structured PDMS stamp to print 140 nm-wide lines with 70 nm periodicity [8]. Along the same lines, others have designed "multivalent inks" that have multiple functional groups capable of binding to the substrate [154]; the enhanced surface adsorption of multivalent inks reduces the spreading of the ink into the noncontact areas of the substrate. Dendrimers have also been particularly useful in this area since, by using dendrimer inks with multiple thioether end groups, it is possible to perform (+)µCP followed by a wet etch with a resolution better than 100 nm (Figure 3.23) [155]. As most biomolecules have a much higher molecular weight than *n*-alkylthiols, their diffusion will be negligible, such that they will be particularly suited for µCP at the submicron scale.

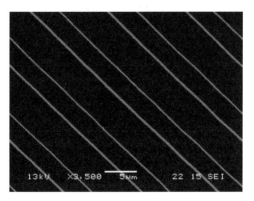

Figure 3.23 High resolution (+)µCP with dendrimer inks; 100 nm gold lines were prepared by (+)µCP of thioether dendrimers for 2 min, dipping in ODT for 6 s, and etching in Fe(III)/thiourea for 2.5 min.

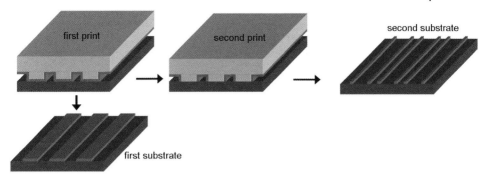

Figure 3.24 The principle of edge transfer printing.

An alternative approach to improve the resolution of μCP is that of *edge transfer lithography* (Figure 3.24) [156–158], in which the edges of micrometer-sized stamps are used to reproduce submicrometer structures. After removing the top layer of the ink that is required to be transferred from the protruding features of a stamp, the stamp is brought in conformal contact with another substrate, whereupon any residual ink at the edges of the features is transferred to the substrate.

In the case of a conventional PDMS stamp with a microrelief surface structure, the selective transfer of ink occurs essentially due to a rapid transfer in the contact area and a slow (ideally, negligible) transfer in the noncontact area. It could be argued that the air-filled voids between the microstructures at the stamp surface pose a diffusion barrier for the ink, since volatile inks can easily cross this barrier but nonvolatile inks cannot. A major advance in the resolution of μCP involves a radically altered design of stamps; instead of exploiting the voids in the microrelief pattern as a diffusion barrier, it is possible to impose a diffusion barrier on a *flat* PDMS stamp [159]. For example, by oxidation of the PDMS surface, a thin silicon oxide film is created, which is essentially impermeable to apolar inks. If the oxidation is directed by a mask, then a flat stamp with a surface pattern of silicon oxide on PDMS will result that can be used for the μCP of alkylthiol, which are transferred exclusively in the nonoxidized area. The properties of the diffusion barrier and stability of the stamp may be improved by coating the silicon oxide film with a fluorinated silane SAM, and even volatile, low-molecular-weight inks can be printed with such chemically patterned flat stamps. Moreover, because the stamp is flat, all problems due to deformation of the microrelief surface structures are circumvented. Hence, the resolution of the stamp is now limited only by the resolution of the oxidation mask, which can be made by conventional photolithography and/or electron beam lithography (EBL). Recently, the resolution of μCP with flat stamps was further improved by using DPN to "write" a nanostructured oxidation mask on the surface of a flat PDMS stamp [118]. Following oxidation, the stamp can be functionalized with hydrophilic and fluorinated silanes. It was demonstrated that the chemical nanopattern on the stamp can be replicated on a gold substrate in the form of a nanopatterned alkylthiol SAM, which can serve as a nanoscale etch mask. Among others, the patterns included a nanoscale map of the USA! Regular arrays of gold dots with a diameter of 80 nm spaced by

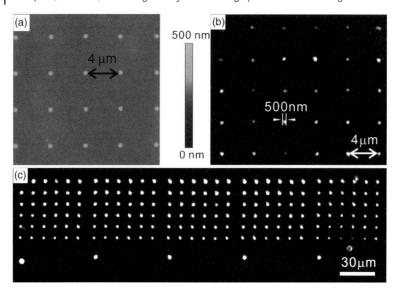

Figure 3.25 High-resolution μCP with a flat PDMS stamp that was nanostructured by DPN. (a) An AFM topography of the PEG pattern used for fabricating a flat stamp for μCP of proteins; (b) A fluorescence image of the printed TRITC-conjugated IgG; (c) A fluorescent image of the printed TRITC pattern on glass. Image reproduced from Ref. [118]; © 2008, Wiley-VCH.

10 μm can be readily obtained using this method. Alternatively, the nanopatterned stamp can be used to print proteins in a nanoscale array on glass (Figure 3.25).

In summary, the resolution of μCP may be substantially better than 100 nm. In particular, the design of chemically patterned, flat elastomer stamps has radically improved the resolution of μCP. Although the nanostructuring of surfaces by μCP is less straightforward than conventional microstructuring by μCP, "nanocontact printing" represents an attractive bench-top method for the preparation of nanoscale patterns of a range of active structures in a parallel manner.

3.8
Conclusions and Outlook

μCP was first developed for the preparation of patterned SAMs of *n*-alkylthiols on gold substrates. Inspired by the pioneering studies of Whitesides and coworkers, many research groups have shown that the nature of the ink, the stamp, and the substrate can be widely modified in order to improve the printing quality and to exploit the possibilities of μCP for a range of applications in materials and life sciences.

μCP has proven to be a valuable method for the preparation of microstructured and nanostructured surfaces, and has emerged as a versatile tool for the preparation of biological microarrays. Interesting methods for the simultaneous μCP of multiple biological inks have recently been reported. The highly selective molecular recognition of biomolecules may also be used in the replication of arrays by μCP. Furthermore, it can be foreseen that surface reactions induced by μCP will provide a straightforward and versatile method for surface chemistry in general, and for the fabrication of (bio)molecular microarrays and nanoarrays in particular.

References

1 Carter, T.F. (1955) *The Invention of Printing in China and its Spread Westward*, Ronald Press Co., New York.

2 Kipphan, H. (2000) *Handbuch der Printmedien: Technologien und Produktionsverfahren*, Springer, Berlin.

3 Adams, J.M., Faux, D.D., and Rieber, J.J. (1996) *Printing Technology*, 4th edn, Delmare Publishers, Albany, NY.

4 Kumar, A. and Whitesides, G.M. (1993) *Appl. Phys. Lett.*, **63**, 2002.

5 Xia, Y., Venkateswaran, N., Qin, D., Tien, J., and Whitesides, G.M. (1998) *Langmuir*, **14**, 363.

6 Li, H., Kang, D.-J., Blamire, M.G., and Huck, W.T.S. (2002) *Nano Lett.*, **2**, 347.

7 Li, H., Muir, B.V.O., Flichet, G., and Huck, W.T.S. (2003) *Langmuir*, **19**, 1963.

8 Ruiz, S.A. and Chen, C.S. (2007) *Soft Matter*, **3**, 168.

9 Perl, A., Reinhoudt, D.N., and Huskens, J. (2009) *Adv. Mater.*, **21**, 2257.

10 Stein, J., Lewis, N.L., Gao, Y., and Scott, R.A. (1999) *J. Am. Chem. Soc.*, **121**, 3693.

11 Bietsch, A. and Michel, B. (2000) *J. Appl. Phys.*, **88**, 4310.

12 Delamarche, E., Schmid, H., Michel, B., and Biebuyck, H. (1997) *Adv. Mater.*, **9**, 741.

13 Hui, C.Y., Jagota, A., Lin, Y.Y., and Kramer, E.J. (2002) *Langmuir*, **18**, 1394.

14 Odom, T.W., Love, J.C., Wolfe, D.B., Paul, K.E., and Whitesides, G.M. (2002) *Langmuir*, **18**, 5314.

15 Schmid, H. and Michel, B. (2000) *Macromolecules*, **33**, 3042.

16 Wilbur, J.L., Kumar, A., Kim, E., and Whitesides, G.M. (1994) *Adv. Mater.*, **6**, 600.

17 Guo, Q., Teng, X., and Yang, H. (2004) *Nano Lett.*, **4**, 1657.

18 Trimbach, D., Feldman, K., Spencer, N.D., Broer, D.J., and Bastiaansen, C.W.M. (2003) *Langmuir*, **19**, 10957.

19 Delamarche, E., Schmid, H., Bietsch, A., Larsen, N.B., Rothuizen, H., Michel, B., and Biebuyck, H. (1998) *J. Phys. Chem. B*, **102**, 3324.

20 Wilbur, J.L., Biebuyck, H.A., MacDonald, J.C., and Whitesides, G.M. (1995) *Langmuir*, **11**, 825.

21 Jeon, N., Finnie, K., Branshaw, K., and Nuzzo, R. (1997) *Langmuir*, **13**, 3382.

22 Brzoska, J.B., Azouz, I.B., and Rondelez, F. (1994) *Langmuir*, **10**, 4367.

23 Allara, D.L., Parikh, A.N., and Rondelez, F. (1995) *Langmuir*, **11**, 2357.

24 Owen, M.J. and Smith, P.J. (1994) *J. Adhes. Sci. Technol.*, **8**, 1063.

25 Hillborg, H., Tomczak, N., Olah, A., Schonherr, H., and Vancso, G.J. (2004) *Langmuir*, **20**, 785.

26 Hu, S., Ren, X., Bachman, M., Sims, C.E., Li, G.P., and Allbritton, N. (2002) *Anal. Chem.*, **74**, 4117.

27 Delamarche, E., Donzel, C., Kamounah, S.S., Wolf, H., Geissler, M., Stutz, R., Schmid-Winkel, P., Michel, B., Mathieu, H.J., and Schaumburg, K. (2003) *Langmuir*, **19**, 8749.

28 Sadhu, V.B., Perl, A., Peter, M., Rozkiewicz, D.I., Engbers, G., Ravoo, B.J., Reinhoudt, D.N., and Huskens F.J. (2007) *Langmuir*, **23**, 6850.

29 Bernard, A., Delamarche, E., Schmid, H., Michel, B., Bosshard, H.R., and Biebuyck, H. (1998) *Langmuir*, **14**, 2225.

30 Bernard, A., Renault, J.-P., Michel, B., Bosshard, H.R., and Delamarche, E. (2000) *Adv. Mater.*, **12**, 1067.

31 Lange, S.A., Benes, V., Kern, D.P., Hoerber, J.K.H., and Bernard, A. (2004) *Anal. Chem.*, **76**, 1641.

32 Auletta, T., Dordi, B., Mulder, A., Sartori, A., Onclin, S., Bruinink, C.M., Peter, M., Nijhuis, C.A., Beijleveld, H., Schonherr, H., Vancso, G.J., Casnati, A., Ungaro, R., Ravoo, B.J., Huskens, J., and Reinhoudt,

D.N. (2004) *Angew. Chem., Int. Ed.*, **43**, 369.

33 Bruinink, C.M., Nijhuis, C.A., Peter, M., Dordi, B., Crespo Biel, O., Auletta, T., Mulder, A., Schönherr, H., Vancso, G.J., Huskens, J., and Reinhoudt, D.N. (2005) *Chem. Eur. J.*, **11**, 3988.

34 Nijhuis, C.A., Sinha, J.K., Wittstock, G., Huskens, J., Ravoo, B.J., and Reinhoudt, D.N. (2006) *Langmuir*, **22**, 9770.

35 Ludden, M.L.W., Mulder, A., Schulze, K., Subramaniam, V., Tampe, R., and Huskens, J. (2008) *Chem. Eur. J.*, **14**, 2044.

36 Kim, Y., Kim, D., Park, J., Shin, G., Kim, G., and Ha, J. (2008) *Langmuir*, **24**, 14289.

37 Wu, X.C., Bittner, A.M., and Kern, K. (2004) *Adv. Mater.*, **16**, 413.

38 Degenhart, G.H., Dordi, B., Schonherr, H., and Vancso, G.J. (2004) *Langmuir*, **20**, 6216.

39 Kohli, N., Dvornic, P.R., Kaganove, S.N., Worden, R.M., and Lee, I. (2004) *Macromol. Rapid Commun.*, **25**, 935.

40 Campbell, C.J., Smoukov, S.K., Bishop, K.J.M., and Grzybowski, B.A. (2005) *Langmuir*, **21**, 2637.

41 Vogelaar, L., Barsema, J.N., van Rijn, C.J.M., Nijdam, W., and Wessling, M. (2003) *Adv. Mater.*, **15**, 1385.

42 Vogelaar, L., Lammertink, R.G.H., Barsema, J.N., Nijdam, W., Bolhuis-Versteeg, L.A.M., van Rijn, C.J.M., and Wessling, M. (2005) *Small*, **1**, 645.

43 Xu, H., Ling, X., van Bennekom, J., Duan, X., Ludden, M.J.W., Reinhoudt, D.N., Wessling, M., Lammertink, R.G.H., and Huskens, J. (2009) *J. Am. Chem. Soc.*, **2**, 797.

44 Allen, C.G., Dorr, J.C., Khandekar, A.A., Beach, J.D., Schick, I.C., Schick, E.J., Collins, R.T., and Kuech, T.F. (2007) *Thin Solid Films*, **515**, 6812.

45 Hidber, P.O., Helbig, W., Kim, E., and Whitesides, G.M. (1996) *Langmuir*, **12**, 1375.

46 Hidber, P.O., Nealey, P.F., Helbig, W., and Whitesides, G.M. (1996) *Langmuir*, **12**, 5209.

47 Kind, H., Geissler, M., Schmid, H., Michel, B., Kern, K., and Delamarche, E. (2000) *Langmuir*, **16**, 6367.

48 Xue, M., Zhang, Z., Zhu, N., Wang, F., Zhao, X., and Cao, T. (2009) *Langmuir*, **25**, 4347.

49 Chen, J., Mela, P., Möller, M., and Lensen, M.C. (2009) *ACS Nano*, **3**, 1451.

50 Whitesides, G.M., and Laibinis, P.E. (1990) *Langmuir*, **6**, 87.

51 Wenzl, I., Yam, C.M., Barriet, D., and Lee, T.R. (2003) *Langmuir*, **19**, 10217.

52 Colorado, R. Jr and Lee, T.R. (2003) *Langmuir*, **19**, 3288.

53 Burleigh, T.D., Gu, Y., Donahey, G., Vida, M., and Waldeck, D.H. (2001) *Corrosion*, **57**, 1066.

54 Jennings, G.K., Yong, T.-H., Munro, J.C., and Laibinis, P.E. (2003) *J. Am. Chem. Soc.*, **125**, 2950.

55 Petrenko, V.F. and Peng, S. (2003) *Can. J. Phys.*, **81**, 387.

56 Leggett, G.J. (2003) *Anal. Chim. Acta*, **479**, 17.

57 Ahn, H.-S., Cuong, P.D., Park, S., Kim, Y.-W., and Lim, J.-C. (2003) *Wear*, **255**, 819.

58 Adams, D.M., Brus, L., Chidsey, C.E.D., Creager, S., Creutz, C., Kagan, C.R., Kamat, P.V., Lieberman, M., Lindsay, S., Marcus, R.A., Metzger, R.M., Michel-Beyerle, M.E., Miller, J.R., Newton, M.D., Rolison, D.R., Sankey, O., Schanze, K.S., Yardley, J., and Zhu, X. (2003) *J. Phys. Chem. B*, **107**, 6668.

59 Salomon, A., Cahen, D., Lindsay, S., Tomfohr, J., Engelkes, V.B., and Frisbie, C.D. (2003) *Adv. Mater.*, **15**, 1881.

60 Aizenberg, J. (2000) *J. Chem. Soc., Dalton Trans.*, 3963.

61 Ostuni, E., Yan, L., and Whitesides, G.M. (1999) *Colloids Surf. B*, **15**, 3.

62 Mrksich, M. (2002) *Curr. Opin. Chem. Biol.*, **6**, 794.

63 Xia, Y., Zhao, X., and Whitesides, G.M. (1996) *Microelectron. Eng.*, **32**, 255.

64 Kumar, A., Biebuyck, H.A., Abbott, N.L., and Whitesides, G.M. (1992) *J. Am. Chem. Soc.*, **114**, 9188.

65 Geissler, M., Schmid, H., Bietsch, A., Michel, B., and Delamarche, E. (2002) *Langmuir*, **18**, 2374.

66 Wolfe, D.B., Love, J.C., Paul, K.E., Chabinyc, M.L., and Whitesides, G.M. (2002) *Appl. Phys. Lett.*, **80**, 2222.

67 Zhao, X.M., Wilbur, J.L., and Whitesides, G.M. (1996) *Langmuir*, **12**, 3257.

68 Love, J.C., Wolfe, D.B., Haasch, R., Chabinyc, M.L., Paul, K.E., Whitesides, G.M., and Nuzzo, R.G. (2003) *J. Am. Chem. Soc.*, **125**, 2597.

69 Carvalho, A., Geissler, M., Schmid, H., Michel, B., and Delamarche, E. (2002) *Langmuir*, **18**, 2406.

70 Michel, B., Bernard, A., Bietsch, A., Delamarche, E., Geissler, M., Juncker, D., Kind, H., Renault, J.P., Rothuizen, H., Schmid, H., Schmidt-Winkel, P., Stutz, R., and Wolf, H. (2001) *IBM J. Res. Dev.*, **45**, 697.

71 Love, J.C., Wolfe, D.B., Chabinyc, M.L., Paul, K.E., and Whitesides, G.M. (2002) *J. Am. Chem. Soc.*, **124**, 1576.

72 Wolf, S. (1990) *Silicon Processing for the VLSI Era*, Lattice Press, Sunset Beach.

73 Kim, E., Whitesides, G.M., Freiler, M.B., Levy, M., Lin, J.L., and Osgood, R.M. (1996) *Nanotechnology*, **7**, 266.

74 Delamarche, E., Geissler, M., Wolf, H., and Michel, B. (2002) *J. Am. Chem. Soc.*, **124**, 3834.

75 Saalmink, M., van der Marel, C., Stapert, H.R., and Burdinski, D. (2006) *Langmuir*, **22**, 1016.

76 Trimbach, D.C., Al-Hussein, M., de Jeu, W.H., Decré, M., Broer, D.J., and Bastiaansen, C.W.M. (2004) *Langmuir*, **20**, 4738.

77 Lee, M.S., Hong, S.-C., and Kim, D. (2004) *Jpn. J. Appl. Phys.*, **43**, 8347.

78 Shah, R.R., Merreceyes, D., Husemann, M., Rees, I., Abbott, N.L., Hawker, C.J., and Hedrick, J.L. (2000) *Macromolecules*, **33**, 597.

79 Tu, H., Heitzman, C.E., and Braun, P.V. (2004) *Langmuir*, **20**, 8313.

80 Huang, S., Dai, L., and Mau, A. (2002) *Physica B*, **322**, 333.

81 Gu, G., Philipp, G., Wu, X., Burghard, M., Bittner, A.M., and Roth, S. (2001) *Adv. Funct. Mater.*, **11**, 295.

82 Argyrakis, P., Teo, L., Stevenson, T., and Cheung, R. (2005) *Microelectron. Eng.*, **78–79** 647.

83 Casimirius, S., Flahaut, E., Laberty-Robert, C., Malaquin, L., Carcenac, F., Laurent, C., and Vieu, C. (2004) *Microelectron. Eng.*, **73–74**, 564.

84 Melosh, N.A., Boukai, A., Diana, F., Gerardot, B., Badolato, A., Petroff, P.M., and Heath, J.R. (2003) *Science*, **300**, 112.

85 Loo, Y.L., Hsu, J.W.P., Willett, R.L., Baldwin, K.W., West, K.W., and Rogers, J.A. (2002) *J. Vac. Sci. Technol. B*, **20**, 2853.

86 Jeon, S., Menard, E., Park, J.-U., Maria, J., Meitl, M., Zaumseil, J., and Rogers, J.A. (2004) *Adv. Mater.*, **16**, 1369.

87 Menard, E., Bilhaut, L., Zaumseil, J., and Rogers, J.A. (2004) *Langmuir*, **20**, 6871.

88 Schmid, H., Wolf, H., Allenspach, R., Riel, H., Karg, S., Michel, B., and Delamarche, E. (2003) *Adv. Funct. Mater.*, **13**, 145.

89 Lasky, J.B. (1986) *Appl. Phys. Lett.*, **48**, 78.

90 Tong, Q.Y. (2001) *Mater. Sci. Eng., B*, **B87**, 323.

91 Zaumseil, J., Meitl, M.A., Hsu, J.W.P., Acharya, B.R., Baldwin, K.W., Loo, Y.-L., and Rogers, J.A. (2003) *Nano Lett.*, **3**, 1223.

92 Loo, Y.L., Willett, R.L., Baldwin, K.W., and Rogers, J.A. (2002) *Appl. Phys. Lett.*, **81**, 562.

93 Loo, Y.L., Lang, D.V., Rogers, J.A., and Hsu, J.W.P. (2003) *Nano Lett.*, **3**, 913.

94 Loo, Y.L., Willett, R.L., Baldwin, K.W., and Rogers, J.A. (2002) *J. Am. Chem. Soc.*, **124**, 7654.

95 Wang, Z., Yuan, J., Zhang, J., Xing, R., Yan, D., and Han, Y. (2003) *Adv. Mater.*, **15**, 1009.

96 Helt, J.M., Drain, C.M., and Batteas, J.D. (2004) *J. Am. Chem. Soc.*, **126**, 628.

97 Wolfe, D.B., Love, J.C., Gates, B.D., Whitesides, G.M., Conroy, R.S., and Prentiss, M. (2004) *Appl. Phys. Lett.*, **84**, 1623.

98 Childs, W.R. and Nuzzo, R.G. (2002) *J. Am. Chem. Soc.*, **124**, 13583.

99 Childs, W.R. and Nuzzo, R.G. (2004) *Adv. Mater.*, **16**, 1323.

100 Jackman, R.J., Duffy, D.C., Cherniavskaya, O., and Whitesides, G.M. (1999) *Langmuir*, **15**, 2973.

101 Jackman, R.J., Duffy, D.C., Ostuni, E., Willmore, N.D., and Whitesides, G.M. (1998) *Anal. Chem.*, **70**, 2280.

102 Sassolas, A., Leca-Bouvier, B.D., and Blum, L.J. (2008) *Chem. Rev.*, **108**, 109.

103 Zhu, H. and Snyder, M. (2003) *Curr. Opin. Chem. Biol.*, **7**, 55.

104 Feizi, T., Fazio, F., Chai, W., and Wong, C.H. (2003) *Curr. Opin. Struct. Biol.*, **13**, 637.

105 Kane, R.S., Takayama, S., Ostuni, E., Ingber, D.E., and Whitesides, G.M. (1999) *Biomaterials*, **20**, 2363.

106 Chen, C.S., Mrksich, M., Huang, S., Whitesides, G.M., and Ingber, D.E. (1997) *Science*, **276**, 1425.

107 (a) Graber, D.J., Zieziulewicz, T.J., Lawrence, D.A., Shain, W., and Turner, J.N. (2003) *Langmuir*, **19**, 5431;(b) LaGraff, J.R. and Chu-LaGraff, Q. (2006) *Langmuir*, **22**, 4685.

108 Tan, J.L., Tien, J., and Chen, C.S. (2002) *Langmuir*, **18**, 519.

109 Renault, J.P., Bernard, A., Bietsch, A., Michel, B., Bosshard, H.R., Delamarche, E., Kreiter, E., Hecht, B., and Wild, U.P. (2003) *J. Phys. Chem. B*, **107**, 703.

110 Yeung, C.K., Lauer, L., Offenhausser, A., and Knoll, W. (2001) *Neurosci. Lett.*, **301**, 147.

111 Park, T.J., Lee, S.Y., Lee, S.J., Park, J.P., Yang, K.S., Lee, K.B., Ko, S., Park, J.B., Kim, T., Kim, S.K., Shin, Y.B., Chung, B.H., Ku, S.J., Kim, D.H., and Choi, I.S. (2006) *Anal. Chem.*, **78**, 7197.

112 Kwak, S.K., Lee, G.S., Ahn, D.J., and Choi, J.W. (2004) *Mater. Sci. Eng. C - Bio.*, **24**, 151.

113 Wilhelm, T. and Wittstock, G. (2002) *Langmuir*, **18**, 9485.

114 Biasco, A., Pisignano, D., Krebs, B., Cingolani, R., and Rinaldi, R. (2005) *Synthetic Met.*, **153**, 21.

115 James, C.D., Davis, R.C., Kam, L., Craighead, H.G., Isaacson, M., Turner, J.N., and Shain, W. (1998) *Langmuir*, **14**, 741.

116 Delamarche, E., Geissler, M., Bernard, A., Wolf, H., Michel, B., Hilborn, J., and Donzel, C. (2001) *Adv. Mater.*, **13**, 1164.

117 Geissler, M., Bernard, A., Bietsch, A., Schmid, H., Michel, B., and Delamarche, E. (2000) *J. Am. Chem. Soc.*, **122**, 6303.

118 Zheng, Z., Jang, J.W., Zheng, G., and Mirkin, C.A. (2008) *Angew. Chem., Int. Ed.*, **47**, 9951.

119 Rozkiewicz, D.I., Brugman, W., Kerkhoven, R.M., Ravoo, B.J., and Reinhoudt, D.N. (2007) *J. Am. Chem. Soc.*, **129**, 11593.

120 Rożkiewicz, D.I., Gierlich, J., Burley, G.A., Gutsmiedl, K., Carell, T., Ravoo, B.J., and Reinhoudt, D.N. (2007) *ChemBioChem*, **8**, 1997.

121 Xu, C., Taylor, P., Ersoz, M., Fletcher, P.D.J., and Paunov, V. (2003) *J. Mater. Chem.*, **13**, 3044.

122 Hovis, J.S. and Boxer, S.G. (2001) *Langmuir*, **17**, 3400.

123 Kung, L.A., Kam, L., Hovis, J.S., and Boxer, S.G. (2000) *Langmuir*, **16**, 6773.

124 Renault, J.P., Bernard, A., Juncker, D., Michel, B., Bosshard, H.R., and Delamarche, E. (2002) *Angew. Chem., Int. Ed.*, **41**, 2320.

125 Jang, C.-H., Tingey, M.L., Korpi, N.L., Wiepz, G.J., Schiller, J.H., Bertics, P.J., and Abbott, N.L. (2005) *J. Am. Chem. Soc.*, **127**, 8912.

126 Tingey, M.L., Wilyana, S., Snodgrass, E.J., and Abbott, N.L. (2004) *Langmuir*, **20**, 6818.

127 Kim, J. and Crooks, R.M. (2007) *Anal. Chem.*, **79**, 7267.

128 Yu, A.A., Savas, T.A., Taylor, G.S., Elie, A.G., Smith, H.I., and Stellacci, F. (2005) *Nano Lett.*, **5**, 1061.

129 Helmuth, J.A., Schmid, H., Stutz, R., Stemmer, A., and Wolf, H. (2006) *J. Am. Chem. Soc.*, **128**, 9296.

130 (a) Love, J.C., Estroff, L.A., Kriebel, J.K., Nuzzo, R.G., and Whitesides, G.M. (2005) *Chem. Rev.*, **105**, 1103;
(b) Onclin, S., Ravoo, B.J., and Reinhoudt, D.N. (2005) *Angew. Chem., Int. Ed.*, **44**, 6282.

131 Ravoo, B.J. (2009) *J. Mater. Chem.*, **19**, 8902.

132 Sullivan, T.P. and Huck, W.T.S. (2003) *Eur. J. Org. Chem.*, 17.

133 (a) Yan, L., Zhao, X.M., and Whitesides, G.M. (1998) *J. Am. Chem. Soc.*, **120**, 6179;
(b) Yan, L., Huck, W.T.S., Zhao, X.M., and Whitesides, G.M. (1999) *Langmuir*, **15**, 1208;(c) Lahiri, J., Ostuni, E., and Whitesides, G.M. (1999) *Langmuir*, **15**, 2055.

134 Sullivan, T.P., van Poll, M.L., Dankers, P.Y.W., and Huck, W.T.S. (2004) *Angew. Chem., Int. Ed.*, **43**, 4190.

135 Rozkiewicz, D.I., Ravoo, B.J., and Reinhoudt, D.N. (2005) *Langmuir*, **21**, 6337.

136 Rozkiewicz, D.I., Kraan, Y., Werten, M.W.T., de Wolf, F.A., Subramaniam, V.,

Ravoo, B.J., and Reinhoudt, D.N. (2006) *Chem. Eur. J.*, **12**, 6290.

137 Rozkiewicz, D.I., Jancewski, D., Verboom, W., Ravoo, B.J., and Reinhoudt, D.N. (2006) *Angew. Chem., Int. Ed.*, **45**, 5292.

138 (a) Rostovtsev, V.V., Green, L.G., Fokin, V.V., and Sharpless, K.B. (2002) *Angew. Chem., Int. Ed.*, **42**, 2596;(b) Tornøe, C.W., Christensen, C., and Meldal, M. (2002) *J. Org. Chem.*, **67**, 3057.

139 Kolb, H.C., Finn, M.G., and Sharpless, K.B. (2001) *Angew. Chem., Int. Ed.*, **40**, 2004.

140 Michel, O. and Ravoo, B.J. (2008) *Langmuir*, **24**, 12116.

141 Li, X.M., Peter, M., Huskens, J., and Reinhoudt, D.N. (2003) *Nano Lett.*, **3**, 1449.

142 Shestopalov, A.A., Clark, R.L., and Toone, E.J. (2007) *J. Am. Chem. Soc.*, **129**, 13818.

143 Snyder, P.W., Johannes, M.S., Vogen, B.N., Clark, R.L., and Toone, E.J. (2007) *J. Org. Chem.*, **72**, 7459.

144 Spruell, J.M., Sheriff, B.A., Rozkiewicz, D.I., Dichtel, W.R., Rohde, R.D., Reinhoudt, D.N., Stoddart, J.F., and Heath, J.R. (2008) *Angew. Chem., Int. Ed.*, **47**, 9927.

145 Hyun, J., Zhu, Y., Liebmann-Vinson, A., Beebe, T.P., and Chilkoti, A. (2001) *Langmuir*, **17**, 6358.

146 Feng, C.L., Vancso, G.J., and Schönherr, H. (2006) *Adv. Funct. Mater.*, **16**, 1306.

147 Nandivada, H., Chen, H.Y., Bondarenko, L., and Lahann F J. (2006) *Angew. Chem., Int. Ed.*, **45**, 3360.

148 Truong, T.T., Lin, R., Jeon, S., Lee, H., Maria, J., Gaur, A., Hua, F., Meinel, I., and Rogers, J.A. (2007) *Langmuir*, **23**, 2898.

149 Yoo, P.J., Choi, S.J., Kim, J.H., Suh, D., Baek, S.J., Kim, T.W., and Lee, H.H. (2004) *Chem. Mater.*, **16**, 5000.

150 Csucs, G., Künzler, T., Feldman, K., Robin, F., and Spencer, N.D. (2003) *Langmuir*, **19**, 6104.

151 Tormen, M., Borzenko, T., Steffen, B., Schmidt, G., and Molenkamp, L.W. (2002) *Microelectron. Eng.*, **61**, 469.

152 Bessueille, F., Pla-Roca, M., Mills, C.A., Martinez, E., Samitier, J., and Errachid, A. (2005) *Langmuir*, **21**, 12060.

153 Libouille, L., Bietsch, A., Schmid, H., Michel, B., and Delamarche, E. (1999) *Langmuir*, **15**, 300.

154 Liebau, M., Huskens, J., and Reinhoudt, D.N. (2001) *Adv. Funct. Mater.*, **11**, 147.

155 Perl, A., Peter, M., Ravoo, B.J., Reinhoudt, D.N., and Huskens, J. (2006) *Langmuir*, **22**, 7568.

156 Wu, X., Lenhert, S., Chi, L., and Fuchs, H. (2006) *Langmuir*, **22**, 7807.

157 Sharpe, R.B.A., Titulaer, B.J.F., Peeters, E., Burdinski, D., Huskens, J., Zandvliet, H.J.W., Reinhoudt, D.N., and Poelsema, B. (2006) *Nano Lett.*, **6**, 1235.

158 Xue, M., Yang, Y., and Cao, T. (2008) *Adv. Mater.*, **20**, 596.

159 Sharpe, R.B.A., Burdinski, D., Huskens, J., Zandvliet, H.J.W., Reinhoudt, D.N., and Poelsema, B. (2005) *J. Am. Chem. Soc.*, **127**, 10344.

4

Advances in Nanoimprint Lithography: 2-D and 3-D Nanopatterning of Surfaces by Nanoimoprint Lithography, Morphological Characterization, and Photonic Applications

Vincent Reboud, Timothy Kehoe, Nikolaos Kehagias, and Clivia M. Sotomayor Torres

4.1
Introduction

The advances in nanofabrication by emerging patterning methods made during the past fourteen years have been dramatic, ranging from laboratory-scale experiments reviewed in 2003 [1] to reports on some of these methods appearing in the road map of the most demanding industry, namely microelectronics [2]. Among these methods, which include self-assembly, microcontact printing, scanning probes and nanoimprint lithography (NIL), attention in this chapter is focused mainly on NIL, since it is perhaps the most mature of the then-emerging nanofabrication methods.

NIL as a nanopatterning process has intrinsically many advantages, since it combines simplicity with a wealth of functional materials based on polymers. At present, one trend is to develop NIL processes to fabricate three-dimensional (3-D) structures, tiered or wood-pile or combinations thereof, among others. There is an enormous demand to replicate polymers with combined micro- and nanometer features that require 3-D nanopatterning. In this chapter, details are provided of the many studies reported to date in 3-D NIL, in addition to those of the present authors' own contributions to the field. It will be seen that whilst 3-D NIL and resolution below 20 nm are still to be met, solid progress is being made nonetheless.

Today, the transition from a laboratory-scale method to a full-scale technology is still in progress, albeit well advanced, with commercial printing equipment available in the market, a preliminary set of NIL processes for specific applications [3], and continued rapid developments in tools, designs, stamps, process simulations, materials and applications. During this transition, the importance of metrology cannot be underestimated since, without nanometrology for the critical dimensions, it would be very difficult to transfer such applications to the production stage. The status of metrology in NIL is also described in the chapter, with an incursion into the physical properties of polymer films thinner than 10 nm. Clearly, there is still a long way to go in this area, and innovative methods are much in demand.

Nanotechnology, Volume 8: Nanostructured Surfaces. Edited by Lifeng Chi
Copyright © 2010 WILEY-VCH Verlag GmbH & Co. KGaA, Weinheim
ISBN: 978-3-527-31739-4

One application of NIL which has experienced major progress due to the functionality offered by polymers when mixed with nanoparticles (whereby they are converted into a nanocomposite), has been in the area of *photonics*. Here, the feature sizes are slightly larger and the tolerances slightly more relaxed than in, for example, electronic applications. Hence, the potential uses of NIL can be illustrated in the field of photonics by two device-like structures, and a perspective offered in this area of applications.

4.2
Three-Dimensional, Nanoimprint-Based Lithography

4.2.1
Background

In this section, an overview is provided of the nanoimprint-based techniques used to fabricate 3-D structures. During the past few years, several next-generation lithography (NGL) techniques have been developed and progressed beyond the 22 nm barrier node. To meet this demand, the semiconductor industry has for example used adapted photolithographic processes with ever-decreasing wavelengths – from optical, to ultraviolet (UV), to deep UV, to extreme UV – in an effort to beat the diffraction limit, but this led to dramatic increases in tool costs. In contrast, imprint-based lithography techniques require neither expensive projection optics, advanced illumination sources, nor specialized resist materials.

There are two basic approaches to imprint lithography (Figure 4.1) based on the use of temperature (thermal NIL) and/or ultraviolet light (UV-NIL) to transfer the

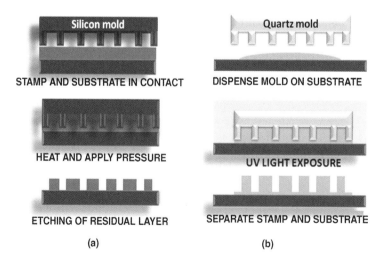

Figure 4.1 Schematic representations of (a) the thermal NIL process and (b) the UV-NIL process.

Table 4.1 Surface energies of common materials used in nanoimprint lithography. Values taken from Ref. [9].

Material	Surface energy (mN m^{-1})
PMMA	41.1
PS	40.7
PTFE	15.6
$-CF3$ and $-CF2$	15–17
Silicon surface	20–26

mold to the imprinted resist. In thermal NIL (Figure 4.1a), as developed by S. Chou *et al.* [4, 5], a hard template (mold/stamp) such as silicon is used to imprint a thermoplastic polymer that is then heated to a temperature above the polymer glass transition temperature (T_g), while applying a relatively high pressure. After a specific time, which depends on the architecture and topography of the template, the polymer is cooled to a temperature below its T_g, at which point the stamp and substrate can be separated. In order to minimize the adhesion between the imprinted resist and the mold, a fluorine-based material is deposited onto the mold surface [6] to serve as an anti-adhesive agent.

The values of surface energy of the most frequently used materials are listed in Table 4.1. Features as small as 5 nm [7] have been reported, while in a separate report 200 mm wafer surfaces have been patterned successfully [8]. These features position NIL as a high-throughput lithographic technique capable of functioning within small- and medium-sized manufacturing companies.

In 1998, a modified nanoimprint process was developed at the University of Texas (UT-Austin) by the group of C.G. Wilson [10]. In this process, which was referred to as step and flash nanoimprint lithography (SFIL), a photo-curable liquid resist was molded in a step-and-repeat manner by applying UV light when the transparent mold was in contact with the resist (see Figure 4.1b). Unlike thermal NIL, the SFIL process was carried out at room temperature and used relatively low pressures, which in turn led to a significant reduction in the imprint time. The latest generation of SFIL tools has a specification for 300 mm wafers [11], with sub-50 nm resolution [12], and today several instruments are available commercially from several suppliers, including the EV Group, Molecular Imprints, Nanonex, Obducat, and Smart Equipment Technology.

The main achievements of thermal and UV-based NIL are summarized and compared in Table 4.2.

In comparison to the photolithography process, NIL-based methods are referred to as "1 × 1 processes"; that is, the resolution of both imprint-based techniques is determined by the resolution of the template. Unfortunately, this advantage of ultimate resolution could in time become a disadvantage, since any unintentional template artifact might be transferred with high fidelity to the molded material. It is for this reason that high-quality (noncontaminated) templates must be fabricated,

Table 4.2 Comparison of the two basic imprint techniques.

Technique	Smallest/ largest features in same print	Minimum pitch (nm)	Largest wafer printed (mm)	Overlay accuracy (nm)	T align, T print, T release, T cycle	No. of times stamp used
NIL	5 nm [13]/N/A	14	200 [14]	500	Minutes, 10 s, Min, 10–15 min	>50
SFIL	25 nm/μm	50	300 [15, 16] stamp size: ~26 × 26 mm^2	50 [17]	20 wafers per hour [18]	800

and nondestructive inspected methods employed to maintain the quality control of the system. An example of a nondestructive, nano-metrological technique is described in the following subsection.

Currently, imprint-based process are investigated for the manufacture of, for example, photonic crystal devices [19], micro- and nano-optical components [20], and media storage devices [21]. Today, one of the most interesting applications and capabilities of NIL techniques is the direct imprinting of multilevel structures; this is of particular interest in the semiconductor industry, as the simultaneous imprinting of multiple device levels can greatly reduce the number of steps (by about 50%) associated with back-end-of-line (BEOL) processing [22].

In 2005, a research group at the University of Texas proposed the use of a dual damascene imprint template, rather than a traditional lithographic method, to build the metal interconnect stack [23]. For such a process a hard template with tiered-like structures was required and, depending on the type of imprint method, either a transparent (UVNIL) or nontransparent (thermal NIL) mold was used. The imprinted material used would then need to be either a UV-curable resist or a thermoplastic film, respectively. Although, in most thermal NIL cases, the template used was of similar size to the imprinted substrate, the production of the mold was always very expensive. Moreover, in UVNIL (and particularly in SFIL mode) the template was much smaller (ca. 2 × 2 cm^2) and the imprint proceeded in a step-and-repeat fashion. This led to an increase in throughput in SFIL, since lower temperatures and pressures were required compared to thermal NIL. However, these lower values also helped to achieve sub-100 nm alignment between the two layers.

A schematic representation of the multilayer imprint process is shown in Figure 4.2. In this procedure, a rigid transparent stamp is first brought into close proximity to, and in alignment with, the substrate. A low-viscosity photocurable resist is then dispensed onto the pre-patterned substrate, most likely using areas with metallic stripes. The stamp and substrate are then brought into contact, followed by UV light exposure when the cavities in the stamps has been filled by the resist. In most cases, the resist used is a low-molecular-weight monomer incorporating

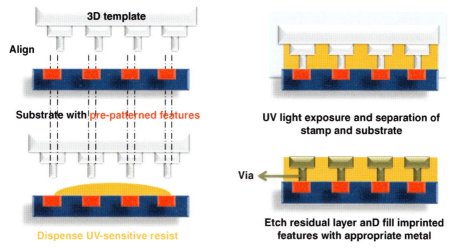

Figure 4.2 Fabrication process of a multilayer interconnection with UVNIL technology.

photoinitiator molecules. When the resist has polymerized the stamp can be removed, leaving behind an inverse patterned replica. As in thermal NIL, a thin residual layer always remains that can be removed by using a classical reactive ion etching (RIE) method. Infiltration of the opened (imprinted) areas is then carried out in order to connect the two levels. Compared to photolithographic methods, the imprint-based strategy for the fabrication of interconnected structures will reduce by half the steps required to wire the adjacent layers.

As described above, alignment of the via and upper wiring level is carried out at the template fabrication stage, such that only one alignment step per metal layer is required during the fabrication sequence [24]. Thus, it becomes clear that one of the most challenging issues of direct multilayer nanopatterning is the fabrication of 3-D stamps (Figure 4.3), and several techniques have been proposed for the creation of such templates. The "pros" and "cons" of each technique, together with representative scanning electron microscopy (SEM) images, are listed in Table 4.3. The data in Table 4.3 indicate that, although direct 3-D patterning can be achieved by NIL with a high throughput, it is still necessary to fabricate the master with a single lithographic technique (though a combination of techniques may sometimes be needed). There appear to be several limiting factors that hinder the use of these techniques for the mass production of 3-D devices, including high cost, low throughput, low resolution, and complexity of procedure.

In order to create more complex structures, several other methods involving a combination of different techniques have been investigated; details of these "nonconventional" 3-D patterning methods are listed in Table 4.4. For applications in photonics, and in particular for the creation of 3-D devices such as photonic crystals, it is important to minimize the number of steps in the stacking process. In this way, the excessive use of lift-off, sacrificial layer removal and etching that is normally performed in planar technologies, can be avoided. Moreover, alignment to

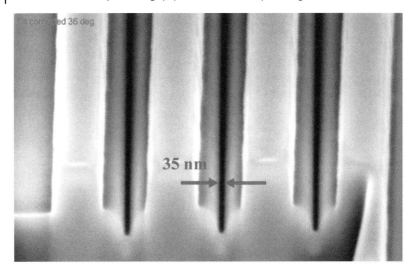

Figure 4.3 Tilted scanning electron microscopy (SEM) image of a tiered-like Si template fabricated by focused ion beam (FIB) lithography.

within $\sim\lambda/20$ is also necessary. One of the most difficult milestones for imprint-based technologies has been is to prove their ability to fabricate 3-D devices at the optical scales. Despite integration in the third dimension requiring compact, fast and cost-efficient device fabrication methods, several modified imprint-based techniques have been described as possible solutions to these problems.

Within the context of 3-D nanofabrication, two alternative fabrication processes have been developed, the details of which are presented below. Whilst both of these (imprint-based) techniques are capable of meeting the important requirements of high resolution and low cost, issues of alignment and reproducibility in large-scale areas have yet to be resolved. Hence, in the following subsections, after a brief discussion of the reversal nanoimprint technique and its potential, the limiting factors responsible for its poor uptake as a method for patterning 3-D device-like structures are outlined. In addition, as an alternative to the reversal imprint technique, a novel method of fabrication is introduced, namely reverse-contact UVNIL.

4.2.2
Reverse NIL

As discussed above, by using NIL it is possible to transfer a wide variety of stamp profiles into a polymer, although the 3-D patterning possibilities are limited. However, recent progress in nanoimprinting techniques has led to the introduction of a new method that is similar to NIL and might provide a solution to this problem. In the so-called "reverse nanoimprint" technique [30] or "bonding" process [31], the

Table 4.3 Conventional direct 3-D patterning techniques, indicating whether the technique is sequential or parallel.

Method	Advantages/Drawbacks	Features fabricated
Electron beam Resist is exposed to a focused electron beam. Two axes of rotation and enhanced control of focus for a true 3-D fabrication are needed (Sequential)	*Advantages:* High-resolution (sub-10 nm) *Drawbacks:* Low throughput Limited exposure depth Limited area Electron scattering in resist and substrate	Sub-100 nm 2-D plasmonic crystal structure made by means of EBL
X-ray lithography Illumination of a X-ray mask. 3-D obtained by multiple exposures of the sample at tilted angles. (Parallel)	*Advantages:* Resolution sub-50 nm Aspect ratio ~20 High throughput *Drawbacks:* Complex process High cost	Photonic crystal [25]
Focused ion beam Direct milling or growth of material by accelerated and focused ions. 3-D achieved by control of ion energy and tilted angles. (Sequential)	*Advantages:* High resolution (sub-20 nm) High aspect ratio ~40 *Drawbacks:* Low throughput Gaussian beam Limited area	Photonic crystal structure with holes of 160 nm diameter
Two-photon lithography Photopolymer is exposed to a focused femtosecond laser beam. (Sequential)	*Advantages:* High resolution Arbitrary shapes In-depth writing *Drawbacks:* Low throughput Complex process	Microbull [26]

(Continued)

Table 4.3 *(Continued)*

Method	Advantages/Drawbacks	Features fabricated
Direct 3-D NIL Deformation of a thermo-plastic polymer by a rigid mold, followed by dry etching (Parallel)	*Advantages:* High resolution (sub-10 nm) High throughput *Drawbacks:* Low aspect ratio $\sim$3 Nonarbitrary shapes	Top view SEM image of direct 3-D structure. Insert shows a schematic of the profile

EBL = electron beam lithography.

polymer film is first spin-coated onto the stamp and then transferred to the substrate; by simply repeating the process on the same substrate, it is then possible to build 3-D polymer structures in a layer-by-layer fashion. Most importantly, the reverse NIL process can be carried out at a much lower temperature ($T_{imp} \sim T_g$) than conventional NIL, which allows the imprint cycles to be shortened. Unfortunately, one problem associated with this technique when using thermoplastic polymers is that each additional layer requires polymers with a progressively lower glass transition temperature (T_g) [32], and this in turn limits the number of layers formed. The reverse nanoimprint process where, depending on the size and density of the stamp features, either a "whole-layer transfer" mode or an "inking" mode can be observed, is shown schematically in Figure 4.4.

In recently conducted reverse imprinting experiments [33], two different transfer modes were observed, depending on the stamp topography. For features above 1 μm, and if the protrusions on the stamp were not too dense – that is, if the stamp presented a protrusion area of about 25% or less – then the "inking" transfer mode was observed. In this case, a positive copy of the stamp remained on the substrate because only the polymer on top of the stamp protrusions was transferred, and as a result no residual layer remained after reverse imprinting. This was due to the fact that spin-coating on such large and separated features created a non-flat film. An example of reverse imprint fabrication using the inking mode is shown in Figure 4.5, where a grating structure was imprinted on a 1 μm-period grating. In this case, even at a pressure of 60 bar, transfer of the top layer did not damage the underlying cured polymer grating.

Recently, Nakajima *et al.* [34] showed that, by controlling the temperatures of the mold and substrate at temperatures above and below T_g, respectively, the reverse imprint technique could be used to fabricate 3-D structures (nanochannels), using the same polymer [poly(methylmethacrylate); PMMA].

Table 4.4 Nonconventional direct 3-D patterning techniques.

Method	Advantage/Drawbacks	Features fabricated
Two-photon lithography and phase mask Photopolymer is exposed to an unfocused laser beam through conformable phase mask. (Parallel)	*Advantages:* Parallel In-depth writing *Drawback:* Complex process	Photonic crystal [27]
Combination of NIL and X-ray lithography X-ray lithography on a substrate pre-patterned by NIL	*Advantages:* Complex shapes High throughput *Drawback:* High cost	Pillars on hemispheres [26]
Combination of lithographic steps and wet etching	*Advantages:* High resolution Complex shapes at a relatively high throughput *Drawbacks:* Complex process Nonarbitrary shapes	Complex 3-D stamp for NIL [28]
Reverse NIL	*Advantages:* Sub-200 nm resolution Suspended structure *Drawbacks:* Alignment issues Reproducibility issues	Wood pile-like structures [29]

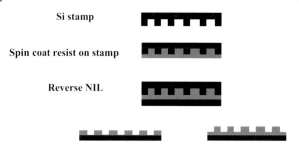

Figure 4.4 Schematics of the reverse nanoimprint process. Top to bottom: A polymer is first spin-coated onto the stamp, and then transferred to the flat or pre-patterned substrate.

4.2.3
Reverse-Contact UVNIL

A combination of the reversed NIL and UVNIL techniques has been shown to generate a promising nanofabrication technique termed reverse contact UVnanoimprint lithography (RUVNIL) [35–37]. This new technique has three main advantages: (i) the stamp does not need to be treated with an anti-adhesive layer; (ii) no residual layer remains after imprinting; and (iii) 3-D device-like structures can be obtained using the same polymer for each layer by repeating the procedure. Potentially, this method could be used to build up structures with several layers suitable, for example, in the fabrication of 3-D periodic structures. These might include photonic crystals with predicted defects, diffractive optical elements, and embedded channels for nano/micro fluidic devices for bioapplications.

This lithography process is illustrated schematically in Figure 4.6. A thin film of resist is first spin-coated onto the stamp (Figure 4.6b); this sacrificial polymer layer is used as an adherence promoter, as a planarization layer, and also to protect the stamp from being contaminated by the photocuring resist. A film of a UV crosslinkable polymer is then spin-coated onto the first layer (Figure 4.6c), after which the polymer bilayer is reverse-imprinted onto a flat or pre-patterned surface (Figure 4.6d). The stamp and substrate are then heated to a temperature above the T_g of mr-NIL 6000 (Figure 4.6e) and exposed to UV light. The stamp and substrate are separated just after a post-baking step (Figure 4.6f), thus ensuring a good adhesion between the polymer and the underlying substrate. Finally, both the unexposed polymer areas and the sacrificial layer are removed, leaving behind the negative features of the original stamp (Figure 4.6g). In this way, the oxygen plasma-etching step which is usually necessary in standard NIL is avoided.

Figure 4.7 shows the SEM images of 3-D structures fabricated by repeating the RUVNIL process described above. In particular, Figure 4.7a shows a cross-sectional SEM image of a bilayer woodpile-like structure, where there is no underflow of the second polymer layer on the first imprinted layer. In this case, 650 nm lines have been

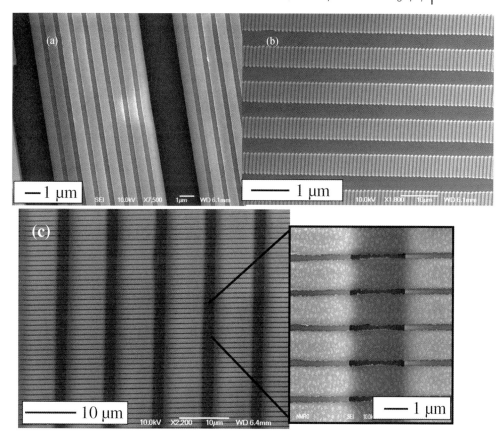

Figure 4.5 Examples of reverse-imprinted features in the whole-layer transfer mode. A 1 μm period grating is reverse-imprinted on a 10 μm period grating, with the lines (a) parallel or (b, c) perpendicular to each other. Depending on the features separation on the substrate, the transfer can be effective only on the protrusions (b) or on the whole surface, forming air-bridged structures (c).

RUVNIL-imprinted on 1 μm grating structures. A top-view SEM image of the same bilayer structure is shown in Figure 4.7b.

4.2.4
The Prospects for 3-D NIL

The mastering of 3-D NIL is expected to unlock an even wider range of applications, including supramolecular ordering and artificial tissues, while diffractive optical elements and complex light-handling curved structures constitute another avenue which is being actively pursued. However, such advances depend heavily on the stamp design and on material developments, as well as monitoring by suitable metrology.

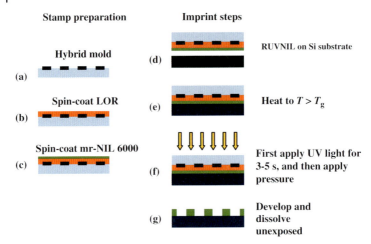

Figure 4.6 (a–c) Schematics of the stamp preparation steps; (d–g) Imprint steps of the RUVNIL technique.

The selective surface functionalization of horizontal or vertical or slopes represents a new challenge to be met in the development of artificial mesomaterials and micromaterials, with nanometer control of their properties – and, therefore, also of their functions.

4.3
Metrology for Nanoimprinting

4.3.1
Introduction

The metrological techniques used for NIL are similar to those that have been developed previously and are currently in use for nanofabrication generally, such as for deep UV optical lithography or electron beam lithography (EBL). Well-established techniques such as SEM [38, 39], atomic force microscopy (AFM) [40] and scatterometry [41] all find good use in characterizing surfaces structured by nanoimprinting. However, there are requirements to measure features that are particular to NIL, such as residual thickness and a complex line profile, and this influences the choice of established techniques which are used. This has also encouraged new developments, such as real-time scatterometry to measure line shape evolution due to reflow or annealing, and diffraction to monitor stamp-filling and detect defects. Polymer physical properties are critical to the nanoimprint process, and these include rheological properties, elastic modulus, and the T_g of the resist. Much effort has gone in to characterizing these at the nanometer scale, to detect changes due to the reduction of size, using methods including nanoindentation, Brillouin scattering, and photoacoustic metrology.

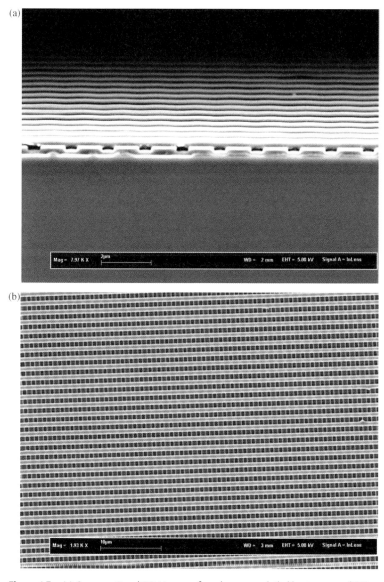

Figure 4.7 (a) Cross-sectional SEM image of a polymer woodpile-like structure; (b) Top view SEM image of the same 3 D cross bar structure (see text for details).

4.3.2
Scanning Electron Microscopy

Scanning electron microscopy is the standard "workhorse" metrology technique for NIL, as it is for all nanoscale structures and fabrication methods, whether biological, chemical, or physical. The latest commercially available field-emission SEM instru-

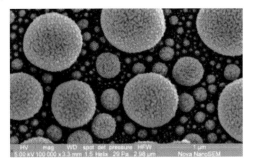

Figure 4.8 A test structure of tin particles, imaged using environmental SEM [43].

ments are capable of a resolution of less than 1 nm when used at high voltage, above 15 kV [42, 43]. High-voltage operation requires that the samples have a conducting surface, so as to remove the relatively large current deposited by the electron beam; consequently, such resolution is only possible when imaging stamp materials such as doped silicon or nickel, or resists made from conducting polymers, as might be used for EBL. The imaging of insulating materials such as quartz or glass (or indeed most of the polymers used as nanoimprint resists) at such high resolution generally requires a conductive coating layer of gold or other metal [44]. Uncoated small polymer structures can also be damaged by the electron beam current [45]; hence, in order to avoid damaging or altering the sample, the insulating surfaces can be imaged directly by using a low accelerating voltage for the electron beam, of approximately 1 kV or less [46], and using a partial vacuum with a low water vapor pressure to help remove the charge. This method, referred to as "environmental SEM" (Figure 4.8) [47], is the most common method by which nanoimprinted structures and processes are characterized [48].

The measurement of width-critical dimensions with SEM (or CD-SEM) requires the use of image-processing algorithms to assign a definite boundary to the gray edges of imaged features [49]. This is especially difficult if the edges themselves are sloped, although it is possible to assign a top and bottom width to features [50].

In order to measure thicknesses or 3-D profiles with SEM, it is necessary to make destructive cross-sections through samples [51]. Whilst this is performed routinely to make use of the excellent resolution of SEM, it leads inevitably to the waste of sample materials.

By using methods developed in the semiconductor fabrication industry, a large number of individual imprints and wafers have been tested, and statistical analyses applied to characterize the reliability of NIL as a large-scale nanofabrication method. This was typified by a recent study conducted at Sematech, the semiconductor industry research and development agency of the USA [52]. Results obtained using a Molecular Imprints Inc. Imprio300 instrument are summarized in Table 4.5. In this case, 300 mm wafers were imprinted with a stamp with a patterned area, or field, of 32 × 26 mm, and measurements made at five locations within each field (upper and lower left and right, and center), of the

Table 4.5 SEM results of thickness measurements of imprinted lines.

		Line 2	Line 4	Line 6
Lower Left	Average	32.4	33.7	31.9
	Min	30.1	30.9	30.2
	Max	33.3	34.7	32.8
	Range	3.2	3.8	2.6
	3 Sigma	1.5	1.6	1.3
Upper Left	Average	33.2	34.5	32.5
	Min	31.4	32.6	31
	Max	33.9	35.5	33.4
	Range	2.6	2.9	2.5
	3 Sigma	1.2	1.2	1.1
Center	Average	30.8	33	32.3
	Min	29	31.5	30.9
	Max	31.6	33.7	32.8
	Range	2.6	2.2	1.9
	3 Sigma	1.1	1	1
Lower Right	Average	32.1	33.7	32
	Min	30.7	32.1	30.4
	Max	32.8	34.4	32.6
	Range	2.1	2.3	2.2
	3 Sigma	1	1.1	0.9
Upper Right	Average	31	30.3	32.8
	Min	29.6	29	31.5
	Max	31.7	31	33.6
	Range	2.1	2	2.1
	3 Sigma	0.9	1	0.9

same three lines (Lines 2, 4, and 6). Of 2400 individual lines measured, across five wafers, the average width recorded was 32.4 nm, with three standard deviations (3σ) of 3.5 nm.

Whilst this represents an excellent degree of uniformity in fabrication, it must be considered in light of the very high standards required for the semiconductor industry. The International Technology Roadmap for Semiconductors (ITRS) sets a requirement of 3σ uniformity of less than 12% of the minimum feature size; hence, for the 32 nm node (which is due to be achieved by 2011 for Flash gate half pitch [53]) there is a uniformity requirement that 99.7% of all structures must be within ±3.8 nm of the 32 nm designed critical dimension. By this criterion, the Sematech NIL results are only just acceptable.

The ability to measure such critical dimension uniformity (0.32 nm) places a requirement on any metrology technique for a measurement repeatability of 10% of this (i.e., 0.32 nm) [54], which is approximately at the limit of what can be achieved by using SEM and scatterometry at present [55, 56]. The need for a metrology tool uncertainty of less than 0.3 nm remains an ongoing challenge, with metrology being pushed closely by the demands of reducing lithography feature sizes.

4.3.3
Atomic Force Microscopy

Atomic force microscopy is probably the most inexpensive method used to obtain nanoscale measurements, with instrument prices beginning at about €20 000 for the simplest designs. Hence, since its invention at IBM in 1986 [57], AFM has become a ubiquitous feature of laboratories. AFM is a powerful method that can be used to map the surface topography of a sample by scanning a probe across the sample's surface. The probe is held by a flexible cantilever, the deflection of which can be monitored, and this allows the relative height of the surface to be recorded. Since the displacement of the probe from the surface is known through the atomic forces between them, if the interaction with the surface is limited to one atom at the apex of the probe tip, then the atomic resolution of the surface can be determined [58].

The method is nondestructive and can be used on any type of surface, from conducting to insulating; moreover, atomic-scale resolution is possible even when used in air [59]. Because the atomic force between the probe and surface can be monitored, and is characteristic of the material present, it is possible to obtain physical, chemical, and dimensional information about the surface. As well as chemically distinguishing individual atoms of a certain material on the surface [60], it is also possible to measure frictional forces, by dragging the probe across the surface, lateral to the cantilever [61]; moreover, by pushing the probe tip into the surface and then withdrawing it, the viscoelastic properties of the material can be calculated from the force versus displacement curve [62]. This is of particular relevance to thermal nanoimprinting and nanoindentation (these are discussed further in Section 4.3.7).

While AFM is capable of extremely high spatial resolution, one drawback of the method is that it is relatively slow, and so is normally limited to imaging only a small part of the sample surface. The speed of the method is limited by the fact that a probe tip must be physically scanned across the surface while maintaining good contact; this allows an image to be built up serially by rastering back and forth across the surface. However, this cannot be achieved as quickly as scanning with an electron beam, or when optical methods, which sample an area of the surface in parallel. As a consequence, AFM has often taken the role of a reference metrology, and used to calibrate and improve the accuracy of other methods (e.g., SEM or scatterometry) being used to characterize a whole wafer [63].

One weakness of AFM is its limited ability to measure the width of high-aspect ratio structures. This stems from the shape of the probe tip, which is roughly pyramidal, and means that whilst at the probe apex one atom may interact with a flat surface, the increasing width of the probe away from the tip prevents access to narrow gaps and corners of features. Currently, this problem can be overcome by extending the probe tip with very high-aspect ratio structures such as carbon nanotubes (CNTs)

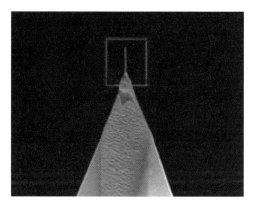

Figure 4.9 A carbon nanotube attached to the tip of an AFM probe [65].

(Figure 4.9) [64]. Curved and flared tips have also been used to improve access to sidewalls [65], while tips can also be tilted with respect to the surface [66], so that accurate 3-D profiles can be generated.

4.3.4
Transmission Electron Microscopy

Although transmission electron microscopy (TEM) is another extremely powerful technique, capable of atomic resolution [67], it requires samples which are thin enough to allow electrons to pass through (this is normally <100 nm, depending on the material). For this reason, the sample preparation – which normally involves cutting a slice of material with a focused ion beam – means that the technique takes a long time, and is destructive [68]. For this reason, TEM is also mainly used in nanofabrication to provide cross-sections as a reference metrology for quicker methods, such as SEM, scatterometry [69], and AFM [70].

4.3.5
Optical Critical Dimension Metrology: Scatterometry

The diffraction limit of light sets a lower bound on the size of what can be imaged optically to approximately half the wavelength of the light used. However, if the properties of the incident light are changed by the structure being investigated, then an image can be recreated from the reflected or scattered light, with resolution far below the diffraction limit [71]. Scatterometry uses the optical signal from an ellipsometer, applied to periodic structures, in which the change of the polarization of the scattered light depends upon the size and shape of the lines or other structures comprising it.

Ellipsometry is a one-dimensional method, used to measure the thickness and optical properties of planar layers, with a resolution of Angstroms, by analyzing the change of polarization of light reflected from the sample. Two curves are generated, based on the S and P polarizations of the reflected light (oscillating perpendicular and parallel to the plane of incidence) as a function either of wavelength, angle, or incident polarization. The curves generated by optical modeling are fitted to these in order to extract the data of layer thicknesses and complex refractive indices [72]. Ellipsometry is often used to establish the refractive index of flat samples of a material, to be used as input data for scatterometry measurements of patterned samples of the same material.

Reflectometry is another optical metrology, in which the light is incident normally on the sample, and the thickness is calculated from the intensity of the reflected light, which depends upon constructive or destructive interference, depending on the layer thickness [73]. Most optical metrology tool manufacturers provide versions of all three techniques [74, 75].

As with optical methods generally, *scatterometry* is both noncontact and nondestructive in nature. It is capable of measuring line widths as small as 20 nm with a resolution of less than 1 nm, depending on how many independent, or floating, variables there are in the analysis [76]. Scatterometry is an indirect measurement technique, in two important ways. Since it analyzes diffracted light, it is usually necessary to fabricate periodic test structures, alongside the structures to be characterized, which usually are not sufficiently periodic themselves [77], and dimensional data are taken from these test structures. Also, the structure is not imaged directly; rather, the dimensional parameters defining it are calculated by a comparison of the measured signal with simulated signals. This usually involves matching the measured data to a library of previously generated data sets, which can take from several seconds to minutes to complete [78]. However, in an effort to speed up the matching process, a variety of mathematical solutions, including neural networks, have been developed [79].

Scatterometry is a genuinely 3-D measurement method, in that the width and height critical dimensions, as well as line shape profile can be measured at the same time, without altering or damaging the sample. This has led to it becoming a reliable method for measuring the width of lines below 50 nm, because at this scale, fabrication processes produce lines the degree of sidewall slope or curvature of which is significant compared to their average width, and so must be properly modeled to produce an accurate width result. In this way, more than five floating parameters can be solved simultaneously, allowing complex 3-D structures to be characterized in a single measurement [80] (Figure 4.10).

4.3.6
Other Methods

Other techniques under development include scatterfield and through-focus optical metrology, both of which use an optical microscope as a nanometrology tool. Scatterfield metrology can be described as a version of variable angle scatterometry, in which an angular scan is achieved by moving an aperture in the back focal plane of the microscope, so that light is incident and re-collected over a small angle through the objective lens [81]. This method is attractive not only

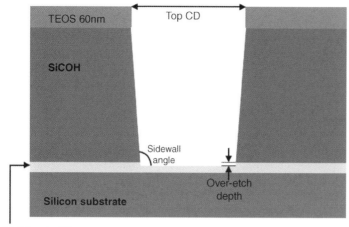

TEOS 60nm

Top CD

SiCOH

Sidewall angle

Over-etch depth

Silicon substrate

Etch barrier 35nm
(SiC or SiN)

Figure 4.10   Multilevel structure measured using scatterometry [81]. See text for details.

because it opens the possibility of using alignment optics for metrology, but also because it enables the use of smaller grating test structures than are required for conventional scatterometry.

In the *through-focus method*, a series of images are recorded, using an optical microscope, of features below the diffraction limit, at different focal distances. The intensity profiles of these are combined to create a 2-D intensity map characteristic of the structures, with a sensitivity to line width changes of 2 nm [82]. One strength of this method is that structures do not have to be periodic in order to be measured.

The short wavelength of X-rays, from approximately 10 to 0.01 nm, can be used in a number of ways for metrology on the nanometer scale. X-ray diffraction (XRD) can be used to provide both 3-D and physical information, such as density and porosity [83]. In critical dimension-small-angle X-ray scattering (CD-SAXS), a beam of X-rays from a synchrotron source is incident normal to the sample, and the transmitted, diffraction pattern analyzed. The line width, pitch, height and line profile can be recreated, as well as the material density, upon which the diffraction of the X-rays also depends [84]. In specular X-ray reflectivity (SXR), X-rays from a Cu Kα source are incident at a grazing angle and the reflected diffracted signal is measured over a range of angles, using a goniometer [85]. With SXR, although the line to space ratio can be measured, in order to calculate the actual line width value it is necessary to have measured the period using another method.

X-ray imaging is currently being investigated for metrology, but is challenging as it requires a good collimated X-ray beam (typically from a synchrotron), and because the resolution is limited not by the wavelength but rather by half the minimum separation in the Fresnel zone plate lenses used to focus the beam. To date, the smallest separation to have been achieved is 20 nm [86].

Optical sub-wavelength diffraction is a technique which can be used to optically characterize structures as small as 50 nm by analyzing the far-field diffraction pattern of line gratings composed of sub-wavelength-sized features. Information can be obtained about the critical dimension, height, and the presence of any defects in the structures. The method uses grating test structures, which have a period greater than the diffraction limit. However, within each period there are features below the diffraction limit which do not affect the angle of diffracted orders, but do affect the relative diffraction efficiency of each order [87].

4.3.7
Physical Properties

A vital part of controlling the nanoimprint process is knowing the physical properties of the polymers used, including viscosity, Young's modulus, and the T_g. Since it is particularly important to measure these parameters at the nanoscale, where physical properties are often different to the bulk values, this has led to the development of existing techniques to measure such small samples.

Elastic modulus measurement at the nanometer scale can be performed by nanoindentation using an AFM tip on polymers [88], as well as other materials [58]. There is some uncertainty regarding this method, due to the difficulty of controlling the tip shape and radius; hence, it has not been used to characterize films of thickness less than 100 nm, and neither has any difference been recorded for Young's modulus measured by nanoindentation from films thicker than 100 nm, and bulk values.

Force and displacement measurements of polystyrene films on the nanometer scale have been made using nanoindentation techniques [89, 90]. These have been used to study the viscoelastic flow of polymers above their T_g under flat and patterned punches, which press the polymer from an initial thickness of 170 nm to a residual thickness of 20 nm, closely recreating the conditions of NIL. The viscoelastic flow of the polymer under a flat punch was found to behave according to bulk models in most cases. One effect of confinement was found for high-molecular-weight polymers (9 000 kDa), which occurs when the thickness of the film is reduced to less than the gyration radius of the polymer, which in this case was approximately 84 nm [91]. For such a thin layer, it was found that deformation of the polymer was accelerated, and this has been termed "confinement thinning."

The most commonly observed effect due to nanoscale dimensions in polymers is a change in the T_g. Typically, the T_g is indicated by a sudden increase in the rate of thermal expansion, taken from thickness measurements made using ellipsometry. For free-standing polystyrene films, a decrease in T_g of up to 80 K has been measured for 20 nm-thick films, compared to the bulk value [92]. The onset in the reduction of T_g begins at a thickness less than approximately 90 nm.

The elastic modulus of polymer structures as thin as 80 nm has been measured by studying the acoustic modes via Brillouin scattering [93]. This is a version of Raman scattering, but with a much higher resolution, achieved by using a Fabry–Perot cavity to resolve peaks within 1 nm of the excitation wavelength, which are characteristic of the energies of phonons confined in nanoscale structures. The Brillouin spectra of lines of thickness 180 to 80 nm, created by deep UV lithography on silicon, were analyzed to derive the speed of sound in the structures, and from this the elastic modulus. No change in the physical properties was measured with respect to bulk values for thicknesses above 80 nm.

The *ultrashort laser pulse photoacoustic method* has been used to characterize the physical properties of layers of PMMA of thicknesses ranging from 586 to 13 nm, spin-coated onto Si wafers. Acoustic speeds, cp, calculated from time of flight and film thicknesses as measured by ellipsometry, were found to increase below approximately 80 nm, with an increase of 20% for a 13 nm sample, compared to the bulk value. This corresponds to an increase in Young's modulus of 44% [94]. The implications of this result for the NIL process are currently under investigation.

4.3.8
Residual Layer Thickness in NIL

Nanoimprint lithography has some features which are particular to it, and occur as a result of the process, including an underlying residual resist layer, and complex line shape profiles, due to the physical forces which deform the resist during and after imprinting.

In order to use the nanoimprinted resist layer for pattern transfer into the substrate, the residual layer must first be etched away. It is essential that the residual layer is uniform across the wafer in order for the fabricated structures to retain the same critical dimensions after this etching step. The most appropriate method to measure residual layer thickness is scatterometry, as it is nondestructive and enables characterization underneath the patterned layer through the transparent resist [95]. Alternatively, samples can be cleaved and a cross-section image made by using SEM, although as the imprinted samples are clearly then sacrificed this is most often used for process development, including methods to ensure a uniform residual layer, such as designing stamps with a uniform array of imprint features [96]. Where large (µm) and small (nm) features are together on the same stamp, the drop dispensing of a precise volume of resist to match the stamp feature sizes [97] has been developed.

Coarse-grain finite difference simulation software has been developed to model the nanoimprinting process over an extended area of several square millimeters, to predict the residual layer thickness, and a very close agreement was found with measured thicknesses [98].

The line shape profile produced by nanoimprinting has been studied using a variety of metrologies, although the most commonly used is scatterometry [99], due to its 3-D measurement capability. In order to enhance the effect of the residual stresses which remain in the polymer structures after imprinting, and which may cause them to deform over time after their release from the mold, one commonly used experiment has been to deliberately cause the lines to reflow by heating them outside of the mould. The resultant line shapes that evolve with time have been measured using AFM [100], while optical diffraction [101] has been used to characterize when the onset of deformation occurs.

4.3.9
Towards An Integrated Metrology

Real-time measurements of polymer line reflow *in situ* of the heating stage have been performed using scatterometry, and compared with *ex situ* measurements of the frozen line shapes by using AFM and SXR, producing very similar results [102]. Each scatterometry measurement takes less than 12 s; however, similar scatterometry measurements, using an optimized library matching method to assign line profile shapes, reduced the individual measurement acquisition times to less than 10 s [103].

These measurements represent progress towards achieving an *in situ* monitoring of the nanofabrication process, which is part of the goal of an integrated metrology. As outlined in the ITRS Roadmap [104], with the reduction in minimum features below 32 nm, and the associated reduction in tolerances to a few nanometers, it is increasingly important to control small variations, or drift, (due to the environmental, instrument or materials) in the fabrication process parameters. This calls for close monitoring of the process, or Advanced Process Control (APC), which requires that metrology be performed either in line with the production, or *in situ*, in the process chamber, so that the time taken for corrective actions can be reduced, and the yield maintained. This is especially relevant to nanoimprinting, as any defect which may occur in the stamp will be replicated in every imprint, and so must be corrected as soon as possible.

Most work in this area has been focused on using optical techniques, as these are nondestructive, can be performed in any atmosphere, and are relatively fast. Scatterometry provides the most complete picture of the fabricated structure [105], while optical diffraction has been used to monitor mold-filling, and to provide a timescale of the imprinting process. However, this is only possible with line widths greater than the diffraction limit – usually approximately 200 nm, with pitches over 400 nm [106]. Recently, scatterometry has been used in optical lithography to make combined measurements of overlay, for double-patterning and critical dimensions [107]. What is a common theme in making use of the simplicity of optical diffraction, or of using the more complex scatterometry for combined measurements, is the need to ensure the maximum value for money from measurements. As integrated metrology requires the deployment of more instruments to monitor each step of the process, the cost is inevitably increased, and so this too requires careful measurement to ensure an efficient fabrication process.

From the above it is clear that new methods are needed, or existing ones need to be developed further, to be used in-line with suitable accuracy and speed. One major issue will inevitably relate to data handling with decreasing feature sizes under production conditions. Furthermore, nanometrology will have to be extended to applications which have tolerances of a few nanometers, and not necessarily in flat but rather on curved substrates. Much remains to be developed in nanometrology in general, and in NIL in particular.

4.4
Two-Dimensional Nanopatterned Polymer Components for Photonic Applications

4.4.1
Overview on Applications Realized by NIL

Optical devices, such as displays, light-emitting components, polarizers, and anti-reflective coatings are used in everyday life in a variety of applications. Currently, NIL offers the capability of a cost-efficient large-scale patterning for polymer photonic components with the requested high resolution and high throughput for such structures. As with common lithography techniques, NIL provides the same tremendous number of applications, which could be separated in two categories: (i) the use of the nanoimprinted polymers as an etch mask to be transferred into the substrate; and (ii) the direct use of the nanoimprinted polymer as devices or components. In both cases, high throughput and high resolution in the nanoscale range are requested over large areas.

With regards to the first category of applications, when using standard NIL techniques it becomes necessary to etch the thin residual layer before transferring the nanostructures into the substrate. This additional step is not critical, and the number of process steps is usually reduced by the use of 3-D imprinting in comparison with standard lithography techniques (see Section 4.2). Moreover, NIL enables potentially relatively cost-efficient nanopatterning if compared to next-generation optical lithography technologies such as deep UV or extreme UV lithography. The latter requires extremely high manufacturing volumes to be economically viable, and it was for this reason that NIL was included in the semiconductor industry roadmap as a possible next-generation lithography to deliver the 32 nm node and beyond [108]. This alternative fabrication method of nanoimprinted mask transfer has already provided applications examples in the fabrication of surface-acoustic-wave generators and filters for mobile phones [109], patterned media for hard-disks [110], and as sub-wavelength polarizers for displays [111]. Although, NIL is currently not limited in resolution for such applications, the main technological issues are the overlay accuracy, defectivity, and critical dimension control (cf. Section 4.3).

The second category of applications concerns the direct patterning in a single step of polymer structures as end products. Nanoscale-patterned polymer films could be tentatively organized into sub-applications categories: the fabrication of organic light-emitting diodes (OLEDs) and plastics electronics; the realization of templates and polymer stamps; biotechnology, including tissue engineering lab-on-a-chip and cell studies; surface modification combined with self-assembled techniques; and 3-D polymer surfaces and the generation of optical components.

In this section, the recent advances in the realization of nanopatterned polymer devices for light control are highlighted. Following by a review of the different optical resonators produced with NIL, examples are provided of optical resonators for lasing applications. Attention is then focused on the use of NIL to pattern functionalized polymers [112]. Active materials can be directly patterned to create lasers [113–115], organic light-emitting devices [116, 117] and conductive organic polymers to realize cost-efficient organics electronics [118]. Specific examples of the direct imprint of nanocomposite polymers to control the emission of light from polymer films will be provided, after which a brief description of nanoimprinted polymer devices will conclude this overview of nanoimprinted photonic components.

4.4.2
Nanoimprinted Optical Resonators

The NIL technique is particularly suitable for the fabrication of integrated polymer optical devices, due to its high resolution and parallel processing of polymer layers. Furthermore, NIL can deliver a surface roughness compatible with the demands of light guiding. Polymer waveguide-type wavelength filters based on a Bragg grating [119, 120], waveguides [121], microring resonator [122, 123], Mach–Zehnder interferometers [124], lasers [125–129], plasmonic components [130, 131], and photonic crystals [132–136] have been recently realized using NIL, and demonstrating its potential as a high-volume and cost-effective patterning technique with sub-10 nm resolution. Optical resonators represent the key components for the spatial confinement and control of light, and the different approaches for creating polymer optical resonators via NIL, associated with their high-quality factors (when applicable), are listed in Table 4.6. (Note: A high-quality factor indicates a long lifetime of the photons in the resonator, leading to a sharp wavelength selection.)

Different optical resonator types can be allocated roughly to three types to achieve optical feedback: (i) specular reflection [137–141]; (ii) ring resonators [142]; and (iii) periodic structures [143–146] (gratings/photonic crystals). Light is coupled in/out to optical resonators in several ways: evanescent field coupling via random scattering from roughness (specular reflection); via a closely spaced waveguides (specular reflection) and standard input/output coupling through gratings (photonic crystals); or by photo-pumping of the imprinted active media, and re-emission. The feedback of resonators based on specular reflection is ensured by reflections on the sidewalls, with incidence angles above the critical angle for total internal reflection. This type of feedback is based on plane waves propagation to minimize losses on reflection, which limits the minimum resonator size to $100 \times 100\,\mu m^2$. There is no obvious input/output coupling mechanism for such resonators, except by evanescent field coupling which can achieved by bringing a waveguide in close proximity ($<\sim$200 nm) to the resonator. The incident angle on one of the sidewalls can be reduced below the critical angle by using a trapezoidal shape instead of a square; coupling-out of the light is then realized, showing multimode laser emission, although the magnitude of

Table 4.6 Polymer optical resonators in polymer fabricated by NIL.

Method	Typical structures	In/Out coupling	Wave-length selectivity	Q factor	Advantage	Drawback
Specular reflection	Ref.s [137–139]	Evanescent	No	NA	Relatively easy fabrication	No wavelength selectivity
	Ref. [140, 141]	Evanescent	Yes	5×10^6	Relatively easy fabrication	No wavelength selectivity
Wave-guide	Ref. [142]	Evanescent	Yes	5800	Relatively easy fabrication	Difficult to optimize Wavelength selectivity

(Continued)

Table 4.6 (*Continued*)

Method	Typical structures	In/Out coupling	Wave-length selectivity	Q factor	Advantage	Drawback
1-D grating	Refs [143, 144]	Built in	Yes	-[a]	Relatively easy fabrication	Light control: 1-D
2-D grating	Ref. [145]	Built in	Yes	1020[a]	Wave-length selectivity Relatively easy fabrication	Light control: 2-D
3-D grating	Refs [146, 147]	Built in	Yes	—	Total control of the light	Difficult fabrication Alignment issue

a) Limited by the resolution of the spectrometer.

the output coupling is difficult to control. A ring resonator coupled to wave-guides [144] acts as Fabry–Pérot showing a Q-factor of 5800, and the device size is limited by the bending loss of the waveguide. The quality of the imprints between the ring and the waveguides is critical to achieve high Q-factors. In order to achieve high Q-values with specular resonators, polymer-imprinted toroidal resonators have been successfully created by using extremely smooth polymer surfaces. Material-limited Q-values of up to 5×10^6 have been measured by bringing a waveguide within close proximity to imprinted toroidal resonators elevated above the substrate. Unfortunately, however, exposure of the surfaces to ambient conditions may cause the resonators to be degraded over time; consequently, it is usually necessary to shield the resonators.

Photonic crystals can be used to produce compacter resonators, with optical feedback being achieved with only a few tens of periods. The wavelength selection is realized by periodically varying the refractive index of the patterned materials (typically a fraction of the optical wavelength); such variation in turn induces a modification of the dispersion relation of propagating modes in the material, and this may lead to the generation of slow group velocity modes and to the opening of photonic band gaps (as the well-known Bragg grating). Photonic bandgaps result in optical feedback in 1-, 2- and 3-D directions. A typical cross-section of a nanoim-printed Bragg grating with 350 nm pitch is shown in Figure 4.11a. Features from the silicon stamp are usually very well reproduced in polymer layers with adequate imprinting parameters; for example, a lines separation of 60 nm is shown in Figure 4.11, and the residual layer is about 120 nm thick in this case. Such structures, known as "Bragg gratings," can be used efficiently to create nanoim-printed polymer optical resonators and to build in the coupling of the light. These optical resonators can be integrated with waveguides to couple in/out light of the resonators in planar geometries. In fact, planar polymer-based resonators can operate by using waveguiding in the polymer. Imprinted waveguides, beam splitters and bent waveguides can be easily obtained using standard imprinting processes [148]. Figure 4.11b and c show current optical microscope images of such structures, where the uniform Newton colors indicate a uniform residual layer. Polymer interferometers can be made with 800 nm separation between the two waveguides (Figure 4.11d and e).

In order to achieve 2-D optical feedback, 2-D periodic structures – called 2-D photonic crystals (PhCs) – are formed, for example, with holes in the imprinted polymer [127]; the light is then controlled in the plane of the substrate. Other advantages of 2-D defect-free PhCs over conventional 1-D feedback gratings include the potentially highly directional vertical emission and a lower lasing threshold. Ideally, 3-D periodic structures which allow the control of the light in the three spatial directions are required, but such structures are particularly complex to fabricate using either holographic lithography [149] or serial layer stacking [150] or self-assembled techniques.

At present, nanoimprinted optical resonators that combine the best control of light in/out coupling, wavelength selection and easiest fabrication by NIL are the 1-D and 2-D grating resonators. Smooth polymer surfaces are required to avoid random

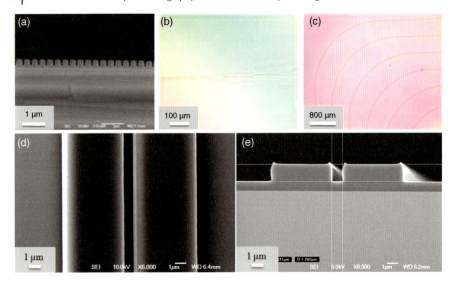

Figure 4.11 (a) SEM cross-section of imprinted polymer grating (pitch: 350 nm, lines separation: 60 nm, residual layer: 120 nm); (b) Optical microscope image of bent waveguides in mr-NIL 6000; (c) Optical microscope image of imprinted beam splitter in mr-NIL 6000; (d) Top-view; (e) Cross-sectional SEM images of the two interfering waveguides.

scattering and to reach respectable Q-factors. Nanoimprint lithography is well suited for the creation of such polymeric structures, since the low degree of roughness of silicon stamps is transferred to the polymers (the transferred roughness can be reduced even further by a control reflow of the polymer [151].).

4.4.2.1 Nanoimprinted Polymeric Band-Edge Lasers

Polymer dye lasers might provide compact and inexpensive coherent light sources for microfluidics and integrated optics in the visible range. The advantages of 2-D defect-free PhCs over the conventional 1-D feedback gratings are, potentially, a less-directional vertical emission and lower lasing thresholds. Such PhCs have been studied to create band-edge lasers in organic media [152, 153], and have shown their potential of integration in planar optical circuits [154]. However, one reason why 2-D PhCs have not yet been produced in mass numbers is that expensive techniques, such as EBL or laser interference lithography, are required for their fabrication. The latter approach offers a higher throughput than the former, but does not yet meet the requirements for mass production [155]. A series of PhCs was directly fabricated in a printable polymer loaded with dye-emitting molecules, and showed lasing oscillation at different photonic band-edge frequencies. For these nanoimprinted band-edge lasers, a dye-doped polymer was used, composed of rhodamine 6G (R6G; from Sigma-Aldrich) directly dissolved at a concentration of $2.5 \times 10^{-3} \, \mathrm{mol \, l^{-1}}$ in the polymer mr-NIL 6000 (from Microresist Technology). It is known that organic emitters degrade when exposed to air at high temperatures, and this results in low light emission efficiency. To minimize the thermal degradation, mr-NIL 6000 was chosen because of its relative low T_g (ca. 45 °C). The active films were spun on a glass substrate at 1500 r.p.m. for 1 min and then baked at 115 °C for 5 min to remove the residual solvent. The measured polymer thickness was 400 nm.

The imprinting process was performed in a 6 cm (2.5 inch) Obducat nanoimprinting machine at 90 °C and under 60 bar pressure for 5 min. After sample cooling, the stamp was separated from the patterned polymer at 40 °C. A reduction of less than 3% in the photoluminescence (PL) intensity was found after patterning with an unstructured silicon stamp, while the refractive index of the doped polymer was measured by ellipsometry to be 1.614 at 550 nm. Stamps with the two lattice constants (460 and 500 nm) have been produced using EBL (Jeol 6000) with a dose of 130 μC cm^{-2} and a beam current of 100 pA, using a 150 nm-thick layer of ZEP 520 resist (Zeon) that had been pre-baked at 120 °C and developed for 30 s in a solution of ZED N50 (Zeon). The silicon stamp was etched 350 nm deep using an inductively coupled plasma (ICP) reactive ion etching system (Surface Technology Systems), with a mixture of SF_6 and C_4F_8 gases. The stamp was subsequently coated with an anti-adhesive monolayer (tridecafluor-1,1,2,2-tetrahydro-octyl trichlorosilane) deposited from the vapor phase, which results in a very low surface energy to facilitate detachment of the stamp from the polymer. The nanoimprinted samples were optically pumped in a vacuum cell with a 0.7 ns frequency-doubled Q-switched Nd : YO4 laser light at 532 nm focused to a 50 μm-diameter spot on the sample surface.

Figure 4.12a shows the SEM image of a silicon stamp and a nanoimprinted photonic crystal in the dye-chromophore-loaded polymer matrix. The 2-D pillar arrays of the silicon stamp were faithfully transferred onto the modified polymer. Figure 4.12b shows the measured emission spectrum of the 2-D PhC with 460 and 500 nm lattice constants. The reduced frequencies were measured as 0.765 ± 0.001 and 0.876 ± 0.001 for the 460 and 500 nm PhCs, respectively. Using a plane-wave algorithm, the reduced frequencies of the three band edges, Γ_1, X_4, were calculated as 0.766 and 0.877, respectively, yielding a very good agreement between the numerical and experimental band edge frequencies. The laser with the 460 nm lattice constant operated at 601.4 ± 0.3 nm, approximately 40 nm away from the maximum of the spontaneous emission peak, and indicating a strong optical feedback provided by the

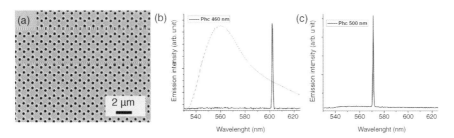

Figure 4.12 (a) SEM image of an imprint in the composite polymer mr-NIL 6000 with rhodamine 6G; (b) Emission spectra of a band edge laser with lattice constants of 460 nm and 500 nm. The dotted line shows the emission spectra of rhodamine 6G in mr-NIL 6000 below the threshold.

Table 4.7 Comparison of 1-D nanoimprinted R6G-doped polymer lasers.

Reference	Threshold (μJ mm^{-2})	Area (μm^2)
[000] (Li et al., 2006)	8	200×4
[156]	8	250×1000
[000] (Pisignano et al., 2004)	6.5	200×200

PhC. The laser surface was 125-fold smaller than those measured for the 1-D nanoimprinted organic feedback grating, made from R6G-doped SU-8 polymer [156]. A laser threshold of $3 \, \mu$J mm^{-2} was obtained. A 1-D nanoimprinted laser doped with R6G is shown for comparison in Table 4.7. No lasing oscillation was observed for areas without a PhC pattern under the same pumping conditions. These results indicated that the direct imprint of a spin-coated, dye-doped polymer with a PhC stamp could be used as a band-edge laser with a relative low degradation of the gain property of the dye.

The lifetime of the lasers as function of the number of excitation pump pulse at $8.5 \, \mu$J mm^{-2} (corresponding to 2.8-fold the laser threshold) was also measured. The laser emission fell exponentially to 10% of its initial values after 8200 pulses, which was comparable to solid-state dye lasers emitting in the visible wavelengths. In order to improve the lifetime of the lasers, one solution might be to replace the dye molecules with semiconductor nanocrystals with optical gain embedded in a printable polymer [137].

4.4.3
Patterning in Functionalized Polymers

NIL presents the unique advantage to pattern polymers in a single step to realize, for example, optical components. In addition, unsurpassed size- and shape-dependent electronic properties of semiconductor and metal nanocrystals (NCs) are extremely attractive as novel structural building blocks for the construction of a new generation of innovative materials and solid-state devices. Recent advances in chemical synthesis have resulted in colloidal NCs with a wide range of compositions, combined with an excellent control of size, shape, and uniformity. As the surfaces of the NCs can be easily engineered by ligand exchange and surface functionalization, they can be placed in almost any chemical environment, although their use in devices for photonic and sensing applications normally requires them to be incorporated into a polymer matrix, in order that their properties can be exploited. A strategy for incorporating NCs into printable polymers, to allow their homogeneous distribution in the polymer matrix, is shown in Figure 4.13a. In this case, the pre-synthesized TOPO-coated (CdSe)ZnS core-shell luminescent nanocrystals are incorporated into a PMMA homopolymer and into a PMMA-based co-polymer. The functionalized polymer acts as a stabilizing and protective layer surrounding every single NC (see Figure 4.13b and c). The

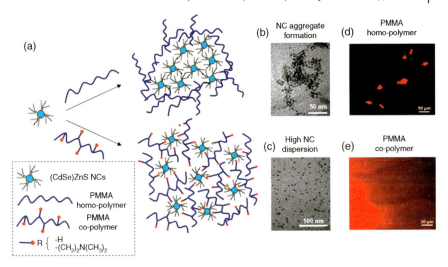

Figure 4.13 (a) Schematic illustration of TOPO-coated (CdSe)ZnS nanocomposites (NCs) in PMMA homopolymer and in functionalized PMMA based co-polymers; (b) TEM images of NCs, revealing aggregation in the case of PMMA homopolymer; (c) High NC dispersion when embedded in functionalized co-polymers; (d, e) Fluorescence microscopy images of (CdSe)ZnS NCs incorporated in (d) PMMA homopolymer and (e) PMMA block co-polymer (PMMA$_{70}$-*co*-DMEAMA$_{30}$). Reproduced from Ref. [134].

fluorescence microscopy image (Figure 4.13d) with the PMMA homopolymer shows a strong aggregation of the NCs whilst, in the case of the PMMA co-polymer block, a homogeneous emission over the whole surface of the polymer film is obtained, showing a high compatibility of the NCs with the host polymer. (The experimental details of these studies can be obtained from Ref. [135].)

The fabrication of 2-D patterned light-emitting structures in this luminescent nanocomposite, using NIL, has been demonstrated. A similar imprint process as that described above has been used to pattern the nanocomposite polymer. Figure 4.14a

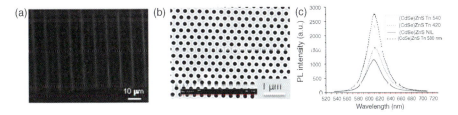

Figure 4.14 (a) Fluorescence image of patterned waveguides obtained by NIL onto the nanocomposite thin films; (b) SEM images of nanoimprinted photonic crystals in a PMMA-based polymer matrix, into which (CdSe)ZnS NCs have been incorporated; (c) PL spectra of unpatterned PMMA-based polymer matrix with (CdSe)ZnS NCs on a Pyrex substrate (solid line) imprinted with a flat stamp, and PL spectra of a 2-D photonic crystal with a 580 nm lattice (dash-dot line). Panels (a) and (b) reproduced from Ref. [134].

shows the fluorescence image of nanoimprinted waveguides, and Figure 4.14b the SEM images of nanoimprinted photonic crystals onto the nanocomposite polymer. The imprinted pattern transfer did not suffer from any unusual roughness or degradation, which meant that the incorporation of (CdSe)ZnS had not caused any deterioration of the duplication fidelity of the stamp in the photoluminescent polymer. The nanoimprinted PhCs could then be optically excited using a CW Ar$^+$ laser at a wavelength of 514.5 nm, with a power of 240 μW focused down to a 10 μm spot, and with the incident beam normal to the surface. The collection cone was defined by a 10× microscope objective with a numerical aperture (NA) of 0.4. The photoluminescence of samples was collected through the same objective of microscope, and analyzed spectrometrically. First, no degradation of the photoluminescence intensity of NCs was observed after patterning by NIL. The ratio between the PL intensities (integrated over 530–750 nm) of the patterned structure and the unpatterned imprinted surface has been measured: the maximum enhancement factor obtained was equal to 2.4 at room temperature for the lattice constant of 580 nm. This extraction enhancement demonstrated that the nanoimprinted photonic crystal slab structure could represent a potential candidate for high-efficiency light-emitting diodes (LEDs), based on polymers.

Whilst it is clear that one solution to solving the light-trapping problem consists of using 2-D photonic crystals fabricated by NIL, another approach would be to increase the spontaneous recombination rate of the emitters. This can be based on the energy transfer between light emitters and surface plasmons (SPs). The results of several investigations of enhanced light emission via SPs have been described [157, 158]. Recently, comparable studies have been conducted with dye-doped organic films [159] and with conjugated polymer films [160] in close proximity to metal surfaces. Similar coupling processes have been observed in both organic and inorganic structures, with important enhancements in the spontaneous emission intensity of the emitters. The two approaches mentioned above can be combined to enhance the light-emission efficiency of organic thin films. As an example, the fabrication of printed nanostructures using a thermoplastic polymer was studied, into which R6G and gold nanoparticles were incorporated, using a previously described strategy [134] to incorporate the nanoparticles. The water-soluble gold nanoparticles were synthesized via a non-seeding method [161], the gold nanoparticle size having been chosen to be close to the plasmon resonance wavelength of the nanoparticles with the emission wavelength of the dye. The R6G was diluted in 1 ml of mr-I PMMA 75 k 300, with a concentration of dye molecules of 5×10^{-4} M. The peak emission of R6G in the polymer was measured at 550 nm, and small amounts of gold nanoparticles in toluene solution were added to the polymer–dye emitting composite (Figure 4.15a). Several nanoparticles concentrations were tested, from 0 to 9.76×10^{-5} M.

Samples of the mixtures of dye with Au nanoparticles in mr-I PMMA (now called the "functionalized polymer") were placed in quartz cuvettes, and the spontaneous emission spectra (obtained by exciting the functionalized polymer at 450 nm) were collected perpendicular to the excitation. In order to pattern the functionalized

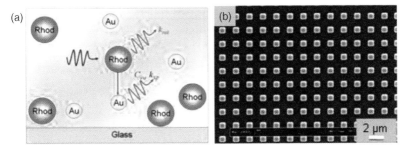

Figure 4.15 (a) Schematics of the coupling between metallic nanoparticles and dye emitters; (b) SEM image of a nanoimprinted grating in mr-I PMMA, in which R6G and Au nanoparticles have been incorporated.

polymer by NIL, the same process as described above was followed. The stamp and polymer were brought into contact at a temperature of 170 °C, and a pressure of 60 bar was applied for 5 min. Separation of the stamp and substrate was performed at 90 °C.

The coupling of SPs to emitters has been tested with metallic nanoparticles. For this, small amounts of Au nanoparticles were added to the solution of R6G in mr-I PMMA, increasing the concentration of nanoparticles in the polymer from 0 to 9.76×10^{-5} M. The PL intensity was then recorded from samples with different nanoparticle concentrations in the mixture. Measurements of the emission intensity, integrated over the range 500 to 750 nm, indicated an increase of up to 175% in the emission of the dye when the Au nanoparticles concentration reached 3.82×10^{-5} M. This enhancement could be attributed to an increased absorption and emission of R6G in the presence of metallic nanoparticles. For an Au nanoparticles concentration below 9×10^{-5} M, the number of absorbed R6G molecules per metallic nanoparticle was expected to exceed one, whereby the gain of the dye compensated for the loss in the localized SPs.

At higher concentrations of Au nanoparticles in the functionalized polymer, the PL intensity decreased due to a too-high number of Au nanoparticles in solution, the losses of which – due to the localized SPS – were no longer compensated. However, the good printability of PMMA as a thermoplastic material confirmed the use of prepared nanocomposite materials for the fabrication of devices for plasmonic applications. In these studies, grating structures and plain films were patterned in the functionalized polymer by using NIL. The SEM image of a nanoimprinted grating in the nanocomposite thin film is shown in Figure 4.15b. The results obtained may lead to a new approach towards new plasmonics devices fabricated using NIL.

4.4.4
Outlook on Nanoimprinted Polymer Devices

It has been seen that NIL is well-suited process to the fabrication of polymeric optical resonators, challenging photonic structures, and polymer devices, combining the unique advantages of patterning with high resolution on large areas, and with a high throughput. Nonetheless, further developments are required in this direction to produce full photonic integrated circuits at low cost, with high degrees of functionality, and also to monitor the lifetime of such imprinted optical components. These studies have been conducted in part to demonstrate how NIL might be developed on 200 mm wafers to allow the fabrication of two optical devices, namely optical encoders [162] and double-sided organic LEDs with enhanced light extraction efficiency [3]. Both, photonic devices [136, 137] and plasmonic [3] devices can be directly fabricated by NIL, using the same materials during the same fabrication step with different functionalities [163]; alternatively, they may be separately fabricated and post-assembled. In addition, roll-to-roll, step-and-flash and step-and-stamp techniques have demonstrated huge potential for mass production, with the roll-to-roll approach having recently been used to fabricate fluidic platforms and organic LEDs [3]. One important area of activity that has developed during recent years has involved electronic printing devices, the target being to create printing methods that can be used for large-area flexible electronic devices [164]. High-resolution patterning techniques have been developed to provide a nanometer-scale separation between the source and drain electrodes of transistors in plastic circuits [165], while NIL methods have proven their ability in the fabrication of polymer devices and photonic components. Yet, there remain three main issues to be solved before NIL can meet the stringent requirements of mass manufacturing: (i) to minimize the number of defects per square centimeter; (ii) to improve the overlay accuracy (a 50 nm overlay accuracy was achieved by using interferometric *in situ* alignment techniques [166]); and (iii) to create a production throughput that would permit many hundreds of wafers to be printed on an hourly basis.

4.5
Conclusions

In reviewing the status of 3-D NIL, the associated nanometrology, and its optical applications, 3-D NIL will surely become increasingly important as novel and highly functional nanostructures are achieved that combine polymers, optically active, and biological materials. Moreover, these methods are nonexhaustive, since magnetic, nonlinear optical and other properties can be utilized, depending on the doping of the printable polymer.

The crucial role of nanometrology in NIL has also been recognized, and how it can be used to unravel nanorheological aspects when polymer thicknesses are on the order of only a few tens of nanometers. The need for new methods was clearly illustrated, as was the need not only to integrate nanometrology into a manufacturing environment, but also to take into consideration the vast amount of data that will be generated via in-line monitoring.

Clearly, the application of NIL to photonics is simply the "tip of the iceberg." By using periodic patterning, it should be possible to enhance certain interactions, such as the slow modes of a photonic crystals and the emitted light from dye chromophores. It is also likely that the interplay between nanophotonic concepts and dispersion relationships in solids for practical polymer photonics structures will be clarified in the very near future.

Acknowledgments

The authors gratefully acknowledge the support of the EC-funded project NaPaNIL (NMP2-LA-2008-214249). The content of these studies is the sole responsibility of the authors.

Mads Brokner Christiansen and Anders Kristensen are sincerely acknowledged for their helpful insight on nanoimprinted optical resonators.

References

1 Sotomayor Torres, C.M. (ed.) (2003) *Alternative Lithography: Unleashing the Potentials of Nanotechnology*, Kluwer Academic Plenum Publishers, New York.

2 http://pubict.itrs.net.

3 Ahopelto, J. and Schift, H. (2008) Library of Processes, www.NAPANIL.org.

4 Chou, S.Y., Krauss, P.R., and Renstrom, P.J. (1995) *Appl. Phys. Lett.*, **67** (21), 3114.

5 Chou, S.Y. and Krauss, P.R. (1997) *Microelectron. Eng.*, **35**, 237–240.

6 Schift, H., Saxer, S., Park, S., Padeste, C., Pieles, U., and Gobrecht, J. (2005) *Nanotechnology*, **16**, 171–175.

7 Austin, M.D., Ge, H., Wu, W., Li, M., Yu, Z., Wasserman, D., Lyon, S.A., and Chou, S.Y. (2004) *Appl. Phys Lett.*, **84**, 5299.

8 Perret, C., Gourgon, C., Lazzarino, F., Tallal, J., Landis, S., and Pelzer, R. (2004) *Microelectron. Eng.*, **73–74**, 172.

9 Brandrup, J., Immergut, E.H., and Grulke, E.A. (1999) *Polymer Handbook (database)*, John Wiley & Sons.

10 Colburn, M., Johnson, S., Damle, S., Bailey, T., Choi, B., Wedlake, M., Michaelson, T., Sreenivasan, S.V., Ekerdt, J., and Willson, C.B. (1999) *Proc. SPIE*, **3676**, 379.

11 Miller, M., Schmid, G., Doyle, G., Thompson, E., and Resnick, D.J. (2006) S-FIL Template Fabrication for Full Wafer Imprint Lithography, in Proceedings NNT 06, San Francisco, US, 15–17 November.

12 Resnick, D.J., Schmid, G., Thompson, E., Stacey, N., Olynick, D.L., and Anderson, E. (2006) Step and Flash Imprint Lithography Templates for the 32 nm Node and Beyond, in Proceedings NNT 06, San Francisco, US 15–17 November.

13 Austin, M.D., Ge, H., Wu, W., Li, M., Yu, Z., Wasserman, D., Lyon, S.A., and Chou, S.Y. (2004) *Appl. Phys. Lett.*, **84**, 5299.

14 Gourgon, C., Perret, C., Tallal, J., Lazzarino, F., Landis, S., Joubert, O., and Pelzer, R. (2005) *J. Phys. D: Appl. Phys.*, **38**, 70.

15 Miller, M., Schmid, G., Doyle, G., Thompson, E., and Resnick, D.J. (2006) Proceedings NNT 06, San Francisco, US 15–17 November.

16 Wu, T.W., Best, M., Kercher, D., Dobisz, E., Bandic, Z., Yang, H., and Albrecht, T.R. (2006) Proceedings NNT 06, San Francisco, US 15–17 November.

17 Sreenivasan, S.V., Schumaker, P., McMackin, I., and Choi, J. (2006) Nano-Scale Mechanics of Drop-On-Demand UV Imprinting, in Proceedings NNT 06, San Francisco, US 15–17 November.

18 Hershey, R., Miller, M., Jones, C., Subramanian, M.G., Lu, X., Doyle, G., Lentz, D., and LaBrake, D. (2006) *Proc. SPIE*, **6337**, 6337M.

19 Vlasov, Y.A., Bo, X.Z., Sturm, J.C., and Norris, D.J. (2001) *Nature*, **414**, 289–293.

20 Seekamp, J., Zankovych, S., Helfer, A.H., Maury, P., Sotomayor-Torres, C., Boettger, M., Liguda, G., Eich, C., Heidari, M., Montelius, B., and Ahopelto, L. (2002) *J. Nanotechnol.*, **13**, 581–586.

21 Cui, B., Zhaoning, Y., Ge, H., and Chou, S.Y. (2007) *Appl. Phys. Lett.*, **90**, 043118.

22 Palmieri, F., Stewart, M.D., Wetzel, J., Hao, J., Nishimura, Y., Jen, K., Flannery, C., Li, B., Chao, H.L., Young, S., Kim, W.C., Ho, P.L., and Willson, C.G. (2006) *Proc. SPIE*, **6151**, 61510J/1–61510J/9.

23 Stewart, M., Wetzel, J., Schmid, G., *et al.* (2005) *Proc. SPIE -Microlithography*, **5751**, 210.

24 Schmid, G.M., Stewart, M.D., Wetzel, J., Palmieri, F., Hao, J., Nishimura, Y., Jen, K., Kim, E.K., Resnick, D.J., Liddle, J.A., and Willson, C.G. (2006) *J. Vac. Sci. Technol. B*, **24** (3), 1283.

25 Romanato, F., Businaro, L., Vaccari, L., Cabrini, S., Candeloro, P., De Vittorio, M., Passaseo, A., Todaro, M.T., Cingolani, R., Cattaruzza, E., Galli, M., Andreani, C., and Di Fabrizio, E. (2003) *Microelectron. Eng.*, **479**, 67–68.

26 Tormen, M., Businaro, L., Altissimo, M., Romanato, F., Cabrini, S., Perennes, F., Proietti, R., Sun, H.-B., Kawata, S., and Di Fabrizio, E. (2004) *Microelectron. Eng.*, **73**, 535–541.

27 Jeon, S., Malyarchuk, V., Rogers, J.A., and Wiederrecht, G.P. (2006) *Opt. Express*, **14**, 2300–2308.

28 Tormen, M., Carpentiero, A., Vaccari, L., Altissimo, M., Ferrari, E., Cojoc, D., and Di Fabrizio, E. (2005) *J. Vac. Sci. Technol. B*, **23**, 2920–2924.

29 Kehagias, N., Zelsmann, M., Pfeiffer, K., Ahrens, G., Gruetzner, G., and Sotomayor Torres, C.M. (2005) *J. Vac. Sci. Technol. B*, **23** (6), 2954–2957.

30 Huang, X.D., Bao, L.-R., Cheng, X., Guo, L.J., Pang, S.W., and Yee, A.F. (2002) *J. Vac. Sci. Technol. B*, **20**, 2872.

31 Borzenko, T., Tormen, M., Schmidt, G., Molenkamp, L.W., and Janssen, H. (2001) *Appl. Phys. Lett.*, **79**, 2246.

32 Bao, L.R., Cheng, X., Huang, X.D., Guo, L.J., Pang, S.W., and Yee, A.F. (2002) *J. Vac. Sci. Technol. B*, **20**, 2881.

33 Kehagias, N., Zelsmann, M., Pfeiffer, K., Ahrens, G., Gruetzner, G., and Sotomayor Torres, C.M. (2005) *J. Vac. Sci. Technol. B*, **23** (6), 2954–2957.

34 Nakajima, M., Yoshikawa, T., Sogo, K., and Hirai, Y. (2006) *Microelectron. Eng.*, **83**, 876–879.

35 Kehagias, N., Reboud, V., Chansin, G., Zelsmann, M., Jeppesen, C., Schuster, C., Kubenz, M., Reuther, F., Gruetzner, G., and Sotomayor Torres, C.M. (2007) *Nanotechnology*, **18**, 175303.

36 Kehagias, N., Chansin, G., Reboud, V., Zelsmann, M., Schuster, C., Kubenz, M., Reuther, F., Gruetzner, G., and Sotomayor Torres, C.M. (2007) *Microelectron. Eng.*, **84**, 921.

37 Kehagias, N., Reboud, V., Chansin, G., Zelsmann, M., Jeppesen, C., Reuther, F., Schuster, C., Kubenz, M., Gruetzner, G., and Sotomayor Torres, C.M. (2006) *J. Vac. Sci. Technol. B*, **24** (6), 3002–3005.

38 Le, Q.T., Claes, M., Conard, T., Kesters, E., Lux, M., and Vereecke, G. (2009) *Microelectron. Eng.*, **86**, 181–185.

39 Klein, M.F.G., Hein, H., Jakobs, P.J., Linden, S., Meinzer, N., Wegener, M., Saile, V., and Kohl, M. (2009) *Microelectron. Eng.*, **86**, 1078–1080.

40 Foucher, J., Pargon, E., Martin, M., Reyne, S., and Dupré, C. (2008) *Proc. SPIE*, **6922**, 69220.

41 Zangooie, S., Sendelbach, M., Angyal, M., Archie, C., Vaid, A., Matthew, I., and Herrera, P. (2008) *Proc. SPIE*, **6922**, 69220.

42 JEOL JSM-7600f, JEOL Ltd., 1-2, Musashino 3-chome Akishima, Tokyo 196–8558, Japan. Available at: http://www.jeol.com/PRODUCTS/ElectronOptics/ScanningElectron MicroscopesSEM/SemiinLensFE/JSM7600F/tabid/519/Default.aspx.

43 Zeiss ULTRA 60, Carl Zeiss NTS GmbH, Carl-Zeiss-Straße 56, 73447 Oberkochen, Germany. Available at:

http://www.zeiss.de/
c1256e4600305472/ContentsFrame/
b7e0976de51e3013c1256e58004f5177.

44 Otto, M., Bender, M., Zhang, J.,
Fuchs, A., Wahlbrink, T., Bolten, J.,
Spangenberg, B., and Kurz, H. (2007)
Microelectron. Eng., **84**, 980–983.

45 Austin, M.D., Zhang, W., Ge, H.,
Wasserman, D., Lyon, S.A., and
Chou, S.Y. (2005) *Nanotechnology*,
16, 1058–1061.

46 Joy, D.C. (2006) *J. Surf. Sci. Nanotechnol.*,
4, 369–375.

47 Vladár, E., Villarrubia, J.S., Cizmar, P.,
Oral, M., and Postek, M.T. (2008) *Proc.
SPIE*, **6922**, 69220.

48 Sasaki, S., Hiraka, T., Mizuochi, J.,
Nakanishi, Y., Yusa, S., Morikawa, Y.,
Mohri, H., and Hayashi, N. (2009) *Proc.
SPIE*, **7271**, 72711.

49 Nasu, O., Sasada, K., Ikeda, M., and
Ezumi, M.O. (2002) *Hitachi Review*,
51 (4), 125–129.

50 Frase, C.G., Buhr, E., and Dirscherl, K.
(2007) *Meas. Sci. Technol.*, **18**, 510–519.

51 Chaix, N., Landis, S., Gourgon, C.,
Merino, S., Lambertini, V.G., Durand, G.,
and Perret, C. (2007) *Microelectron. Eng.*,
84, 880–884.

52 Litt, L.C. and Malloy, M. (2009) *Proc.
SPIE*, **7271**, 72711.

53 International Technology Roadmap for
Semiconductors, Executive Summary
2007 Ed., p. 14. Available at: http://public.
itrs.net/.

54 International Technology Roadmap for
Semiconductors, 2007 Ed., Metrology,
Table MET3a. Available at: http://public.
itrs.net/.

55 Pritschow, M., Butschke, J., Irmscher, M.,
Parisolib, L., Oba, T., Iwai, T., and
Nakamura, T. (2009) *Proc. SPIE*, **7271**,
72711.

56 Ke, C.M., Hu, J., Wang, W., and Huang, J.
(2009) *Proc. SPIE*, **7272**, 72720.

57 Binnig, G., Quate, C.F., and Gerber, Ch.
(1986) *Phys. Rev. Lett.*, **56** (9), 930.

58 Giessibl, J. (2005) *Mater. Today*, **8**,
32–41.

59 Veeco Dimension Icon, Veeco
Instruments Inc., Terminal Drive,
Plainview, NY 11803, USA. Available at:
http://www.veeco.com/default.aspx.

60 Sugimoto, Y., Pou, P., Abe, M., Jelinek, P.,
Perez, R., Morita, S., and Custance, O.
(2007) *Nature*, **446**, 64–67.

61 Meyer, G. and Amer, N.M. (1990) *Appl.
Phys. Letts.*, **57**, 2089–2091.

62 Delobelle, P., Guillon, O., Fribourg-
Blanc, E., Soyer, C., Cattan, E., and
Remiens, D. (2004) *Appl. Phys. Lett.*,
85 (22), 5185–5187.

63 Ukraintsev, V.A. (2009) *Proc. SPIE*,
7272, 727205.

64 Park, B.C., Choi, J., Ahn, S.J., Kim, D.H.,
Lyou, J., Dixson, R., Orji, N.G., Fu, J., and
Vorburger, T.V. (2007) *Proc. SPIE*, **6518**,
651819.

65 Muruyama, K., Gonda, S., Koyanagi, H.,
Terasawa, T., and Hosaka, S. (2006) *Jpn. J.
Appl. Phys.*, **45** (7), 5928–5932.

66 Orji, N.G., Dixson, R.G., Bunday, B.D.,
and Allgair, J.A. (2008) *Proc. SPIE*, **6922**,
692208.

67 Bartela, T.P., Kisielowski, C., Specht, P.,
Shubina, T.V., Jmerik, V.N., and Ivanov,
S.V. (2007) *Appl. Phys. Lett.*, **91**, 101908.

68 Giannuzzia, L.A. and Stevie, F.A. (1999)
Micron, **30**, 197–204.

69 Sendelbach, M., Zangooie, S., Vaid, A.,
Herrera, P., Leng, J., and Kim, I. (2008)
Proc. SPIE, **6922**, 69220.

70 Dahlen, G.A., Liu, H.C., Osborn, M.,
Osborne, J.R., Tracy, B., and del
Rosario, A. (2008) *Proc. SPIE*, **6922**,
69220.

71 Huang, H.T. and Terry, F.L. Jr (2004) *Thin
Solid Films*, **455–456**, 828–836.

72 Herzinger, M., Johs, B., McGahan,
W.A., Woollam, J.A., and Paulson,
W. (1998) *J. Appl. Phys.*, **83** (6),
3323–3336.

73 Clement, T., Ingole, S., Ketharanathan,
S., Drucker, J., and Picrauxa, S.T. (2006)
Appl. Phys. Lett., **89**, 163125.

74 R. Nanometrics Incorporated, 1550
Buckeye Drive, Milpitas, CA 95035 USA.
Available at: http://www.nanometrics
com/products.html.

75 KLA-Tencor Corporation, One
Technology Drive, Milpitas, California
95035, USA. Available at: http://www.
kla-tencor.com.

76 Germer, T.A., Patrick, H.J., Silver, R.M.,
and Bunday, B. (2009) *Proc. SPIE*, **7272**,
72720.

77 Zhou, W., l Hsieh, M., Koh, H., and Zhou, M. (2008) *Proc. SPIE*, **6922**, 69223.

78 Pundaleva, H., Nam, D., Han, H., Lee, D., and Han, W. (2006) *Proc. SPIE*, **6152**, 61520.

79 Gereige, T., Robert, S., Thiria, S., Badran, F., Granet, G., and Rousseau, J.J. (2008) *J. Opt. Soc. Am. A*, **25** (7), 1661–1667.

80 Silver, R.M., Zhang, N.F., Barnes, B.M., Zhou, H., Heckert, A., Dixson, R., Germer, T.A., and Bunday, B. (2009) *Proc. SPIE*, **7272**, 727202.

81 Patrick, H.J., Attota, R., Barnes, B.M., Germer, T.A., Dixson, R.G., Stocker, M.T., Silver, R.M., and Bishop, M.R. (2008) *J. Micro/Nanolith. MEMS MOEMS*, **7** (1), 013012.

82 Attota, R., Silver, R., and Barnes, B.M. (2008) *Proc. SPIE*, **6922**, 69220.

83 Lee, H.J., Soles, C.L., Ro, H.W., Jones, R.L., Lin, E.K., Wu, W., and Hines, D.R. (2005) *Appl. Phys. Lett.*, **87**, 263111.

84 Jones, R.L., Hu, T., Soles, C.L., Lin, E.K., Reano, R.M., Pang, S.W., and Casa, D.M. (2006) *Nano Lett.*, **6** (8), 1723–1728.

85 Lee, H.J., Soles, C.L., Liu, D.W., Bauer, B.L., and Wu, W.L. (2002) *J. Polym. Sci., Part B: Polym. Phys.*, **40**, 2170.

86 Jefimovs, L., Vila-Comamala, J., Pilvi, T., Raabe, J., Ritala, M., and David, C. (2007) *Phys. Rev. Lett.*, **99**, 264801.

87 Kehoe, T., Bryner, J., Reboud, V., Kehagias, N., Landis, S., Gourgon, C., Vollmann, J., Dual, J., and Sotomayor Torres, C.M. (2008) *Proc. SPIE*, **6921**, 69210.

88 VanLandingham, M.R., Villarrubia, J.S., Guthrie, W.F., and Meyers, G.F. (2001) *Macromol. Symp.*, **167**, 15–43.

89 Rowland, H.D., King, W.P., Cross, G.L.W., and Pethica, J.P. (2008) *Am. Chem. Soc.*, **2** (3), 419–428.

90 Cross, G.L.W., Connell, B.S.O., Pethica, J.B., Rowland, H., and King, W.P. (2008) *Rev. Sci. Instrum.*, **79**, 013904.

91 Rowland, H.D., King, W.P., Pethica, J.P., and Cross, G.L.W. (2008) *Science*, **322**, 720–724.

92 Dalkoni-Veress, K., Forrest, J.A., Murray, C., Gigault, C., and Dutcher, J.R. (2001) *Phys. Rev. E*, **63**, 031801.

93 Hartschuh, R., Kisliuk, A., Novikov, V., Sokolov, A.P., Heyliger, P.R., Flannery, C.M., Johnson, W.L., Soles, C.L., and Wu, W.L. (2005) *Appl. Phys. Lett.*, **87**, 173121.

94 Kehoe, T., Bryner, J., Reboud, V., Vollmann, J., and Sotomayor Torres, C.M. (2009) *Proc. SPIE*, **71**, 72711.

95 Fuard, D., Perret, C., Farys, V., Gourgon, C., and Schiavone, P. (2005) *J. Vac. Sci. Technol. B*, **23** (6), 3069–3074.

96 Landis, S., Chaix, N., Gourgon, C., Perret, C., and Leveder, T. (2006) *Nanotechnology*, **17**, 2701–2709.

97 Brooks, C., Schmid, G.M., Miller, M., Johnson, S., Khusnatdinov, N., LaBrake, D., Resnick, D.J., and Sreenivasan, S.V. (2009) *Proc. SPIE*, **7271**, 72711.

98 Kehagias, N., Reboud, V., Sotomayor Torres, C.M., Sirotkin, V., Svintsov, A., and Zaitsev, S. (2008) *Microelectron. Eng.*, **85** (5–6), 846–849.

99 Al-Assaad, R.M., Regonda, S., Tao, L., Pang, S.W., and Hu, W. (2007) *J. Vac. Sci. Technol. B*, **25**, 2396–2401.

100 Leveder, T., Landis, S., Davoust, L., Soulan, S., and Chaix, N. (2007) *Proc. SPIE*, **6517**, 65170.

101 Ding, Y., Ro, H.W., Germer, T.A., Douglas, J.F., Okerberg, B.C., Karim, A., and Soles, C.L. (2007) *ACS Nano*, **1** (2), 84–92.

102 Patrick, H.J., Germer, T.A., Ding, Y., Ro, H.W., Richter, L.J., and Soles, C.L. (2009) *Proc. SPIE*, **7271**, 727128.

103 Soulan, S., Besacier, M., Leveder, T., and Schiavone, P. (2007) *Proc. SPIE*, **6617**, 661713.

104 International Technology Roadmap for Semiconductors, 2008 Update, Overview, Table MET1. Available at: http://public.itrs.net/.

105 Levin, T., Livne, M., and Gillespie, R.M. (2007) *Proc. SPIE*, **6518**, 651855.

106 Yu, Z., Gao, H., and Chou, S.Y. (2007) *Nanotechnology*, **18**, 065304.

107 Li, J., Liu, Z., Rabello, S., Dasari, P., Kritsun, O., and Volkman, C. (2009) *Proc. SPIE*, **7272**, 727207.

108 International Technology Roadmap for Semiconductors (April 4 2005). Available at: http://public.itrs.net/.

109 Cardinale, G.F., Skinner, J.L., Talin, A.A., Brocato, R.W., Palmer, D.W., Mancini, D.P., Dauksher, W.J., Gehoski, K., Le, N., Nordquist, K.J., and Resnick, D.J. (2004) *J. Vac. Sci. Technol. B*, **22**, 3265–3270.

110 McClelland, G.M., Hart, M.W., Rettner, C.T., Best, M.E., Carter, K.R., and Terri, B.D. (2002) *Appl. Phys. Lett.*, **81**, 1483–1485.

111 Ahn, S.W., Lee, K.-D., Kim, J.S., Kim, S.H., Lee, S.H., Park, J.D., and Yoon, P.W. (2005) *Microelectron. Eng.*, **78–79**, 314–318.

112 Sotomayor Torres, C.M., Zankovych, S., Seekamp, J., Kam, A.P., Clavijo Cedeño, C., Hoffmann, T., Ahopelto, J., Reuther, F., Pfeiffer, K., Bleidiessel, G., Gruetzner, G., Maximov, M.V., and Heidari, B. (2003) *Mater. Sci. Eng. C*, **23**, 23–31.

113 Nilsson, D., Nielsen, T., and Kristensen, A. (2004) *Rev. Sci. Instrum.*, **75**, 4481–4486.

114 Nilsson, D., Balslev, S., and Kristensen, A. (2005) *J. Micromech. Microeng.*, **15**, 296–300.

115 Reboud, V., Lovera, P., Kehagias, N., Zelsmann, M., Reuther, F., Gruetzner, G., Redmond, G., and Sotomayor Torres, C.M. (2007) *Appl. Phys. Lett.*, **91**, 151101.

116 Wang, J., Sun, X., Chen, L., and Chou, S.Y. (1999) *Appl. Phys. Lett.*, **75**, 2767–2769.

117 Cheng, X., Hong, Y., Kanicki, J., and Guo, L.J. (2002) *J. Vac. Sci. Technol. B*, **20**, 2877–2880.

118 Clavijo Cedeno, C., Seekamp, J., Kam, A.P., Hoffmann, T., Zankovych, S., Sotomayor Torres, C.M., Menozzi, C., Cavallini, M., Murgia, M., Ruani, G., Biscarini, F., Behl, M., Zentel, R., and Ahopelto, J. (2002) *Microelectron. Eng.*, **61–62**, 25–31.

119 Seekamp, J., Zankovych, S., Helfer, A.H., Maury, P., Sotomayor Torres, C.M., Bottger, G., Liguda, C., Eich, M., Heidari, B., Montelius, L., and Ahopelto, J. (2002) *Nanotechnology*, **13**, 581–586.

120 Ahn, S.W., Lee, K.D., Kim, J.S., Kim, S.H., Park, J.D., Lee, S.H., and Yoon, P.W. (2005) *Nanotechnology*, **16**, 1874.

121 Kehagias, N., Zankovych, S., Goldschmidt, A., Kian, R., Zelsmann, M., Sotomayor Torres, C.M., Pfeiffer, K., Ahrens, G., and Gruetzner, G. (2004) *Superlattices and Microstructures*, **36**, 201–210.

122 Chao, C.Y. and Guo, L.J. (2002) *J. Vac. Sci. Technol. B*, **20** (6), 2862–2866.

123 Kim, D.H., Im, J.G., Lee, S.S., Ahn, S.W., and Lee, K.D. (2005) *IEEE Photonic. Tech. L.*, **17**, 11.

124 Paloczi, G.T., Huang, Y., Yariv, A., Luo, J., and Jen, A.K.Y. (2004) *Appl. Phys. Lett.*, **85** (10), 1662–1664.

125 Meier, M., Dodabalapur, A., Rogers, J.A., Slusher, R.E., Mekis, A., Timko, A., Muray, C.A., Ruel, R., and Nalamasu, O. (1999) *J. Appl. Phys.*, **86** (7), 3502–3507.

126 Pisignano, D., Persano, L., Visconti, P., Cingolani, R., and Gigli, G. (2003) *Appl. Phys. Lett.*, **83** (13), 2545–2547.

127 Reboud, V., Lovera, P., Kehagias, N., Zelsmann, M., Schuster, C., Reuther, F., Gruetzner, G., Redmond, G., and Sotomayor Torres, C.M. (2007) *Appl. Phys. Lett.*, **91**, 151101.

128 Arango, F., Christiansen, M.B., Gersborg-Hansen, M., and Kristensen, A. (2007) *Appl. Phys. Lett.*, **91**, 223503.

129 Chen, Y., Li, Z., Zhang, Z., Psaltis, D., and Scherer, A. (2007) *Appl. Phys. Lett.*, **91** (5), 051109.

130 Reboud, V., Kehagias, N., Zelsmann, M., Fink, M., Reuther, F., Gruetzner, G., and Sotomayor Torres, C.M. (2007) *Opt. Express*, **15**, 12, 7190.

131 Reboud, V., Kehagias, N., Striccoli, M., Placido, T., Panniello, A., Curri, M.L., Zelsmann, M., Reuther, F., Gruetzner, G., and Sotomayor Torres, C.M. (2007) *J. Vac. Sci. Technol. B*, **25**, 2642.

132 Schift, H., Park, S., Jung, B., Choi, C.G., Kee, C.S., Han, S.P., Yoon, K.B., and Cobrecht, J. (2005) *Nanotechnology*, **16**, S261–S265.

133 Belotti, M., Torres, J., Roy, E., Pepin, A., Chen, Y., Gerace, D., Andreani, L.C., and Galli, M. (2006) *Microelectron. Eng.*, **83** (4–9), 1773–1777.

134 Tamborra, M., Striccoli, M., Curri, M.L., Alducin, J.A., Mecerreyes, D., Pomposo,

J.A., Kehagias, N., Reboud, V., Sotomayor Torres, C.M., and Agostian, A. (2007) *Small*, **3**, 822.

135 Reboud, V., Kehagias, N., Zelsmann, M., Striccoli, M., Tamborra, M., Curri, M.L., Agostiano, A., Fink, M., Reuther, F., Gruetzner, G., and Sotomayor Torres, C.M. (2007) *Appl. Phys. Lett.*, **90**, 011114.

136 Reboud, V., Lovera, P., Kehagias, N., Zelsmann, M., Schuster, C., Reuther, F., Gruetzner, G., Redmond, G., and Sotomayor Torres, C.M. (2007) *Appl. Phys. Lett.*, **91**, 151101.

137 Sasaki, M., Li, Y., Akatu, Y., Fujii, T., and Hane, K. (2000) *Jpn. J. Appl. Phys*, **39**, 7145–7149.

138 Li, Y., Sasaki, M., and Hane, K. (2001) *J. Micromech. Microeng.*, **11**, 3, 234–238.

139 Kragh, P. and Kristensen, A. (2003) *Proc. of the 17th Conference on Solid-State Transducers, Eurosensors*, 380.

140 Armani, M., Srinivasan, A., and Vahala, K.J. (2007) *Nano Lett.*, **7**, 6.

141 Armani, K., Kippenberg, T., Spillane, S.M., and Vahala, K.J. (2003) *Nature*, **421**, 925–929.

142 Jay Guoa, L.Y. (2002) *J. Vac. Sci. Technol. B*, **20**, 2862.

143 Balslev, S., Rasmussen, T., Shi, P., and Kristensen, A. (2005) *J. Micromech. Microeng.*, **15**, 2456–2460.

144 Balslev, S., Nielsen, R.B., Petersen, D.H., and Kristensen, A. (2006) *J. Vac. Sci. Technol. B*, **24**, 3252–3257.

145 Reboud, V., Lovera, P., Kehagias, N., Zelsmann, M., Schuster, C., Reuther, F., Gruetzner, G., Redmond, G., and Sotomayor Torres, C.M. (2007) *Appl. Phys. Lett.*, **91**, 151101.

146 Kehagias, N., Reboud, V., Chansin, G., Zelsmann, M., Jeppesen, C., Schuster, C., Kubenz, M., Reuther, F., Gruetzner, G., and Sotomayor Torres, C.M. (2007) *Nanotechnology*, **18**, 17, 175303.

147 Kehagias, N., Reboud, V., Chansin, G., Zelsmann, M., Jeppesen, C., Reuther, F., Schuster, C., Kubenz, M., Gruetzner, G., and Sotomayor Torres, C.M. (2006) *J. Vac. Sci. Technol. B*, **24** (6), 3002–3005.

148 Kehagias, N., Zelsmann, M., and Sotomayor Torres, C.M. (2005) *Proc. SPIE*, **5825**, 654.

149 Sharp, D.N., Campbell, M., Dedman, E.R., Harrison, M.T., Denning, R.G., and Turberfield, A.J. (2002) *Opt. Quantum Electron.*, **34**, 3, 3–12.

150 Kehagias, N., Reboud, V., Chansin, G., Zelsmann, M., Jeppesen, C., Reuther, F., Schuster, C., Kubenz, M., Gruetzner, G., and Sotomayor Torres, C.M. (2006) *J. Vac. Sci. Technol. B*, **24** (6), 3002–3005.

151 Chao, C.Y., and Guo, L.J. (2004) *IEEE Photonics Technol. Lett.*, **16**, 1498–1500.

152 Cho, C.O., Jeong, J., Lee, J., Kim, I., Jang, D.H., Park, Y.S., and Woo, J.C. (2005) *Appl. Phys. Lett.*, **87**, 161102.

153 Kwon, S.H., Ryu, H.Y., Kim, G.H., Lee, Y.H., and Kim, S.B. (2003) *Appl. Phys. Lett.*, **83**, 3870.

154 Joannopoulos, J.D., Villeneuve, P.R., and Fan, S. (1997) *Nature*, **386**, 143.

155 Byeon, K.J., Hwang, S.Y., and Lee, H. (2007) *Appl. Phys. Lett.*, **91**, 091106.

156 Christiansen, M.B., Schøler, M., and Kristensen, A. (2007) *Opt. Express*, **15**, 3931.

157 Köck, A., Gornik, E., Hauser, M., and Beinstingl, W. (1990) *Appl. Phys. Lett.*, **57**, 2327–2329.

158 Barnes, W.L. (1999) *J. Lightwave Technol.*, **17**, 2170–2182.

159 Reboud, V., Kehagias, N., Zelsmann, M., Fink, M., Reuther, F., Gruetzner, G., and Sotomayor Torres, C.M. (2007) *Opt. Express*, **15**, 12, 7190.

160 Neal, T.D., Okamoto, K., Scherer, A., Liu, M.S., and Jen, A.K.-Y. (2006) *Appl. Phys. Lett.*, **89**, 221106.

161 Jana, N.R. (2005) *Small*, **1**, 875.

162 Merino, S., Retolaza, A., Schift, H., and Trabadelo, V. (2007) *Microelectronic Eng.*, **84**, 848.

163 Hu, W., Lu, N., Zhang, H., Wang, Y., Kehagias, N., Reboud, V., Sotomayor Torres, C.M., Hao, J., Li, W., Fuchs, H., and Chi, L. (2007) *Adv. Mater.*, **19**, 2119.

164 Rogers, J.A. (2001) *Science*, **291**, 1502–1503.

165 Behl, M., Seekamp, J., Zankovych, S., Sotomayor Torres, C.M., Zentel, R., and

Ahopelto, J. (2002) *Adv. Mater.*, **14** (8), 588–591.

166 Fuchs, A., Vratzov, B., Wahlbrink, T., Georgiev, Y., and Kurz, H. (2004) *J. Vac. Sci. Technol. B*, **22**, 3242.

167 Li, Z., Zhang, Z., Emery, T., Scherer, A., and Psaltis, D. (2006) *Opt. Express*, **14**, 696.

168 Christiansen, M., Schøler, M., and Kristensen, A. (2007) *Opt. Express*, **15**, 3931.

169 Pisignano, D., Persano, L., Gigli, G., Visconti, P., Stomeo, T., De Vittorio, M., Barbarella, G., Favaretto, L., and Cingolani, R. (2004) *Nanotechnology*, **15**, 766.

Part Two
Bottom-Up Strategy

Nanotechnology, Volume 8: Nanostructured Surfaces. Edited by Lifeng Chi
Copyright © 2010 WILEY-VCH Verlag GmbH & Co. KGaA, Weinheim
ISBN: 978-3-527-31739-4

5
Anodized Aluminum Oxide

Günter Schmid

5.1
Introduction

Aluminum is, like titanium, zirconium, hafnium, vanadium, niobium, tantalum or magnesium, a so-called "gate metal" [1]. Gate metals have special electrochemical properties, and are distinguished by the formation of insulating oxide layers if they are used as anodes in electrochemical redox reactions. The current is based on ion transport, and is closed down at a temperature- and voltage-dependent material-specific limit; this occurs due to a reduction of the electric field by the increasing oxide layer. In contrast, the cathodic use of a gate metal results in the evolution of hydrogen. The formation of oxide layers is, of course, only possible if a solvent is used in which the oxide is not soluble. In contrast to most other metals, gate metals form compact, strongly adhering oxide layers that protect the metal beneath then from further oxidation. Due to its electrode potential of -1.662 V, aluminum is readily oxidized by contact with air to give oxide layers that are 1 to 10 nm thick [2], and this protective oxide layer can be extended up to 1 μm by anodic oxidation in neutral electrolytes [3]. This behavior, combined with its low specific weight, makes aluminum a particularly valuable material, and it is used preferentially in aircraft and automobile construction.

The electrolytic oxidation of aluminum has long been known as the Eloxal process, and this has been applied on a practical basis to generate homogeneous oxide layers on aluminum materials. Aluminum oxide is a typical insulator, with a band gap of 7–8 eV [1]. The electronic charge transport is very small and is, at high field strengths, exceeded by the ion conductivity. In anodically generated layers the charge transport is mainly determined by existing space charges [3–6] that are generated during the anodizing process in the barrier layer between metal and metal oxide, and additionally between the metal oxide and electrolyte. These are generated by Al^{3+} cations and by O^{2-} anions, as well as by electrolyte anions.

Porous aluminum oxide is generated by the anodic oxidation of aluminum surfaces in electrolytes that are able to dissolve the formed oxide. Anodized aluminum oxide (AAO), when equipped with nanopores with diameters varying between a few nanometers up to several hundreds of nanometers, is a most valuable

Nanotechnology, Volume 8: Nanostructured Surfaces. Edited by Lifeng Chi
Copyright © 2010 WILEY-VCH Verlag GmbH & Co. KGaA, Weinheim
ISBN: 978-3-527-31739-4

material for many reasons. Although porous alumina surfaces are *per se* interesting nanostructured materials, the pores can also be used as templates to generate nanowires, nanotubes or nanoparticles of different materials such as metals or semiconductors. Moreover, they can also serve as imprinting tools for the fabrication of nanostructured surfaces of various materials, and equipped with nanosticks that correspond to the pore size of the AAO-surface. One very special development during recent years has been the generation of AAOs with ordered pore-structures.

These aspects, relating in particular to nanoporous AAOs, will be discussed in detail in the following sections.

5.2
Fundamentals of Aluminum Oxide Formation

5.2.1
Barrier Oxide Layers

During the anodizing of high-purity aluminum foils or plates in neutral or weak acidic electrolytes, compact, nonporous so-called "barrier oxide" layers are formed. Examples of such electrolytes include boric acid, phosphate, ammonium borate, or tartrate solutions [1–3]. If a voltage is applied between an aluminum anode and an appropriate cathode, the current intensity I drops exponentially with time, corresponding to Eq. (5.1) [1–3].

$$I = I_0 \, e^{\beta E} \tag{5.1}$$

where I_0 and β are temperature-dependent material constants, and E is the electric field strength in the oxide.

Since the electric field strength E decreases with increasing oxide layer thickness d, [corresponding to Eq. (5.2)]:

$$E = \Delta U / d \tag{5.2}$$

where ΔU is the voltage drop and the current I falls exponentially. Hence, oxide formation will be closed down depending on the voltage applied. The ratio of the resultant thickness of the oxide layer and the anodizing voltage lies between 0.8 and 1.4 nm V^{-1} [1, 3, 7, 8]. Depending on the type of electrolyte, transport of the current occurs mainly via Al^{3+} cations and protons (phosphate-containing electrolytes) or by anions such as OH$^-$, O^{2-} and electrolyte anions (borate-containing electrolytes) [2]. The qualitative relationship between current density and time is shown in Figure 5.1 [3].

The formation of compact barrier layers can be explained by the so-called "High Field Law." This starts out from the fact that charge transport in aluminum oxide layers at high field strengths (up to 10^9 V m^{-1}) is dominated by ion conductivity. The electronic conductivity is very small, and only relevant at low field strengths due to tunneling processes and deposited foreign ions [1, 2, 4–6]. This residual current is the

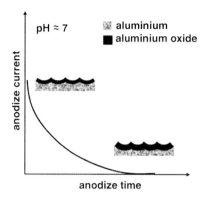

Figure 5.1 Current density–time course of barrier oxide formation.

reason why the current density at the end of the anodizing process is not zero. At high field strengths electronic conductivity can be neglected. The law also presumes that the diffusion of ions in the opposite direction to the electric field at sufficiently high field strengths can be excluded. The ionic conductivity is caused by the ions hopping from regular lattice positions and interstitial positions to neighbored fault points, due to the high electric field strength. These hopping steps require a distinct activation energy W in the field-free space, and W increases with the hopping distance, and can be varied by applying an electric field. The relationship between the activation energy and the electric field is shown graphically in Figure 5.2 [1].

Hence, the activation energy for a hopping process in the opposite direction of the electric field direction increases [Eq. (5.3)] and decreases if hopping occurs in the direction of the electric field [Eq. (5.4)]:

$$W_{\leftarrow} = W + (1-\alpha)a\,z\,F\,E \tag{5.3}$$

$$W_{\rightarrow} = W - \alpha\,a\,z\,F\,E \tag{5.4}$$

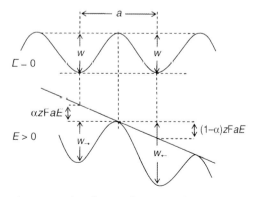

Figure 5.2 The influence of an electric field on the activation energy [1].

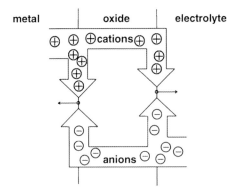

Figure 5.3 Formalized sketch of aluminum oxide growth at both boundary layers [1].

where α is the transfer coefficient which describes the symmetry of the activation barrier, z is the charge number, a the hopping distance, E the electric field strength, and F is Faraday's constant.

Typical values for the activation energies lie between 0.9 and 1.7 eV [1].

Since the transport numbers of the cations during oxide formation lie between 0.2 and 0.4, and may even be 0.5 at high field strengths, both the anions and cations are responsible for oxide formation at the metal/metal oxide boundary layer as well as at the metal oxide/electrolyte boundary layer. This occurs due to the simultaneous migration of the anions and cations [1, 3, 9, 10]. The process is summarized in Figure 5.3.

About one-half of the metal ions generated at the metal/metal oxide boundary layer move to the metal oxide/electrolyte boundary layer, where they react with OH^- and O^{2-} ions to produce a new oxide and, as a consequence the metal oxide/electrolyte boundary layer will be moved in the direction of the electrolyte. The other half of the metal ions react at the metal/metal oxide boundary layer with correspondingly moved O^{2-} ions to form fresh oxide, thus shifting the metal/metal oxide boundary layer in the direction of the metal. The mobile charge carriers are generated exclusively at the boundaries rather than inside the oxides, since the activation energy that is necessary for ion hopping is much lower than the energy needed for the formation of Schottky or Frenkel defects [1].

5.2.2
Formation of Nanoporous Aluminum Oxide

5.2.2.1 Mechanism of Formation

The anodic switching of aluminum foils or plates in alkaline (and especially in acid) electrolytes results in the formation of porous oxide layers that consist of two components – a thin barrier layer, which is comparable to that discussed above, and a porous layer. The thickness of the barrier layer is only 0.8–1.0 nm V^{-1}, due to a continuous dissolution of the oxide by the electrolyte [2, 3, 11]; consequently, a continuous anodic current passage is possible. The conductivity of the barrier layer is

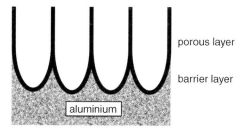

porous layer

barrier layer

aluminium

Figure 5.4 The sequence of aluminum, the barrier layer, and the porous aluminum oxide layer.

based on ion transport phenomena (see Section 5.2.1), with the adjacent porous oxide layer being characterized by pores that run perpendicular to the surface. The formation of pores is the consequence of several factors, including the voltage, temperature, the type of electrolyte, and the electrolyte concentration. The typical construction of the barrier and porous layers is shown schematically in Figure 5.4.

There exist two major models that describe the mechanism of porous oxide formation. In the model of O'Sullivan and Wood [11], it is assumed that the aluminum surface has a nanometer-scale roughness, while on top of the heights the current density is increased such that oxide formation at these positions is also increased. Due to the high field strength (up to $10^9\,\mathrm{V\,m^{-1}}$), polarization of the oxide lattice sets in, and this is accompanied by a favored dissolution of aluminum oxide by the electrolyte. As the electric field strength at positions with thin oxide layers is higher, the oxide dissolves faster here than at the elevated positions, with the result that concave structures and, finally, pores are formed. The formation of a surface which is saturated with nanometer-sized irregularities can be initiated by a so-called "electropolishing process." To achieve this, an anodization process is carried out at high temperature, high current, and under very low or very high pH conditions, linked with a continuous dissolution of the formed oxide. This results in a surface of nanosized irregularities as the best conditions in which to grow AAOs.

The course of the pore formation, starting with the generation of the barrier layer, is shown schematically in Figure 5.5. Here, the starting situation A changes to B, after which an interplay between the chemical dissolution and the electric field-assisted pore growth begins (C). This ends in a steady-state plateau region as a function of the barrier layer thickness (D) which is, in part, a function of the applied voltage.

The model of Macdonald [8] starts out from the presumption that cationic vacancies in the aluminum oxide layer diffuse to the surface under the influence of the electric field, with interruption of the electric contact and followed by formation of small elevations on the aluminum surface. From here on, the process follows the steps described by O'Sullivan and Wood. Hence, the two models only differ in their very early stages, which are responsible for different current densities linked with different dissolution behaviors.

The pore diameters, pore densities and thicknesses of the membranes have been shown to depend on the experimental conditions (see Table 5.1 for details). Clearly, pore diameters ranging from about 10 nm to several hundred nanometers are possible, depending on the voltage. Logically, the thickness of the oxide layer

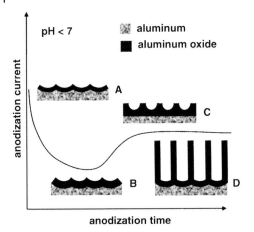

Figure 5.5 Relationship between anodization current and anodization time in acidic electrolytes, with the formation of pores.

corresponds with the anodizing time, but may vary from a few nanometers up to several hundred micrometers. In order to generate pores of a constant diameter through the whole oxide layer, a constant voltage must be maintained during the generation process. The linear correlation between the applied voltage and pore diameter is shown graphically in Figure 5.6.

Based on transmission electron microscopy (TEM) investigations, a linear regression of the measured values and the specific pore diameter d_{TEM} results in [13]:

$$d_{TEM} = 1.37 \text{ nm V}^{-1} \, U + 0.36 \text{ nm} \qquad (5.5)$$

Based on other TEM investigations, it also follows that the pore density is linearly proportional to the reciprocal square of the applied voltage (see Figure 5.7). A similar

Table 5.1 Parameters for anodized aluminum oxide (AAO) formation for some frequently used polyprotic electrolytes (Source [12]).

Anodization parameters for common polyprotic electrolytes						
% Electrolyte (w/w)	Temperature (°C)	Potential (V)	Duration (h)	Thickness (μm)	Pore diameter (nm)	Pore density (N cm^{-2})
4% H_3PO_4	0	130	8	50	200	1.3×10^8
1% H_2CO_4	−5	90	2	40	120	2.2×10^9
1% H_2CO_4	0	70	3	30	86	4.3×10^9
1% H_2CO_4	0	40	6	40	60	1.2×10^{10}
4% H_2CO_4	2	30	10	25	52	1.4×10^{10}
10% H_2SO_4	0	20	4	20	32	3.7×10^{10}
10% H_2SO_4	5	15	6	15	22	8.0×10^{10}
15% H_2SO_4	8	10	3	5	10	3.8×10^{11}
20% H_2SO_4	20	2	1	<1	~5	1.5×10^{12}

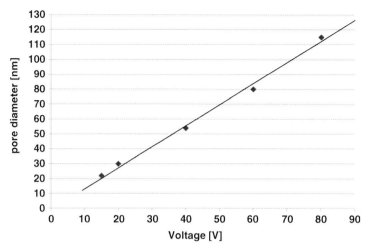

Figure 5.6 Relationship between the applied voltage and the resultant pore diameter.

relationship can be deduced via investigations using atomic force microscopy (AFM) [13].

One important aspect of AAO fabrication is a perfect detachment of the membranes from the aluminum substrates, where they are generated. Among several routes employed to detach the porous layer from the substrate, a stepwise 10% voltage reduction at completion of the process was shown to be the most efficient. Due to the voltage reduction, proportionally smaller pores are formed in the barrier layer, and this is linked with a corresponding thinning of the barrier layer. Finally, hydrogen evolution begins due to an interaction of the acidic electrolyte solution and the

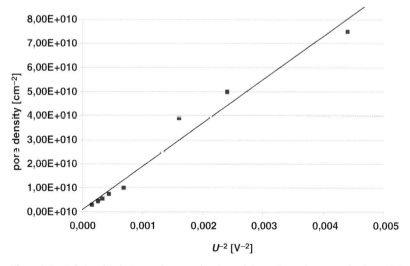

Figure 5.7 Relationship between the pore density and the reciprocal square of voltage [13].

aluminum metal. As the hydrogen gas is formed, it bubbles between the oxide layer and the aluminum, so as to detach the AAO film.

Another frequently applied method of detachment involves the use of mercuric chloride, which reacts with the aluminum support to form an amalgam, causing separation of the AAO from the surface. In both cases, the wet oxide film can be removed carefully from the solution, rinsed, dried and, if necessary, transferred to a crystalline membrane.

One final point with regards to AAO formation concerns the order of the pores. Under the conditions described above, the generated pores are predominantly dense-packed but do not show any real highly ordered structure. However, highly ordered pore structures can be fabricated by applying a two-step process [14] that starts with a 24 h anodization process, followed by dissolution of the oxide layer in a strong acid, such that an aluminum surface is formed that is well prepared for a second anodization procedure. This second anodization results in perfect hexagonally ordered pores that have no branches which can often be observed under "normal" conditions. Another pretexturing process involves the use of a single-crystal silicon carbide mold to imprint aluminum foils before anodization. and by using this method defect-free areas in the millimeter range can be generated [15]. Highly ordered pores can also be obtained by means of a two-dimensional (2-D) array of monodisperse nanoparticles (e.g., Fe_2O_3) as a template [16]. In this case, an aluminum layer is first sputtered onto the particles and then removed, producing a perfect template for the subsequent anodization process.

5.2.2.2 Chemical Composition

The as-formed "aluminum oxide" layers do not really consist of pure Al_2O_3; rather, they are characterized by a complex mixture of amorphous hydrated aluminum–oxygen compounds, including incorporated electrolyte ions [2, 8, 11, 17]. Within a porous layer, it is possible to distinguish three main areas (see Figure 5.8). The pores themselves are enclosed by an amorphous electrolyte-containing layer, followed by an aluminum oxide hydrate (AlOOH) layer, which is free of electrolyte. The latter layer

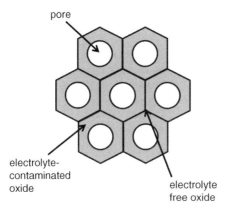

Figure 5.8 The approximate chemical composition of a porous alumina layer.

corresponds in the ideal case to a Böhmit stoichiometry [1–3, 18]. The thickness of the electrolyte-free region varies with the nature of the electrolyte, and increases from sulfuric acid, oxalic acid, phosphoric acid, to chromic acid. The yield of electrolyte in the contaminated layer may be up to 14% in the case of sulfate.

The hydrothermal treatment of such layers results in crystalline Bömit species; thermal treatment from 450 °C upwards produces nonstable γ-aluminum oxide, whilst at temperatures in excess of 1200 °C stable α-aluminum oxide layers are formed [18].

5.3
Characterization of Nanoporous Aluminum Oxide Membranes

During recent years, two main methods have been successfully developed to image and characterize nanoporous aluminum oxide layers on aluminum, or detached as membranes, namely electron microscopy (EM) and AFM. Whether applied as TEM or scanning electron microscopy (SEM), EM can provide valuable complementary information to AFM, and the simultaneous use of both techniques is generally advantageous when investigating membrane samples.

5.3.1
Electron Microscopy

Generally, the layer thickness of AAO membranes does not allow direct imaging by TEM, and samples must often be prepared using an ion-etching process, despite this resulting in very thin layers. A TEM image of the surface of a well-ordered membrane with a pore size of 53 ± 10 nm is shown in Figure 5.9. In this case, the fabrication was carried out at 40 V in 4% oxalic acid over 46 h, and the pore density (p) was 10^{10} cm^{-2} [19].

As can be seen from Figure 5.9a, highly ordered hexagonal areas were apparent over the entire image, while the membrane structure, with its pores, electrolyte-containing intermediate layer and dark hexagons of pure oxide (see Figure 5.8) could be clearly seen in a magnified area (Figure 5.9b).

Typically, SEM is also well-suited to imaging not only the surfaces of membranes, but also their cross-sections, from which the pores – which run perpendicular to the surface – can be visualized. A minor disadvantage of SEM is that nonconducting surfaces such as aluminum oxide must first be coated with a thin metal film in order to avoid electrostatic charging. In fact, if this is not very carefully carried out, the pores can become fully or partially become closed and the images falsified. The major advantage of SEM is that the AAOs do not require any previous treatment, by ion-etching. The SEM images of 15 V and 40 V membrane surfaces, equipped with pores of about 20 nm and 50–60 nm, are shown respectively in Figures 5.10 and 5.11 [13]. In Figure 5.11, some of the pores appear either partially or totally closed.

From about 60 V upwards, the pore structures are normally less well developed when compared to the 40 V membranes, with both pore geometry and distribution

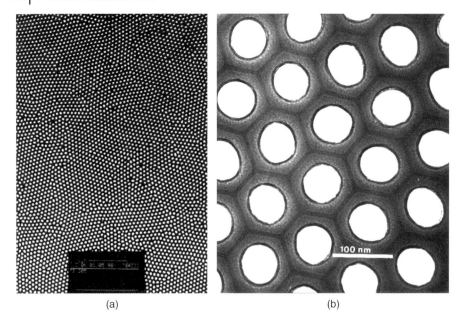

(a)   (b)

Figure 5.9 Transmission electron microscopy image of a 40 V aluminum oxide membrane. (a) Highly ordered hexagonal areas; (b) Magnified cutout indicating the electrolyte-containing intermediate layer and hexagons of pure oxide (dark regions). Panel (b) was reproduced with permission from Springer.

being of poorer quality. An enlargement of a portion of membrane generated at 150 V is shown in Figure 5.12 [13].

The cross-sectional imaging of membranes with SEM allows an insight into both pore structure and quality. Although, normally, the pores run parallel through the membrane, occasional embranchments may be observed, especially in membranes

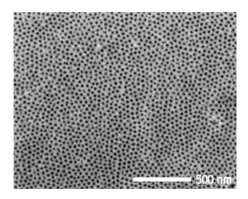

Figure 5.10 Scanning electron microscopy image of a 15 V membrane surface with pores of about 20 nm.

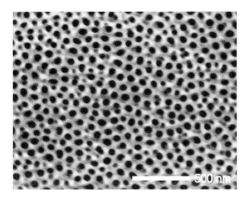

Figure 5.11 Scanning electron microscopy image of a 40 V membrane with 50–60 nm pores.

where the pores are very small. A cross-sectional SEM image of a 60 nm pore membrane with perfect parallel pores of uniform size is shown in Figure 5.13.

SEM has also been applied to demonstrate the existence of the barrier layer beneath the membranes [20].

5.3.2
Atomic Force Microscopy (AFM)

Since its discovery, AFM, together with scanning tunneling microscopy (STM) and other scanning probe microscopy techniques, have undergone continuous development to a point where they now represent unrenouncable tools for the characterization of all types of surface. In contrast to SEM, AFM is based on the forces between a tip and the surface atoms, without the need for any electronic interactions, so that both conductive and nonconductive surfaces can be investigated [21, 22]. The resolution depends firstly on the quality of the tip. At the so-called contact-modus, the forces between the tip and the surface are repulsive, whereas in the noncontact modus technique the forces are of an attractive nature. The best results for AAO

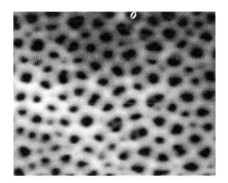

Figure 5.12 Scanning electron microscopy image of a 150 V membrane, indicating the reduced quality compared to 40 V membranes.

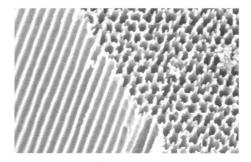

Figure 5.13 Scanning electron microscopy image of a cross-sectioned membrane with 60 nm pores. Reproduced with permission from A. Heilmann, Fraunhofer Institute, Halle, Germany.

surfaces are obtained when they are pretreated by ion beam milling. Comparisons between EM and AFM measurements have indicated a small difference in pore diameter, of about $0.18\ nm\ V^{-1}$, the reason for this being seen as a method-specific image fault, with nanometer-sized structures on surfaces becoming enlarged while the cavities appear reduced in extension. The reasons for this well-known phenomenon are explained in Figures 5.14 and 5.15, where the numbers 1 to 3 indicate typical positions of the tip's route over the surface. Compared to the size of the object, the curvature radius of the tip is larger. As a consequence, the lateral extension of an isolated object may appear to be too large, whereas the height of the particle can be measured more or less correctly.

The pores in AAOs can be considered as the negatives of particles. Depending on the tip radius, the tip will enter too late into the pore space and be repelled too early, due to contact of the tip wall with the pore wall (see Figure 5.15).

In the case of ion beam-milled surfaces, an additional special effect must be considered since, due to the low angle at which the ion beam meets the surface, the upper areas of the pore walls will be additionally thinned and alter the detail of the AFM (see Figure 5.16) [13].

The scanning curve is characterized by two steps, caused first by the thinner pore wall and then by the original wall; this can be seen from a cross-section through an AFM image of an ion beam-milled surface (Figure 5.17). Occasionally, the step from the thinned upper pore wall to the original wall can be identified by additional shoulders in the cross-section line.

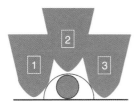

Figure 5.14 Schematic depiction of the scanning line of an atomic force microscopy (AFM) tip over an isolated particle on a smooth surface. The numbers 1 to 3 indicate typical positions of the tip's route over the surface.

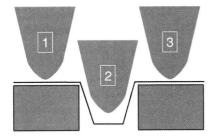

Figure 5.15 Sketch of the AFM tip motion in contact with a nanopore.

Hence, AFM images can become falsified not only by the unavoidable imaging problem of the method, but additionally by any preceding treatment of the surface. An AFM image of a hexagonally ordered 40 V pore structure after ion beam milling is shown in Figure 5.18.

AFM has also been applied to image the reverse side of AAO membranes with an intact barrier layer, and this can be achieved by the oxidative dissolution of the aluminum carrier. An AFM image of a membrane lower side, indicating the polyhedral round forms of the barrier layer (see also Figure 5.4) is shown in Figure 5.19 [13].

The differences in pore diameter for TEM and AFM characterizations and eventual pretreatments are summarized in Table 5.2.

5.4
Aluminum Oxide Membranes as Templates

One of the most attractive applications of nanoporous alumina membranes is in using the ordered pores as templates, to generate correspondingly ordered arrays of 2-D wires, tubes, or particles. As a result, numerous activities have emerged during the past decade, with polymers [23], carbon [24–27], semiconductors [28–30],

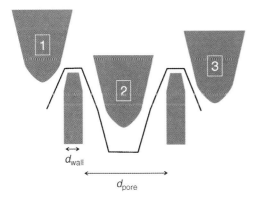

Figure 5.16 Sketch of the AFM tip motion in contact with ion beam-milled surfaces in detail.

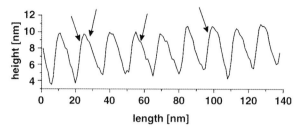

Figure 5.17 Cross-section through an ion beam-milled 40 V anodized aluminum oxide (AAO) membrane. The arrows indicate steps from the thinned upper pore wall to the original wall (cf. Figure 5.16.

metals [31–33] and various other materials having been arranged in the pores of AAOs [34]. In general, the tubes or wires generated can be separated from the alumina template by dissolving the latter with an acid or a base.

The variability of the pore diameters and pore lengths is of enormous advantage when tuning the products. However, if membranes with barrier layers are used as templates, then the resultant wires or tubes cannot be positioned directly on a surface in an upright position. However, this does become possible if membranes that are open on both sides are used, and this can be achieved either by removing the oxide barrier layer with a phosphoric acid solution [35], or by ion beam milling. In the following sections, examples are provided where tubes, wires or dots are placed on supports, leading to the creation of novel nanostructured surfaces (as the title of this book might suggest!).

5.4.1
Carbon Nanotubes and Nanowires

Highly ordered arrays of carbon nanotubes (CNTs) can be fabricated by the pyrolysis of acetylene on cobalt catalysts, inside hexagonally ordered pores of aluminum oxide membranes at 650 °C [25]. In this way, large-scale arrangements of densely packed CNTs become available, with diameters ranging from 10 nm to several hundred nanometers, and lengths of up to 100 μm. CNT arrangements of such quality are of

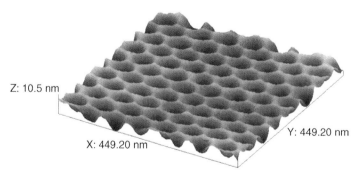

Figure 5.18 Atomic force microscopy image of a perfectly ordered hexagonal AAO surface.

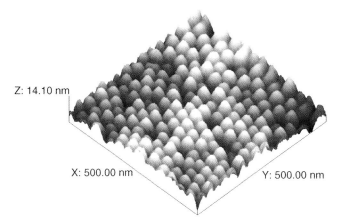

Z: 14.10 nm

X: 500.00 nm

Y: 500.00 nm

Figure 5.19 Atomic force microscopy image of the reverse side of a barrier layer, generated at 25 V.

general interest for future applications in nanoelectronics, such as data storage, field emission displays, or sensors.

In contrast to the above-described bodies, CNTs as well as wires of diamond structure may become available if microwave plasma-assisted chemical vapor deposition (CVD) is used with acetone as the carbon source, instead of the simple thermal decomposition described above [27]. Diamond tubes and wires exhibit totally different properties compared to CNTs consisting of graphitic structures, with the high stability and the negative electron affinity allowing novel applications in both nano- and microelectronics. The creation of low-field emitters [36–38] or cold cathode flat-panel displays [39, 40] has been proposed by using such diamond species.

Both, aligned polycrystalline diamond nanowires and diamond-like nanotubes can be created using AAO membranes as templates, the main advantage being their variability. The anodization of a 0.15 mm Al sheet in 0.3 M H_3PO_4 at 1 °C under a voltage of 190 V for 70 min resulted in pores which were about 7 μm long and 300 nm wide. In order to open the down-side of the membrane, the aluminum is first dissolved with $HgCl_2$, after which the barrier layer is removed using phosphoric acid [35]. Such through-hole membranes are perfectly suited for the generation of diamond tubes or wires, the individual production steps of which are depicted in Figure 5.20.

Table 5.2 Observed diameters (d) depending on the method of investigation and pretreatment by ion beam milling [13].

Method	Diameter (d) (nm)
TEM	$1.37\,\text{nm V}^{-1} \cdot U + 0.36\,\text{nm}$
AFM, untreated	$0.72\,\text{nm V}^{-1} \cdot U + 0.07\,\text{nm}$
AFM, untreated (ion beam)	$1.19\,\text{nm V}^{-1} \cdot U + 0.02\,\text{nm}$

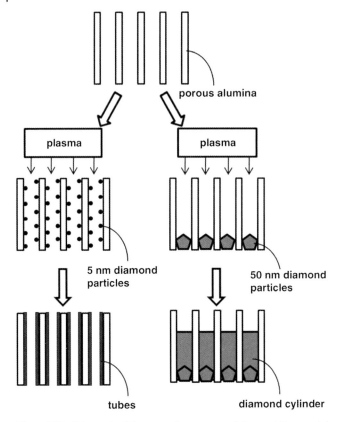

Figure 5.20 Schematic of the generation process of diamond-like nanotubes (left) and nanowires (right).

The first step consists of depositing ultrasonically dispersed 5 nm diamond particles on the pore walls to create tubes, and of about 50 nm diamond particles at the bottom of the pores to create wires. In both cases, the deposited diamond particles serve as seeds for the growth of further particles, resulting in tubes and cylinders, respectively. The as-prepared alumina membranes are then placed into a microwave plasma chamber whereby, at a microwave power of 3 kW, 80 Torr with hydrogen as carrier gas and temperatures of about 1000 °C are achieved. A reaction time of 8 h leads to an arrangement of parallel tubes or wires with an outer diameter of 300 nm, corresponding to the pore diameters, with both the tubes and cylinders standing upright and parallel on the substrate after dissolution of the alumina with concentrated phosphoric acid. The substrate also consists of a diamond film formed during the deposition process on the membrane. The SEM image of diamond-like nanotubes is shown in Figure 5.21, whereas Figure 5.22a shows a cross-sectional field of parallel diamond nanowires, and Figure 5.22b shows the wire arrangement from the top, indicating a clear hexagonal arrangement [27].

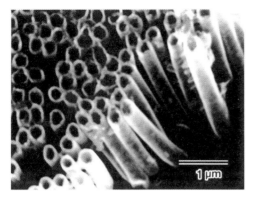

Figure 5.21 Scanning electron microscopy image of diamond-like nanotubes of 300 nm diameter and about 7 μm length [27].

As already mentioned, diameters and lengths of tubes and wires can be varied along with the pore geometries. Based on the Raman spectra of diamond wires, a broad signal at 1440 cm^{-1} indicates the presence of some sp^2 carbon, whereas the diamond peak is observed at 1334 cm^{-1}, as expected.

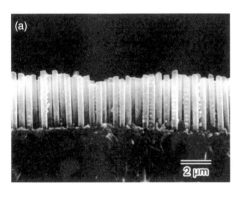

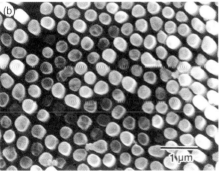

Figure 5.22 Scanning electron microscopy image of diamond nanowires visualized (a) from the side and (b) from the top. The diameter (300 nm) and length (7 μm) correspond to the alumina pores [27].

The procedure also allows doping of the diamond wires, for instance with boron. In this case, the originally colorless and transparent wires become dark blue.

5.4.2
Metal Nanotubes and Nanowires

Whereas, the simple filling of porous aluminum oxide membranes by using electrochemical or chemical techniques is relatively well known, the fabrication of free-standing aligned metal nanotubes on substrates remains very limited. However, by applying appropriate templates and synthesis procedures, several examples have been identified in recent years, some of which are discussed in the following subsections.

Well-ordered, 35 μm-long Ni nanotubes can be generated by electrodeposition using commercially available alumina membranes (Anapore) [41], although to achieve this the pore walls must first be chemically modified with methyl-γ-diethy-lenetriaminopropyl-dimethoxysilane; this allows nickel to be deposited preferentially onto the walls, as a result of strong interactions between the metal and the amino groups. Without such pretreatment of the pore walls, Ni nanowires would be formed instead of tubes. At current densities of 0.6 mA cm^{-2} and Ni^{2+} ions from NiSO$_4$ in a boronic acid-containing aqueous solution, Ni nanotubes of outer diameter 160 ± 20 nm can be generated. However, as the length of the tubes and their wall thickness will depend on the experimental conditions employed, and can vary over a wide range, it is possible to obtain pore wall thicknesses ranging from 30 nm to 60 nm. Moreover, if the membrane material is removed by aqueous NaOH, then arrays of Ni nanotubes are obtained, as shown in Figure 5.23.

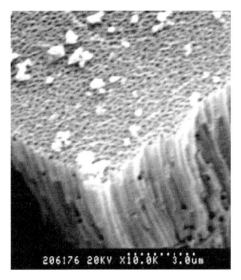

Figure 5.23 Scanning electron microscopy image of free-standing, densely packed Ni nanotubes of 160 ± 20 nm outer diameter [41].

Magnetic measurements of these Ni nanotube arrangements with aspect ratios of ~200 indicate enhanced coercivities compared to the bulk nickel. Strong inter-tube interactions are also observed.

Various metal nanotubes can also be synthesized by a different procedure in AAOs [33]. In contrast to the above method with chemically modified pore walls, the alternative consists of the pre-deposition of CNTs onto the pore walls of the alumina membranes via the pyrolytic decomposition of ethyne [42]. By using a gold film on one side of the membrane as an electric contact, the electrodeposition of Ni first results in the formation of Ni wires with CNT walls. The next step comprises a thermal treatment of these AAO/CNT/Ni systems at 400 °C in air, so as to oxidize the Ni wires to NiO; an increase in temperature to 600 °C then burns up the CNTs. As a result of this procedure, highly ordered nanochannels of the former CNT dimension are yielded. In this way, various metals such as Pt, Au, Bi, In, and Ni can be electrodeposited into the annular nanochannels, and this will result in a coaxial sandwich system with NiO cores and metal walls inside the aluminum oxide membrane. The NiO and Al$_2$O$_3$ can then be chemically dissolved to leave the free-standing metal nanotubes. The different reaction steps, from the alumina membrane to the nanotube array, are shown schematically in Figure 5.24.

By having CNT diameters of 50 nm and a wall thickness of 10 nm, it is possible to produce metal nanotubes of the same dimensions; an SEM image of such Pt nanotubes of 30 μm length is shown in Figure 5.25.

The deposition of metal nanowires in the pores of alumina membranes usually occurs if a direct current (DC) is used. However, the first step involves a detachment

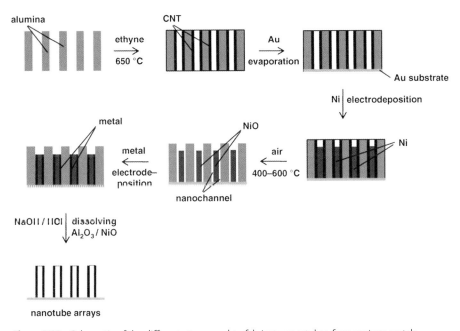

Figure 5.24 Schematic of the different steps used to fabricate nanotubes from various metals.

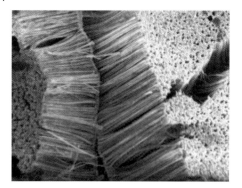

Figure 5.25 Scanning electron microscopy image of aligned Pt nanotubes, with wall thickness ca. 10 nm, and total diameter ca. 50 nm [33].

of the membrane from the aluminum support, and etching of the barrier layer (as discussed above). Since a metallic contact must be created on one side of the membrane, the latter must be thick enough to be free-standing [43, 44]. Another procedure involves the use of an alternating deposition potential, which causes the metal nanowires to be deposited on the barrier layer of the membrane, thus avoiding any membrane pretreatment [45–48]. This method has recently been adopted by using highly ordered alumina membranes [31]. Pore arrays of a high aspect ratio are fabricated by using an appropriately long anodization [35, 49] whereby, after generating the membrane, the barrier layer and pore walls are thinned by isotropic chemical etching, followed by two current-limited anodization steps. The remaining aluminum support can then be used as an electric contact for the electrodeposition of metals from metal salt solutions [31].

Pulsed electrodeposition under a modulated voltage control has been shown to produce the best results if compact metal nanowires are fabricated in the membranes [31, 50–53]. Despite the creation of numerous metal nanowires inside the aluminum oxide membranes, only a limited number of examples exists, where parallel and free-standing wires on a support have been obtained after detachment of the membrane material, representing a nanostructured surface. Rather, in most cases randomly oriented wires, lying on the support, are produced. On the other hand, numerous other methods to generate ordered metal or semiconductor nanowires on surfaces have been developed, albeit via other methods that are not the object of this chapter (e.g., see Ref. [54]). Two examples of metal nanowires plated substrates by means of AAO membranes are discussed in the following subsections.

Perfect 2-D arrays of Cu nanowires on silicon supports have been prepared by the anodization of an Al film sputtered onto a Si/SiO_2 substrate (step a → b in Figure 5.26). The aluminum oxide membrane was then etched away with phosphoric acid/chromic acid so as to produce an array of nanoholes in the Al film (step b → c in Figure 5.26). In a second anodization step, carried out at 40 V until the aluminum was totally oxidized, the final perfect pore structure was formed [55] (steps c → d in Figure 5.26). Deposition of Cu in the pores proceeds best by nonselective electroless plating (step d → e).

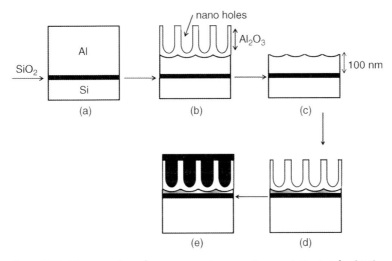

Figure 5.26 The generation of copper nanowires on a Si support. See text for details.

The deposition of Cu in the pores succeeds best via nonselective electroless plating. In this case, after having activated the alumina surface by $PdCl_2$, copper is deposited from $CuSO_4 \cdot 5H_2O$, while the pores are completely filled with Cu if the aspect ratio is 2.5. As the Cu nanowires are connected by a copper film on top, this film can be delaminated with the wires, using a Scotch tape and pulling from the Si substrate.

A similar generation of free-standing copper nanowires has succeeded via nano-porous AAO membranes on top of a metallic substrate, followed by the deposition of copper inside the pores from a plating bath of specific formulation and dissolution of the AAO template [56].

Antimony nanowires can be fabricated in anodic alumina membranes by pulsed electrodeposition under modulated voltage control at 40 V [57]. In this case, the aluminum support and barrier layer could be removed chemically, followed by the sputtering of a gold film onto one side of the membrane as the working electrode. As an antimony precursor $SbCl_3$ was used, the upper part of the alumina was dissolved with NaOH solution following electrodeposition of the Sb wires.

5.4.3
Semiconductor Nanowires

The application of nanoporous alumina membranes is, of course, not limited to the fabrication of carbon or metal nanotubes and nanowires, but has been extended to semiconductors and to other materials (see Section 5.4.4). Some examples of typical semiconductor nanowires are provided in the following subsections.

The generation of silicon nanowires can, among others, be based on a so-called vapor–liquid–solid (VLS) growth [58]. In this case, a gaseous Si source (SiH_4 or $SiCl_4$) is thermally decomposed at an appropriate temperature by contact with a metal catalyst (such as Au), and then diffuses into the metal to produce a liquid alloy. On

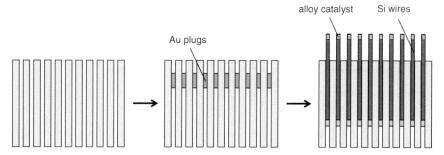

Figure 5.27 Schematic representation of the fabrication of Si nanowires on top of an alumina membrane.

reaching supersaturation, the Si nanowires begin to precipitate and grow underneath the liquid alloy droplet. Whilst the principle of this process has long been known [59–64], it can also be applied by using nanoporous alumina membranes as templates [58], whereby membranes of various pore diameters, equipped with a thin Ag film on the top side, are used to electrodeposit Au plugs inside the pores, and to act as catalysts for the VLS process. When the VLS process is started the Si wires grow first inside and finally outside of the pores, such that the membrane is decorated with Si nanowires. The principle of the system is depicted in Figure 5.27, and an example of such a nanostructured surface is shown in Figure 5.28.

Currently, TiO_2 is of increasing interest with regards to its semiconductor properties, most recently in photochemical solar cells. As TiO_2 nanowires are believed to play a special role in these developments, the routine production of TiO_2 nanowires *per se* and nanowires decorating different supports continues to attract increasing attention. Indeed, nanoporous aluminum oxide membranes might again play an important role in routine fabrications, with 40 V membranes being applied to TiO_2 production via a sol–gel process [65]. In this case, a TiO_2 sol can be prepared from tetrabutyl titanate, ethanol, acetic acid, and water. A through-hole 40 V membrane, generated by etching the Al support by $HgCl_2$ and dissolving the barrier layer with phosphoric acid, is then immersed gradually in the gel, followed by heat treatment. Temperatures of up to 650 °C finally cause the TiO_2 to be transferred to anatase quality. Previously, free-standing nanowires of up to 20 μm have been created by dissolving part of the membrane material from one side with phosphoric acid.

Cadmium chalcogenides belong to the most attractive – and therefore increasingly investigated – group of materials in nanotechnology; CdS is representative of this group. Whereas, CdS films and nanoparticles are well-known objects of research, CdS nanowire arrays have undergone much less development, due mainly to their more complicated fabrication. Yet, aluminum oxide membranes represent a good opportunity to close that gap. By following a long-recognized method for preparing CdS from Cd^{2+} and elemental sulfur [66] in dimethyl sulfoxide (DMSO), CdS nanowires can be generated in AAO pores by electrochemical deposition [28]. For this, membranes with pore diameters between 9 and 35 nm, together with the original Al support, are used as the working electrode, with graphite as the

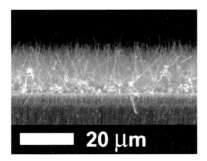

Figure 5.28 Scanning electron microscopy image of Si nanowires grown from the pores of a 50 V alumina membrane.

counter-electrode, using an alternating current. However, if the Al support and the barrier layer are removed by the above-mentioned methods, then a metal electrode can be positioned, after which a direct current electrodeposition would become possible [67, 68]. Detachment of the alumina material by NaOH has resulted in free-standing wires with diameters that corresponded to the pore diameters, and lengths of up to 1 µm.

5.4.4
Other Materials

Besides carbon, metals and semiconductors (as discussed above), a series of other materials can be used to create nanotubes or nanowires in the pores of alumina membranes. Boron nitride (BN), a typical nonconductor, is briefly described as an example in the following subsection. By using trichloroborazine, polycrystalline BN nanotubes were prepared, using CVD, when gaseous borazine was pyrolyzed at 750 °C over the open pores of commercially available membranes (Anodisc) [29]. In the case of borazine (which has the advantage of already having the correct B : N ratio), the nanotubes were able to reach lengths of up to 20 µm with, as usual, parts of the membrane material being dissolved in NaOH to produce free-standing nanotubes on the alumina support.

Coaxial C/BN/C nanotubes can be generated by the sequential pyrolysis of acetylene and trichloroborazine. The filling of BN nanotubes with metals has also been shown possible via an electrochemical deposition of copper into BN tubes that resulted in the production of BN-coated Cu nanowires [68].

5.4.5
Nanoparticles

Clearly, in addition to fabricating nanotubes or nanowires of various materials, it is also possible to generate assemblies of nanoparticles by the use of nanoporous alumina membranes. Although a recent report has described much of the detail relating to this subject [69], the discussion here will relate only to certain principles, as the technical procedures for preparing nanoparticle arrangements rather than nanowires are only marginally different. For example, separately fabricated ultra-thin through-hole alumina membranes can be used equally well as can membranes generated directly on the smooth surfaces of interest and coated in advance with a thin aluminum film [70]. Consequently, semiconductor, metal or metal oxide nanoparticles can each be deposited through the short pores on the substrates, followed by dissolution of the alumina masks (as per usual). Generally, the arrangement of pores in pre-prepared membranes is of a better quality than that produced by connected Al films. In fact, the best results with connected membranes have been achieved using rather thick Al films (20 μm), though this is a clear disadvantage for the subsequent deposition of nanoparticles. Thinner Al films (0.8 μm) can be used if pre-texturing with SiC or Si_3N_4 is carried out in advance [71, 72], such that the formed concave imprints serve as nucleation points in the subsequent anodization process. The use of such connected membranes means that the removal of any barrier layer between the pores and substrate must first be mastered, although several procedures have been described to overcome such a problem [31, 71–77].

Currently, most deposition procedures are based on vapor-phase techniques such as electron-beam evaporation, sputtering, molecular beam epitaxy, CVD, or pulsed laser deposition [69]. The use of membrane masks, directly fabricated onto a substrate, allows also wet chemical procedures such as electrochemical and electroless deposition to be carried out, due to their strong connection with the underlying substrate.

5.5
Nanoporous Alumina Membranes as Imprinting Tools

Among the principal techniques to fabricate micro- and nanostructured surfaces, which include lithography, self-assembly, controlled deposition, size reduction or replication by physical contact, the lithographic methods play a major role in the semiconductor industry [78–80]. Although lithographic methods are generally limited by the wavelength of the applied irradiation, the so-called "nanolithographic" techniques have meanwhile opened the door to higher-quality nanostructured surfaces by providing the to write structures on surfaces, using an AFM tip [81].

Among these various techniques for fabricating micro- or nanostructured surfaces, imprinting processes with stiff masks play a dominant role. The expression "imprinting" infers that a mask is pressed into a substrate to form an inverse 1 : 1 image. For instance, compact discs (CDs) are produced by imprinting polycarbonate discs by nickel matrices [82]. In another example of a successful imprinting process, a SiO_2-covered Si wafer is structured with EBL, and then used to imprint a poly (methylmethacrylate) (PMMA)-coated Si wafer. The holes produced can then be filled by metals, followed by dissolution of the PMMA, such that a surface with metal islands results [83].

Replication techniques which use nanoporous aluminum oxide membranes as an imprinting tool are details in the following subsections.

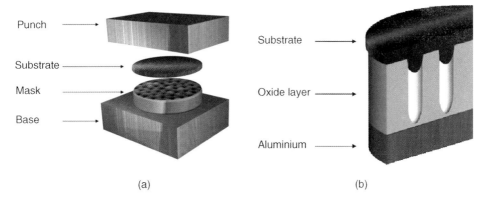

Figure 5.29 (a) Schematic of the imprinting device; (b) Material flow into the nanopores. Note: the pores shown on the mask in panel (a) were enlarged in order to render them visible.

5.5.1
Imprinting Techniques and Conditions

The alumina membranes can be applied as stamps in different forms, with sheets, discs, or foils each suited to imprinting other materials. Whilst one-sided anodized discs can be used directly as stamps, foils must be placed on a stamp of another material. However, foils have the advantage of being more flexible than hard discs, and so cracking of the porous layer can better be avoided; in fact, even re-use is possible. Details of the imprinting process are shown in Figure 5.29a and b [84, 85]. In this case, the alumina mask and substrate to be imprinted are positioned between the punch and the base of the press device. The material flow into the pores is shown in Figure 5.29b. Usually, the surface to be nanostructured is softer than the alumina, but if this is not the case then raising the temperature may help to achieve an appropriate softness.

The perfect 1 : 1 transfer of a porous stamp onto a surface can best be visualized if some irregularities exist, as is the case with the example in Figure 5.30. Here, a 150 V membrane with some fractures and other defects has been used to imprint a Pd

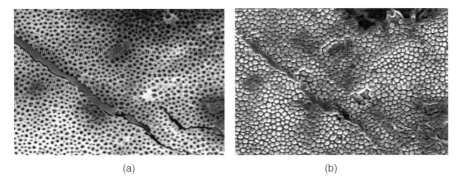

Figure 5.30 Scanning electron microscopy images of (a) a nonperfect 150 V alumina membrane, and (b) an imprinted Pd surface, showing the same defects.

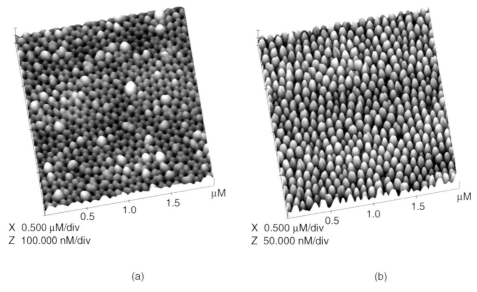

X 0.500 µM/div
Z 100.000 nM/div

(a)

X 0.500 µM/div
Z 50.000 nM/div

(b)

Figure 5.31 Atomic force microscopy image of (a) a 40 V (50 nm) alumina membrane, and (b) the corresponding imprinted PMMA surface.

surface. It can easily be seen that, besides the pores themselves, all defects of the membrane are transferred to the Pd surface [84].

By using a high-quality membrane for imprinting a PMMA surface at 110 °C, combined with a pressure of 80 MPa for 60 s, the result was a near-perfect inverse image of the pore structure (see Figure 5.31), where the hexagonal structure of the pores is seen to be transferred to the PMMA surface. Whereas, the pore and the pillar density, the diameters and the distances between membrane and PMMA surface agree quite well, the heights of the PMMA pillars deviate characteristically from the lengths of the pores. This can be followed from height profiles [84]. This effect is not caused by a break of the PMMA pillars during the separation of the mask from the substrate, but rather is due to an incomplete filling of the pores by the polymer. The average pillar height in this case lies between 40 and 50 nm, giving an aspect ratio of approximately 1.

The results of imprinting depend mainly on the mechanical properties of the masks and substrates. The mechanical properties of metals are given by a series of characteristic values, such as hardness, breaking tension, break constriction, breaking strain, pressure resistance, and bending strength. These values relate to well-known properties such as toughness, ductility, brittleness and wear resistance, and provide information regarding the general properties of a material. If an external force is applied at a metal stick, it is elastically elongated in a reversible process that is described by Hooke's law:

$$\sigma = E \cdot \varepsilon \tag{5.6}$$

where σ is the tension (in Pa), E is the elasticity module (in Pa), and ε is the elongation ($\Delta l / l$) [86].

If the so-called "flow limit" is overcome by an external force, a metal stick would be irreversibly deformed and Hooke's law no longer valid, such that finally the break point would be reached. The special ductility of metals is a consequence of the bonding situation in metals, characterized by the existence of freely mobile electrons (electron gas). The mechanical properties of the metals that have been used for imprinting (see Section 5.5.2) are summarized in Table 5.3 [87–89].

As can be seen from these data, properties such as flow limit, breaking strain or hardness can vary for the same metal, depending on its pretreatment. The metals used in the processes described below for imprinting are classified as "hard" due to their pretreatment. In spite of certain differences in their mechanical properties, the metals used behave in identical fashion with respect to the irreversibility of the imprinting-determined structures. The ductility of all metals used is sufficient for their surfaces to be imprinted at room temperature.

In contrast, the mechanical properties of polymers differ greatly from each other compared with metals, due to their chemical composition. As the polymer chains of thermoplasts are not linked among each other (in contrast to elastomers and duromers), thermoplasts should be better suited for imprinting. Above the glass-point the mechanical stability decreases rapidly; however, as the glass-point depends not only on the molecular masses but also on the crystallinity, technical polymer products usually do not have a distinct glass-point but rather a transition region. This

Table 5.3 Mechanical properties of the metals used for imprinting with alumina membranes.

Metal	Flow limit (MPa)	Breaking strain (MPa)	Modulus of elasticity (GPa)	Hardness (Vickers)
Aluminum (99.999%)	10–35 (soft) 110–170 (hard)	50–90 (soft) 130–195 (hard)	70.6	21 (soft) 35–48 (hard)
Aluminum (99.5%)	—	68–127	—	—
Aluminum (99.0%)	—	98–157	—	—
Lead	5.5	12	16.1	5
Iron	120–150	180–210	211.4	—
Copper	54 (soft) 270 (hard)	224 (soft) 314 (hard)	129.8	49 (soft) 87 (hard)
Brass	300–700	—	110–115	—
Nickel	150 (soft) 480 (hard)	400 (soft) 600 (hard)	199.5	75
Palladium	34.5 (soft) 205 (hard)	140–195 (soft) 325 (hard)	121	40 (soft) 100 (hard)
Platinum	14–35 (soft) 185 (hard)	125–150 (soft) 200–300 (hard)	170	40 (soft) 100 (hard)
Silver	—	172 (soft) 330 (hard)	82.7	25 (soft) 95 (hard)
Zinc	—	37	104.5	30

Table 5.4 Mechanical properties of the polymers used for imprinting.

Polymer	Elongation at break (%)	Breaking strain (MPa)	Modulus of elasticity (MPa)
PC	100–150	55–75	2.3–2.4
PE	—	15–40	0.5–1.2
PMMA	1.5–4.0	80	2.4–3.3
PTFE	400	7–20	0.3–0.8

PC = polycarbonate; PE = polyethylene; PMMA = poly(methylmethacrylate);
PTFE = polytetrafluoroethylene.

can be seen from the data in Table 5.4, in which the mechanical data of the investigated polymers are collected [87].

Compared to metals, the elasticity moduli and breaking strains of polymers are smaller. Indeed, there are considerable differences in the plasticity of polymers at room temperature; for example, polytetrafluoroethylene (PTFE) can be formed at room temperature, whereas PMMA will break unless it is warmed up.

Besides the mechanical properties of the materials to be imprinted, those of the imprinting mask (in this case, aluminum oxide) are equally important. The hardness of nanoporous alumina layer lies between 320 and 360 (Vickers), which is much higher than that of the materials to be imprinted. In contrast, the brittleness of ceramics is generally high, and therefore oxide layers may be destroyed under pressure if this is not carefully adjusted.

Finally, the behavior of alumina stamps is also dependent on their mechanical constitution. For example, anodized aluminum discs, when used at 100 MPa for imprinting PTFE over a 20 s period will become deformed to some extent, thus reducing the pressure to 70 MPa [84]. As a consequence, the numerous fractures that have formed will be transferred to the substrate (see Figure 5.32).

Bursting of the oxide layer can occur for different reasons, one of which is a lack of perfect coplanarity at any position if extended stamps and substrates are used. A

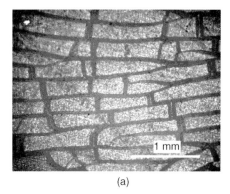
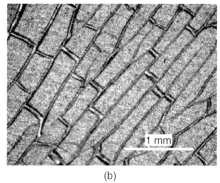

(a)   (b)

Figure 5.32 Light microscopy images of (a) an anodized aluminum disc (70 V) after imprinting, and (b) and an imprinted PTFE surface.

material which is capable of flowing can equilibrate such unevenness, but not in the case of a thick disc. The main reason for such roughness is the use of insufficiently pretreated technical aluminum surfaces. However, even electropolishing cannot fully prevent such defects, and in fact even if perfectly smooth surfaces are used, crack formation may occur if the flow limit of aluminum is exceeded. The consequent flow of the metal beneath the oxide layer causes tensions to be built up, and this results in crack formation.

Such disadvantages of aluminum discs can be prevented to a large extent if aluminum foils, oxidized on one side, are used for imprinting [84]. In this case, not only will the flow processes be reduced, but so too will the tendency towards crack formation of the oxide layer.

Alumina membranes that have been detached from the aluminum substrate and then used as stamps are not suited for imprinting processes, as the membrane usually fractures under pressure.

5.5.2
Imprinting of Metal Surfaces

The hardness of alumina allows the imprinting of many metals and alloys and, as noted above, the quality of the structured surfaces depends heavily on their pretreatment.

Aluminum can be imprinted by its own oxide. The surface quality is best pre-prepared by electropolishing, with Al sheets and discs being polished by anodization at 75 °C in highly concentrated electrolyte solutions for 10 min, whereas for Al foils (75 μm) only 1 min at 10 V is required. Due to the elevated temperature, the oxide layers are removed continuously from the surfaces, after which any traces of aluminum oxide are dissolved using chromic acid and phosphoric acid [84, 85]. Despite this careful smoothening of the Al surfaces to be imprinted, a nanosized roughness can still be observed. The AFM images of an as-prepared Al surface, before and after imprinting at 250 MPa, are shown in Figure 5.33. Here, the aluminum pillars have an average height of 200–230 nm and an aspect ratio of about 1. The pillars on the imprinted surface (Figure 5.33b) clearly show an additional fine structure, caused by the nanosized roughness of the electropolished surface. In fact, for applications where large surfaces are advantageous (as in catalysis), this effect might be very welcome.

This example demonstrates how the substrate surface influences the imprinting process. Although the flow limit of the metals has been exceeded, the locally different distributions of pressure have resulted in different degrees of transformation.

Lead surfaces may also be prepared, although problems in obtaining smooth surfaces have produced poor results. Due to the special ductility of lead, its surfaces may become partially cracked under high pressure, as identified from SEM images [84].

The transition metals *iron, nickel, palladium,* and *platinum* can be nanostructured at pressures of between 1000 and 1500 MPa, while *copper* and *silver* have been successfully nanostructured by 50 nm and 150 nm pore masks at 985 MPa [84, 85].

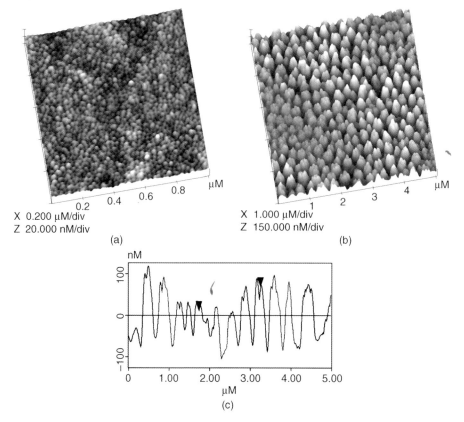

X 0.200 μM/div
Z 20.000 nM/div

(a)

X 1.000 μM/div
Z 150.000 nM/div

(b)

(c)

Figure 5.33 Atomic force microscopy images of an electropolished Al surface (a) before and (b) after imprinting with about 180 nm pores, at a pressure of 250 MPa; (c) A cross-section, indicating the multiple tips of the Al pillars.

An AFM image of a silver foil, imprinted with a 50 nm pore alumina mask, is shown in Figure 5.34, where this has resulted in Ag pillars with aspect ratios of between 0.8 and 1.5.

In the case of *zinc* and *brass*, Zn can be easily imprinted at 500 MPa, whereas brass (which is much harder) requires a pressure of 985 MPa to be imprinted with 200 nm pore masks. An AFM image and the corresponding gray-scale shading image of an imprinted brass surface with pillars of an aspect ratio of 0.8–1.4 are shown in Figure 5.35a and b [84]. Here, the gray-scale image (Figure 5.35b) results from the deviation S_x of the height h in the scanning direction x (arrow). The 3-D impression results from the fact that the structure heights, which increase in the scanning direction, appear light (right side), whereas decreasing structure heights on the opposite side become dark (left side). Although, from such images the topography can better be perceived, this type of imaging does not provide any information regarding the structure heights.

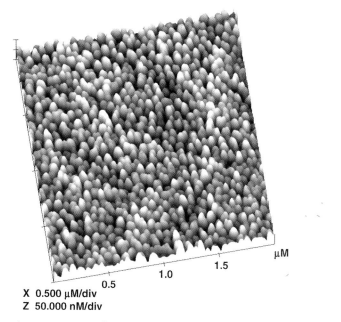

X 0.500 µM/div
Z 50.000 nM/div

Figure 5.34 Atomic force microscopy image of a nanostructured Ag surface (mask: 50 nm pores).

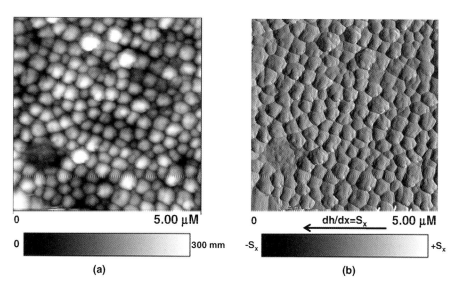

Figure 5.35 Atomic force microscopy image of (a) an imprinted brass surface, and (b) the gray-scale shading image deduced from it.

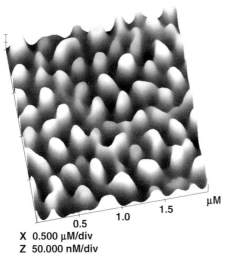

X 0.500 μM/div
Z 50.000 nM/div

Figure 5.36 Atomic force microscopy image of a polycarbonate surface, imprinted by a 180 nm pore mask.

5.5.3
Imprinting of Polymers

Polymers can usually be imprinted at lower pressures compared to metals, and an image of a perfect transfer of the mask structure on PMMA was shown in Figure 5.31.

Polycarbonate (PC) can be imprinted using 180 nm pore masks at 200 MPa at room temperature [84, 85]; the result is shown in Figure 5.36, and heights of 80–90 nm and aspect ratios of about 0.5 result under these conditions.

Polyethylene (PE) gives corresponding results.

Polytetrafluoroethylene (PTFE) is a technically important, high-temperature-resistant thermoplastic with a low surface energy and friction coefficient. It is easily deformable, tends to creep, and is mechanically only scarcely loadable; hence, it is often used as anti-adhesive material. These properties become visible during imprinting experiments, and for imprinting alumina foils are better suited than either sheets or disks. An AFM image of a PTFE surface, imprinted by a 50 nm pore mask at 130 MPa and at room temperature, is shown in Figure 5.37. In this case, the superimposed roughness can be traced back to the material's properties.

Additional damages may also occur during separation of the mask from the substrate, and this is especially the case at high temperatures. Variations in the imprinting time, between 10 and 300 s, had no significant influence on the quality of the imprinted surfaces.

Polymer-coated metals are of major practical relevance for many reasons, but notably for hydrophobizing the surfaces (this effect may be improved by nanostructuring, and is discussed in Section 5.6). Metal sheets, when coated with two different commercially produced silicon polyesters, Silikoftal HTL 2 and Silikoftal NS 60 (Degussa), were used for imprinting with nanoporous alumina. As these polymers

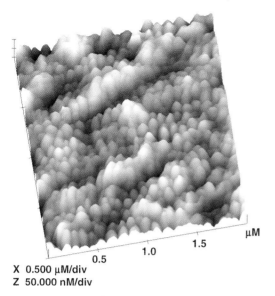

X 0.500 μM/div
Z 50.000 nM/div

Figure 5.37 Atomic force microscopy image of a PTFE surface, imprinted by a 50 nm pore mask at 130 MPa, at room temperature.

become very hard and brittle if fully polymerized, imprinting is best carried out before polymerization. Although four different states were tested [84], imprinting of the softest coating (10 min at 100 °C) with about 200 nm pore masks (foils) produced good results for both polymers at a pressure of 130 MPa, with aspect ratios of 0.5 to 0.8. An increased hardness (10 min at 160 °C and 10 min at 250 °C) still allowed imprinting, but with decreasing aspect ratios. After the fourth polymerization step (2 min at 300 °C) the somewhat softer material NS 60 could still be structured, and with good results (see Figure 5.38).

5.5.4
Special Techniques to Imprint Hard Materials

The metals and polymers discussed above are each softer than the imprinting material, aluminum oxide. The problem of nanostructuring surfaces which are harder than alumina can be solved by treating via indirect routes. This can be demonstrated by a process which results in the production of a nanostructured silicon, which cannot be used directly for imprinting. The various steps in nanostructuring a silicon surface by using a 50 nm alumina membrane are shown schematically in Figure 5.39 [90]. In this case, aluminum discs of 30 mm diameter and 6 mm thickness (step A2) are fabricated at 40 V and 0 °C for 60 min, after preanodization. The Si surface to be nanostructured is coated with a 70 nm-thick PMMA film by spin-coating a PMMA solution in chlorobenzene (step A1). Subsequently, imprinting occurred at 10^7–10^8 Pa, at temperatures between 140 and 160 °C (step B), and a thin film of PMMA remained after imprinting (step C) which was removed by

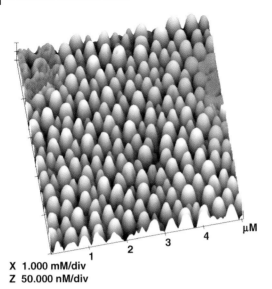

X 1.000 mM/div
Z 50.000 nM/div

Figure 5.38 Imprinting result (AFM) of Silikoftal NS 60-coated metal sheet after hardening at 300 °C for 2 min. The aspect ratio was 0.3–0.6.

an anisotropic oxygen plasma (step D). Structuring of the Si surface was then followed by reactive ion etching (RIE) with CF_4/H_2 plasma (step E). AFM images of the imprinted PMMA surface before and after RIE are shown in Figure 5.40a and b, respectively.

As can be seen from Figure 5.40b, the plasma attacks not only the residual PMMA film but also to some extent the PMMA pillars, the original height of which (160 nm) was reduced to about 80 nm, although the base diameter was unchanged. The result of the final etching step can be seen in Figure 5.41, where the PMMA pillar structure was transferred into the Si surface, resulting in Si pillars of about 50 nm in height. The SEM image in Figure 5.41a shows a larger area of the structured surface, whereas an AFM image of the magnified cut-out (top right-hand corner) is shown in Figure 5.41b.

5.6
Properties of Nanoimprinted Polymer Surfaces

The altered properties of nanoimprinted surfaces can be illustrated by means of polymers.

5.6.1
Optical Properties

The light transmission of transparent polymers is of considerable practical relevance. The minimum reflection of light (i.e., maximum transparency) is a situation where polymer windows can be used, for example, to cover electronic devices in

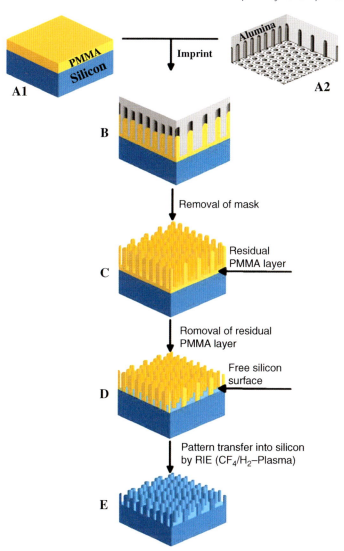

Figure 5.39 Schematic of the procedure to nanostructure a Si surface. Reproduced with permission from Ref. [95]; © 1996, Royal Chemical Society, London.

automobiles, mobile telephones, and solar cells. The elimination of light reflection has also been developed by nature; the so-called "moth-eye effect" causes the invisibility of night-active insects and, due to their high transparency, an optimized light efficiency for animals. The process is based on the nanostructured surface of the eyes where, due to the existence of building blocks that are smaller than the wavelength of visible light (200–300 nm) on the surface, the classical reflection of light when it is transmitted between air and a more dense medium is almost eliminated [91, 92]. Rather, the sharp transition between air and the material on a

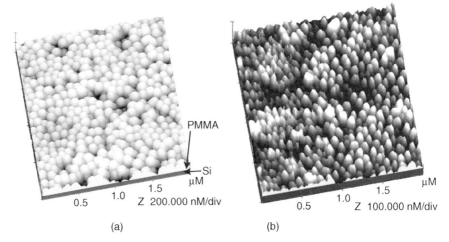

(a)   (b)

Figure 5.40   (a) Atomic force microscopy image of an imprinted PMMA film; (b) After reactive ion etching to remove the residual film on the Si surface. Reproduced with permission from Ref. [95]; © 1996, Royal Chemical Society, London.

smooth surface is substituted by a series of reflections, and this results in a gradient with a continuously increasing refractive index between the air and the surface.

PMMA, as a representative of the imprinted polymers, has been studied with respect to its transparency change, from a nonimprinted to an imprinted state [85]. In

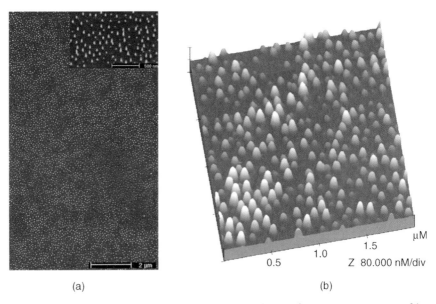

(a)   (b)

Figure 5.41   (a) Scanning electron microscopy and (b) and atomic force microscopy images of the final nanostructured Si surface. Reproduced with permission from Ref. [95]; © 1996, Royal Chemical Society, London.

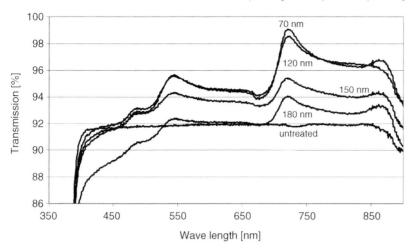

Figure 5.42 UV-visible transmission spectra of PMMA windows, imprinted with 180, 150, 120, and 70 nm pore masks. An untreated sample is shown for comparison.

a series of nanostructured probes with decreasing structure size, transmission was shown to increase in line with decreasing structure units. The UV-visible transmission spectra of PMMA windows imprinted with 180 to 70 nm pore alumina masks, are shown in Figure 5.42 [85]. Here, compared to a nonimprinted sample, there was a clear increase in transparency, especially at 520, 720, and 870 nm, all in the visible region. In the case of the 70 nm PMMA pillars, the transparency reached 99%. Whereas, the moth-eye effect functions best with structure units of about 300 nm, in this case the maximum value was observed with 70 nm pillars, which in turn suggests the need for a somewhat modified explanation, namely the formation of a surface layer with a low refractive index.

5.6.2
Wetting Properties

The wettability of a surface depends on the chemical nature of the material, and of its surface structure. Again, nature demonstrates this phenomenon in the so-called "Lotus effect", which keeps clean not only Lotus leaves but also numerous other biological surfaces, such as butterfly wings [93–95]. The effect is based on the increased hydrophobicity of a material with a low surface tension by a micro- and/or nanostructured surface. Whereas, metals exhibit high surface tensions, linked with a good wettability, glass and plastics show low surface tensions. The wettability of a surface is measured via the contact angle θ, which is the angle between a solid surface and the tangent, set on a liquid droplet. It can be calculated by using the Young equation [96]:

$$s_{sg} - \sigma_{sl} = \sigma_{lg} \cdot \cos(\theta) \tag{5.7}$$

where σ_{sl} is the interfacial tension solid/liquid, σ_{sg} is the interfacial tension solid/gas, σ_{lg} is the interfacial tension liquid/gas, and θ is the contact angle solid/liquid.

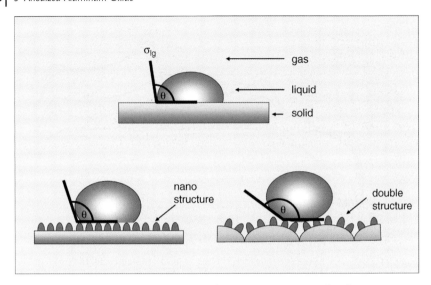

Figure 5.43   Increase of the contact angle (θ) by a micro/nanostructured surface.

Both, microstructured and/or nanostructured hydrophobic surfaces decrease wettability due to an additional reduction in the surface tension, and an increase of the contact angle. The differences in contact angles between a flat structure, and between nanostructured and a micro/nanostructured surfaces, are shown schematically in Figure 5.43. Here, the combination of micro- and nanostructured surfaces results in large contact angles, a situation which is especially realized in Lotus leaves. In this case, a contact angle of 0° corresponds to a perfect wettability, and an angle of 180° to a perfect hydrophobicity; however, neither value is reached in practice.

PTFE surfaces show increasing contact angles for water droplets with increasing structure size [85]. The results obtained with pore diameters ranging between 50 and 200 nm are listed in Table 5.5. Compared to nontreated surfaces, the contact angle was increased from 112° to 146°.

The reality can be shown via light microscopic images of water droplets on variously structured PTFE surfaces (Figure 5.44). Here, the contact surface corre-

Table 5.5   Measured contact angles (θ) depending on structure size on PTFE surfaces.

Pore diameters of the masks (nm)	Calculated structural distances (nm)	θ (°)
—	—	112 ± 3
50	106 ± 6	128 ± 5
75	159 ± 9	126 ± 3
120	212 ± 12	132 ± 2
120	265 ± 15	140 ± 5
180	398 ± 23	145 ± 2
200	451 ± 26	146 ± 3

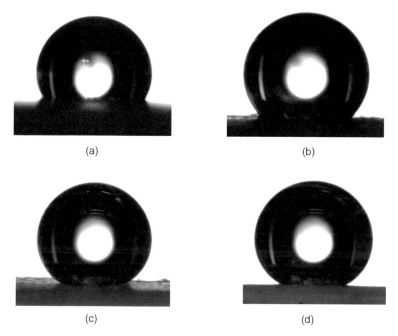

Figure 5.44 Light microscopy images of water droplets on different imprinted PTFE surfaces. (a) Nonimprinted; (b) 50 nm pores; (c) 120 nm pores; (d) 170 nm pores.

sponds with the real wetted area, which can be calculated from the measured contact angle [97]. The proportions of these areas vary from 50% (50 nm) to 25% (200 nm).

5.7
Surfaces with Nanoholes

To date, the use of nanoporous aluminum oxide membranes has been targeted exclusively towards the creation of nanoparticles, nanowires or nanotubes on surfaces. However, nanoporous alumina membranes can also be applied to fabricate surfaces with nanohole arrays. Of course, many other techniques have been developed to structure surfaces with nanoholes where, again, the use of (very thin) alumina membranes offers considerable advantages. This is because, in addition to a high pore regularity, it is also possible to create extended arrays. Diamond, semi-conductor and metal surfaces can each be treated by using alumina membranes as masks for various etching processes. Nanohole-structured surfaces are of practical interest for similar reasons, such as nanowire- or nanodot-structured materials. Here again, the thickness of the membranes is a decisive factor for success since, if they are too thick, then shadowing effects of the pore walls will reduce their quality. As the membranes are also etched, too-thin membranes can partially be destroyed, with membranes of 300–700 nm thickness eventually providing the best results [98, 99].

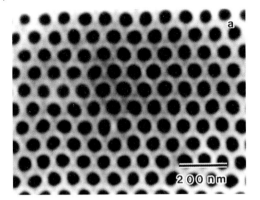

Figure 5.45 Scanning electron microscopy image of a diamond surface with ordered nanoholes, produced by polyethylene (PE) [104].

In any case, the etching rate of the membrane should be less than that of the corresponding surface.

The dominating etching technique is RIE, followed by plasma etching (PE) and fast atom beam etching (FAB), while ion milling (IM) plays a secondary role. Previously, RIE techniques have been applied for etching semiconductor surfaces such as Si [100], GaAs [98, 101, 102], GaN [101] and InP [99], whilst PE is more suited to the etching of Si [103], diamond [104–106], GaN [73, 107] and Al [102]. In the case of FAB, etching has been applied to Si [108], diamond [109], and GaAs [110].

Typically, a variety of etching gases can be used. For RIE processes, Cl_2 and Br_2 as well as BCl_3 and $SiCl_4$ are common, whereas for PE gases such as CF_4, $CBrF_3$, O_2 and also Cl_2 can be applied. In addition to O_2 and Cl_2, SF_6 has been used for FAB techniques.

Due to the slow simultaneous etching of the pore walls, the holes on the substrates will have a more or less expressed conical structure, depending on the etching time. As an example, a diamond surface with ordered holes generated by O_2 plasma etching through an alumina membrane is shown in Figure 5.45 [104].

Similar to surfaces decorated with wires, dots or tubes, surfaces with nanohole arrangements demonstrate interesting physical properties [69], although these will not be discussed at this point. Nonetheless, these include the antireflection of Si [103, 108], the photonic crystal behavior of GaN [110], and the increase of capacitance of porous diamond films by a factor of 400 [105, 106].

5.8
Summary and Outlook

Aluminum plays a special role among the so-called "gate metals," as it forms the most qualified nanopores during anodization, with variations in pore diameter, ranging from about 10 nm to several hundred manometers, easily being arranged. Furthermore, aluminum foils, which frequently are used as starting materials, are cheap and easily available. Besides routine anodization, special techniques have been developed to generate highly ordered pore arrays, and the mechanism of such formation is well understood. Previously, many applications have been developed, and many are foreseen for the near future. Two of these (as discussed in this chapter) include: (i) pore filling with very different materials, which results in wires, tubes or particles of variable dimensions; and (ii) the use of nanoporous alumina surfaces for imprinting numerous surfaces of metals and polymers. In both cases, nanostructured surfaces are formed, leading to the creation of materials with novel physical and chemical properties. Yet, such early promise must be developed further to permit imprinting processes for extended surfaces, perhaps in the meter range. Pore walls, chemically modified by catalytically active metals, have been tested in gas-phase catalysis [111], and the first attempts to apply a pore-size specific release of chemical compounds (i.e., drugs) have initiated novel developments in slow but continuous rates of drug delivery [112]. Yet, numerous other future applications can be foreseen, including optics, electronics and magnetism, to name but a few.

Nanoporous alumina membranes are also used as matrices for the fabrication of surfaces with nanoholes, including various etching techniques. Such concave, nanostructured surfaces offer interesting properties compared to nontreated materials.

Taken together, nanoporous alumina membranes represent a unique family of materials which, despite having experienced impressive progress during the past two decades, will surely continue to play major roles in many further scientific and practical developments.

References

1 Lohrengel, M.M. (1993) *Mater. Sci. Eng.*, **6**, 241.

2 Thompson, G.E. and Wood, G.C. (1983) *Treatise on Materials Science and Technology*, **23**, 205.

3 Diggle, J.W., Downie, T.C., and Goulding, C.W. (1969) *Chem. Rev.*, **69**, 365.

4 Parkhutik, V.P. and Shershulskii, V.I. (1986) *J. Physics D: Appl. Phys.*, **19**, 623,

5 Valand, T. and Heusler, K.E. (1983) *J. Electroanal. Chem.*, **149**, 71.

6 Hurlen, T., Lian, H., and Ödegard, O.S. (1984) *Electrochim. Acta*, **29**, 579.

7 Keller, F., Hunter, M.S., and Robinson, D.L. (1953) *J. Electrochem. Soc.*, **100/9**, 411.

8 Macdonald, D.D. (1993) *J. Electrochem. Soc.*, **140/3**, L27.

9 Siejika, J. and Ortega, C. (1977) *J. Electrochem. Soc.*, **124/6**, 883.

10 Thompson, G.E., Furneauax, R.C., and Wood, G.C. (1978) *Nature*, **272**, 433.

11 O'Sullivan, J.P. and Wood, G.C. (1970) *Proc. R. Soc. London*, **317**, 511.

12 Hornyak, G.L., Dutta, J., Tibbals, H.F., and Rao, A.K. (eds) (2008) *Introduction to Nanoscience*. CRC Press.

13 Sawitowski, T. (1999) Neue Nano-komposite. Goldcluster, Goldkolloide und Silizium in Aluminiumoxid-membranen – Struktur und Eigenschaften. PhD thesis, University of Essen, Germany.

14 Asoh, H., Nishio, K., Nakao, M., Tamamura, T., and Masuda, H. (2001) *J. Electrochem. Soc.*, **148**, B152.

15 Masuda, H., Yamada, H., Satoh, M., and Asoh, H. (1997) *Appl. Phys. Lett.*, **71**, 2770.

16 Matsui, Y., Nishio, K., and Masuda, H. (2006) *Small*, **2**, 522.

17 Randon, J., Mardilovich, P.P., Govyadinov, A.N., and Paterson, R. (1995) *J. Colloid Interface Sci.*, **169**, 335.

18 Wefers, K. and Misra, C. (1987) Company Report. Alcoa Laboratories.

19 Schmid, G., Bäumle, M., Heim, I., Kröll, M., Müller, F., and Sawitowski, T. (1999) *J. Cluster Sci.*, **10**, 223.

20 Furneaux, R.C., Rigby, W.R., and Davidson, A.P. (1989) *Nature*, **337**, 147.

21 Binnig, G., Gerber, Ch., Stoll, E., Albrecht, T.R., and Quate, C.F. (1987) *Europhys. Lett.*, **3/12**, 1281.

22 Rugar, D. and Hansma, P. (1990) *Physics Today*, **10**, 23.

23 Lu, Q., Gao, F., Komarneni, S., and Mallouk, T.E. (2004) *J. Am. Chem. Soc.*, **126**, 8650.

24 Che, G.L., Lakshmi, B.B., Fischer, E.R., and Martin, C.R. (1998) *Nature*, **393**, 346.

25 Li, J., Papadopoulos, C., Xu, J.M., and Moskovits, M. (1999) *Appl. Phys. Lett.*, **75**, 367.

26 Li, C., Papadopoulos, J., and Xu, J.M. (1999) *Nature*, **402**, 253.

27 Masuda, H., Yanagishita, T., Yasui, K., Nishio, K., Yagi, I., Rao, N., and Fujishima, A. (2001) *Adv. Mater.*, **13**, 247.

28 Routkevitch, D., Bigioni, T., Moskovits, M., and Xu, J.M. (1996) *J. Phys. Chem.*, **100**, 14037.

29 Shemilov, K.B. and Moskovits, M. (2000) *Chem. Mater.*, **12**, 250.

30 Lei, Y., Zhang, L.D., and Fan, J.C. (2001) *Chem. Phys. Lett.*, **338**, 231.

31 Nielsch, K.M., Müller, F., Li, A.P., and Gösele, U. (2000) *Adv. Mater.*, **12**, 582.

32 Cao, H.Q., Xu, Z., Sang, H., Sheng, D., and Tie, C.Y. (2001) *Adv. Mater.*, **13**, 121.

33 Mu, C., Yn, X.Y., Wang, R.M., Wu, K., Xu, D.S., and Guo, G.L. (2004) *Adv. Mater.*, **16**, 1550.

34 Schneider, J.J., Popp, A., and Engstler, J. (2008) Fundamentals and Functionality of Inorganic Wires, Rods and Tubes, in *Nanotechnology. Principles and Fundamentals*, vol. 1 (ed. G. Schmid), Wiley-VCH, Weinheim, pp. 97–138.

35 Masuda, H., Yada, K., and Osaka, A. (1998) *Jpn. J. Appl. Phys.*, **37**, L1340.

36 Okano, K., Yamada, T., Ishihara, H., Koizumi, S., and Itoh, J. (1997) *Appl. Phys. Lett.*, **70**, 2201.

37 Shiomi, H. (1997) *Jpn. J. Phys. Lett.*, **36**, 7745.

38 Kornienko, O., Reilly, P.T.A., Whitten, W.B., and Ramsey, J.M. (2000) *Anal. Chem.*, **72**, 559.

39 Geis, M., Efremow, N.N., Krohn, K.E., Twichell, J.C., Lyszcarz, T.M., Kalish, R., Greer, J.A., and Tabat, M.D. (1998) *Nature*, **393**, 431.

40 Grill, A. (1999) *Diamond Relat. Mater.*, **8**, 428.

41 Bao, J., Tie, C., Xu, Z., Zhou, Q., Shen, D., and Ma, Q. (2001) *Adv. Mater.*, **13**, 1631.

42 Gao, H., Wang, F., Xu, D.S., Wu, K., Xie, Y.C., Liu, S., Wang, E.G., Xu, J., and Yu, D.P. (2003) *J. Appl. Phys.*, **93**, 5602.

43 Masuda, H., Yotsuy, M., and Ishida, M. (1998) *Jpn. J. Appl. Phys.*, **37**, L1090.

44 Jessensky, O. (1997) Untersuchungen zum Porenwachstum in 6H-Siliziumkarbid und anodischem Aluminiumoxid. PhD thesis, Martin-Luther-University of Halle, Germany.

45 Al Mawlavi, D., Coombs, N., and Moskovits, M. (1991) *J. Appl. Phys.*, **70**, 4421.

46 Li, F., Metzger, M., and Doyle, W.D. (1997) *IEEE Trans. Magn.*, **33**, 3715.

47 Routkevitch, D., Tager, A.A., Haruyama, J., Almawlawi, D., Moskovits, M., and Xu, J.M. (1996) *IEEE Trans. Electron Devices*, **147**, 1646.

48 Sautter, W., Ibe, G., and Meier, J. (1974) *Aluminium*, **50**, 143.

49 Li, A.P., Müller, F., Birner, A., Nielsch, K., and Gösele, U. (1999) *Adv. Mater.*, **11**, 483.

50 Dobrev, D., Vetter, J., Angert, N., and Neumann, R. (1999) *Appl. Phys. A*, **69**, 233.

51 Dobrev, D., Vetter, J., Angert, N., and Neumann, R. (2001) *Appl. Phys. A*, **72**, 729.

52 Choi, K.H., Kim, H.S., and Lee, T.H. (1998) *J. Power Sources*, **75**, 230.

53 Sun, M., Zangari, G., Shamsuzzoha, M., and Metzger, F.R.M. (2001) *Appl. Phys. Lett.*, **78**, 2964.

54 Fan, H.J., Werner, P., and Zacharias, M. (2006) *Small*, **2**, 700.

55 Shingubara, S., Okino, O., Sayama, Y., Sakaue, H., and Takahagi, T. (1999) *Solid State Electron.*, **43**, 1143.

56 Taberna, P.-L., Mitra, S., Poizot, P., Simon, P., and Tarascon, J.-M. (2006) *Nat. Mater.*, **5**, 567.

57 Zhang, Y., Li, G., Wu, Y., Zhang, B., Song, W., and Zhang, L. (2002) *Adv. Mater.*, **14**, 1227.

58 Bogart, T.E., Dey, S., Lew, K.-K., Mohney, S.E., and Redwing, J.M. (2005) *Adv. Mater.*, **17**, 114.

59 Wagner, R.S. and Ellis, W.C. (1964) *Appl. Phys. Lett.*, **4**, 89.

60 Wagner, R.S., Ellis, W.C., Jackson, K.A., and Arnold, S.M. (1964) *J. Appl. Phys.*, **35**, 2993.

61 Cui, Y., Lauhorn, L.J., Gudiksen, M.S., Wang, J., and Lieber, C.M. (2001) *Appl. Phys. Lett.*, **78**, 2214.

62 Westwater, J., Gosain, D.P., and Usui, S. (1997) *Jpn. J. Appl. Phys. Part 1*, **36**, 6204.

63 Westwater, J., Gosain, D.P., Tomiya, S., Usui, S., and Ruda, H. (1997) *J. Vac. Sci. Technol. B*, **15**, 554.

64 Westwater, J., Gosain, D.P., and Usui, S. (1998) *Phys. Status Solidi A*, **165**, 37.

65 Lei, Y., Zhang F L.D., Meng, G.W., Li, G.H., Zhang, X.Y., Liang, C.H., Chen W., and Wange S.X. (2001) *Appl. Phys. Lett.*, **78**, 1125.

66 Baranski, A.S. and Fawcett, W.B. (1980) *J. Electrochem. Soc.*, **127**, 766.

67 Klein, J.D., Herrich, R.D. II, Palmer, D., Sailor, M.J., Brumlik, C.J., and Martin, C.R. (1993) *Chem. Mater.*, **5**, 902.

68 Charkarvarti, S.K. and Vetter, J. (1993) *J. Micromech. Microeng.*, **3**, 57.

69 Lei, Y., Cai, W., and Wilde, G. (2007) *Prog. Mater. Sci.*, **52**, 465.

70 Masuda, H. and Satoh, H. (1996) *Jpn. J. Appl. Phys.*, **35**, L126.

71 Masuda, H., Yasui, K., Sakamoto, Y., Nakao, M., Tamamura, T., and Nishio, K. (2001) *Jpn. J. Appl. Phys.*, **40**, L1267.

72 Choi, J., Sauer, g., Goering, P., Nielsch, K., Wehrspohn, R.B., and Gösele, U. (2003) *J. Mater. Chem.*, **13**, 1100.

73 Wang, Y.D., Chua, S.J., Sander, M.S., Chem, P., Tripathy, S., and Fonstad, C.G. (2004) *Appl. Phys. Lett.*, **85**, 816.

74 Sander, M.S. and Tan, L.S. (2003) *Adv. Funct. Mater.*, **13**, 393.

75 Rabin, O., Herz, P.R., and Lin, Y.M. (2003) *Adv. Funct. Mater.*, **13**, 631.

76 Tian, M.L., Yu, S.Y., Wang, J.G., Kumar, N., Wertz, E., and Li, Q. (2005) *Nano Lett.*, **5**, 697.

77 Choi, J., Sauer, g., Nielsch, K., Wehrspohn, R.B., and Gösele, U. (2003) *Chem. Mater.*, **15**, 776.

78 Xia, Y., Rogers, J.A., Paul, K.E., and Whitesides, G.M. (1999) *Chem. Rev.*, **99**, 1823.

79 Xia, Y. and Whitesides, G.M. (1998) *Angew. Chem., Int. Ed.*, **37**, 550.

80 Wallraff, M. and Hinsberg, W.D. (1999) *Chem. Rev.*, **99**, 1801.

81 Piner, R.D., Zhu, J., Xu, F., Hong, S., and Mirkin, C.A. (1999) *Science*, **183**, 661.

82 Emmelius, M., Pawlowski, G., and Vollmann, H.W. (1989) *Angew. Chem., Int. Ed.*, **28**, 1445.

83 Chou, S.Y., Krauss, P.R., and Renstrom, P.J. (1995) *Appl. Phys. Lett.*, **67**, 3114.

84 Levering, M. (2003) Strukturierung von Oberflächen mit nanoporösem Aluminiumoxid. PhD thesis, University of Essen, Germany.

85 Schmid, G., Levering, M., and Sawitowsky, T. (2007) *Z. Anorg. Allg. Chem.*, **633**, 2147.

86 Beyer, B. (1971) *Werkstoffkunde NE-Metalle*, VEB Deutscher Verlag, Grundstoffindustrie, Leipzig, Germany, p. 340.

87 Goodfellow (2002) *Datenblätter*, Goodfellow, Bad Nauheim, Germany.

88 Merkel, M. and Thomas, K.H. (1998) *VEB Fachbuchverlag Leipzig*, Germany, p. 340.

89 Ross, R.B. (1980) *Metallic Materials Handbook*, 3rd edn, E. & F. N. Spon Ltd.

90 Kruse, M., Frankza, S., and Schmid, G. (2003) *Chem. Commun.*, 1333.

91 Macleod, B. and Sonetz, G. (1999) *Laser Focus World*, **8**, 1–55.

92 Aydin, C., Zaslavsky, A., Sonek, G.J., and Goldstein, J. (2002) *Appl. Phys. Lett.*, **80**, 2242.

93 Wagner, T., Neinhuis, C., and Barthlott, W. (1996) *Acta Zool.*, **77**, 213.

94 Wolter, M., Barthlott, W., Knoch, M., and Noga, G.J. (1988) *Angew. Bot.*, **62**, 53.

95 Barthlott, W., Neinhuis, C., Jetter, R., Bourauel, T., and Riederer, M. (1996) *Flora*, **191**, 169.

96 Israelachvili, I. (1995) *Intermolecular & Surfaces Forces*, Academic Press, London.

97 Chen, W., Fadeev, A.Y., Hsieh, M.C., Öner, D., Youngblood, J., and McCarthy, T. (1999) *Langmuir*, **15**, 3395.

98 Cheng, G.S. and Moskovits, M. (2002) *Adv. Mater.*, **14**, 1567.

99 Nakao, M., Oku, S., Tamamura, T., Yasui, K., and Masuda, H. (1999) *Jpn. J. Appl. Phys.*, **38**, 1052.

100 Crouse, D., Lo, Y.H., Miller, A.E., and Crouse, M. (2000) *Appl. Phys. Lett.*, **76**, 49.

101 Liang, J.Y., Chik, H., Yin, A.J., and Xu, J. (2002) *J. Appl. Phys.*, **91**, 2544.

102 Menon, L., Ram, K.B., Patibandla, S., Aurongzeb, D., Holtz, M., and Yun, J. (2004) *J. Electrochem. Soc.*, **151**, C492.

103 Tian, L., Ram, K.B., Ahmad, I., Menon, L., and Holtz, M. (2005) *J. Appl. Phys.*, **97**, 026101.

104 Masuda, H., Watanabe, M., Yasui, K., Tryk, D.A., Rao, T.N., and Fujishima, A. (2000) *Adv. Mater.*, **12**, 444.

105 Honda, K., Rao, T.N., Tryk, D.A., Fujishima, A., Watanabe, M., and Yasui, K. (2000) *J. Electrochem. Soc.*, **147**, 659.

106 Honda, K., Rao, T.N., Tryk, D.A., Fujishima, A., Watanabe, M., and Yasui, K. (2001) *J. Electrochem. Soc.*, **148**, A668.

107 Wang, J.D., Chua, S.J., Tripathy, S., Sander, M.S., Chen, P., and Fonstad, C.G. (2005) *Appl. Phys. Lett.*, **86**, 071917.

108 Kanamori, Y., Hane, K., Sai, H., and Yugami, H. (2001) *Appl. Phys. Lett.*, **78**, 142.

109 Ono, T., Konoma, C., Miyashita, H., Kananmori, Y., and Esashi, M. (2003) *Jpn. J. Appl. Phys.*, **42**, 3867.

110 Nakao, M., Oku, S., Tanaka, H., Shibata, Y., Yokoo, A., and Tamamura, T. (2002) *Opt. Quantum Electron.*, **34**, 183.

111 Kormann, H.-P., Schmid, G., Pelzer, K., Philippot, K., and Chaudret, B. (2004) *Z. Anorg. Allg. Chem.*, **630**, 1913.

112 Kipke, S. and Schmid, G. (2004) *Adv. Funct. Mater.*, **14**, 1184.

6
Colloidal Lithography

Gang Zhang and Dayang Wang

6.1
Introduction

The advent of nanoscience and nanotechnology has, in recent years, led to a tremendous enthusiasm among the research groups of different scientific disciplines such as physics, chemistry, and biology, their common aim being to utilize nanostructures with the intent of pursuing the innovative properties derived from nanometer dimensions. In this context, the fabrication of nanostructures has today become an increasing demand. Clearly, low-throughput and expensive maskless lithography represents a less-accessible choice for chemists, physicists, material scientists, and biologists. The successful extension of mask-assisted lithography beyond microelectronics workshops have been largely limited by problems of mask design and preparation. Recently, much effort has been expended towards the development of nonconventional lithographic techniques, especially those that are integrated with a bottom-up nanochemical procedure for surface patterning with a low-cost, flexible processing capability, and a high throughput. Most of the nonconventional lithographic techniques developed to date, however, require the assistance of conventional lithographic techniques, such as photolithography, to design and make the masks or masters. Hence, in attempting to address this challenge, an increasing amount of attention has been paid to the use of self-assemblies of molecules and colloidal particles for the development of ingenious, cheap, and nonlithographic methods of masking.

Monodisperse colloidal particles with sizes that range from tens of nanometers to tens of micrometers, can be easily synthesized via wet chemistry approaches such as emulsion polymerization and sol–gel synthesis. Due to the size and shape monodispersity, these particles can self-assemble into both two-dimensional (2-D) and three-dimensional (3-D) extended periodic arrays, which usually are referred to as "colloidal crystals." The latter are usually characterized by a brilliant iridescence arising from the Bragg reflection of light by their periodic structures. Despite such beauty, the iridescent color has recently inspired the explosive study of fabrication of 3-D colloidal crystals or inverse opals – that is, a 3-D inverted replication of the

Nanotechnology, Volume 8: Nanostructured Surfaces. Edited by Lifeng Chi
Copyright © 2010 WILEY-VCH Verlag GmbH & Co. KGaA, Weinheim
ISBN: 978-3-527-31739-4

crystals for pursuing a complete energy bandgap to manipulate electromagnetic waves, similar to the situation with electrons in semiconductors. Before being used as photonic materials, both the ordered arrays of solid particles and those of the interstices between the particles of colloidal crystals, have already been used as masks or templates for surface patterning, for example via etching or the deposition of materials. This bottom-up masking methodology has recently attracted more attention for surface patterning due to the processing simplicity, the low cost, the flexibility of extending on various substrates with different surface chemistries (and even curvatures), and the ease of scaling down the feature size to below 100 nm. In this chapter, the various surface-patterning processes based on the use of colloidal crystals as masks – referred to hereafter as colloidal lithography (CL) – will be discussed, the processing principles reviewed, and recent advances in the area surveyed.

6.2
Colloidal Crystallization: The Bottom-Up Growth of Colloidal Masks

The success of using colloidal crystals as masks for surface patterning is determined by the ability to directing the self-assembly of colloidal particles and to manipulate the crystal packing structures. Provided that their size and shape are monodisperse, colloidal particles can be readily self-assembled into long-range ordered arrays with a hexagonal packing, driven simply by entropic depletion and gravity. Subsequent evaporation of the solvent leads to thermodynamically and mechanically stable face-centered cubic (*fcc*) or hexagonally close-packed (*hcp*) extended crystals. Until now, a range of colloidal crystallization techniques – with and without the aid of templates – has been successfully developed to implement colloidal crystallization in a controlled fashion [1–3]. However, due to the vast number of reports made on colloidal crystallization, the immense diversity of the crystallization techniques described, and taking into account the fact that colloidal lithography relies on the masking of single or double layers of colloidal crystals, attention in this section will be centered mainly on the currently available techniques for 2-D colloidal crystallization.

6.2.1
Sedimentation

Sedimentation represents a natural pathway for colloidal crystallization since, when dispersed in a liquid, colloidal particles tend to settle out of the fluid under gravity and to accumulate and precipitate on a wall – a process which can be described by Stokes' law. This sedimentation process can be used to grow colloidal crystals of high quality, while the crystal thickness can be fine-tuned by adjusting the particle concentration. Unfortunately, however, as the sedimentation time may be up to several hundreds of hours, time-consumption represents the major drawback of this technique [4]. It is possible to accelerate the rate of sedimentation by applying centrifugal force, but this is undertaken at the cost of reducing the quality of the colloidal crystals obtained. Neither does sedimentation carried out under centrifugal forces allow the formation of 2-D colloidal crystals. An additional drawback of sedimentation in colloidal crystallization results from the intermediate stage during solvent evaporation, at which the colloidal particles are not in close contact but rather are interspaced by water necks. If a complete evaporation of the solvent is then carried out, this will cause cracks to form that are difficult not only to prevent but also to manage [5, 6].

During the early 1990s, Nagayama's group began a systematic study of the sedimentation of colloidal particles in the presence of strong attractive capillary forces [7]. By using optical microscopy and a Teflon ring to confine the dispersions of colloidal particles, the particle sedimentation dynamics on a solid substrate could be directly observed. The observations made by Nagayama and colleagues suggested the existence of a two-stage mechanism for 2-D colloidal crystallization:

- *Nucleation*, which led to the particles becoming trapped on the substrate due to attractive capillary forces between the particles and the surrounding solvents. This occurred especially when the solvent layer thickness was comparable to the diameter of the particles during solvent evaporation.
- *Crystal growth*, whereby convective flux caused the particles to be moved to the existing ordered domains, as a result of water evaporation from the meniscus between the particles (Figure 6.1) [7].

Subsequently, Micheletto and coworkers fabricated 2-D colloidal crystals on a solid substrate through sedimentation, by tilting the substrate through about 9° and maintaining a constant system temperature with a Peltier cell [8]. The procedure used by Micheletto *et al.* allowed the growth of 2-D colloidal crystals that were composed of particles less than 100 nm in size, which was not possible via the Nagayama protocol. However, when the 2-D colloidal crystals obtained via

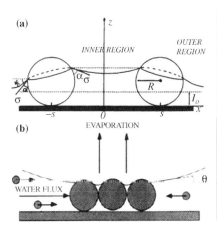
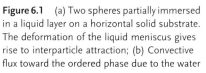
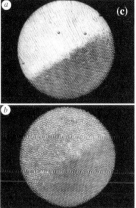

Figure 6.1 (a) Two spheres partially immersed in a liquid layer on a horizontal solid substrate. The deformation of the liquid meniscus gives rise to interparticle attraction; (b) Convective flux toward the ordered phase due to the water evaporation from the menisci between the particles in the 2-D array; (c) Photographs of 2-D crystal growth. Reproduced with permission from Ref. [7].

Micheletto's procedure were compared to those obtained via Nagayama's method, they proved to be of a much poorer quality, especially in terms of their surface coverage and degree of long-range ordering.

6.2.2
Vertical Deposition

When a supporting substrate is held vertically in a suspension of colloidal particles, moving the front of the suspension flow – either by evaporating the solvent or by withdrawing the substrate from the suspension – can cause the colloidal particles to be pinned onto the substrates (the process of nucleation) and also a convective transfer of the particles from the bulk phase to the drying front (the process of crystallization) (Figure 6.2) [9]. The thickness of the colloidal crystals obtained by vertical deposition depends on the ratio between the thickness of the liquid films that remain to support the substrates and the diameter of the colloidal particles [9]. When this ratio is much greater than 1, 3-D colloidal crystals are obtained of high quality, and the crystal thickness can be fine-tuned by adjusting the particle

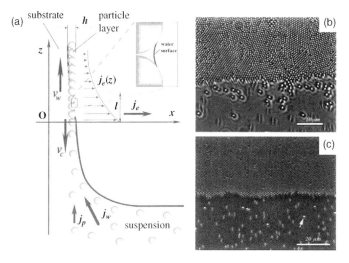

Figure 6.2 (a) Sketch of the particle and water fluxes in the vicinity of monolayer particle arrays growing on a substrate plate that is being withdrawn from a suspension. The inset shows the menisci shape between neighboring particles. Here, v_w is the substrate withdrawal rate, v_c is the array growth rate, j_w is the water influx, j_p is the respective particle influx, j_e is the water evaporation flux, and h is the thickness of the array; (b, c) A part of the leading edge of a growing monolayer particle array. The upper-halves of the photographs show the formations of (b) differently oriented small domains of ordered 814 nm particles, and (c) a single domain of ordered 953 nm particles. The lower halves show particles being dragged by the water flow towards the forming monolayer. Because of the high velocity on a microscale $(v_p = 100\,\mathrm{m\,s^{-1}})$, the particles are seen as short, fuzzy lines. The particles (one is indicated by an arrow in panel b) seen as bright spots have a large diameter (compared to average values) and are wedged into the wetting film. Reproduced with permission from Ref. [9].

concentration [10]. However, when the ratio is similar to or less than 1, 2-D colloidal crystals are obtained [9]. Vertical deposition may also allow the formation of crack-free colloidal crystals, provided that the suspensions of colloidal particles wet support the substrates well, that there is no interaction between the particles and the substrates, the suspensions are sufficiently stable, and the solvent evaporation is well controlled [9].

Dip-coating is a rapid and dip-coater assisted variant of vertical deposition [11]. A number of techniques have also been developed to improve the efficiency and quality of colloidal crystallization via vertical deposition, such as variable-flow deposition [12], isothermal heating evaporation-induced self-assembly [13], two-substrate deposition [14], reduction of the humidity fluctuation [15], adjustment of the meniscus shape [16], temperature-induced convective flow [17] and vertical deposition with a tilted angle [18]. The maximal size of the colloidal particles used for vertical deposition is limited by the sedimentation of the colloidal particles; these sizes are typically 400–500 nm for silica particles and 1 μm for polystyrene particles. In aiming to compete with sedimentation, Kitaev and Ozin used a low pressure to accelerate the solvent evaporation, and successfully grew large-area 2-D binary colloidal crystals, where the diameter ratio of the large to small particles was in the range of 0.175 to 0.225 (Figure 6.3) [19].

Vertical deposition has recently been extended to the stepwise growth of 2-D colloidal crystals with large and small colloidal particles on a substrate [20, 21]. In this procedure, the 2-D colloidal crystals of the large particles first formed on the substrate are used as a template to grow 2-D colloidal crystals of the small particles. Then, by deliberately tuning the concentration of the small particle suspension, it is possible to construct binary colloidal crystals with stoichiometric ratios of large to small particle sizes of 1 : 2, 1 : 3, 1 : 4, or 1 : 5 [20, 21].

6.2.3
Spin Coating

Spin coating was the first technique used to grow 2-D colloidal crystal masks for colloidal lithography, due to the fact that it allows easy and quick crystal formation over large areas [22]. The long-range ordering degree of 2-D colloidal crystals obtained by spin coating can be improved by increasing the wetting of the suspensions of colloidal particles on the supporting substrates, for example by adding ethylene glycol to the suspensions [23]. Unfortunately, the spin coating process is far more complicated than it first appears, and the underlying mechanism remains in debate. When Relig and Higgins conducted a theoretical analysis of the physics governing the spin coating of a colloidal particle suspension on a planar substrate, they proposed that:

- The functional relationship between the suspension viscosity and the particle concentration plays a much more significant role during the spin coating of a colloidal particle suspension, especially in the case of a non-hard sphere suspension, than in the spin coating of polymer solutions.

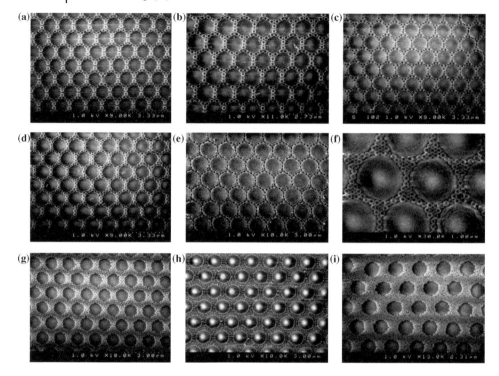

Figure 6.3 Library of surface micropatterns produced by accelerated evaporation coassembly of binary dispersions of monodisperse microspheres with a large size ratio and imaged using field-emission scanning electron microscopy. The larger spheres of all binary dispersions were PS latex of size, $d_L = 1.28\,\mu m$, while their volume fraction (ϕ_L) and the volume fraction (ϕ_S) and size (d_S) of smaller spheres were as follows: (a) $\phi_L = 0.017$, $\phi_S = 3.4 \times 10^{-4}$, $d_S = 290\,nm$ silica; (b) $\phi_L = 0.014$, $\phi_S = 2.5 \times 10^{-4}$, $d_S = 260\,nm$ silica; (c) $\phi_L = 0.014$, $\phi_S = 2.1 \times 10^{-4}$, $d_S = 225\,nm$ silica; (d) $\phi_L = 0.017$, $\phi_S = 3.8 \times 10^{-4}$, $d_S = 260\,nm$ silica; (e) $\phi_L = 0.014$, $\phi_S = 2.7 \times 10^{-4}$, $d_S = 225\,nm$ PS latex; (f) $\phi_L = 0.017$, $\phi_S = 3.0 \times 10^{-4}$, $d_S = 145\,nm$ silica; (g) $\phi_L = 0.017$, $\phi_S = 4.3 \times 10^{-4}$, $d_S = 205\,nm$ silica; (h) $\phi_L = 0.017$, $\phi_S = 4.1 \times 10^{-4}$, $d_S = 145\,nm$ silica; (i) $\phi_L = 0.017$, $\phi_S = 5.6 \times 10^{-4}$, $d_S = 145\,nm$ silica. Reproduced with permission from Ref. [19].

- The time scale associated with the spin coating of colloidal particle suspensions is rather different from that associated with the spin coating of polymer solutions.
- The inter-particle interaction should be taken into account to elucidate the packing ordering of the particles, the porosity of the particle films, and the functional relationship between the coated film thickness and the substrate angular velocity, although this is difficult to model.
- In order to minimize the secondary Marangoni instability for striation-free and uniform films of colloidal particles, a rapid substrate acceleration, high spinning speed, and reduced evaporation speed are needed [24].

Jiang and Mcfarland were successful in fabricating wafer-scale long-range ordered and non-close-packed 2-D and 3-D colloidal crystals by the spin coating of a highly viscous triacrylate suspension of silica particles and the subsequent polymerization of triacrylate, followed by a partial removal of the polymer matrices [25, 26]. Wang and Möhwald have developed a stepwise spin-coating protocol to consecutively deposit large and small colloidal particles in binary colloidal crystals, in which the interstitial arrays in the 2-D colloidal crystal of the large particles are used to template the deposition of small particles, due to their spatial and depletion entrapment (Figure 6.4) [27].

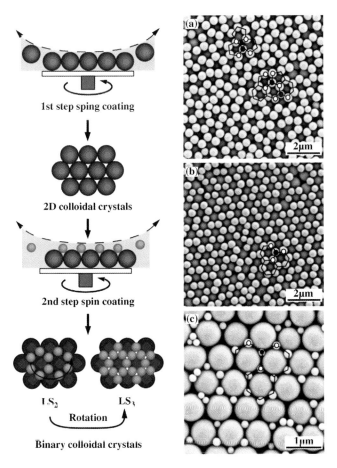

Figure 6.4 Left column: Schematic diagram of the procedure used to fabricate binary colloidal crystals by stepwise spin coating. Right column: Scanning electron microscopy images of the binary colloidal crystals produced by stepwise spin coating at a spin speed of 3000 rpm, in which 519 nm (a) , 442 nm (b) , and 222 nm silica spheres (c) were confined within the interstices between hexagonal close-packed 891 nm silica spheres. The closed or open circles mark locations of small spheres, while the polygon frames highlight their patterns. Reproduced with permission from Ref. [27].

6.2.4
Colloidal Crystallization at the Water/Air Interface

During recent years, extensive investigations have been conducted into the use of a water/air interface as a platform for molecular self-assembly. In particular, the Langmuir–Blodgett (LB) technique has proved to be a powerful and versatile method of organizing amphiphilic molecules at macroscopic monolayer films at the water/air interface, and to transfer these films to solid substrates in a controlled manner [28]. It has also been shown, but recognized to a lesser degree, that in a biphasic system such as water/oil, colloidal particles behave in rather similar fashion to amphiphilic molecules, in that from a thermodynamic standpoint they prefer to attach to the interface [29]. Based on this analogy, the water/air interface has been extended to support the self-assembly of colloidal particles. For example, when Pieranski conducted the first deliberate microscopic observation of 2-D colloidal crystallization at the water/air interface, it was hypothesized that there was a repulsive interaction between the dipoles of colloidal particles trapped at the interface, and that this was due to the asymmetric charge distribution on the particle surface driving the particles to self-assemble in an ordered array (Figure 6.5) [30]. Later, Park *et al.* developed the technique of *heat-assisted interfacial colloidal crystallization*, the success of which relied

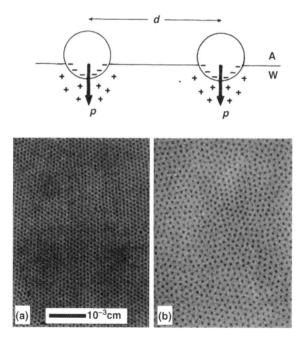

Figure 6.5 Upper panel: Schematic of the model of interaction of colloidal particles at the water (W)/air (A) interface. Lower panel: Photographs of polystyrene spheres (black dots) trapped at water/air interface. (a) Crystalline structure; (b) Disordered structure. Reproduced with permission from Ref. [30].

on the convective flow generated during heating rather than on the interface activity of the colloidal particles [31]. Once 2-D colloidal crystals have been formed at the water/air interface, the LB technique can be used to transfer them onto different substrates [32–35]. Significantly, the LB technique allows a repetition of the transfer of 2-D colloidal crystals onto a substrate into 3-D colloidal crystals with precisely defined layer numbers [35].

In comparison with the water/air interface, a water/oil interface represents a much better platform to trap colloidal particles, due to the relatively low interfacial tension [29]. Thus, water/oil interfaces have been used to grow 2-D colloidal crystals [36, 37], while transfer of the resultant 2-D colloidal crystals to solid substrates remains problematic. In addition to water/air interfaces, air/water/air interfaces have also been used for colloidal crystallization. For example, Velikov and colleagues have studied colloidal crystallization in thinning foam films [38], whilst by using air/water/air interfaces for crystallization Wang and coworkers have successfully obtained free-standing and crack-free colloidal crystal films with sizes in excess of several square millimeters [39]. In another study, rather than use a water/air interface, Zental and coworkers used the interface between melted germanium and air for colloidal crystallization, and obtained crack-free colloidal crystals [40].

6.3
Top-Down Modification of Colloidal Masks

As discussed above, many techniques have been developed to produce 2-D colloidal crystals of high quality. However, in order to increase the structural complexity of the surface patterns obtained via CL, the as-prepared 2-D colloidal crystals can be either etched or deformed, using physical or chemical methods, to tune the size and geometry of the interstices between the solid particles in the crystals. An overview of the strategies developed to modify colloidal crystals is provided in the following subsections.

6.3.1
Controlled Deformation

In general, polymers undergo a second-order phase transition from hard glassy state to a soft rubbery state above a glass transition temperature (T_g), due to the free-volume change between the polymer chains. Therefore, annealing slightly above the T_g can cause the deformation of spherical polymeric beads. It has been shown that, compared to heating in an oven, microwave radiation can provide a much more precise control of such deformation, since its intensity can be easily adjusted [41]. Giersig and coworkers have recently developed a new annealing technique in which a microwave pulse is used to heat polystyrene (PS) microspheres, in a mixture of good and poor solvents for PS. This allowed not only a reduction in the sizes of the interstices of 2-D PS colloidal crystals, but also a deformation of their geometry, from triangular to rodlike, while preserving the interparticle spacing and packing order of

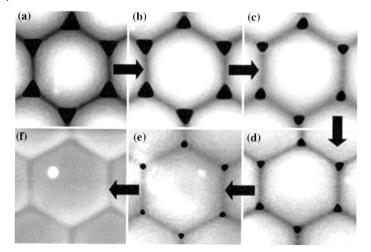

Figure 6.6 Precise control of the degree of annealing is achieved via adjustment of the number of microwave exposures. A 540 nm polystyrene latex mask annealed in 25 ml of water/EtOH/acetone mixture by (a) 1, (b) 2, (c) 4, (d) 6, (e) 7, and (f) 10 microwave pulses. Reproduced with permission from Ref. [42].

the original crystals (Figure 6.6) [42]. Recently, Yang *et al.* described a photolithographic process for the production of hierarchical arrays of nanopores or nanobowls by using colloidal crystals of photoresist particles [43]. In this case, the major difference in T_g between the crosslinked (UV-exposed) and non-crosslinked (UV-screened) particles was the most favorable factor for producing a high contrast in interstitial pore sizes during the baking stage. Although, in the case of inorganic particles, deformation is difficult to achieve by thermal annealing, Polman and colleagues have successfully deformed silica@Au core-shell microspheres into oblate ellipsoids by using high-energy ion irradiation. Such transition occurred due to the fact that the ion-induced deformation of the silica core was counteracted by the mechanical constraint of the gold shell (Figure 6.7) [44]. Vossen and coworkers recently reported that silica particles could undergo an anisotropic deformation under ion bombardment, due to an expansion in the plane perpendicular to the ion beam [45].

6.3.2
Reactive Ion Etching

During the early 1980s, Deckmann and Dunsmuir pioneered investigations into the etching of a colloidal crystal into a textured surface, using a reactive ion beam [46]. Since then, reactive ion etching (RIE) has been widely used to interdependently reduce the particle sizes and thus widen the interstitial space in 2-D colloidal crystal masks; this eventually led to the close-packing structures of the crystals to become non-close-packing (*vide infra*). In 3-D colloidal crystals, RIE is an anisotropic process,

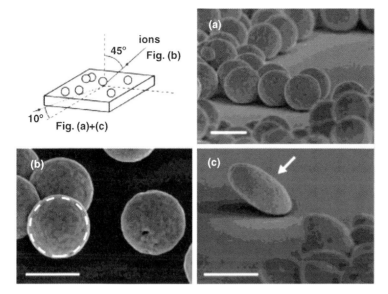

Figure 6.7 Scanning electron microscopy (SEM) images of silica-core/Au-shell colloids on a silicon substrate. (a) Unirradiated; (b, c) Irradiated with 30 MeV Cu ions at 45° and at 77 K, to a fluence of 5×10^{14} ions cm^{-2}, viewing angle parallel (b) or almost perpendicular (c) to the ion-beam direction. The scheme shown at the upper-left shows the ion-beam direction and the SEM viewing angles. Scale bars = 500 nm. Reproduced with permission from Ref. [44].

as the upper layers act as shadow masks for etching the lower layer particles. Such anisotropic RIE can cause spherical particles to become nonspherical particles, while the particle shapes and hierarchical nanostructures obtained will depend heavily on the stacking sequence of the colloidal crystals, the crystal orientation relative to the substrate, the number of colloidal layers, and the RIE conditions employed (Figure 6.8) [47]. Of greatest significance is the fact that the anisotropic RIE can provide a new method for machining the surfaces of the colloidal particles. First, the double layers of PS colloidal crystals were partially filled with silica nanoparticles, such that removal of the top layer PS particles left behind an ordered macroporous silica matrix with regularly arranged openings, beneath which were located the bottom layer particles. The macroporous silica matrices were then used as masks for further RIE of the PS particles beneath. The nanopores, which were arranged in threefold or fourfold symmetry depending on the crystalline orientation of the original colloidal crystals, were then machined on the PS particles [48]. Together, the integration of an anisotropic RIE protocol, the use of binary colloidal crystals composed of PS and silica particles with identical or different sizes as masks, and the use of macroporous matrices as masks represented a powerful method of sculpting spherical particles to multifaceted and nanobored particles [49, 50]. The morphologies of the resultant PS particles were largely dependent on the crystal orientation with respect to the etchant flow, the number of colloidal layers, the size ratio of silica to PS microspheres, the etching angle in the RIE process, the stacking sequence of

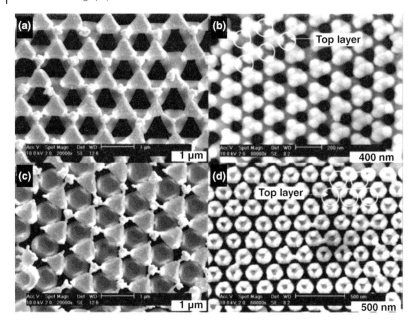

Figure 6.8 Modification of a mask using reactive ion etching (RIE) for the fabrication of binary and ternary particle arrays with nonspherical building blocks. (a, b) Triangle arrays using binary and ternary colloidal spheres with an *hcp* arrangement; (c, d) Polygonal structures produced from colloidal layers with the (111) plane and the (100) plane of the face-centered-cubic structure, respectively. Reproduced with permission from Ref. [47].

the binary colloidal layers, and the tilt angle of the substrate and the orientation angle of the crystal plane with respect to the etchant flow in the RIE process.

6.4
Colloidal Lithography

6.4.1
Colloidal Mask-Assisted Etching

When a 2-D colloidal crystal is formed on a solid substrate, the interstices between the solid particles can used as masks for reactive ions to create patterned bumps or pores on the substrate. Forests of silicon pillars with diameters less than 500 nm and an aspect ratio of up to 10 were fabricated by first, conducting an O_2 RIE to turn close-packed PS particle monolayers into non-close-packed layers, and subsequently conducting a "Bosch" process to etch the supporting silicon wafers [51]. Subsequent scanning electron microscopy (SEM) imaging showed that the etching rate of the resultant structures decreased in line with the increased aspect ratio, which suggested that the etching process was limited by the chemical transport rate. The reactive plasma can be dispersed by a particle in a point-contact with a substrate, which leads to the induction of so-called "underetching" of the colloidal mask and eventually produces a dome structure of the substrate. Underetching can be avoided by modifying the shape, size, and coverage of the colloidal mask. Sow *et al.* have demonstrated the characteristic features of a RIE silicon substrate using a PS colloidal crystal mask, and produced a double-dome structure by a simultaneous etching of the mask and the regions beneath the particles [52]. When compared to conventionally used polymer masks, such as photoresists removed by organic developers, colloidal masks can be removed easily by sonication, thereby causing very little damage to the nanostructured substrates obtained via RIE. Ordered arrays of polyacrylic acid domes have been fabricated by using 2-D PS colloidal crystals as masks for the O_2 RIE of polymeric films; removal of the PS masks caused no damage to the surface chemistry and the structure of the resultant polymeric domes, thus enabling the conjugation of proteins [53]. Previously, 2-D PS colloidal crystals have also been used as masks for the dry etching of SiO_2 slides so as to create periodic arrays of nanoplates that can be transferred onto polymer films by imprinting [54]. By using colloidal crystals as masks for catalytic etching, Zhu *et al.* have fabricated large-scale periodic arrays of silicon nanowires, the diameters, heights and center-to-center distances of which could be accurately controlled (Figure 6.9) [55]. In a similar study, by using colloidal crystals as masks to create arrays of nanopores on supporting solid substrates via RIE, followed by the consecutive deposition of gold films and removal of the colloidal masks, Ong *et al.* fabricated 2-D ordered arrays of gold nanoparticles nested in the nanopores of the templated substrate [56]. One potential extension of having gold nanoparticles confined in nanopores would be their use as catalysts for the growth of nanowires composed of other materials, such as ZnO.

6.4.2
Colloidal Mask-Assisted Chemical Deposition

By combining microcontact printing with colloidal crystal masking, Xia *et al.* were able to develop a simple method, termed edge-spreading lithography (ESL), that could be used to generate mesoscopic structures on substrates [57]. As the name suggests, ESL utilizes the edges of masks – the perimeters of the footprint of particles on substrates – to define the features of the resultant structures. The ESL procedure begins with the formation of 2-D colloidal crystals of silica beads on the surfaces of gold or silver thin films. Silica beads are used for several reasons: (i) they are inert to most organic solvents; (ii) they are commercially available as monodispersed samples in a range of sizes; (iii) they can be readily assembled into ordered arrays over large areas; (iv) they are mechanically more robust than most polymer beads of equivalent size; and (v) their hydrophilic surfaces support the spreading of the thiols [57]. As shown in Figure 6.10a, typically, a planar polydimethylsiloxane (PDMS) stamp bearing a thin film of the ethanol solution of an alkanethiol was placed on a 2-D silica colloidal crystal. The thiol molecules were then released from the stamp to the silica particle during contact, and subsequently transferred to the substrate along the

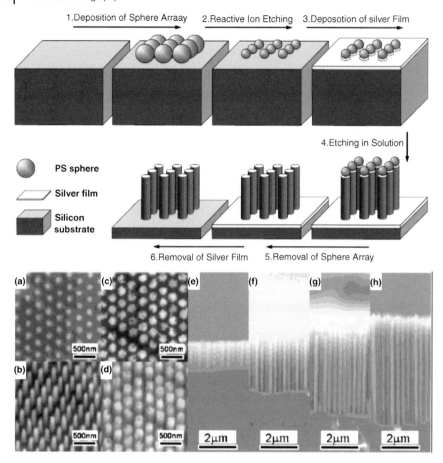

Figure 6.9 Upper panel: Schematic depiction of the fabrication process. Lower panel: SEM images of samples where PS spheres with a nominal diameter of 260 nm have been used. Plane-view and title-view (ca. 15°) images of samples fabricated using PS spheres with a reduced diameter of (a, b) 100 nm and (c, d) 180 nm; (e–h) Cross-sectional SEM images of samples after etching for (e) 4 min, (f) 8 min, (g) 12 min, and (h) 16 min. Reproduced with permission from Ref. [55].

surfaces of the silica particles; this led to the creation of a self-assembled monolayer (SAM) that encircled the footprint of each silica particle. The area of the thiol SAM was able to expand laterally via reactive spreading, as long as the thiols were continuously supplied, such that the width of the thiol SAM rings could be varied between 30 and 340 nm. Following removal of the stamp and bead lift-off, the ring pattern was developed by wet-etching with aqueous Fe^{3+}/thiourea, using the patterned SAM as a resist [57]. The most important point here was that ESL allowed the generation of concentric rings of different alkanethiol SAMs by successive printing with different thiol inks, while removal of the silica particle templates and selective etching yielded concentric gold rings (Figure 6.10b) [58].

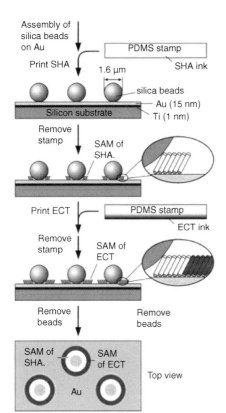

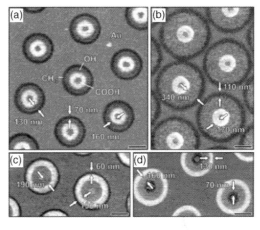

Figure 6.10 Left column: Schematic illustration of the edge-spreading lithography (ESL) procedure used for side-by-side patterning of sulfanylhexadecanoic acid (SHA) and eicosanethiol (ECT) monolayer rings on a gold substrate. The process involves two successive prints that are performed on a 2-D array of silica beads supported on a thin film of gold. In the first step, SHA molecules (white) are guided from a planar stamp to the gold surface, where they assemble into a monolayer, as directed by the circular footprint of each bead and lateral spreading. In the second step, ECT molecules (black) are applied in a similar fashion, thus forming a self-assembled monolayer (SAM) that emerges from the edges of the SHA monolayer. Removal of the beads yields an array of concentric rings of SHA and ECT SAMs on the surface. Right column: Lateral force microscopy (LFM) images of concentric rings of carboxy- (bright), hydroxy- (gray), and methyl-terminated (dark) thiolate monolayers on gold. (a) The rings were fabricated under the following conditions: 1 min for SHA, 1.5 min for 12-hydroxydodecanethiol (HDDT), and 3 min for ECT; (b) An increase in the printing times for HDDT and ECT to 3.5 and 4 min, respectively, resulted in wider rings for these two monolayers; (c, d) The position of each monolayer in the concentric structure could be varied by changing the printing order. The pattern in (c) was generated by printing HDDT for 1.5 min, followed by printing of SHA and ECT for 3 min each. The sample shown in (d) was prepared by printing both ECT and HDDT for 1 min, and SHA for 2 min. All scale bars = 500 nm. Reproduced with permission from Ref. [58].

Shin *et al.* have developed an alternative means of integrating colloidal masking and contact printing, termed contact area lithography (CAL), which can be used for the direct generation of periodic surface chemical patterns at the sub-100 nm scale [59, 60]. In contrast to ESL, CAL relies on the self-assembly of octadecyltrichlorosilane (OTS). Following the formation of a 2-D colloidal crystal of silica on a silicon wafer, the SAM of OTS was grown homogeneously both on the silica particles and on the supporting silicon wafer, via a sol–gel process. The removal of silica particles left behind a periodically arranged array of openings in the OTS SAM, with the same symmetry as that of the 2-D colloidal crystals. The openings were subsequently used as masks, either for the growth of ordered arrays of nanoparticles (e.g., of titania), or for the selective etching of ordered arrays of silica cavities on the silicon wafer. In the case of titania growth, nucleation proved to be rather site-selective due to significant differences in surface energy between the growing and surrounding surfaces [60].

6.4.3
Colloidal Mask-Assisted Physical Deposition: Nanosphere Lithography

In 1981, Fischer and Zingsheim were the first to use 2-D colloidal crystals as masks for contact imaging with visible light [22], whilst a year later Deckman and Dunsmuir demonstrated the feasibility of using 2-D colloidal crystals as masks for both the physical deposition of materials and, in turn, patterning the surfaces of the supporting substrates (Figure 6.11) [61]. Consequently, the latter authors coined the term "natural lithography" to describe this process, since "naturally" assembled single layers of latex particles were used as masks rather than lithographic masks. Later, the capabilities of natural lithography were expanded, with the RIE process in particular

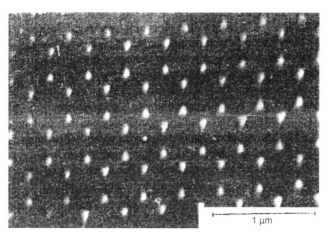

Figure 6.11 Triangular silver posts fabricated using a lift-off process. Silver was evaporated over a densely packed array of 0.4 μm spheres, and the spheres were dissolved in methylene chloride. Reproduced with permission from Ref. [61].

being developed to increase the structural complexity of 2-D colloidal crystal masks [46]. Since then, the group of Van Duyne has expended much effort towards developing patterning techniques that used colloidal crystals as masks for metallic vapor deposition [23, 62–64]. In the context of nanoscience, the term "natural lithography" was changed to "nanosphere lithography" (NSL), and its use explored over a variety of experimental parameters, notably of the incident angle that would lead to a diversification of the patterns obtained. The same group also extended single-layer masking to double-layer masking and, perhaps most importantly, conducted intensive investigations into the plasmon resonance properties of metallic patterns obtained via NSL. In this case, the correlation with feature morphology was of particular interest, the intention being ultimately to develop highly sensitive biosensors based on surface-enhanced Raman spectroscopy (SERS) [65]. Following the seminal studies of Van Duyne and colleagues, colloidal crystals came to be identified as being low-cost, flexible, and easily adoptable masks for the growth of new nanostructures with a diverse structural complexity. The uses of NSL and their variants for surface patterning on planar substrates, and especially on microparticles, are summarized in the following subsections.

6.4.3.1 Surface Patterning on Planar Substrates

In the NSL procedure, a 2-D colloidal crystal is used as a mask for the physical deposition of a material, the latter being freely chosen without any limitations, and often including various metals such as gold and silver. The projection of the interstices between ordered close-packed particles defines the shape of the nanodots deposited on substrates; the dots usually show a quasi-triangular shape, and are arranged in a P_{6mm} array due to the hexagonal packing of the colloidal crystal mask (Figure 6.12a–c). The dot size is about one-fourth of the particle diameter, while the distance between nearest-neighbor dots is about one-half of the sphere diameter. The dot height is controlled by the physical deposition conditions, notably the deposition time. Van Duyne *et al.* have extended colloidal crystal masking from single layers of hexagonally close-packed particles to double layers [23]. Since overlapping of the interstices between the upper and lower layers leads to an hexagonal array of quasi-hexagonal projections on a substrate, the use of a double-layer colloidal crystals as a mask will yields an hexagonal array of quasi-hexagonal nanodots (Figure 6.12d and e).

In a general NSL procedure, the substrate to be patterned is positioned normal to the direction of material deposition. The in-plane shape of the nanodots and spacing of the nearest-neighbor dots derived from NSL are then dictated by a projection of the interstices of single or double layers of colloidal crystals on the substrates. These can be fine-tuned by varying the projection geometry of the interstices on substrates, for example by tilting the masks with respect to the incidence of the vapor beam. This approach has inspired the development of angle-resolved NSL (AR-NSL), as pioneered by the group of Van Duyne [64].

In the AR-NSL process, the incident angle of the propagation vector of the material deposition beam with respect to the normal direction of the colloidal mask (θ) and/or the azimuth angle of the propagation vector with respect to the nearest-neighbor

(a)   **(d)**

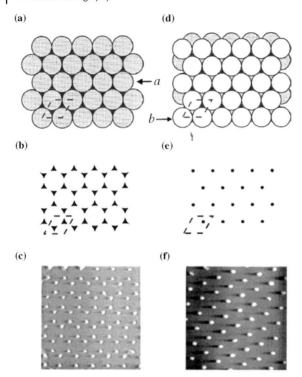

(b)   **(e)**

(c)   **(f)**

Figure 6.12 Schematic diagrams of single-layer (SL) and double-layer (DL) nanosphere masks and the corresponding periodic particle array (PPA) surfaces. (a) *a* (111) SL mask, dotted line = unit cell, *a* = first layer nanosphere; (b) SL PPA, two particles per unit cell; (c) 1.7 × 1.7 μm constant-height AFM image of a SL PPA with M = Ag, S = mica, $D = 264$ nm, $d_m = 22$ nm, $r_d = 0.2$ nm s^{-1}; (d) *a* (e) $p(1 \times 1)$-*b* DL mask, dotted line = unit cell, *b* = second layer nanosphere; (f) DL PPA, one particle per unit cell; (g) 2.0 × 2.0 μm constant-height AFM image of a DL PPA with M = Ag, S = mica, $D = 264$ nm, $d_m = 22$ nm, $r_d = 0.2$ nm s^{-1}. Reproduced with permission from Ref. [23].

particles in the colloidal masks (φ) – the mask registry with respect to the vector of the material deposition beam – have been used to reduce the size of the nanodots obtained and, at the same time, to elongate their triangular shape (Figure 6.13). By rotating substrates, Giersig and coworkers have recently found that AR-NSL can generate much more complicated metallic nanostructures, and they referred to this process as "shadow NSL" [42, 66, 67]. Due to rotation of the colloidal mask, the shadow NSL process is resolved by the azimuth angle (φ) of the incidence deposition beam rather than the incident angle (θ).

An elegant extension of AR-NSL was to conduct a stepwise physical vapor deposition (PVD) of identical or different materials, but at different angles of incidence. In this case, the group of Van Duyne succeeded in growing surface-patterning features composed of two triangular nanodots that were either overlapped or separated by two deposition steps at $\theta = 0°$ and $\theta > 0°$, respectively [63]. The

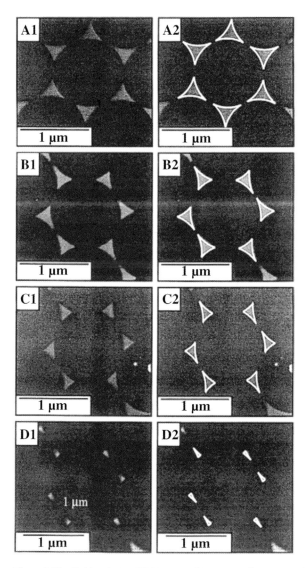

Figure 6.13 Field-emission SEM images of AR NSL-fabricated gold nanodot arrays and images with simulated geometry superimposed, respectively. (A1, A2) $\theta = 108°$, $\psi = 288°$, (D1, B2) $\theta = 208°$, $\phi = 28°$, (C1, C2) $\theta = 268°$, $\phi = 168°$, and (D1, D2) $\theta = 408°$, $\phi = 28°$. All samples were Cr-deposited onto Si(111) substrates. Original magnification of images $= \times 40\,000$. θ is the incidence angle and ϕ the azimuth angle. Reproduced with permission from Ref. [64].

overlapping or spacing between the two nanodots was seen to depend on the incident angle at the second step of deposition. When three deposition steps at three different incident angles – zero, tilted forward and tilted backward – were conducted, chains of triangular dots were obtained. although the registry of colloidal crystal masks – the azimuth of the incident deposition beam (φ) – was changed only minimally. Giersig *et al.* have also developed a stepwise shadow NSL protocol to deposit different materials at different incident angles when the colloidal masks were rotating, and have succeeded in encapsulating the metallic structures so as to protect them against oxidation [67].

Recently, Zhang and Wang demonstrated the feasibility of consecutively depositing two different metals, such as gold and silver, at two different incident angles, in order to construct ordered binary arrays of gold and silver nanoparticles [68]. This approach was seen to be independent of the sphere sizes of the colloidal masks and the chemical nature of materials deposited, but did demonstrate a profound dependence on the registry of colloidal masks with respect to the incident vapor beam and the incident angle. When the projection of the incident beam onto the substrates was coincident with the vector between the nearest-neighbor particles, triangular gold and silver nanodots were obtained, interspaced by a tiny gap, and each of these was arranged in an array with P_{6mm} symmetry (Figure 6.14). However, when the projection of the incident beam on the substrates was coincident with the vector between the next-nearest-neighbor particles, then triangular gold nanodots, triangular silver nanodots, and rectangular nanodots composed of triangular gold and silver nanodots were obtained, each of which was arranged in an hexagonal array.

Prior to PVD, colloidal crystal masks can undergo RIE to reduce the sizes of the particles and widen the interstitial spaces, thus increasing the dimensions of the triangular nanodots obtained via NSL. Increasing the RIE time can also cause

(a)

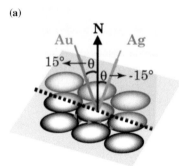

(b)

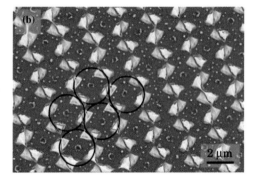

Figure 6.14 (a) Schematic illustration of depositing gold and silver onto a hexagonally close-packed sphere monolayer at incident angles (θ) of 15° and −15°, respectively. The colloidal mask is registered so that the vector between nearest-neighbor spheres is in line with the projection of the incidence beam on the mask, highlighted by a black dotted line. The incidence beams of gold and of silver, and the normal direction of the colloidal template are highlighted by yellow, blue, and black arrows, respectively. The incident angles (θ) of the vapor beam with respect to the normal direction of the colloidal masks are marked as red; (b) SEM image of the resultant heterogeneous binary array. The mask is a monolayer of hexagonally close-packed 830 nm PS spheres. The original location of PS spheres, gold nanoparticles (NPs), and silver NPs are highlighted by black circles, yellow triangles, and blue triangles, respectively. Reproduced with permission from Ref. [68].

close-packed colloidal crystal masks to become non-close-packed, which in turn leads to thin films with hexagonally arranged pores [69, 70]. Wang *et al.* have recently integrated AR-NSL with the use of RIE-modified colloidal crystals as masks, to diversify the structural complexity of the patterning feature derived from NSL from triangular (or deformed) nanodots to nanorods and nanowires [71]. After modification via O_2 RIE, 2-D colloidal crystal masks were registered so that the projection of the metal vapor beam on the colloidal mask was coincident with the vector between the nearest-neighbor particles. When PVD was conducted at the incident angle of 45°, zigzag nanowires were obtained that were well separated and aligned in parallel. However, when the projection of the metal vapor beam on the colloidal mask was adjusted in line with the vector between the next-nearest-neighbor particles, only nanorods were obtained and these were arranged in an hexagonal array. A stepwise rotation of the colloidal crystal masks by 120°, to deposit identical or different materials, led to quasi-3-D grids of nanowires or nanorods with a defined vertical, and especially lateral, heterogeneity (Figure 6.15). The lateral arrangement of different nanowires into a periodic array with a defined alignment is difficult to implement by other means, whether conventional lithographic or self-assembly techniques.

Wang *et al.* have recently extended the RIE process for the modification of double layers of colloidal crystals for AR-NSL [72]. By using O_2 plasma-etched bilayers of hexagonally packed particles as masks for gold deposition, it was possible to fabricate highly ordered binary arrays of gold nanoparticles of various shapes, including a shuttlecock-shaped array composed of small, crescent-shaped nanoparticles, and a large fan-shaped array (see Figure 6.16). The size and shape of both the small and large nanoparticles obtained could be manipulated by altering the plasma-etching period and the incident angle of the Au vapor flow. When compared to the corresponding bulk materials, the melting point of the nanoparticles was much lower, and they were much more sensitive to the surface tension. As the large curvature caused a high surface tension, annealing of the non-round nanoparticles might give rise to a retraction of their apexes, and eventually the creation of a round shape [73]. Wang *et al.* have successfully transformed the shape of Au nanoparticles obtained from crescent- or fan-like array to a round form, with a rather narrow distribution in terms of size and shape (Figure 6.17) [72].

Dmitriev *et al.* have extended colloidal crystal masking from a use for material deposition to one of controlled etching, and have developed an interesting variant of NSL, termed hole-mask colloidal lithography (HCL) [74]. HCL differs from conventional NSL in that the substrate and colloidal crystal mask are interspaced by a sacrificial layer. After PVD, removal of the colloidal mask leads to a thin film mask with nanoholes. This so-called "hole-mask" is subsequently used for vapor deposition and/or etching steps to further define a patterning feature on the substrate. Removal of the sacrificial layer, along with the hole-mask, leaves behind the substrate with a predesigned surface pattern composed of, for instance, discs, ellipsoids, and cores (Figure 6.18). HCL displays several advantages over NSL, notably a large area coverage, a high fabrication speed (the fabrication time does not scale with area), an independent control over the feature size and spacing, and processing simplicity

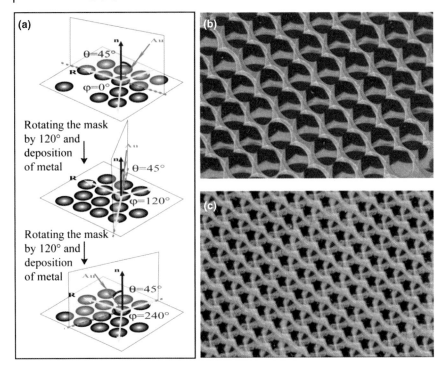

Figure 6.15 (a) Schematic depiction of constructing quasi-3-D grids of multiplex zigzag nanowires by stepwise rotation of the colloidal mask by 120° with respect to the reference vector (R) between nearest-neighboring spheres over the course of metallic vapor deposition. The projection of metal vapor on the mask was set coincidence with the reference vector (R), namely $\varphi = 0°$. SEM images of quasi-3-D grids of multiplex zigzag nanowires obtained by stepwise depositing gold, silver, and nickel at $\varphi = 0°$, $\varphi = 120°$, and $\varphi = 240°$, using plasma-etched close-packed 830 nm PS sphere monolayers as masks. The structure obtained by two and three deposition steps are shown in panels (b) and (c), respectively. The plasma etching time was 20 min, θ was 45°, and the deposition time 30 min. Reproduced with permission from Ref. [71].

(the nanofabrication process is reduced to conventional material deposition and RIE). Moreover, HCL can be applied to a wide range of materials, including Au, Ag, Pd, Pt, and SiO_2.

6.4.3.2 Surface Patterning on Particles

Various colloidal spheres, whether organic and inorganic, can be produced that are exceedingly monodisperse in terms of their size and shape. Nevertheless, their surfaces remain chemically homogeneous or heterogeneous in an undefined way, despite there being well-established methods for their modification. As this surface chemistry renders the coupling of spheres spatially isotropic, it is difficult to spatially direct the organization of the spheres, and they tend to self-assemble only into simple and energy-favorable *fcc* or *hcp* structures. Controlling the surface properties of

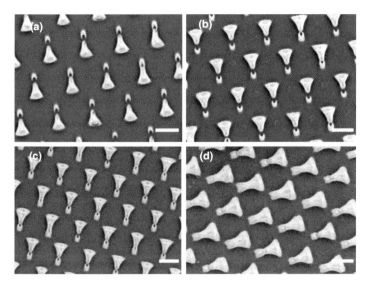

Figure 6.16 SEM images of hexagonally arranged Au nanoshuttlecocks obtained by using bilayers of hexagonal close-packed 925 nm PS spheres, etched by O_2-plasma for 10 (a), 20 (b), 25 (c), and 30 min (d), as masks for Au vapor deposition. The incidence angle of Au vapor flow was set as 15°. Scale bars = 500 nm. Reproduced with permission from Ref. [72].

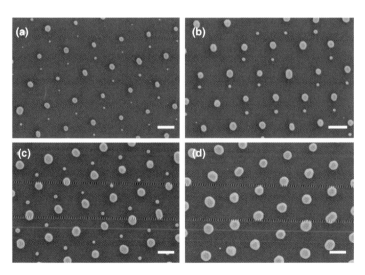

Figure 6.17 SEM images of the hexagonal binary arrays obtained by annealing the Au nanoshuttlecock arrays derived from the hexagonal close-packed 925 nm PS sphere bilayers etched for 10 (a), 20 (b), 25 (c), and 30 min (d). The SEM images of the original shuttlecock arrays are shown in Figure 6.16. Scale bars = 500 nm. Reproduced with permission from Ref. [72].

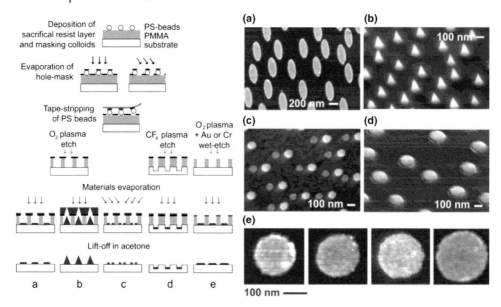

Figure 6.18 Left column: Diagram illustrating the basic process steps and resultant structures produced with HCL nanofabrication. Right column: SEM images of the five different nanostructure types produced by HCL. (a) Array of identically oriented elliptical Au nanostructures; (b) Au nanocone array; (c) Binary arrays of Au–Ag nanodisc pairs (note the slightly different imaging conditions for Au and Ag nanodiscs in each pair; Au is imaged brighter); (d) Embedded nanodiscs; (e) Discs with fine-tuned diameters, where the disc size increases from left to right. Reproduced with permission from Ref. [74].

colloidal particles is one of the oldest and, at the same time, the most vital topics in colloid science and physical chemistry. Patchy particles – that is, particles with more than one patch or patches that are less than 50% of the total particle surface – should present the next generation of particles for assembly [75–77]. However, patterning the surface of colloidal particles with sizes of micrometers or submicrometers represents a formidable challenge, due to the lack of a proper mask.

When 2-D colloidal crystals are used as masks for PVD, it is expected that only the upper surfaces of the colloidal particles (which are exposed directly to the vapor beam) will be coated with the new materials. This leads to the creation of two spatially well-separated halves on the colloidal particles – coated and noncoated – with two distinct surface chemical functionalities [78, 79]. Such particles are usually referred to as *Janus particles*. By embedding a monomer of close-packed colloidal particles in a photoresist layer, Bao *et al.* managed to tune the surface areas of the colloidal particles exposed to the vapor beam during material deposition, by etching the photoresist layer with O_2 plasma; this in turn led to a good control of the domain sizes deposited on the particles [80]. When a monolayer of close-packed colloidal particles is constructed at the water/air interface or the wax/liquid interfaces, a selective modification can be implemented in either of the two phases, and this leads to the production of Janus particles [81, 82]. Shin *et al.* have recently extended the CAL procedure to decorate silica particles with ordered arrays of titania nanoparticles by selective removal of the upper layer particles [60].

Wang *et al.* pioneered the use of upper single layers of colloidal crystals as masks for the lower layer particles during PVD [83]. By using the upper single layer of a colloidal crystal as masks for gold vapor deposition, various Au patterns were embossed on the upper halves of the particles in the second layer, such as triangles, squares, and bow-ties, the size and shape of which were predominantly manipulated by orientation of the template crystals. Most importantly, the methodology reported by Wang *et al.*, which used colloidal crystals for self-masking, was independent of the curvature and chemical composition of the surfaces (Figure 6.19). This would clearly

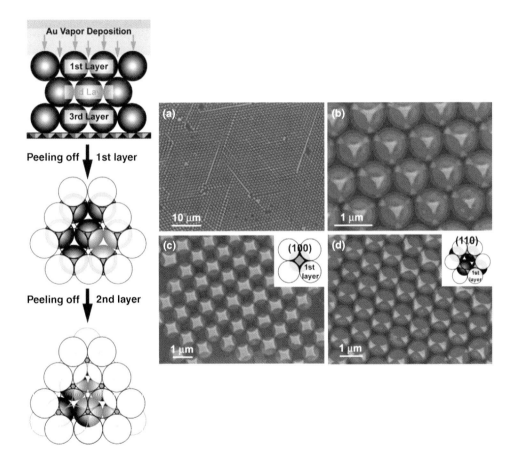

Figure 6.19 Left column: Schematic illustration of the procedure to create colloidal spheres with Au-patterned surfaces by the combination of Au vapor deposition and using the top mono- or bilayers of colloidal crystals with (111) facets parallel to the substrates as masks. Right column: (a) Low-magnification and (b–d) high-magnification SEM images of 925 nm polystyrene (PS) spheres with Au-patterned surfaces, generated by templating the top monolayers of colloidal crystals with (b) (111), (c) (100), and (d) (110) facets parallel to the substrates. Reproduced with permission from Ref. [83].

provide a versatile way in which to pattern highly curved surfaces, a situation that is difficult to achieve by using routine lithographic techniques. By using O_2 plasma to etch the colloidal crystal templates (mainly the top layer) and conducting PVD at the non-zero incident angle, Wang *et al.* also found that the size and shape of the patterns obtained on the second layer particles showed a pronounced dependence on the plasma etching time and the incident angle [84]. Pawar and Kretzschmar have recently extended the use of colloidal crystals for self-masking for glancing angle deposition [85]. During PVD at a glancing incident angle, the shadow effects caused by neighboring particles were used for surface patterning particles with the same particle monolayer. This differed from Wang's strategy, where the upper layers were used as masks for surface patterning the particles in the lower layers. The size and shape of the resultant patterns were determined by the incident angle and monolayer orientation, such that the smallest patch produced via glancing angle deposition was 3.7% of the particle surface.

Wang *et al.* have recently used the upper double layers as masks for patterning particles in the third layers, via PVD [86]. Whilst the smaller interstices in the upper bilayers cause a nonuniform diffusion of the Au vapor, the dimension and features of the Au dots obtained previously were neither uniform nor clear-cut when compared to patterns derived from single-layer masking. In order to achieve an homogeneous diffusion of the vapor through the upper double layers to reach the deeper layers in a colloidal crystal, the crystal was made to undergo RIE with O_2 plasma, which widened the interstitial spaces between the particles. The use of RIE-treated colloidal crystals as a mask has greatly improved the uniformity of the patterns generated on the third layer particles. Notably, widening the interstitial spaces allows more vapor to diffuse into and through an RIE-treated colloidal crystal. Any excess vapor that is scattered or reflected by the spheres beneath the third layer or the substrate would be envisioned to condense into a round dot on the lower half of each sphere in the third layer, opposite to the Au vapor flow. As a consequence, Wang *et al.* succeeded in the stereo-decoration of colloidal particles with two, three, four, or five nanodots. The number of dots per sphere was proved to depend on the crystalline structure of the colloidal crystal masks, the plasma etching time, and the incident angle. The nanodots decorated on particles were arranged in a linear, trigonal, tetrahedral, or right-pyramidal fashion, which provided nanoscale analogues of sp-, sp^2-, and sp^3-hybridized atomic orbitals of carbon (Figure 6.20). The Au nanodots obtained on microspheres, therefore, could be recruited as the bonding site to dictate the integration of the spheres, thus paving a new approach to colloidal self-assembly – colloidal valent chemistry of spheres [87] – to create hierarchical and complicated "supraparticles" [75].

6.4.3.3 Extension of Nanosphere Lithography

One extension of NSL is to use the surface patterns obtained as templates to grow nanostructures of a variety of materials, via bottom-up self-assembly. Mulvaney's group has grown monolayer and multilayer films of semiconductor quantum dots on surface patterns derived from NSL, leading to nanostructured luminescent thin films (Figure 6.21) [88, 89]. Valsesia *et al.* have used ordered arrays of polyacrylic acid

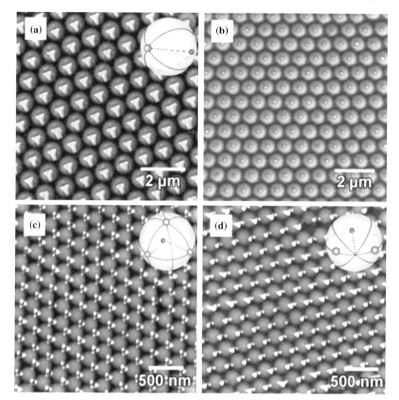

Figure 6.20 (a) SEM image of the gold patterns deposited on the upper halves of 925 nm PS spheres in the third layer, obtained by using their colloidal crystals, and etched by plasma for 10 min, as templates; (b) SEM image of the Au patterns obtained on the lower halves of these spheres; (c, d) SEM images of the gold Au patterns on the upper halves of 270 nm PS spheres by using their colloidal crystals, etched by plasma for 3 min, as templates constructed. The incident angle of the gold vapor was 0° (c) and 10° (d). The insets show schematic illustrations of the spatial configuration of gold nanodots decorated on the microspheres. Reproduced with permission from Ref. [86].

domes derived via NSL to selectively couple with bovine serum albumin [53]. By using NSL-derived surface patterns as templates to grow proteins, Sutherland *et al.* showed that the surface topography could enhance the binding selectivity of fibrinogens to platelets [90].

A second extension is to use NSL-derived surface patterns as etching masks to create surface topography. In this case, Chen *et al.* have fabricated silicon nanopillar arrays with diameters as small as 40 nm and aspect ratios up to 7 [91]. The size and shape of the nanopillars could be controlled by the size and shape of the sputtered aluminum mask, with both parameters being again determined by the feature size of the colloidal mask and the number of the colloid layers. Nanopillars of different shapes can also be fabricated by adjusting the RIE conditions, such as the gas species, bias voltage, and exposure duration for an aluminum mask with a given shape. The

(a)

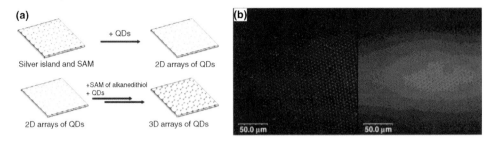

Silver island and SAM   2D arrays of QDs

2D arrays of QDs   3D arrays of QDs

Figure 6.21 (a) Scheme of formation of 3-D quantum dot structures, using a multiple SAM technique based on CL; (b) Photoluminescence and transmission images of QD642 (quantum dots emitting at 642 nm) arrays made with a partially completed bilayer of 5.46 μm PS mask; scan size: 200 × 200 μm. Reproduced with permission from Ref. [89].

as-prepared nanopillar arrays could then be used to imprint a layer of PMMA above its T_g (Figure 6.22) [92]. Similarly, Weekes *et al.* have fabricated ordered arrays of cobalt nanodots for patterned magnetic media [93]. By introducing intermediary layers of SiO_2 between the colloidal crystal masks and substrates, this etching strategy could be applied to a wide range of materials, without too much concern for the surface hydrophilicity of the targeted substrates. By using a similar protocol, large-area ordered arrays of 512 nm pitch holes, and with vertical and smooth sidewalls, have been successfully formed on GaAs substrates [94].

A third extension is to use NSL-derived surface patterns to template or catalyze the growth of other functional materials. Here, Zhou *et al.* have successfully used ordered arrays of gold nanodots derived from NSL as seeds to create highly aligned single-walled carbon nanotubes (CNTs), laid on quartz and sapphire substrates [95]. This method has great potential for the production of CNT arrays, with a simultaneous control over nanotube orientation, position, density, diameter, and even chirality. As a consequence, these CNTs may function as building blocks in future nanoelectronics and ultra-high-speed electronics applications [96]. Wang *et al.* have used gold nanodot arrays as seeds for hexagonally arranged arrays of zinc oxide nanorods, aligned perpendicularly to the substrates [97]. Similarly, Fuhrmann *et al.* have produced ordered arrays of Si nanorods by using the gold nanodots as seeds for molecular beam epitaxy (Figure 6.23) [98], while discretely ordered arrays of organic light-emitting nanodiodes (OLEDs) have been fabricated based on NSL-derived surface patterns [99]. These are not feasible via any other route, as conventional masking techniques may damage the organic heterostructure of the OLED layers.

6.5
Applications of CL

Surface patterns derived via CL, and especially via NSL, are normally composed of metals such as gold and silver, with their primary technical application being highly

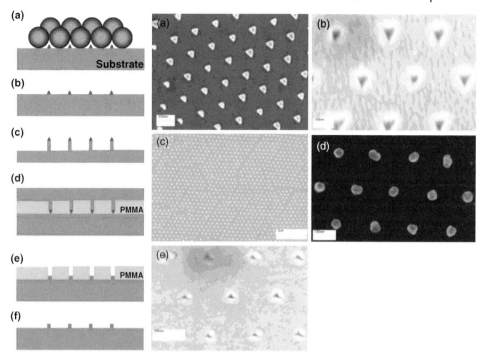

Figure 6.22 Left column: Schematic of the fabrication of large-area periodic nanostructures by a combination of double-layer nanosphere lithography and nanoimprint lithography. (a) The silicon substrate is coated with a double layer of polystyrene spheres and a metal film is deposited on top of the polystyrene beads; (b) After dissolving the polystyrene beads in CH_2Cl_2, periodic metallic arrays are formed on the surface; (c) The silicon substrate is etched using the periodic metal arrays as an etching mask; (d) The silicon nanopillar arrays are used as an imprinting stamp, which is pressed against a PMMA film on a silicon wafer above the polymer's glass transition temperature, (e) The stamp is removed and the desired material deposited; (f) After lift-off, periodic arrays of the desired material are obtained. Right column: (a) SEM image of a nanoimprint stamp fabricated using a 350 nm polystyrene template; (b) The imprinted patterns on PMMA. The base of the triangular hole is about 55 nm; (c) Large-area image of periodic metal dots formed by nanoimprint lithography; (d) SEM image of nanodots formed by nanoimprint lithography. The diameter of the nanodots is about 50 nm; (e) SEM image of the imprinted patterns using a stamp treated with chromium etchant. The lateral dimension of the triangular hole is about 30 nm. Reproduced with permission from Ref. [92].

sensitive biosensors that rely on the localized-surface plasmon resonance (LSPR) of metallic nanostructures [65]. During intensive investigations of the LSPR of metallic nanostructures composed of gold rings [100] and disks [101] and obtained via NSL, it was found that the LSPR could be tuned by varying either the diameter of the disks (at a constant disk height) or the ring thickness. The subsequent shape-dependent red shift originated from the electromagnetic coupling between the inner and outer ring surfaces, and this led to energy shifts and the splitting of degenerate modes [102]. NSL has been also used to create nanocaps and nanocups, the LSPR

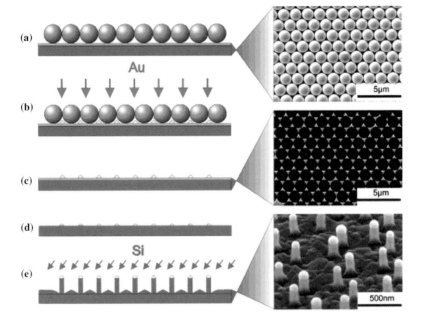

Figure 6.23 Steps of Si nanowire fabrication by NSL. (a) Deposition of a mask of polystyrene particles; (b) deposition of gold by thermal evaporation; (c) removal of the spheres; (d) thermal annealing and cleaning step to remove the oxide layer; (e) Si deposition and growth of nanowires by MBE. The corresponding SEM images at the right show the wafers at the different fabrication steps. Reproduced with permission from Ref. [98].

behavior of which has been studied [103]. For example, by using NSL, Lee *et al.* created gold crescent-moon structures which had a sub-10 nm sharp edge and exhibited a very strong SERS [104]. Moreover, the field emitted on the circular sharp edge of the nanocrescent moon (the "hot spot") could be enhanced more than 1000-fold when illuminated at 785 nm with a near-infrared diode laser. Interestingly, when 1 µM of rhodamine 6G was adsorbed onto the single gold nanocrescent moon it could be detected by a recognizable difference in the SERS spectrum. Such high sensitivity was considered due to the sharp edge of the nanostructure that had been created from the colloidal template.

Besides the exploitation of CL, and the patterns thus obtained via LSPR-assisted sensing, the magnetic properties of CL-derived nanostructures have continued to attract attention. In general, nanoscale magnetic materials often exhibit super-paramagnetic behavior, and an ordered nanostructure of magnetic materials is required when conducting investigations into the mesoscopic effects induced when magnetic materials are confined within nanoscale domains [105]. As the magnetic properties depend heavily on the domain size and inter-domain distances, Weekes *et al.* set out to create ordered arrays of isolated magnetic nanodots via NSL [93]. In this case, the coercivity and switching width of the isolated nanodot arrays were enhanced when compared to those of continuous magnetic films. In addition, well-organized arrays of magnetic nanorings over a large area have been prepared via NSL, and have demonstrated a stable vortex state due to the absence of a destabilizing vortex core. Such findings should hold promise for applications in vertical magnetic random access memories [106, 107]. Albrecht *et al.* have also shown that Co/Pd multilayers on a colloid surface exhibited a pronounced magnetic anisotropy (Figure 6.24) [108].

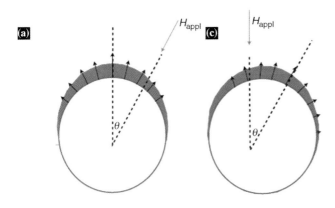

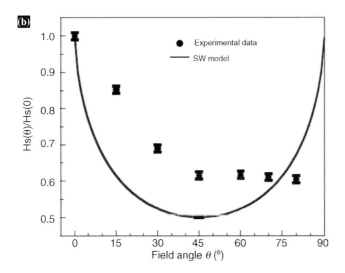

Figure 6.24 (a) Schematic of a magnetic film deposited on a nanosphere, showing the anisotropy distribution indicated by arrows; (b) Switching field as a function of applied field angle for an array with 50 nm particles (black dots). The angular dependence based on the Stoner–Wohlfarth (SW) model is shown as a solid line for comparison. The error bars are the standard deviation of the measurement; (c) The average anisotropy axis can be tuned to the required angle by changing the deposition direction. Reproduced with permission from Ref. [108].

6.6
Summary

The recent development of CL, and especially the integration of etching the colloidal mask, altering the incident angle, and the stepwise and regular changes in mask registry, have led to the creation of a powerful nanochemical patterning tool which is inexpensive (in terms of both capital and operation), has a high throughput, and can easily be adopted on various planar and curved surfaces, including microparticles. Unlike conventional mask-assisted lithographic processes, where the mask design and production tend to pose a challenge when scaling down the feature size and diversifying the feature shape, CL embodies a simple approach to masking, namely the self-assembly of monodisperse microspheres on a targeted substrate. As a consequence, the feature size may easily be shrunk below 100 nm, simply by reducing the diameter of the microspheres used, and according to a simple correlation between the interstice size and the sphere diameter. Likewise, the feature shape can be easily modified by changing the crystalline structure of a colloidal crystal mask, the time of anisotropic etching of the mask, the incident angle of the vapor beam, and the mask registry (the azimuth angle of the vapor beam). Currently, CL permits the fabrication of complicated 2-D and 3-D nanostructured features, such as multiplex nanostructures, with a clear-cut lateral and vertical heterogeneity. These several new nanostructures have proven difficult to implement by conventional lithographic techniques, and cannot be implemented in some cases. Hence, CL provides both a nanochemical and complementary tool for conventional and fully top-down lithographic techniques and, as a result, continues to show immense promise in the field of surface patterning.

Despite the great progress in colloidal crystallization, CL remains at a very early stage of development, and represents a formidable challenge for the creation of defect-free single crystals with defined crystalline faces. The presence of defects dramatically reduces the patterning precision of CL. For instance, the random orientation of polycrystalline crystalline domains in a colloidal mask is disastrous when collimating the mask registry, and in this respect the template-assisted epitaxy for colloidal crystallization shows great promise, as it allows the growth of colloidal crystals with defined packing structures and orientations. As a patterned substrate is a prerequisite for colloidal epitaxy, its applicability to patterning is limited. The ability to transfer a colloidal crystal, derived from such colloidal epitaxy, onto different substrates without causing any deterioration in crystal quality represents an important task for CL. The fabrication of large-area monolayers of periodically close-packed microspheres less than 100 nm in size is also a clear challenge that will involve reducing feature sizes to less than 10 nm, via the process of CL. Unfortunately, in a CL patterning process the feature size and interspace size between features cannot be separately manipulated, since both are directly proportional to the sphere size in a colloidal mask, and this greatly limits the patterning capabilities of CL.

Acknowledgments

D.W. was supported financially by the Max Planck Society, and in part by a DFG grant (WA 1704/4-1) and an EU-FP6 grant (BONSAI, LSHB-CT-2006-037639). G.Z. thanks the NSFC (No. 50703015) and MOST (No. 2007CB936402) for financial support. The authors also thank Dr. W. Li for his role in the preparation of the chapter, and Prof. G. Schmid for his organization of the present themed monograph with Wiley.

References

1 Wang, D. and Möhwald, H. (2004) Template-directed colloidal self-assembly – the route to 'top-down' nanochemical engineering. *J. Mater. Chem.*, **14**, 459–468.

2 Xia, Y., Gates, B., Yin, Y., and Lu, Y. (2000) Monodisperse colloidal particles: old materials with new applications. *Adv. Mater.*, **12**, 693–713.

3 Leunissen, M.E., Christova, C.G., Hynninen, A.-P., Royall, C.P., Campbell, A.I., Imhof, A., Dijkstra, M., van Roij, R., and van Blaaderen, A. (2005) Ionic colloidal crystals of oppositely charged particles. *Nature*, **437**, 235–240.

4 Mayoral, R., Requena, J., Moya, J.S., López, C., Cintas, A., Miguez, H., Meseguer, F., Vazquez, L., Holgado, M., and Blanco, A. (1997) 3D long-range ordering in and SiO$_2$ submicrometer-sphere sintered superstructure. *Adv. Mater.*, **9**, 257–260.

5 Miguez, H., Meseguer, F., López, C., Mifsud, A., Moya, J.S., and Vazquez, L. (1997) Evidence of FCC crystallization of SiO$_2$ nanospheres. *Langmuir*, **13**, 6009–6011.

6 Miguez, H., López, C., Meseguer, F., Blanco, A., Vazquez, L., Mayoral, R., Ocaña, M., Fornes, V., and Mifsud, A. (1997) Photonic crystal properties of packed submicrometric SiO$_2$. *Appl. Phys. Lett.*, **71**, 1148–1150.

7 Denkov, N.D., Velev, O.D., Kralchevsky, P.A., Invanov, I.B., Yoshimura, H., and Nagayama, K. (1992) Mechanism of formation of 2D crystals from latex-particles on substrates. *Langmuir*, **8**, 3183–3190.

8 Micheletto, R., Fukuda, H., and Ohtsu, M. (1995) A simple method for the production of a 2D ordered array of small latex-particles. *Langmuir*, **11**, 3333–3336.

9 Dimitrov, A.S. and Nagayama, K. (1996) Continuous convective assembling of fine particles into 2D arrays on solid surfaces. *Langmuir*, **12**, 1303–1311.

10 Jiang, P., Bertone, J.F., Hwang, K.S., and Colvin, V.L. (1999) Single-crystal colloidal multilayers of controlled thickness. *Chem. Mater.*, **11**, 2132–2140.

11 Gu, Z.-Z., Fujishima, A., and Sato, O. (2002) Fabrication of high-quality opal films with controllable thickness. *Chem. Mater.*, **14**, 760–765.

12 Zhou, Z. and Zhao, X.S. (2004) Flow-controlled vertical deposition method for the fabrication of photonic crystals. *Langmuir*, **20**, 1524–1526.

13 Wong, S., Kitaev, V., and Ozin, G.A. (2003) Colloidal crystals films: advances in universality and perfection. *J. Am. Chem. Soc.*, **125**, 15589–15598.

14 Chen, X., Chen, Z., Fu, N., Lu, G., and Yang, B. (2003) Versatile nanopatterned surfaces generated via 3D colloidal crystals. *Adv. Mater.*, **15**, 1413–1417.

15 Chung, Y.W., Leu, I.C., Lee, J.H., and Hon, M.H. (2006) Influence of humidity on the fabrication of high-quality colloidal crystals via a capillary-enhanced process. *Langmuir*, **22**, 6454–6460.

16 Kim, M.H., Im, S.H., and Park, O.O. (2005) Rapid fabrication of two- and three-dimensional colloidal crystal films via confined convective assembly. *Adv. Funct. Mater.*, **15**, 1329–1335.

17 Cheng, Z., Russel, W.B., and Chaikin, P.M. (1999) Controlled growth of hard-sphere colloidal crystals. *Nature*, **401**, 893–895.

18 Im, S.H., Kim, M.H., and Park, O.O. (2003) Thickness control of colloidal crystals with a substrate dipped at a tilted angle into a colloidal suspension. *Chem. Mater.*, **15**, 1797–1802.

19 Kitaev, V. and Ozin, G.A. (2003) Self-assembled surface patterns of binary colloidal crystals. *Adv. Mater.*, **15**, 75–78.

20 Velikov, K.P., Christova, C.G., Dullens, R.P.A., and van Blaaderen, A. (2002) Layer-by-layer growth of binary colloidal crystals. *Science*, **296**, 106–109.

21 Kim, M.H., Im, S.H., and Park, O.O. (2005) Fabrication and structural analysis of binary colloidal crystals with 2D superlattices. *Adv. Mater.*, **17**, 2501–2505.

22 Fischer, U.C. and Zingsheim, H.P. (1981) Submicroscopic pattern replication with visible light. *J. Vac. Sci. Technol.*, **19**, 881–885.

23 Hulteen, J.C. and van Duyne, R.P. (1995) Nanosphere lithography-a materials general fabrication process for periodic particle array surfaces. *J. Vac. Sci. Technol. A.*, **13**, 1553–1558.

24 Rehg, T.J. and Higgins, B.G. (1992) Spin coating of colloidal suspensions. *AIChE*, **38**, 489–501.

25 Jiang, P. and McFarland, M.J. (2004) Large-scale fabrication of wafer-size colloidal crystals, macroporous polymers and nanocomposites by spin-coating. *J. Am. Chem. Soc.*, **126**, 13778–13786.

26 Jiang, P. and McFarland, M.J. (2005) Wafer-scale periodic nanoholes arrays templated from 2D non-close-packed colloidal crystals. *J. Am. Chem. Soc.*, **127**, 3710–3711.

27 Wang, D. and Möhwald, H. (2004) Rapid fabrication of binary colloidal crystals by stepwise spin-coating. *Adv. Mater.*, **16**, 244–247.

28 Ulman, A. (1991) *An Introduction to Ultrathin Organic Films: FROM LANGMUIR-Blodgett to Self-Assembly*, Academic Press, Boston.

29 Binks, B.P. (2002) Particles as surfactants-similarities and differences. *Curr. Opin. Colloid Interface Sci.*, **7**, 21–41.

30 Pieranski, P. (1980) Two dimensional interfacial colloidal crystals. *Phys. Rev. Lett.*, **45**, 569–572.

31 Im, S.H., Lim, Y.T., Suh, D.J., and Park, O.O. (2002) 3D self-assembly of colloids at a water-air interface: A novel technique for the fabrication of photonic bandgap crystals. *Adv. Mater.*, **14**, 1367–1369.

32 Kondo, M., Shinozaki, K., Bergström, I., and Mizutani, N. (1995) Preparation of colloidal monolayers of alkoxylated silica particles at the air-liquid interface. *Langmuir*, **11**, 394–397.

33 Fulda, K.-U. and Tieke, B. (1994) Langmuir films of monodisperse 0.5 μm spherical polymer particles with a hydrophobic core and a hydrophilic shell. *Adv. Mater.*, **6**, 288–290.

34 van Duffel, B., Ras, R.H.A., De Schryver, F.C., and Schoonheydt, R.A. (2001) Langmuir-Blodgett deposition and optical diffraction of two dimensional opal. *J. Mater. Chem.*, **11**, 3333–3336.

35 Reculusa, S. and Ravaine, S. (2003) Synthesis of colloidal crystals of controllable thickness through the Langmuir-Blodgett technique. *Chem. Mater.*, **15**, 598–605.

36 Goldenberg, L.M., Wagner, J., Stumpe, J., Paulke, B.-R., and Grnitz, E. (2002) Simple method for the preparation of colloidal particle monolayers at the water/alkane interface. *Langmuir*, **18**, 5627–5629.

37 Reynaert, S., Moldenaers, P., and Vermant, J. (2006) Control over colloidal aggregation in monolayers of latex particles at the oil-water interface. *Langmuir*, **22**, 4936–4945.

38 Velikov, K.P., Durst, F., and Velev, O.D. (1998) Direct observation of the dynamics of latex particles confined inside thinning water-air films. *Langmuir*, **14**, 1148–1155.

39 Gu, Z.-Z., Wang, D., and Möhwald, H. (2007) Self-assembly of microspheres at the air/water/air interface into free-standing colloidal crystal films. *Soft Matter*, **3**, 68–70.

40 Griesebock, B., Egen, M., and Zental, R. (2002) Large photonic films by crystallization on fluid substrates. *Chem. Mater.*, **14**, 4023–4025.

41 Hanarp, P., Kall, M., and Sutherland, D.S. (2003) Optical properties of short range ordered arrays of nanometer gold disks prepared by colloidal lithography. *J. Phys. Chem. B*, **107**, 5768–5772.

42 Kosiorek, A., Kandulski, W., Glaczynska, H., and Giersig, M. (2005) Fabrication of nanoscale rings, dots, and rods by combining shadow nanosphere lithography and annealed polystyrene nanosphere masks. *Small*, **1**, 439–444.

43 Moon, J.H., Kim, W.-S., Ha, J.-W., Jang, S.G., Yang, S.-M., and Park, J.K. (2005) Colloidal lithography with crosslinkable particles: Fabrication of hierarchical nanopore arrays. *Chem. Commun.*, 4107–4109.

44 Peninkhof, J.J., Graf, C., van Dillen, T., Vredenberg, A.M., van Blaaderen, A., and Polman, A. (2005) Angle-dependent extinction of anisotropic silica/Au core/shell colloids made via ion irradiation. *Adv. Mater.*, **17**, 1484–1488.

45 Vossen, D.L.J., Fific, D., Penninkhof, J., Van Dillen, T., Polman, A., and Van Blaaderen, A. (2005) Combined optical tweezers/ion beam technique to tune colloidal masks for nanolithography. *Nano Lett.*, **5**, 1175–1179.

46 Deckmann, H.W. and Dunsmuir, J.H. (1983) Applications of surface textures produced with natural lithography. *J. Vac. Sci. Technol. B*, **1**, 1109–1112.

47 Choi, D.-G., Yu, H.K., Jang, S.G., and Yang, S.-M. (2004) Colloidal lithographic nanopatterning via reactive ion etching. *J. Am. Chem. Soc.*, **126**, 7019–7025.

48 Yang, S.-M., Jang, S.G., Choi, D.-G., Kim, S., and Yu, H.K. (2006) Nanomachining by colloidal lithography. *Small*, **2**, 458–475.

49 Choi, D.-G., Jang, S.G., Kim, S., Lee, E., Han, C.-S., and Yang, S.-M. (2006) Multifaceted and nanobored particle arrays sculpted using colloidal lithography. *Adv. Funct. Mater.*, **16**, 33–40.

50 Zheng, Y., Wang, Y., Wang, S., and Huan, C.H.A. (2006) Fabrication of nonspherical colloidal particles via reactive ion etching of surface-patterned colloidal crystals. *Colloids Surf. A*, **277**, 27–36.

51 Cheung, C.L., Nikolić, R.J., Reinhardt, C.E., and Wang, T.F. (2006) Fabrication of nanopillars by nanosphere lithography. *Nanotechnology*, **17**, 1339–1343.

52 Tan, B.J.-Y., Sow, C.-H., Lim, K.-Y., Cheong, F.-C., Chong, G.-L., Wee, A.T.-S., and Ong, C.-K. (2004) Fabrication of a two-dimensional periodic non-close-packed array of polystyrene particles. *J. Phys. Chem. B*, **108**, 18575–18579.

53 Valsesia, A., Colpo, P., Silvan, M.M., Meziani, T., Ceccone, G., and Rossi, F. (2004) Fabrication of nanostructured polymeric surfaces for biosensing devices. *Nano Lett.*, **4**, 1047–1050.

54 Wang, B., Zhao, W., Chen, A., and Chua, S.-J. (2006) Formation of nanoimprinting mould through use of nanosphere lithography. *J. Crystal Growth*, **288**, 200–204.

55 Huang, Z., Fang, H., and Zhu, J. (2007) Fabrication of silicon nanowire arrays with controlled diameter, length, and density. *Adv. Mater.*, **19**, 744–748.

56 Tan, B.J.Y., Sow, C.H., Koh, T.S., Chin, K.C., Wee, A.T.S., and Ong, C.K. (2005) Fabrication of size-tunable gold nanoparticles array with nanosphere lithography, reactive ion etching, and thermal annealing. *J. Phys. Chem. B*, **109**, 11100–11109.

57 McLellan, J.M., Geissler, M., and Xia, Y. (2004) Edge spreading lithography and its application to the fabrication of mesoscopic gold and silver rings. *J. Am. Chem. Soc.*, **126**, 10830–10831.

58 Geissler, M., McLellan, J.M., Chen, J., and Xia, Y. (2005) Side-by-side patterning of multiple alkanethiolate monolayers on gold by edge-spreading lithography. *Angew. Chem., Int. Ed.*, **44**, 3596–3600.

59 Bae, C., Shin, H., Moon, J., and Sung, M.M. (2006) Contact area lithography (CAL): A new approach to direct formation of nanometric chemical patterns. *Chem. Mater.*, **18**, 1085–1088.

60 Bae, C., Moon, J., Shin, H., Kim, J., and Sung, M.M. (2007) Fabrication of monodisperse asymmetric colloidal clusters by using contact area lithography (CAL). *J. Am. Chem. Soc.*, **129**, 14232–14239.

61 Deckmann, H.W. and Dunsmuir, J.H. (1982) Natural lithography. *Appl. Phys. Lett.*, **41**, 377–379.

62 Hulteen, J.C., Treichel, D.A., Smith, M.T., Duval, M.L. Jensen, T.R., and Van Duyene, R.P. (1999) Nanosphere lithography: size-tunable silver nanoparticle and surface cluster arrays. *J. Phys. Chem. B*, **103**, 3854–3863.

63 Haynes, C.L. and Van Duyne, R.P. (2001) Nanosphere lithography: A versatile nanofabrication tool for studies of size-dependent nanoparticle optics. *J. Phys. Chem. B*, **105**, 5599–5611.

64 Haynes, C.L., McFarland, A.D., Smith, M.T., Hulteen, J.C., and Van Duyne, R.P. (2002) Angle-resolved nanosphere lithography: Manipulation of nanoparticle size, shape, and interparticle spacing. *J. Phys. Chem. B*, **106**, 1898–1902.

65 Willets, A. and Van Duyne, R.P. (2007) Localized surface plasmon resonance spectroscopy and tension. *Annu. Rev. Phys. Chem.*, **58**, 267–297.

66 Giersig, M. and Hilgendorff, M. (2005) Magnetic nanoparticle superstructures. *Eur. J. Inorg. Chem.*, 3571–3583.

67 Kosiorek, A., Kandulski, W., Chudzinski, P., Kempa, K., and Giersig, M. (2004) Shadow nanosphere lithography: Simulation and experiment. *Nano Lett.*, **4**, 1359–1363.

68 Zhang, G. and Wang, D. (2008) Fabrication of heterogeneous binary arrays of nanoparticles via colloidal lithography. *J. Am. Chem. Soc.*, **130**, 5616–5617.

69 Weekes, S.M. and Ogrin, F.Y. (2005) Torque studies of large-area Co arrays fabricated by etched nanosphere lithography. *J. Appl. Phys.*, **97** (10), J503.

70 Choi, D.-G., Kim, S., Jang, S.G., Yang, S.-M., Jeong, J.-R., and Shin, S.-C. (2004) Nanopatterned magnetic metal via colloidal lithography with reactive ion etching. *Chem. Mater.*, **16**, 4208–4211.

71 Zhang, G., Wang, D., and Möhwald, H. (2007) Fabrication of multiplex quasi-three-dimensional grids of one-dimensional nanostructures via stepwise colloidal lithography. *Nano Lett.*, **7**, 3410–3413.

72 Zhang, G., Wang, D., and Möhwald, H. (2007) Ordered binary arrays of Au nanoparticles derived from colloidal lithography. *Nano Lett.*, **7**, 127–132.

73 Habenicht, A., Olapinski, M., Burmeister, F., Leiderer, P., and Boneberg, J. (2005) Jumping nanodroplets. *Science*, **309**, 2043–2045.

74 Fredriksson, H., Alaverdyan, Y., Dmitriev, A., Langhammer, C., Sutherland, D.S., Zäch, M., and Kasemo, B. (2007) Hole-mask colloidal lithography. *Adv. Mater.*, **19**, 4297–4302.

75 Edwards, E.W., Wang, D., and Möhwald, H. (2007) Hierarchical organization of colloidal particles: from colloidal crystallization to supraparticle chemistry. *Macromol. Chem. Phys.*, **208**, 439–445.

76 Zhang, H., Edwards, E.W., Wang, D., and Möhwald, H. (2006) Directing the self-assembly of nanocrystals beyond colloidal crystallization. *Phys. Chem. Chem. Phys.*, **8**, 3288–3299.

77 Glotzer, S.C. and Solomon, M.J. (2007) Anisotropy of building blocks and their assembly into complex structures. *Nat. Mater.*, **6**, 557–562.

78 Fujimoto, K., Nakahama, K., Shidara, M., and Kawaguchi, H. (1999) Preparation of unsymmetrical microspheres at the interfaces. *Langmuir*, **15**, 4630–4635.

79 Lu, Y., Xiong, H., Jiang, X., Xia, Y., Prentiss, M., and Whitesides, G.M. (2003) Asymmetric dimers can be formed by dewetting half-shells of gold deposited on the surfaces of spherical oxide colloids. *J. Am. Chem. Soc.*, **125**, 12724–12725.

80 Bao, Z., Chen, L., Weldon, M., Chandross, E., Cherniavskaya, O., Dai, Y., and Tok, J. (2002) Toward controllable self-assembly of microstructures: Selective functionalization and fabrication of patterned spheres. *Chem. Mater.*, **14**, 24–26.

81 Perro, A., Reculusa, S., Ravaine, S., Bourgeat-Lami, E., and Duguet, E. (2005) Design and synthesis of Janus micro- and nanoparticles. *J. Mater. Chem.*, **15**, 3745–3760.

82 Hong, L., Cacciuto, A., Luijten, E., and Granick, S. (2006) Clusters of charged Janus spheres. *Nano Lett.*, **6**, 2510–2514.

83 Zhang, G., Wang, D., and Möhwald, H. (2005) Patterning microsphere surfaces by templating colloidal crystals. *Nano Lett.*, **5**, 143–146.

84 Zhang, G., Wang, D., and Möhwald, H. (2006) Nanoembossment of Au patterns on microspheres. *Chem. Mater.*, **18**, 3985–3992.

85 Pawar, A.B. and Kretzschmar, I. (2008) Patchy particles by glancing angle deposition. *Langmuir*, **24**, 355–358.

86 Zhang, G., Wang, D., and Möhwald, H. (2005) Decoration of microspheres with gold nanodots—giving colloidal spheres valences. *Angew. Chem., Int. Ed.*, **44**, 7767–7770.

87 Nelson, D.R. (2002) Toward a tetravalent chemistry of colloids. *Nano Lett.*, **2**, 1125–1129.

88 Pacifico, J., Gómez, D., and Mulvaney, P. (2005) A simple route to tunable two-dimensional arrays of quantum dots. *Adv. Mater.*, **17**, 415–418.

89 Pacifico, J., Jasieniak, J., Gómez, D.E., and Mulvaney, P. (2006) Tunable D-3 arrays of quantum dots: Synthesis and luminescence properties. *Small*, **2**, 199–203.

90 Sutherland, D.S., Broberg, M., Nygren, H., and Kasemo, B. (2001) Influence of nanoscale surface topography and chemistry on the functional behaviour of an adsorbed model macromolecule. *Macromol. Biosci.*, **1**, 270–273.

91 Kuo, C.-W., Shiu, J.-Y., and Chen, P. (2003) Size- and shape-controlled fabrication of large-area periodic nanopillar arrays. *Chem. Mater.*, **15**, 2917–2920.

92 Kuo, C.-W., Shiu, J.-Y., Cho, Y.-H., and Chen, P. (2003) Fabrication of large-area periodic nanopillar arrays for nanoimprint lithography using polymer colloid masks. *Adv. Mater.*, **15**, 1065–1068.

93 Weekes, S.M., Ogrin, F.Y., and Murray, W.A. (2004) Fabrication of large-area ferromagnetic arrays using etched nanosphere lithography. *Langmuir*, **20**, 11208–11212.

94 Han, S., Hao, Z., Wang, J., and Luo, Y. (2005) Controllable two-dimensional photonic crystal patterns fabricated by nanosphere lithography. *J. Vac. Sci. Technol. B*, **23**, 1585–1588.

95 Ryu, K., Badmaev, A., Gomez, L., Ishikawa, F., Lei, B., and Zhou, C. (2007) Synthesis of aligned single-walled nanotubes using catalysts defined by nanosphere lithography. *J. Am. Chem. Soc.*, **129**, 10104–10105.

96 Park, K.H., Lee, S., Koh, K.H., Lacerda, R., Teo, K.B.K., and Milne, W.I. (2005) Advanced nanosphere lithography for the areal-density variation of periodic arrays of vertically aligned carbon nanofibers. *J. Appl. Phys.*, **97**, 024311.

97 Wang, X., Summers, C.J., and Wang, Z.L. (2004) Large-scale hexagonal-patterned growth of aligned ZnO nanorods for nano-optoelectronics and nanosensor arrays. *Nano Lett.*, **4**, 423–426.

98 Fuhrmann, B., Leipner, H.S., Höche, H.-R., Schubert, L., Werner, P., and Gösele, U. (2005) Ordered arrays of silicon nanowires produced by nanosphere lithography and molecular beam epitaxy. *Nano Lett.*, **5**, 2524–2537.

99 Veinot, J.G.C., Yan, H., Smith, S.M., Cui, J., Huang, Q., and Marks, T.J. (2002) Fabrication and properties of organic light-emitting "nanodiode" arrays. *Nano Lett.*, **2**, 333–335.

100 Aizpurua, J., Hanarp, P., Sutherland, D.S., Kall, M., Bryant, G.W., and Garcia de Abajo, F.J. (2003) Optical properties of gold nanorings. *Phys. Rev. Lett.*, **90**, 057401.

101 Hanarp, P., Kall, M., and Sutherland, D.S. (2003) Optical properties of short range ordered arrays of nanometer gold disks prepared by colloidal lithography. *J. Phys. Chem. B*, **107**, 5768–5772.

102 Lamprecht, B., Schider, G., Lechner, R.T., Ditlbacher, H., Krenn, J.R., Leitner, A., and Aussenegg, F.R. (2000) Metal nanoparticle gratings: Influence of dipolar particle interaction on the plasmon resonance. *Phys. Rev. Lett.*, **84**, 4721–4724.

103 Liu, J., Maaroof, A.I., Wieczorek, L., and Cortie, M.B. (2005) Fabrication of hollow metal "nanocaps" and their red-shifted optical absorption spectra. *Adv. Mater.*, **17**, 1276–1281.

104 Lu, Y., Liu, G.L., Kim, J., Mejia, Y.X., and Lee, L.P. (2005) Nanophotonic crescent moon structures with sharp edge for ultrasensitive biomolecular detection by local electromagnetic field enhancement effect. *Nano Lett.*, **5**, 119–124.

105 Moser, A., Takano, K., Margulis, D.T., Albrecht, M., Sonobe, Y., Ikeda, Y., Sun, S., and Fullerton, E.E. (2002) Magnetic recording: advancing into the future. *J. Phys. D*, **35**, R157–167.

106 Zhu, J., Zheng, Y., and Prinz, G.A. (2000) Ultrahigh density vertical magnetoresistive random access memory. *J. Appl. Phys.*, **87**, 6668–6673.

107 Zhu, F., Fan, D., Zhu, X., Zhu, J.-G., Cammarata, R.C., and Chien, C.-L. (2004) Ultrahigh-density arrays of ferromagnetic nanorings on macroscopic areas. *Adv. Mater.*, **16**, 2155–2159.

108 Albrecht, M., Hu, G., Guhr, I.L., Ulbrich, T.C., Boneberg, J., Leiderer, P., and Schatz, G. (2005) Magnetic multilayers on nanospheres. *Nat. Mater.*, **4**, 203–206.

7
Diblock Copolymer Micelle Nanolithography: Characteristics and Applications

Theobald Lohmueller and Joachim P. Spatz

7.1
Introduction

Materials at the nanoscale show remarkable physical and chemical properties as a consequence of their small size, and this makes them useful for a wide range of conceivable new applications and technologies [1]. In 1959, Richard P. Feynman announced the issue for the future of "...manipulating and controlling things on a small scale" [2]. Since that time, nanotechnology has indeed evolved to become an important topic with enormous scientific and industrial interest [3], and this has resulted in increasing progress in terms of the development of novel micro- and optoelectronic components, with a subsequent high impact on everyday life. The most famous, yet impressive, example of this rapid evolution was expressed by Moore's law, which stated that the number of components per integrated circuit on a microprocessor would double approximately every two years [4]. Although dating back to the 1970s and aimed at predicting the increase of processing power and data storage capacity in computer technology, this forecast remains valid today, and greatly emphasizes the current vitality of this field of research. Today, nanotechnology enfolds a broad interdisciplinary area in the applied sciences, and is used for the investigation of various fundamental questions in physics, chemistry, and biology [1,3,5].

Two strategies for nanofabrication can be identified, namely "top-down" and "bottom-up":

- Top-down methods comprise photo- [6, 7], X-ray [8, 9], as well as electron (e-beam) [10] and focused ion beam (FIB) [11, 12] lithography, where nanostructured surfaces are generated either by exposing a sensitive material to UV-light or X-ray radiation, or by "writing" a nanopattern with a focused beam of electrons or ions [13]. For patterning, a sample is covered with a photosensitive resist and illuminated through a mask, in close proximity to the substrate. The final structure is developed by subsequent treatment of the substrate with a selective solvent or etching agent; this enables surface patterning with high resolution, depending on the wavelength of the irradiation. Consequently,

Nanotechnology, Volume 8: Nanostructured Surfaces. Edited by Lifeng Chi
Copyright © 2010 WILEY-VCH Verlag GmbH & Co. KGaA, Weinheim
ISBN: 978-3-527-31739-4

photolithography is currently the most widely used technology in the semi-conductor industry where, by using state-of-the-art systems with deep-ultraviolet (DUV) excimer lasers (e.g., ArF: 193 nm) it is possible to pattern structures smaller than 50 nm [14, 15]. No mask is needed in the case of e-beam and FIB lithography, since the pattern is generated directly by a focused beam of electrons and ions, rather than by irradiating the whole sample at once. Although, when using these methods it is possible to achieve resolutions down to only a few nanometers, because they represent a serial process they have the main disadvantages of low processing rates and the need for expensive equipment.

- Bottom-up approaches are the competing concept for nanofabrication, with the idea of the self-organization of small components into larger materials and devices, without any external intervention [16–18]. As a concept for the materials sciences, self-assembly based methods are particularly attractive as they represent an inexpensive and widely applicable fabrication technology, with possible resolution down to a single nanometer. Several strategies have been developed and shown to be capable for patterning of materials at the nanoscale; these include self-assembled monolayers (SAMs) [19, 20], block copolymer lithography [21–23], and colloidal lithography [24, 25], all of which provide cheap and fast processing technologies that produce nanometer-scale resolution. Whilst the applicability of the bottom-up methods is limited by a greater demand on the complexity of the nanopattern, strategies to overcome these drawbacks include placing the molecules directly into an aperiodic topology, as is the case for microcontact printing (μCP) [18, 26, 27] and dip-pen lithography (DPN) [28, 29]. Here, the desired molecules are used as an "ink" which can either be layered (in DPN) or stamped (in μCP) on top of a solid-state substrate. The SAM itself can then be used as a lithographic resist for further modification. Examples of this approach include chemical lithography and scanning probe lithography-based technologies, such as nanografting [30, 31] and near-field scanning optical lithography (NSOM) [32].

The aim of this chapter is to introduce block copolymer micelle nanolithography (BCML) as a versatile bottom-up approach, to generate extended arrays of metallic nanoparticles, and to provide some examples of its related applications [33, 34]. Block copolymers are compounds of separate polymer chains (or blocks respectively), where each block is built up from individual types of monomer. In the case of diblock copolymers, for instance, one molecule contains two polymer chains (or blocks), which are linked by a covalent bond. For entropic reasons, the two blocks do not mix in solution, and thus show a strong tendency to segregate into microphase-separated morphologies, depending on the molecular weight, the segment sizes, and the strength of the molecular interactions between the respective blocks [35, 36]. How structural parameters such as the lateral particle spacing and particle size can be controlled on the substrate, with single-nanometer precision, will be examined in the following subsections. Two intriguing examples will also be provided of how these nanoparticle patterns can be used to mimic materials found in nature, such as the antireflective corneal lens of moths, and artificial extracellular interfaces in the study of cell adhesion.

7.2
Block Copolymer Micelle Nanolithography

7.2.1
Introduction

The underlying principle of BCML relates to the spontaneous formation of amphiphilic block-copolymers to from microphase-separated morphologies [35], and the transfer of these units into nanometer-scale patterns on top of rigid substrates such as silicon wafers or glass coverslips. When diblock copolymers of polystyrene (PS) and polyvinylpyridine (PVP) chains are dissolved in toluene at low concentration, they are present in the form of single chains. However, above their critical micelle concentration (CMC), these molecules begin to segregate while the number of individual free chains in solution remains constant [37–39]. As toluene is a more selective solvent towards PS, the PS block will form the outer micellar shell, surrounding the less-soluble PVP block which builds up the core [40]. This core–shell configuration can be considered as a nanoscopic reactor that allows the selective dissolution of metal precursor salts into the micelle [41]. The distribution of precursor salt per micelle varies only within narrow limits [42], and the incorporation of metal salts into the micellar core has certain effects on the micellar stability of the micelles in solution, compared to the neutral case. Due to increasing interactions between the different copolymer blocks, the CMC shifts towards lower concentrations [43, 44]. The amount of metal salt inside each micelle is adjustable, depending on the ratio of the neutralized number of vinylpyridine versus the total number of vinylpyridine units:

$$m_{metal} = \frac{m_{PS-P_2VP} M_{metal} [VP]_n L}{M_{PS-P_2VP}}$$

where L depicts the loading ratio $L = n(\text{HAuCl}_4)/n(\text{PS-PVP})$ and $1 \geq L \geq 0$. A nanopattern is formed by either spin-coating or dipping a rigid substrate into the polymer solution. Dip-coating is more favorable as it enables a uniform decoration of plain as well as curved substrates over a total area of up to several square centimeters, within a short period of time, and with high accuracy. During substrate retraction, the micelles assemble into a quasi-hexagonal ordered monolayer on top of the surface, the driving force for which process is the evaporation of solvent at the immersion edge. Subsequent plasma treatment can then be applied to remove the whole polymer matrix and to induce the formation of pure metal particles on the surface of the substrate. A schematic overview of the process, together with relevant scanning electron microscopy (SEM) images of the different nanoparticle arrays, are shown in Figure 7.1.

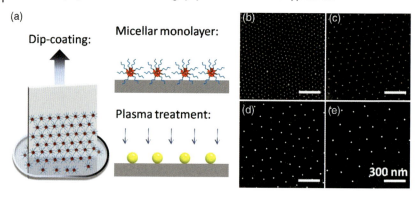

Figure 7.1 Schematic description of the dip-coating process. (a) Diblock copolymer micelles self-assemble into a hexagonal-ordered film when a rigid substrate is dragged out of the toluene solution. Gold nanoparticles are generated by subsequent plasma treatment of the substrate. The distance between individual particles on top of the substrate is a result of the diameter of the micelles, the concentration of the micelle solution, and the dipping velocity. Examples of gold nanoparticle pattern with different spacing: (b) 50 nm; (c) 100 nm; (d) 150 nm; (e) 200 nm.

The particles formed from one polymer solution during the process are all of similar size and shape, and aligned hexagonally on the surface (Figure 7.1b-e). The only major requirement arising from the fabrication process is that the substrate must be resistant against the solvent, and stable during the plasma process. The technique thus offers a great applicability, and has been successfully applied to pattern different materials such as glass, silicon, diamond, sapphire, $SrTiO_3$, and mica, with various different particle compositions. A literature overview dealing with the concept of BCML is provided in Table 7.1.

Table 7.1 A literature overview of block copolymer micelle nanolithography.

Parameter	Component/technique	Reference(s)
Metallic NP	• Au, Pt, Pd	[33, 45, 107]
	• TiO_2	[108]
	• Fe_xPt_y	[109]
Particle size	• Intramicellar electroless deposition	[107]
Particle spacing	• Concentration and velocity dependence	[34, 61, 62]
	• Spacing gradients	[63]
Lateral order		[110–112]
Micro- nanopatterning	• E-beam lithography	[71, 72]
	• Photoresist e-beam; Photolithography	[70, 74]
	• FIB	[73]
	• Micro-contact printing	[113]
Transfer lithography	• PDMS, Polystyrene, PEGDA 700	[106]

The great flexibility of BCML makes it an ideal tool for nanopatterning, with the advantage of high-throughput sample processing but only a minimal need for highly technical (and expensive) equipment [45]. A more detailed description as to how nanoparticle patterns can be characterized, and how experimental parameters such as the lateral order, the interparticle distance, and nanoparticle spacing can be controlled in a large frame, are outlined in the following subsections. A brief overview is also provided on the synthesis of micro-nanopatterned surfaces, using a combination of BCML and conventional top-down lithography.

7.2.2
Characterization on Nanoparticle Arrays

7.2.2.1 Scanning Electron Microscopy (SEM)
Scanning electron microscopy (SEM) represents a powerful tool for sample imaging with nanoscale spatial resolution [46]. During such measurements, the surface of a conductive sample is imaged by scanning the surface topology with a focused electron beam. Nonconductive substrates such as glass or polymeric materials must be covered with a metal or carbon layer prior measurements. Although state-of-the-art SEM systems show a resolution power of less than 1 nm, the theoretical limit is impaired by aberrations of the electron lenses and the interaction volume of the electron beam with the substrate material. Atomic-level resolution can be achieved by using transmission electron microscopy (TEM), in which case the detector is located beneath the sample, such that those electrons transmitted *through* the sample are analyzed. Hence, very thin sample materials are required for these measurements. Consequently, although TEM imaging is currently recognized as the most accurate method for characterizing the size and shape of individual particles, even with atomic resolution, is not practical consider nanoparticle arrays fabricated on large area samples such as glass coverslips or whole silica wafers. Several types of signal are generated by interactions between the electron beam and the probe material, and this provides both topographic and chemical information concerning the sample. The most important of these signals are secondary electrons (SEs), back-scattered electrons (BSEs) and low-energy X-rays. Whereas, secondary and back-scattered electrons provide information concerning surface morphology and material contrast, the chemical composition of the specimen can be analyzed via its characteristic X-ray emission, using energy-dispersive X-ray (EDX) spectroscopy. SEM imaging is particularly advantageous for the characterization of extended nanoparticle arrays, since it is possible to carry out rapid imaging of large areas at several positions on the sample, so as to reveal accurate information concerning the separation distances between individual particles and the particle diameter in-plane. Unfortunately, SEM images provide very little information relating to the nanoparticle height.

7.2.2.2 Atomic Force Microscopy (AFM)
Atomic force microscopy (AFM) is a high-resolution imaging technique used to measure the attractive or repulsive forces between a sharp tip brought into proximity to the surface of a sample [47]. The tips used for AFM are typically fabricated from

silicon or silicon nitride, and have a diameter of between 10 and 50 nm. The available spring constants range from 0.01 to 100 N m^{-1}, with resonant frequencies between 5 and 350 kHz.

When taking measurements, the microscope is used to mechanically scan a certain area of the sample, and is operated in either *contact mode* or *tapping mode*:

- While operating in *contact mode*, the AFM tip is actually in contact with the surface, so that any topographic features encountered will cause the tip to undergo a vertical deflection; these deflections are translated into a feedback signal that carries information about the surface. The tip deflection is monitored by following a laser spot that is reflected from the top of the cantilever, using a photodiode.
- In *tapping mode*, the cantilever oscillates close to its resonance frequency, so that it is barely touching the substrate surface. With increasing tip-to-sample proximity the oscillation amplitude and phase, as well as the resonance frequency of the cantilever are damped, and the damping movements then provide information regarding the surface morphology. Tapping mode is commonly used to measure soft samples, where friction and lateral forces should be minimized.

In general, AFM displays several advantages over SEM, the most notable being that there are virtually no limitations regarding the substrate composition. The samples do not need to be conductive, and the measurements can be performed under atmospheric conditions. The image of the sample also represents a true three-dimensional profile of the surface, with a resolution that is comparable to that of SEM. The main drawbacks of AFM are a high sensitivity to environmental noise, and a low scanning size of approximately 100 μm^2. One other problem is that a convolution of the tip size with the surface topology can create image artifacts in-plane (xy). Thus, in order to provide a complete characterization of the height and spatial orientation of a nanopatterned substrate, a combination of both AFM and SEM should ideally be utilized [48].

7.2.2.3 Spacing and Order of Nanoparticle Arrays

The lateral geometry of a nanoparticle array can be considered to be in a state between crystalline or completely random [49]. When perfectly ordered, crystalline systems are defined by the long range order of their spatial pattern. In case of a 2-D hexagonal lattice, each particle is surrounded by an infinite number of equally distributed neighbors with a constant spacing period. In contrast, a random, amorphous system does not show any long-range order, and all of the pattern features are uniformly distributed with no specific positional information. The perfect pattern geometry is usually affected by defects and deformations, notably dislocations and disclinations as a consequence of the self-assembly process. Disclinations occur if a particle is surrounded for example by five or seven instead of six nearest-neighbors, causing a dislocation of the hexagonal orientation. A model system which is used to identify the quality of a nanoparticle array from an SEM image, compares the structure with the order transition during the melting of a 2-D crystal [49, 50]. A theoretical approach to describe such 2-D melting is known as the Kosterlitz–Thouless–Halperin–Nelson–Young (KTHNY) theory [51–54], where a perfect crystalline phase is disrupted with increasing temperature until the state of complete disorder is reached. Following this model, the translational order of any symmetric lattice during the phase transitions can be described by an order parameter $\psi_{\vec{G}}(\vec{r})$ of the form [55]:

$$\psi_{\vec{G}}(\vec{r}) = \exp(i\vec{G}\vec{r})$$

where $\vec{G}$ is the reciprocal lattice vector of the hexagonal array. For both, disclinations and dislocations, the crystalline order is disrupted and $\psi_{\vec{G}}(\vec{r})$ falls to zero. However, there is a qualitative difference when considering the local-range and long-range order of a crystalline structure. Whereas dislocations cause a translational displacement that does not affect the local hexatic orientation, both translational and long-range orientational orders are impaired by disclinations. Thus, in order to quantify the bond-to-bond orientation of a whole hexagonal lattice, a complement to $\psi_{\vec{G}}(\vec{r})$, the global bond-orientational order parameter $\psi_6(\vec{r}_i)$ must be introduced:

$$\psi_6(\vec{r}_i) = \left| \frac{1}{N} \sum_j \sum_k \exp(6i\theta_{jk}) \right|$$

where θ_{ik} is the orientation angle of the connecting sides (or neighboring particles) j and k relative to ($\vec{r}_i$). The influence of dislocations and disclinations can be distinguished by their influence on $\psi_{\vec{G}}(\vec{r})$ and $\psi_6(\vec{r}_i)$. For an array of nanoparticles, ψ_6 reaches a value between one and zero:

$$0 \leq \psi_6 \leq 1$$

where ψ_6 equals 1 for a perfect hexagonal lattice, but falls to zero with increasing disorder. By calculating the sixfold global order parameter, the average nanoparticle spacing and the corresponding standard error can be derived from all individual particles from a single SEM or AFM image.

7.2.3
Tuning the Pattern Properties

7.2.3.1 Controlling the Nanoparticle Spacing
The precise adjustment of the nanoparticle spacing represents one of the most important issues to realize a broad applicability for BCML. Several experimental parameters may influence the particle separation on the surface. A rather small effect is observed by the amount of metal salt added to the solution. The diameter of the micelles is increased depending on the metal salt loading, and this results in a lowered packing density of the micellar monolayer on the substrate. As a consequence, the hydrodynamic radius of the micelles is also increased, and this is reflected by a lower packing density following transfer to the substrate [43]. The spacing can be adjusted within a few nanometers, but only at the expense of the particle size, which is generally not desirable.

The most obvious way to achieve reproducible and robust control over a distance between single particles is to alter the length of the diblock-copolymer chain, since a longer polymer will result in a bigger micelle [34, 56, 57]. A broad range of lateral

Table 7.2 Examples of spacing values for different diblock copolymer solutions.

Diblock copolymer	c (mg ml^{-1})	L	MnPS – (g mol^{-1})	MnPVP – (g mol^{-1})	Mw/Mn	Spacing (nm)	Order (△)
PS(190)-b-P$_2$VP(190)	5	0.2	19 900	21 000	1.09	28 ± 5	0.54
PS(500)-b-P$_2$VP(270)	5	0.5	52 400	28 100	1.05	58 ± 7	0.50
PS(990)-b-P$_2$VP(385)	5	0.5	103 000	40 500	1.07	73 ± 8	0.39
PS(1350)-b-P$_2$VP(400)	5	0.5	140 800	41 500	1.11	85 ± 9	0.42
PS(1824)-b-P$_2$VP(523)	3	0.5	190 000	55 000	1.10	91 ± 1	0.63
PS(990)-b-P$_2$VP(385)	3	0.5	103 000	40 500	1.07	110 ± 1	0.61
PS(1824)-b-P$_2$VP(523)	2	0.5	190 000	55 000	1.10	139 ± 2	0.71
PS(5348)-b-P$_4$VP(713)	1.5	0.2	557 000	75 000	1.07	176 ± 5	0.40
PS(5348)-b-P$_4$VP(713)	1	0.2	557 000	75 000	1.07	222 ± 7	0.50

distances can be realized by simply varying the molecular weight, as shown in Table 7.2 (the dipping velocity in each case was 12 mm min^{-1}).

For a certain micelle size, it has been shown experimentally that the separation distance between the nanoparticles is also influenced by the concentration of the polymer solution (cf. Table 7.2). Although for higher concentrations the micelles are packed more closely, interestingly the same results are observed for different velocities during the dip-coating process. This is a particularly important finding, since varying either the polymer concentration or the retraction velocity will allow the creation of a broad range of different nanoparticle densities from a single polymer solution, and thus a complete decoupling of the metal salt loading and particle size. By accelerating the velocity during retraction of the substrate, it might even be possible to generate a continuous nanoparticle gradient over the range of several tens of nanometers. The gradient slope can be adjusted between a few micrometers and several millimeters, depending on the acceleration. Consequently, nanoparticle gradients with separation distances of between 80 and 250 nm can be achieved by using only three different polymer solutions, as shown in Figure 7.2.

As depicted in the graphs of Figure 7.2, the interparticle spacing on the samples is smaller for higher retraction velocities. To explain this observation, it is necessary to consider the influence of the retraction velocity of the deposition process during dip-coating. As reported by Darhuber *et al.* [58], the height of the adsorbed film deposited during the dip-coating of a substrate perpendicular to the fluid interface depends on the retraction speed at which the sample is withdrawn from the solution. The dependency between velocity and film thickness can be expressed as [58, 59]:

$$h_\infty = 0.946 \sqrt{\frac{\sigma}{\varrho g}} Ca^{2/3}$$

where Ca denotes the capillary number $Ca = \mu U / \sigma$, and where μ, σ, and ϱ represent the solution viscosity, the surface tension, and the density of the polymer solution respectively; g denotes gravitational acceleration. This expression is only valid for

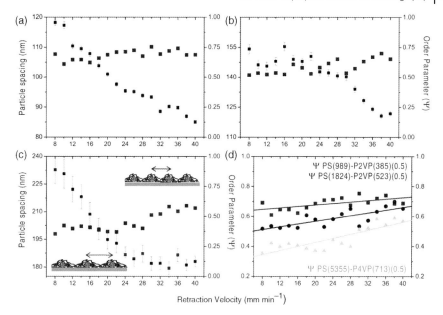

Figure 7.2 Particle spacing realized from three different diblock copolymer solutions as a function of the retraction speed. The retraction velocity is adjusted between 8 and 40 mm min^{-1} in all cases. (a) 3 mg ml^{-1} PS(990)-*b*-P2VP(385) (0.5); (b) 2 mg ml^{-1} PS(1824)-*b*-P2VP(523) (0.5); (c) 1 mg ml^{-1} PS(5348)-*b*-P4VP(713) (0.5). For high retraction velocities above 30 mm min^{-1}, an almost constant value of the interparticle distance was observed for the PS (5348)-*b*-P4VP(713)(0.5) polymer; (d) Linear fit of the corresponding order parameters for all three polymers as a function of the dipping velocity. A trend towards a higher order parameter was observed for smaller interparticle spacings.

very low capillary numbers ($Ca << 1$), which can be estimated in the present system (due to the very low capillary number for pure toluene [60, 62]. According to this equation, the film thickness h_∞ is dependent on the viscosity of the polymer solution and the dipping velocity. With increasing polymer concentration, the viscosity of the solution will therefore also increase. The optimum thickness h_∞ of the micellar film for a constant dipping velocity can thus be expressed by:

$$h_\infty \propto \frac{\mu^{2/3}}{(\varrho g)^{1/2}\sigma^{1/6}}$$

At the same time, assuming a constant number of micelles in solution for a constant polymer concentration, h_∞ is proportional to the dipping velocity U according to:

$$h_\infty \propto U^{2/3}$$

As the film thickness is proportional to the dipping velocity, the number of micelles per area is also proportional to h_∞. As the micelles are all of the same size, the maximum number on the surface will reach a saturation value for high dipping speeds, where the interparticle spacing is almost constant and the nanopattern displays the highest packing density at this point. This is shown in Figure 7.2c, where the interparticle spacing of the PS(5348) polymer is unchanged between 32 and 40 mm min^{-1}. It is important to note that the order parameter is affected depending on the separation distance and the corresponding retraction velocity, and this is especially the case for polymers with a high molecular weight. As the viscosity of the solution increases with higher polymer concentrations, both parameters will influence the dipping process in the same way.

To recapitulate, the spacing period can be controlled by three parameters: (i) the molecular weight of the diblock copolymer; (ii) the concentration of the polymer solution [61]; and (iii) the dipping velocity [61–64]. The latter two points are advantageous for the fabrication of particle arrays, as same type of diblock copolymer can be used for a certain loading parameter, and the particle size is therefore independent of the particle density. However, by neglecting the influence of the order parameter, a wide range of different interparticle spacings can be covered with a single diblock-copolymer by choosing appropriate conditions.

7.2.3.2 Controlling the Particle Size

The particle size is restricted to the amount of metal salt that can be loaded inside each micelle, and is therefore limited to a small range (typically 1–15 nm), depending on the loading ratio and the number of PVP units per micelle. In order to control the size over a wider range, the gold nanoparticles may be used as a seed for an additional growing step by "hydroxylamine seeding" [65, 66]. Here, the metal particles act as catalytic nuclei for the electroless deposition of metal ions from solution by hydroxylamine (NH$_2$OH). As the kinetics for the reduction of adsorbed metal ions exceeds the rate of reduction in solution, the nucleation of new particles is prevented and all of the ions will take part in the production of larger colloids [67, 68]. Unfortunately, this technique cannot be adapted to nanoparticulate substrates as the particles would lift off and the pattern geometry would be destroyed during the growth procedure.

The pattern geometry is preserved during the growth procedure by either: (i) embedding the nanoparticles into a SAM [69, 107]; or (ii) by using the polymer matrix as a stabilizing template [107]. A schematic overview of both strategies is shown in Figure 7.3.

In this case, the glass coverslips were patterned over the whole area below the dotted line. In the first approach, the bare glass area between the gold particles was functionalized by a monolayer of hexadecyltrimethoxysilane (HTMS) to form a stabilizing environment for the gold particles. The formation of a SAM in this system was caused by the selective silanization of the surface by forming a covalent Si$-$O$-$Si bond. The average particle height on the unmodified glass coverslip was revealed (via AFM measurements) to be 6.5 ± 0.4 nm, while the height of the particles embedded in the HTMS monolayer was 4.0 ± 0.4 nm. The difference of 2.5 ± 0.8 nm corresponded to the thickness of the monolayer, and was responsible for the lateral stabilization of the particles on the surface. The substrates were then immersed into an aqueous seeding solution of hydroxylamine and gold acid. Prior to the electroless

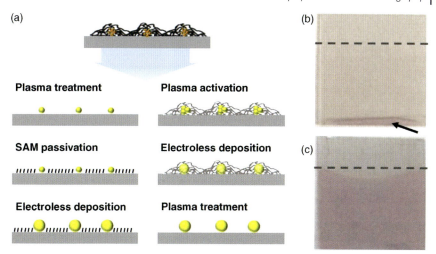

Figure 7.3 Schematic of the particle growth strategies. (a) Formation of a micellar monolayer by dip-coating. The particles are either stabilized by embedding them into a hexadecyltrimethoxysilane (HTMS) layer, or the micelles themselves act as a template at the surface to keep the particles in position; (b, c) Photographs of glass coverslips (size 20×20 mm) before (b) and after (c) particle enlargement. Both samples were decorated up to the dipping edge with nanoparticles (indicated by the dotted line). The successful reaction is made apparent by the homogeneous red color of the structured part of the substrate. For small particles, the appearance of the nanostructure is only visible at the dripping edge (arrow).

deposition process, the initial particle size of about 6 nm was too small to observe plasmon absorbance by the naked eye. The presence of gold particles, however, soon became evident by presence of a red stripe at the bottom of the dipping edge; this was an area of total disorder where multilayer formation and the agglomeration of small particles had led to a dense layer of gold clusters being formed after the plasma treatment. The course of the reaction was detectable after only a few seconds of immersion, as the patterned part of the substrate turned red due to increasing particle plasmon absorbance (Figure 7.3c), while the homogeneous red color of the sample indicated a uniform growth of the particles. Varying the metal type of the seeding solution and the interparticle distance enabled the precise preparation of highly ordered single and bimetallic core–shell nanostructures. Unfortunately, it was necessary to modify the sample by applying a stabilizing monolayer, though this was not always wanted – nor even possible – depending on the substrate chemistry. Notably, as the micellar technique was seen to be adaptive to a broad range of different substrate materials, its versatility was clearly limited.

In a second approach, the polymer shell of the micelles itself was used as a stabilizing matrix surrounding the metal core. In order to enable hydroxylamine reduction, the precursor salt inside each micelle must be reduced to generate a seed of the pure metal, and this was achieved by a short hydrogen plasma activation of the micellar films. The formation of elemental particles in the micelles occurred within

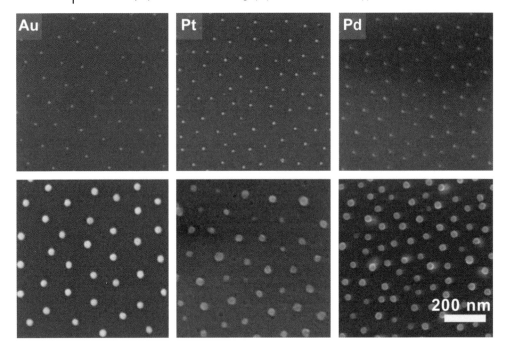

Figure 7.4 Au, Pt, Pd particles grown by intramicellar electroless deposition. Scanning electron microscopy (SEM) images of Au, Pt and Pd particles on glass coverslips before (top; 7 nm initial size) and after (bottom; 25 nm) particle growth. The initial particle size in all cases was ca. 6 nm. All particles were enlarged by intramicellar electroless deposition up to a size of ca. 25 nm, using different immersion times and conditions: Au (0.1% HAuCl$_4$/0.2 mM NH$_3$OHCl, 60 s); Pt (1% H$_2$PtCl$_6$/2 M NH$_3$OHCl, 20 h); Pd (0.1% Pd (Ac)$_2$/200 mM NH$_3$OHCl, 18 h). Adapted from Ref. [107].

the first few minutes, during which activation step some parts of the polymer matrix were etched, although the reaction time was not long enough to remove the polymer film completely [46]. The activated samples were dipped into the particular seeding solution, and the reaction then stopped by rinsing the substrates in ultrapure water. Finally, the samples were exposed to hydrogen plasma to remove the complete polymer residuals. Figure 7.4 shows the SEM images of the Au, Pt, and Pd particles arrays before (upper row) and after (lower row) the metal deposition.

The initial particle size in all cases was 6 nm, and all particles were enlarged by intra-micellar electroless deposition up to a size of 25 nm, using different immersion times and conditions. The geometry of the nanopattern was not affected by the seeding procedure. It should be noted that the experimental parameters for the electroless deposition of Au, Pt or Pd are very different. For example, the deposition time for platinum and palladium particles is much longer than for gold, and the seeding solution must be more concentrated. As a result of working with higher concentrations and longer reaction times, the size distribution of the enlarged platinum particles was less homogeneous than that of gold particles.

When comparing both strategies, the intra-micellar approach had the advantage that the enlargement step could be applied directly to the activated micellar film, which translated as a broader applicability. Particles with a diameter greater than 50 nm not only began to lift off from the surface, but also had a much more disperse size distribution. The latter effect may have been due to the polymer shell surrounding the particles and, in turn, affecting the particle size. Although the stabilization of particles by a SAM required additional modification of the substrate materials, it also allowed the controlled preparation of metal core–shell clusters.

7.2.3.3 Micro-Nanopatterned Interfaces

Besides varying the particle spacing, micro-nanopatterned morphologies represent an additional means of controlling the nanoparticle density. A combination of BCML with conventional "top down" technology enables the generation of aperiodic micro-/nanopatterned surfaces, and the directed location of nanometer-sized features. A schematic overview of these different strategies is shown in Figure 7.5.

Micro-nanopatterned interfaces may be fabricated by either a direct modification of the adsorbed micelles by irradiation with UV-light [70], with e-beam lithography [71, 72], or low-dose FIB milling [73]. In the simplest case, the monomicellar film itself can be used as a negative resist for e-beam lithography on conductive as well as nonconductive substrates. This allows the deposition of single submicron particle patches, or even single gold nanoparticles in an aperiodic pattern on conductive and nonconductive substrates. The micelles are pinned on the substrates as a result of the

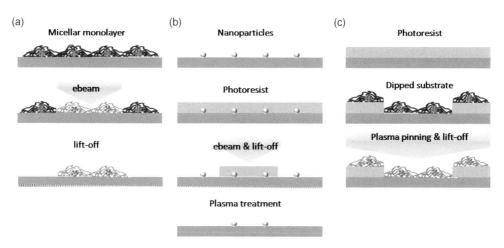

Figure 7.5 Schematic overview of different micro-nanopatterning strategies. (a) The micellar monolayer itself may be used as a resist for electron-beam lithography; (b) Alternatively, the gold nanoparticle array may be covered with a photosensitive resist; (c) By preparing nanoscopic cavities using top-down lithography, it is possible to trap individual micelles inside the prepatterned structure by dip-coating. The micro- nanopatterned substrate is generated by plasma-pinning the micelles to the surface, removal of the photoresist, and a final plasma treatment.

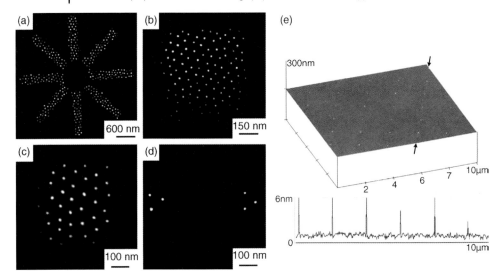

Figure 7.6 (a–d) Micro-nanopatterned particles arrays fabricated by e-beam lithography. (a) Gold nanoparticles arranged in a star pattern; (b, c) Squares patch side length of (b) ca. 600 nm and (c) ca. 200 nm side length; (d) Three single gold particles separated by ca. 400 nm; (e) By preparing separated photoresist cavities and subsequent deposition of single micelles, single particles can be precisely separated over 1 μm apart in a square pattern. Panels (a–d) adapted from Ref. [71]; Panel (e) adapted from Ref. [75].

interaction of the polymer film and the electron beam; subsequent immersion of the substrate into an organic solvent reveals the exposure pattern. The polymer shell of the tethered micelles can then be removed by a subsequent plasma process that is analogous to the normal protocol.

Whilst e-beam lithography has the advantage of high feature resolution, it suffers from the disadvantage of being a serial and time-consuming process. Nonetheless, it can be accelerated by using a combination of standard lithography and subsequent nanoparticle removal (Figure 7.5b) [74]. In this case, although the entire substrate with its gold particles is coated with a photoresist, only certain areas will be illuminated and the final pattern can be generated by removing any unmodified resist and the appropriate underlying particles. Moreover, this approach can be transferred to photolithography, which has the advantage that a large area can be patterned in one step. The major advantage with this combined method is that photolithography is capable of generating aperiodic microstructures, while the high-resolution nanopattern is generated by the micelles via a rapid and simple self-assembly process. Hence, the combination of these methods represents an intriguing approach to nanopatterning that can be conducted considerably faster and simpler than by using a conventional "top-down" approach. In a variation of this strategy, micelles can be deposited either into prestructured cavities (Figure 7.5c) or directly, using μCP [113]. The use of this approach has made possible the generation of linear and circular configurations of gold nanoparticles, and the deposition of single nanoparticles separated by several micrometers [35, 75].

7.3
Applications of Nanopatterned Materials

7.3.1
Moth Eye Antireflective Surfaces

The faceted eye of dawn-active moths is equipped with a periodic array of sub-wavelength-structured protuberances, which behaves as a gradation of the refractive index between the air/cornea interface [76]. In the experiments described here, gold nanoparticles were used as a shadow mask for the subsequent reactive ion etching (RIE) of glass coverslips and fused silica substrates, with the aim of generating a nanometer-sized surface texture similar to the biological example.

The reduction of Fresnel reflections at optical interfaces is a topic of enormous interest for a wide range of applications [77]. The performance of the projection optics of both photographic and microscopy units is greatly affected by the reflection and transmission of light at optical interfaces. In the case of semiconductors, the reflection loss of light in the visible and near-infrared spectral regions may reach 40%, due to the high refractive indices of these materials [78]. Today, state-of-the-art antireflection (AR) coatings are most frequently based on multilayer interference structures with alternating high and low refractive indices [79, 80]. Unfortunately, however, such layer systems tend to perform suboptimally in many aspects, with thin-film coatings suffering from both adhesion problems and radiation damage if the optical device is used over a broad thermal range, or in high-power laser applications. Typical light sources for DUV illumination include excimer lasers such as KrF (248 nm) and ArF (193 nm). The number of available materials with a suitable refractive index to realize broadband antireflection coatings in this spectral region is greatly limited. Whilst thin-film coatings are commonly used to reduce the reflection of optical components in the visible range, similar technologies in the DUV spectral region are difficult to implement, and extremely expensive [81]. One alternative to these multilayer films would be to use subwavelength or antireflective structured surfaces [82] which, in nature, are found on the eyes of nocturnal insects. The compound eye of an insect consists of an arrangement of identical units, the *ommatidia*, each of which represents an independent eye with its own cornea and lens to focus light on the subjacent photoreceptor cells. In the case of nocturnal moths, the surface of each cornea is equipped with a hexagonal array of cuticular protuberances. This structure was first discovered by Bernhard [83], who proposed that the function of these "nipple arrays" might be to suppress reflections from the faceted eye surface in order to avoid fatal consequences for the moth if the reflection were to be detected by a bird or any other predator. The optical properties of a "moth eye" surface can, in principle, be understood as a gradation of the refractive index between air and the corneal material [84, 85]. Some SEM images of the surface

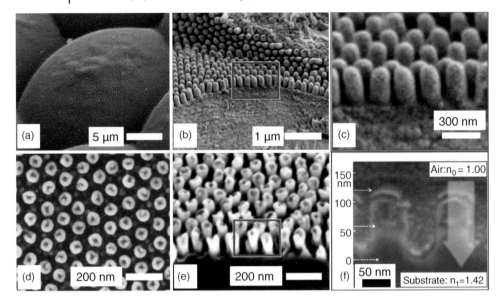

Figure 7.7 (a–c) Scanning electron microscopy (SEM) images of the surface of a genuine moth eye. The insect compound eye consists of microarrays of several thousand single lenslets. The lens of a single ommatidia is equipped with a fine array of protuberances with a structural period smaller than the wavelength of the incoming light. This special profile leads to a continuous increase of material density at the air/cornea interfaces, which results in a gradation of the refractive index; (d–f) SEM images of the "moth eye" structure on fused silica. Note: panel (c) is an enlargement of the box in panel (b); (d) Top-view SEM images of the structure displaying the quasi-hexagonal arrangement; (e) Side-view image of the pillar array measured with a tilt angle of 45°; (f) Focused ion beam (FIB) cross-section through the antireflective structure. The air/material transition is schematically implemented in the micrograph. The pillars have a diameter of 60 ± 4 nm and a lateral spacing of 114 ± 3 nm (center to center), respectively. The height of the structure was measured as 120 ± 5 nm, which corresponds to the effective thickness of the antireflective layer. A cone-type hole is etched into each pillar tip to approximately half of the pillar height. Adapted from Ref. [86].

patterns of a moth eye are shown in Figure 7.7 (details of the eyes of different butterfly species are available in Ref. [76]).

As the distance between the pillars is sufficiently small, the structure cannot be resolved by the incident light. Hence, transition between the air/material interface will appear as a continuous boundary, with the effect of a decreased reflection and improved transmittance of all light with a wavelength larger than the spacing period. Several characteristics of antireflective structured surface offer distinct advantages compared to layers of thin dielectric films. For example, thin-film coatings suffer from problems of mechanical stability, such as layer ablation and tensile stress, while appropriate coating materials with suitable refractive indices barely exist. Moreover, whereas common single- and multi-layer configurations are applicable only within a small wavelength range and normal incidence of light, moth eye structured materials show a reduced and angle-independent reflectance over a broad spectral bandwidth [84].

Artificial "moth eye" antireflective structures can be created by the RIE of prepatterned fused silica samples [86], such that the gold nanoparticles function as a protective resist due to their higher stability against the plasma treatment compared to the underlying material. Remarkably, the tips of the pillars on top of the fused silica sample are hollow, and pores are formed at spots where the gold particles had been placed originally. During the plasma process the reactive ions of the plasma are focused to the contact area of the metallic nanoparticles with the underlying fused silica substrate. This causes a strong depletion of the plasma-generated reactive ion concentration around the metal islands, which in turn causes the particles to act as an etching mask for the processing of hollow, cone-like pillars oriented perpendicular to the substrate. During the etching process, the particles sink into the material. As the RIE process represents an unselective physical ion bombardment of the sample, the gold particles are continuously reduced in size until completely used up, at which point the whole surface is considered to be uniformly etched.

The optical properties of the fabricated samples were observed via wavelength-dependent transmission measurements, and compared to an unstructured reference substrate. As indicated by the SEM images, the topology of the fused silica sample was similar to the corneal surface of a real moth. However, the moth eye lens showed a superior optical performance compared to many non-natural materials, as the overall reflection was reduced whilst the transmission of light in the visible range was increased. The optical properties of plane-fused silica samples were investigated by wavelength- and angle-dependent transmission and reflection measurements, and the data compared to theoretical values for unstructured reference samples (Figure 7.8).

An increase in total transmission was observed over a spectral range from 300 to 800 nm, with a maximum value of transmittance of 99.0%, while the reflectivity of the same sample was damped to 0.7%. As the improved transmission was in accordance

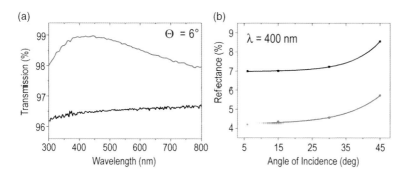

Figure 7.8 Broadband antireflective properties with varying incidence angles. (a) Wavelength-dependent transmission and reflectivity of a "moth eye" fused silica sample (upper line) compared to a reference (lower line); (b) Reflectance of a "moth eye"-structured (lower line) and a reference (upper line) sample as a function of the incident angle. The increase in transmission corresponds to an equivalent decrease in reflection. Adapted from Ref. [86].

with a reduced reflectance, however, it seemed apparent that the light-scattering defects or absorption losses were negligible.

As noted above, AR-structured surfaces enjoy certain advantages over layer-coating configurations, since the reflection is reduced for the omnidirectional incidence of light. This effect was revealed by ellipsometry measurements in which the non-polarized spectral reflection $(R_s + R_p)/2$ was investigated for different angles of incidence. When the reflectance data were compared with calculations of the reflectance of light from nonstructured fused quartz interfaces, the reflectivity of the subwavelength-structured interface was reduced to about 3% over the whole spectral region for incidence angles up to 45° (Figure 7.8b).

In order to demonstrate the excellent applicability of the method to nonplanar optical components, the convex side of a fused silica lens was processed and characterized by sub-300 nm transmission measurements. The planar-convex lens had a diameter of 22.4 mm and a focal distance of 100 mm, which corresponded to a radius of curvature of 50 mm. The reduced reflectivity of the structured part of the lens surface is shown in Figure 7.9a, where the dipping edge is indicated by a white arrow that corresponds to the border line between the antireflective-structured and nonstructured regions. More intense light reflectivity was seen above the dipping edge, whereas the antireflective part of the lens appeared less bright. When transmission in the DUV range was measured between 185 and 300 nm (Figure 7.9b), the performance was improved over the entire DUV spectral region, by 5% for 193 nm and 3% for 248 nm at the excimer laser wavelengths of ArF and KrF, respectively. This increase in transmission, of about 5%, was considered to relate to a virtual elimination of reflection at the modified optical interface.

Besides their remarkable optical properties, these structures offer additional advantages compared to thin-film coatings, in terms of mechanical stability and

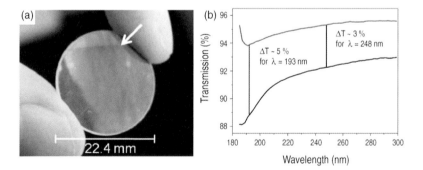

Figure 7.9 The optical properties of a "moth eye"-structured lens. (a) Photograph of the processed lens, demonstrating the antireflective effect. The borderline between the structured (below) and unstructured area is indicated by the white arrow; (b) Transmission spectra of the same lens before (lower line) and after (upper line) processing. An increase in transmission was observed over the whole DUV range, from 185 nm to 300 nm. The improved transmission values at the excimer laser wavelengths 193 nm (ArF) and 248 nm (KrF) are shown as examples. Adapted from Ref. [86].

durability. Moth-eye structured devices can also be used over a broad thermal range, as they are essentially free from adhesion problems and tensile stress between the substrate and the AR layer.

7.3.2
Cells on Nanostructured Interfaces

During recent years, increasing efforts have been made to acquire a deeper understanding of how cells interact with their environment, and in this respect nanopatterned substrates have been identified as powerful tools to engineer cellular environments to study cell-c interaction and adhesion [88]. These experiments, the main aims of which have been to mimic biological interfaces with defined chemical and physical properties, represent some of the most striking examples of the use of gold nanoparticle substrates [87]. For such nanoparticles, the adjustable separation distance of between 20 and 250 nm is within the size range of the nanoscopic subunits of the extracellular matrix (ECM), such as collagen [89]. These findings have underlined the initial proposal that biological processes occur at the nanoscale [90], while the artificial platforms designed specifically for biological applications have permitted identification of the details of cellular functions such as adhesion, migration [63, 91–93], proliferation [94], and differentiation [95], and also confirmed that these functions are regulated on the molecular level. Indeed, the site-controlled immobilization of bioactive molecules on nanoparticle patterns has opened the door to a variety of biologically active templates [96, 97], and such well-defined systems have provided insights into the density effects and spatial organization of cell membrane receptors. Arrays of micro- and nanopatterned adhesion molecules have also been used to investigate how tiny structural differences of only a few nanometers can influence the fate of a cell, whether it lives or dies [98, 99]. Clearly, these experiments have together provided important information regarding the mechanisms involved in cell–cell and cell–ECM interactions.

The adhesion of cells to the ECM is mediated by a class of transmembrane receptors of the integrin family. One important recognition sequence for the $\alpha_v\beta_3$ integrin is RGD, a peptide sequence that consists of arginine, glycine, and aspartic acid and is found in many ECM components [100].

In these experiments, gold nanoparticles were used as anchor points to tether cyclic RGD molecules c(RGDfK)-thiol to the gold nanoparticles on top of a glass coverslip (the set-up is shown schematically in Figure 7.10a). In order to avoid any unspecific binding of proteins to the substrate, and unspecific interactions of the cell with the glass substrate, the area between the nanoparticles must be passivated by either covalent [101] or electrostatic [102] functionalization with poly(ethylene glycol) (PEG). When MC3T3 osteoblasts were seeded onto the nanopattern, the cells showed a sensitive response depending on the separation distance of the RGD ligands on the surface (Figure 7.11); a particle size of 6–8 nm matched the size of a single integrin membrane receptor. When the cells were spread normally on a 58 nm patterned substrate, very few became attached and the spreading area was reduced on a sample where the RGD sequence was tethered more than 73 nm apart. Weak adhesion forces

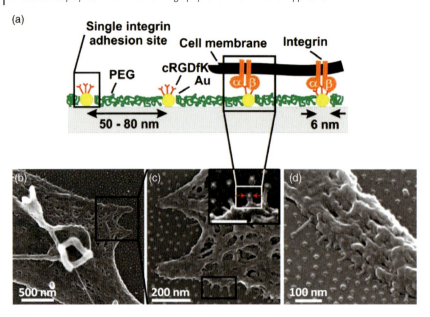

Figure 7.10 (a) Schematic of the biofunctionalized substrate. c(-RGDfK-) molecules are tethered to gold particles, which serve as adhesive anchor points for single integrin membrane receptors of living cells. Note that the particle diameter matches the structural dimensions of the integrin receptors itself. The bare glass surface between the gold nanoparticles is functionalized with a PEG monolayer to avoid protein adsorption and unspecific cell adhesion; (b–d) Scanning electron microscopy images of critical point-dried MC3T3 osteoblasts plated for 21 h on nanopatterned glass substrates. The particle spacing is set to ca. 60 nm. Close-up imaging of the cell rims reveals the interactions of cell protrusions with individual gold nanoparticles, underlining the sensitivity of the cells to communicate with the artificial substrate Adapted from Ref. [63].

were also measured on a nanopattern with a spacing larger than 58 nm [103]. Subsequent high-resolution SEM imaging of the fixed cells showed them to have formed nanoscopic protrusions that were attached to single nanoparticles. The results of these experiments confirmed that cell spreading and focal adhesion formation was impaired above a distance of 58 nm between two neighboring RGD motifs, despite the cells being sensitive enough to attach to individual particle islands. This, in turn, emphasized the fact that clustering of the $\alpha_v\beta_3$ integrin was necessary for the formation of focal adhesions [104, 105]. However, if a gradient nanopattern was presented to the cells, they migrated actively to areas with a lower separation distance between the adhesion motifs [63].

Remarkably, these cell-spreading experiments were conducted with several cell types, each of which showed a similar behavior. Similar experiments were carried out using micro-nanopatterned interfaces, and each produced similar results. Although the overall RGD density on a 58 nm pattern within micrometer-sized squares was lower than in the case of an homogeneous array with a 73 nm separation distance, focal adhesions were formed preferably on the finer-spaced substrates.

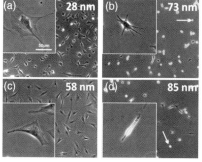
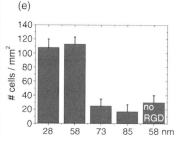

Figure 7.11 Phase-contrast microscopy images of MC3T3 osteoblasts seeded on nanopatterned surfaces, with interparticle distances of: (a) ~28 nm; (b) ~58 nm; (c) ~73 nm; and (d) ~85 nm. While cells spread very well on the 28 and 58 nm pattern, impaired cell spreading is observed on substrates with a interparticle distance >73 nm. Motionless cells appear round (arrows), while migrating cells show long extensions, sensing their environment (b, d). The number of cells attached to substrates with a spacing greater than 73 nm falls to almost the same level found on reference samples with no RGD Adapted from Ref. [98].

This confirmed that cell adhesion was indeed a consequence of the structural parameters on a nanoscopic length scale, rather than an overall ligand-density effect.

Recent developments have shown that the nanopattern can also be transferred to soft materials such as polydimethylsiloxane (PDMS), polystyrene, and hydrogels by the process of "transfer nanolithography" [106]. In addition, it is possible to create curved and complex, 3-D environments that are more closely related to the ECM of a cell *in vivo*. An example of this, using nanostructured hydrogel microtubes, is shown in Figure 7.12. In this case, the hydrogel-tubes were prepared by embedding nanopatterned glass fibers with diameters between 60 and 500 μm into a matrix of polyethylene glycol diacrylate (PEGDA). In order to ensure a complete transfer, the gold particles were functionalized with propene thiol linker molecules. After crosslinking the PEGDA, the glass fiber was dissolved with hydrofluoric acid, which resulted in a channel structure decorated internally with gold nanoparticles, as revealed by cryo-SEM imaging (Figure 7.12b and c). Nanopatterned soft materials offer the additional advantage of controlling the surface stiffness and viscoelastic properties of the substrate. This ability is especially advantageous when investigating the spatiomechanical properties of cell–ECM interactions.

7.4
Conclusions

Block copolymer micelle nanolithography is a rapid and highly reproducible technique for large-scale nanopatterning on the basis of pure self-assembly. In this

(a)

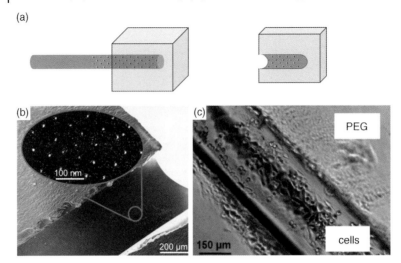

Figure 7.12 Formation of nanostructured hydrogel microtubes. (a) Nanoparticles are transferred from glass microfibers into PEGDA 700 block by using a transfer linker. Removal of the glass fiber resulted in a nanopatterned hydrogel tube; (b) Cryo-SEM image of a PEGDA 700 hydrogel channel decorated with gold nanoparticles; (c) HeLa cells cultured in PEGDA 700 hydrogel channels. The particles at the inside of the tube are functionalized with c(-RGDfK-). Adapted from Ref. [106].

chapter, aspects for characterizing nanoparticle arrays have been discussed, and the experimental conditions presented for controlling the separation distance and size of noble metal particles on top of solid substrates such as glass or silicon wafers. For this, Au, Pt, and Pd nanoparticles were grown homogeneously up to 50 nm and more on the basis of electroless deposition. The micellar approach can also be combined with a conventional top-down technology to prepare micro-nanopatterned interfaces.

The nanoparticle interfaces serve as a platform for biomimetic applications. As the structural period between the particles is of wavelength range, and less than that of visible light, pillar arrays fabricated via RIE demonstrate remarkable antireflective properties. When applied to optical functional materials, this approach represents a rapid, inexpensive and reproducible means of creating highly light-transmissive, antireflective optical devices for use as display panels and projection optics, and also for heat-generating microscopic and excimer laser applications.

Gold particles arrays may also serve as anchor points for the selective binding of extracellular proteins, with such biomimetic environments presenting a striking experimental platform for the investigation of cell adhesion. Application of the high-resolution spatial positioning of signaling molecules to inorganic or polymeric supports will allow the creation of a unique artificial environment for examining the important aspects of spatioregulated cell behavior such as cell attachment, spreading, and migration under molecular control.

References

1 Royal Society and Royal Academy of Engineering, London (2004) *Nanoscience and Nanotechnology: Opportunities and Uncertainties*, The Royal Society and The Royal Academy of Engineering, London.

2 Feynman, R.P. (1960) *Eng. Sci.*, **23**, 22.

3 Whitesides, G.M. (2005) *Small*, **1**, 172.

4 Moore, G.E. (1965) *Electronics*, **38**, 4 pages.

5 Whitesides, G.M. (2003) *Nat. Biotechnol.*, **21**, 1161.

6 Moreau, W.M. (1988) *Semiconductor Lithography: Principles and Materials*, Plenum, New York.

7 Brambley, D., Martin, D., and Prewett, P.D. (1994) *Adv. Mater. Opt. Electron.*, **4**, 55.

8 Feldman, M. and Sun, J. (1992) *J. Vac. Sci. Technol. B*, **10**, 3173.

9 Silverman, J.P. (1997) *J. Vac. Sci. Technol. B*, **15**, 2117.

10 McCord, M.A. (1997) *J. Vac. Sci. Technol. B*, **15**, 2125.

11 Matsui, S., Kojima, Y., Ochiai, Y., and Honda, T. (1991) *J. Vac. Sci. Technol. B.*, **9**, 2622.

12 Melngailis, J. (1987) *J. Vac. Sci. Technol. B.*, **5**, 469.

13 Ito, I. (2004) *Dekker Encyclopedia of Nanoscience and Nanotechnology*, Marcel Dekker Ltd, New York, Vol. 1, pp. 2413–2422.

14 Smith, B.W. (2009) *Proc. SPIE*, 7274.

15 Holmes, S.J., Mitchell, P.H., and Hakey, M.C. (1997) *IBM J. Res. Dev.*, **41** (1 & 2), 7–20.

16 Philip, D. and Stoddart, J.F. (1996) *Angew. Chem., Int. Ed.*, **35**, 1155.

17 Whitesides, G.M. and Grzybowski, B. (2002) *Science*, **295**, 2418.

18 Gates, B.D., Xu, Q., Love, J.C., Wolfe, D.B., and Whitesides, G.M. (2004) *Annu. Rev. Mater. Res.*, **34**, 339.

19 Love, C.J., Estroff, L.A., Kriebel, J.K., Nuzzo, R.G., and Whitesides, G.M. (2004) *Chem. Rev.*, **105**, 1103.

20 Ulman, A. (1996) *Chem. Rev.*, **96**, 1533.

21 Park, M., Harrison, C., Chaikin, P.M., Register, R.A., and Adamson, D.H. (1997) *Science*, **276**, 1401.

22 Black, C.T. *et al.* (2007) *IBM J. Res. Dev.*, **51**, 605.

23 Hamley, I.W. (2003) *Nanotechnology*, **14**, 39.

24 Xia, Y., Gates, B., Yin, Y., and Lu, Y. (2000) *Adv. Mater.*, **12**, 693.

25 Yang, S.M., Jang, S.G., Choi, D.G., Kim, S., and Yu, H.K. (2006) *Small*, **2**, 458.

26 Xia, Y., Rogers, J.A., Paul, K.E., and Whitesides, G.M. (1999) *Chem. Rev.*, **99**, 1823.

27 Xia, Y. and Whitesides, G.M. (1998) *Angew. Chem.*, **110**, 569.

28 Piner, R.D., Zhu, J., Xu, F., Hong, S., and Mirkin, C.A. (1999) *Science*, **283**, 661.

29 Salaita, K. *et al.* (2006) *Angew. Chem., Int. Ed.*, **45**, 7220–7223.

30 Wadu-Mesthrige, K., Xu, S., Amro, N.A., and Liu, G. (1999) *Langmuir*, **15**, 8580.

31 Xu, S., Miller, S., Laibinis, P.E., and Liu, G. (1999) *Langmuir*, **15**, 7244.

32 Herndon, M.K., Collins, R.T., Hollingsworth, R.E., Larson, P.R., and Johnson, M.B. (1999) *Appl. Phys. Lett.*, **74**, 141.

33 Spatz, J.P. *et al.* (2000) *Langmuir*, **16**, 407.

34 Glass, R., Moeller, M., and Spatz, J.P. (2003) *Nanotechnology*, **14**, 1153.

35 Leibler, P. (1980) *Macromolecules*, **13**, 1602.

36 Bates, F.S. and Fredrickson, G.H. (1990) *Annu. Rev. Phys. Chem.*, **41**, 525–557.

37 Israelachvili, J. (1992) *Intramolecular and Surface Forces*, 2nd edn, Academic Press, London.

38 Israelachvili, J. (1994) *Langmuir*, **10**, 3774.

39 Gao, Z. and Eisenberg, A. (1993) *Macromolecules*, **26**, 7353.

40 Izzo, D. and Marques, C.M. (1993) *Macromolecules*, **26**, 7189.

41 Spatz, J.P., Roescher, A., Sheiko, S., Krausch, G., and Moeller, M. (1995) *Adv. Mater.*, **7**, 731.

42 Spatz, J.P., Moessmer, S., and Moeller, M. (1996) *Chem. Eur. J.*, **2**, 1552.

43 Spatz, J.P., Sheiko, S., and Moeller, M. (1996) *Macromolecules*, **29**, 3220.

44 Moessmer, S. *et al.* (2000) *Macromolecules*, **33**, 4791.

45 Kaestle, G. *et al.* (2003) *Adv. Funct. Mater.*, **13**, 853.

46 Heimendahl, M.V. (1980) *Electron Microscopy of Materials: An Introduction*, Academic Press, San Diego, USA.

47 Bhushan, B. (2004) *Springer Handbook of Nanotechnology* (ed. B. Bhushan), Springer-Verlag, Heidelberg, Germany.

48 Grabar, K.C. *et al.* (1997) *Anal. Chem.*, **69**, 471.

49 Angelescu, D.E., Harrison, C.K., Trawick, M.L., Register, R.A., and Chaikin, P.M. (2005) *Phys. Rev. Lett.*, **95**, 025702.

50 Murray, C.A. and Van Winkle, D.A. (1987) *Phys. Rev. Lett.*, **58**, 1200.

51 Kosterlitz, J.M. and Thouless, D.J. (1972) *J. Phys. C*, **6**, 1181.

52 Halperin, B.I. and Nelson, D.R. (1978) *Phys. Rev. Lett.*, **41**, 121.

53 Nelson, D.R. and Halperin, B.I. (1979) *Phys. Rev. B*, **19**, 2457.

54 Young, A.P. (1979) *Phys. Rev. B*, **19**, 1855.

55 Murray, C.A. and Grier, D.G. (1996) *Annu. Rev. Phys. Chem.*, **47**, 421.

56 Spatz, J.P., Roescher, A., and Moeller, M. (1996) *Adv. Mater.*, **8**, 337.

57 Förster, S. and Plantenberg, T. (2002) *Angew. Chem., Int. Ed.*, **114**, 712.

58 Darhuber, A.A., Troian, S.M., Davis, J.M., Miller, S.M., and Wagner, S. (2000) *J. Appl. Phys.*, **88**, 5119.

59 Landau, L.D. and Levich, B. (1942) *Acta Physicochem.*, **17**, 42.

60 Wilson, S.D.R. (1982) *J. Eng. Math.*, **16**, 209.

61 Krishnamoorthy, S., Raphaël, P., Brugger, J., Heinzelmann, H., and Hinderling, C. (2006) *Adv. Funct. Mater.*, **16**, 1469–1475.

62 Bansmann, J. *et al.* (2007) *Langmuir*, **23**, 10150.

63 Arnold, M. *et al.* (2008) *Nano Lett.*, **8**, 2063.

64 Moeller, M. *et al.* (2004) *Polym. Mater. Sci. Eng.*, **90**, 255–256.

65 Brown, K.R. and Natan, M.J. (1998) *Langmuir*, **14**, 726.

66 Sheffer, M. *et al.* (2001) *Langmuir*, **17**, 1713.

67 Stremsdoerfer, G., Martin, J.R., and Clechet, P. (1992) *Electrochem. Soc. Proc.*, **92–93**, 305.

68 Schlesinger, M. (2000) *Modern Electroplating* (ed. M. Schlesinger), John Wiley & Sons, Inc., New York, Weinheim.

69 Resch, R. *et al.* (2001) *Langmuir*, **17**, 5666.

70 Gorzolnik, B., Mela, O., and Moeller, M. (2006) *Nanotechnology*, **17**, 5027.

71 Glass, R. *et al.* (2004) *New J. Phys.*, **6** (101), 17 pages.

72 Glass, R. *et al.* (2003) *Adv. Funct. Mater.*, **13**, 569.

73 Mela, P. *et al.* (2007) *Small*, **3**, 1368–1373.

74 Aydin, D. *et al.* (2009) *Small*, **5**, 1014.

75 Spatz, J.P. *et al.* (2002) *Adv. Mater.*, **14**, 1827.

76 Stavenga, D.G., Foletti, S., Palasantzas, G., and Arikawa, K. (2006) *Proc. Biol. Sci.*, **273**, 661.

77 Kikuta, H., Toyota, H., and Yu, W.i. (2003) *Opt. Rev.*, **10**, 63.

78 Singh, J. (2003) *Electronic and Optoelectronic Properties of Semiconductor Structures*, Cambridge University Press, Cambridge, UK.

79 Sandrock, M. *et al.* (2004) *Appl. Phys. Lett.*, **84**, 3621.

80 Xi, J.Q. *et al.* (2007) *Nat. Photonics*, **1**, 176.

81 Ullmann, J. *et al.* (2000) *Proc. SPIE*, **3902**, 514.

82 Brunner, R. *et al.* (2008) *Proc. SPIE*, **7057**, 707705-1–705705-10.

83 Bernhard, C.G. (1967) *Endeavour*, **26**, 79.

84 Clapham, P.B. and Hutley, M.C. (1973) *Nature*, **244**, 281.

85 Wilson, S.J. and Hutley, M.C. (1982) *Opt. Acta*, **7**, 993.

86 Lohmueller, T., Helgert, M., Sundermann, M., Brunner, R., and Spatz, J.P. (2008) *Nano Lett.*, **8**, 1429.

87 Spatz, J.P. and Geiger, B. (2007) *Methods Cell Biol.*, **83**, 89.

88 Stevens, M.M. and George, J.H. (2005) *Science*, **310**, 1135.

89 Meller, D., Peters, K., and Meller, K. (1997) *Cell Tissue Res.*, **288**, 111–118.

90 Niemeyer, C. and Mirkin, C.A. (2004) *NanoBiotechnology: Concepts, Applications and Perspectives* (eds C. Niemeyer and C.A. Mirkin), Wiley-VCH, Weinheim.

91 Koo, L.Y., Irvine, D.J., Mayes, A.M., Lauffenburger, D.A., and Griffith, L.G. (2002) *J Cell Sci.*, **115**, 1423.

92 Jiang, X.Y., Bruzewicz, D.A., Wong, A.P., Piel, M., and Whitesides, G.M. (2005)

Proc. Natl Acad. Sci. USA, **102** (4), 975–978.

93 Cavalcanti-Adam, E.A. *et al.* (2006) *Eur. J. Cell Biol.*, **85**, 219.

94 Yima, E.K.F. *et al.* (2005) *Biomaterials*, **26**, 5405.

95 Yim, E., Pang, S., and Leong, K. (2007) *Exp. Cell Res.*, **313**, 1820.

96 Wolfram, T., Belz, F., Schön, T., and Spatz, J.P. (2007) *Biointerphases*, **2**, 44.

97 de Mel, A., Jell, G., Stevens, M.M., and Seifalian, A.M. (2008) *Biomacromolecules*, **9**, 2969–2979.

98 Arnold, M. *et al.* (2004) *ChemPhysChem*, **4**, 872.

99 Chen, C.S., Mrksich, M., Huang, S., Whitesides, G.M., and Ingber, D.E. (1997) *Science*, **276**, 1425.

100 Geiger, B., Bershadsky, A., Pankov, R., and Yamada, K. (2001) *Nat. Rev. Mol. Cell Biol.*, **2**, 793–805.

101 Bluemmel, J. *et al.* (2007) *Biomaterials*, **22**, 4739.

102 Kenausis, G.L. *et al.* (2000) *J. Phys. Chem. B*, **104**, 3298–3309.

103 Walter, N., Selhuber, C., Kessler, H., and Spatz, J.P. (2006) *Nano Lett.*, **6**, 4380.

104 Cavalcanti-Adam, E.A. *et al.* (2007) *Biophys. J.*, **92**, 2964.

105 Geiger, B., Spatz, J.P., and Bershadsky, A.D. (2009) *Nat. Rev. Mol. Cell Biol.*, **10**, 21.

106 Graeter, S.V. *et al.* (2007) *Nano Lett.*, **7**, 1413.

107 Lohmueller, T., Bock, E., and Spatz, J.P. (2008) *Adv. Mater.*, **20**, 2297.

108 Spatz, J.P. *et al.* (1998) *Adv. Mater.*, **10**, 473.

109 Ethirajan, A. *et al.* (2007) *Adv. Mater.*, **19**, 406.

110 Yun, S.H., Yoo, S.I., Jung, J.C., Zin, W.C., and Sohn, B.H. (2006) *Chem. Mater.*, **18**, 5646.

111 Park, S., Kim, B., Yavuzcetin, O., Tuominen, M.T., and Russell, T.P. (2008) *ACS Nano.*, **2**, 1363–1370.

112 Park, S. *et al.* (2009) *Science*, **20**, 1030.

113 Chen, J., Mela, P., Moeller, M., and Lensen, M.C. (2009) *ACS Nano.*, **3**, 1451–1456.

8
The Evolution of Langmuir–Blodgett Patterning

Xiaodong Chen and Lifeng Chi

8.1
Introduction

During recent years, surface patterning with nano- or microscopic structures has attracted increasing scientific and technological interest in the research areas of materials science, chemistry, biology, and physics. For instance, patterned surfaces can be used to control the crystal nucleation and to manipulate crystallographic orientation [1], or to guide the self-assembly of polymers [2]. In addition to their uses in templates, patterned surfaces are essential to the development of a number of existing and emerging technologies, such as ultrahigh-density information storage [3]. The ability to fabricate patterned surfaces on the micrometer or nanometer scale also guarantees a continuation in the miniaturization of functional devices, such as the patterned assembly of integrated semiconductor devices [4] and the patterned luminescence of organic light-emitting diodes (LEDs) [5] in microelectronics. Likewise, direct liquid flow on a selectively patterned surface is important for the development of microfluidic systems, and for the miniaturization of flow devices [6]. Active efforts are also under way, for example, to develop micropatterned cell and/or protein arrays for biosensors [7, 8], for microliter chromatography [9], for biological recognition processes [10], and for DNA separation [11, 12]. An easy access to, and cost-effective large-area nanopatterning of, biocompatible films is also important for gene and drug delivery systems, and for tissue engineering [13, 14]. The ability to fabricate patterned surfaces on the microscale or nanoscale also allows for the manipulation of surface wettability [15].

In almost all applications of patterned surfaces, nanostructure fabrication represents the first – perhaps also the most significant – challenges to their realization. Until now, many strategies have been developed for fabricating patterned surfaces, including: (i) photolithography; (ii) electron beam (e-beam) lithography; (iii) scanning probe-based lithography, including dip-pen nanolithography (DPN) [16, 17]; (iv) nanoimprinting lithography (NIL) [18]; and (v) soft lithography [19]. These methods are normally classified as "top-down" approaches, and have demonstrated a high spatial resolution. In contrast, the concepts of self-assembly and self-organization provide an alternative and simple means of realizing small features over large areas via so-called "bottom-up" approaches. These rely on the interactions of building

Nanotechnology, Volume 8: Nanostructured Surfaces. Edited by Lifeng Chi
Copyright © 2010 WILEY-VCH Verlag GmbH & Co. KGaA, Weinheim
ISBN: 978-3-527-31739-4

blocks (such as molecules or nanoparticles) that assemble spontaneously into nano/microstructures. A variety of strategies based on self-assembly, including block copolymer-based lithography, have been demonstrated and subsequently used to fabricate patterned structures [20–22]. Among many of these self-assembly techniques, the Langmuir–Blodgett (LB) technique consists of a series of efficient and parallel processes by which to build up patterned structures on solid surfaces that are chemically or physically differentiated on the micro to submicron scale [23]. A unique property of the LB technique is its ability to provide control over nanoscale assembly by tuning macroscopic properties such as the surface pressure, the molecular composition of monolayer, transfer velocity, and the temperature, subphase, and substrate.

The aim of this chapter is to provide a comprehensive description of the development of the LB technique, as used to fabricate and pattern nanostructures on solid substrates. After a description of the technique's history, controlled LB pattern formation based on small organic molecules and macromolecules is discussed, followed by details of the patterning of nanoparticles and nanowires using the LB method. The applications of nanostructures fabricated via the LB technique are summarized.

8.2
The LB Technique in Retrospect: From Homogeneous Film to Lateral Features

The history of the LB technique can be traced back to experiments conducted by Benjamin Franklin in 1773, when he dropped a teaspoon of oil onto the water surface of a pond [24]. Over a century later, Lord Rayleigh [25] and Agnes Pockels [26] quantified the oil film on the water surface, providing details of its thickness (~ 0.16 nm) and molecular area coverage (~ 0.2 nm^2). Based on these data, Irving Langmuir noted during the early twentieth century that the monolayers of fatty acids could be compressed into a solid-like ordered state on the surface of water, and this led to the development of the Langmuir trough [27]. Subsequently, Langmuir and his student, Katharine Blodgett, showed that the fatty acid monolayers on the water surfaces could be transferred onto a solid support by passing a solid substrate vertically through the air/water interface [28]. Today, this general process is referred to as the LB technique.

Since the 1960s, many stimulating studies have been carried out by Hans Kuhn and others, using LB films, that have led to applications in the fields of electronics, optics, and biology [29, 30]. Yet, within the past two decades the field has undergone a revolution, due mainly to the development of novel experimental techniques or to the enhancement of traditional techniques, including synchrotron X-ray diffraction [31], fluorescence microscopy [32], and Brewster angle microscopy (BAM) [33, 34], each of which can be used to observe monolayers directly on the water surface. Together, these techniques can be used to demonstrate the phase transition behavior and morphological features in Langmuir monolayers, that cannot be observed directly in classical isotherm measurements [35, 36]. Furthermore, the development of atomic force microscopy (AFM) has provided a means of directly imaging the morphology of the monolayer, when transferred onto a solid substrate, with resolution down to the molecular scale [37, 38]. These findings broke the traditional concept that the LB technique could be used only to create homogeneous and defect-free ultrathin films. However, with the introduction of modern experimental methods and their understanding, the LB method has developed into a high-throughput, low-cost, easily integrated method for the controlled assembly and patterning of building blocks that forms the basis of this chapter.

8.3
LB Patterning of Organic Molecules

8.3.1
Direct Transfer of Featured Structures Onto Solid Substrates

Traditionally, the LB technique has proved to be a highly versatile tool for the fabrication of homogeneous organic films on solid substrates, by transferring the closely packed monolayer onto the substrate itself. In contrast, through a rational molecular design, the organic molecules can form either nanostructures or microstructures on the water surface, and these can be transferred onto a solid substrate using the LB technique. As an example, whereas partially fluorinated long-chain fatty acids can form sharply monodisperse circular nanostructures on water surfaces during their spreading [39], normal fatty acids do not behave in this way. The mismatch between hydrocarbon segments and fluorinated segments is responsible for the formation of clusters. In one circular nanostructure, the hydrocarbon segments are packed due to van der Waals attractive interactions, although the packing is restricted by thick and stiff rods of perfluoroalkane helix chains. Semi-fluorinated phosphonic acids can also form stable nanoscale clusters on substrates, with similar behavior [40–42]. Furthermore, Krafft *et al.* found that semifluorinated alkanes (FnHm), diblock molecules with one hydrocarbon segment and one perfluorinated segment, can form nanopatterned structures on water surfaces [43]. The semifluorinated alkanes do not behave as typical amphiphiles, which normally contain one hydrophobic chain with one hydrophilic headgroup. Krafft *et al.* confirmed that the hydrocarbon segments of the semifluorinated alkane molecules were directed towards the substrate, while the fluorinated segments pointed outwards, towards the air. Moreover, the size of these nanostructures could be controlled by the density mismatch between the fluorinated and hydrogenated segments, which was originally due to an adjustment of the intermolecular interactions. Depending on the molecular structure of the FnHm diblocks, the nanostructures were either circular or elongated; however, increasing the FnHm length favored the formation of elongated nanostructures, albeit at the expense of the circular forms (see Figure 8.1) [41, 42].

Liu *et al.* found that the properties of nanostructures could easily be tuned through a rational molecular design and deposition condition [44, 45]. Initially, it was found that the achiral molecules could form chiral superstructures, depending on the

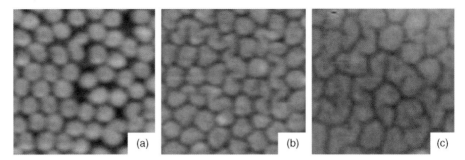

Figure 8.1 Atomic force microscopy images (250 × 250 nm) of transferred monolayers of (a) F8H16, (b) F8H18, and (c) F8H20 transferred onto silicon wafers at 5 mN m^{-1}. Reproduced with permission from Ref. [42].

surface pressure [44]. For example, an achiral amphiphilic derivative of barbituric acid (BA) could form two-dimensional (2-D) spiral structures at a low surface pressure (7 mN m^{-1}), but not at a higher surface pressure (20–30 mN m^{-1}) [44]. The spiral structures showed a clear Cotton effect for the circular dichroism (CD) measurements when they were transferred onto solid substrates. It was suggested that the large aromatic rings of the head groups, together with hydrogen bonding between the BA molecules, might be responsible for a preferential tilting of neighboring molecules in the packed films, and that spiral structures were produced due to the directionality of the hydrogen bonding interactions. Moreover, the morphology of the superstructure was found to play an important role in the properties of the structures [45]. For example, an anthracene derivative would form nanocoils at the water surface with a lower surface pressure (9 mN m^{-1}), but form straight nanoribbons at a higher surface pressure (20 mN m^{-1}). In addition, the straight nanoribbons showed an effect called "photoswitching," whereby their conductivity would change when they were exposed to light. The property of photoswitching arises because the molecules are arranged with their benzene rings stacked almost directly on top of one another, which causes the molecular orbitals of the π-electrons to overlap, leading to a more efficient charge transport. As the coiled nanoribbons had a less efficient stacking, they did not demonstrate photoswitching (Figure 8.2).

The shape of the superstructures (Figure 8.3a) can also be extensively controlled by the subphase conditions. For example, a chiral amphiphilic molecule, C12-(L)Cys-(L)Cys-C18, which consists of two short cysteine peptides as hydrophilic heads and two hydrophobic alkyl chains as tails, can form chiral domains at the air/water interface, owing to intermolecular hydrogen-bonding and hydrophobic interactions [46]. However, when the subphase contained 10^{-8} M CdCl$_2$, the superstructure was changed to a spiral structure, and the size of the structure greatly reduced. Alternatively, when the subphase contained 10^{-6} M CdTe nanoparticles, the superstructure was changed to linear nanostructures (Figure 8.3b) [47]. The reasons for this include: (i) that the addition of electrolytes might reduce the molecular interaction; or (ii) that the presence of thiol groups within the hydrophilic heads of the C12-(L)Cys-(L)Cys-C18 molecule allowed the complexation of metal or semiconductor nanocrystals

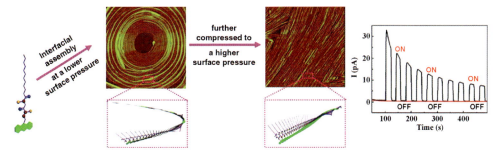

Figure 8.2 Atomic force microscopy image of monolayer on mica deposited at 9 mN m^{-1} (left) and 20 mN m^{-1} (right). The graph at the right shows the photoswitching characteristics of the two-end devices based on the films of BA by white light for the films deposited at 9 mN m^{-1} (red) and 20 mN m^{-1} (green); the scheme for the formation of nanocoils and straight nanoribbons. Reproduced with permission from Ref. [45].

(NCs), which might also change the molecular interaction. In this case, by simply changing the subphase, it would be possible to construct controlled lateral structures from the sub-micrometer scale down to the nanometer scale, simply by adjusting the subtle balance of the molecular interactions (with one or more chemical components). A second example is that the lanthanide ion could induce the stripe formation of phospholipid monolayers through the dynamic binding of subphase lanthanide ions to the phosphocholine headgroups at the air/water interface [48]. Competitive dipole–dipole and electrostatic interactions between the lanthanide-bound and free phospholipid molecules might then have produced long-range ordered arrays of phospholipid stripes, with periodicities of 1.7–1.8 μm.

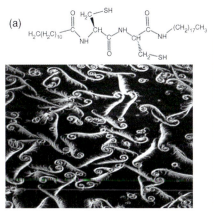

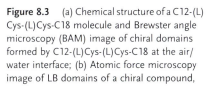

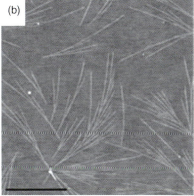

Figure 8.3 (a) Chemical structure of a C12-(L)Cys-(L)Cys-C18 molecule and Brewster angle microscopy (BAM) image of chiral domains formed by C12-(L)Cys-(L)Cys-C18 at the air/water interface; (b) Atomic force microscopy image of LB domains of a chiral compound, C12-(L)Cys-(L)Cys-C18, transferred onto a silicon substrate with the subphase containing 10^{-6} M of a CdTe nanoparticle. Scale bar = 2 μm. Panel (a) reprinted with permission from Ref. [46]; panel (b) reprinted with permission from Ref. [47].

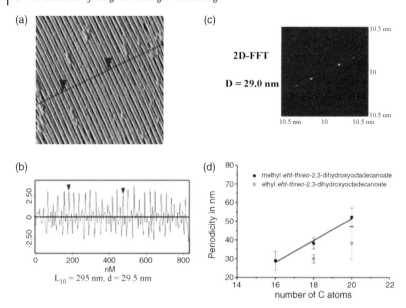

Figure 8.4 (a) Supermolecular periodic structures in a monolayer of ethyl-ent-*threo*-2,3-dihydroxyoctadecanoate. The periodicity was measured as 29 nm, evaluated from (b) the line section of the image or (c) 2-D-FET of the image; (d) The variation in periodicity by changes in chain length or head group. Reproduced with permission from Ref. [49].

The methyl and ethyl esters of ent-*threo*-2,3-dihydroxy fatty acids can also form periodic nanometer-sized structures, as observed with AFM after being transferred onto solid substrates (Figure 8.4) [49]. The ordered structures were not formed by the regular packing of single molecules, but rather by molecular assemblies. Here, it was found that the periodicity could be adjusted by varying the alkyl chain length or head group. For example, in the case of ethyl ent-*threo*-2,3-dihydroxyoctadecanoate, the periodicity was 30 nm, but this was changed to 38 nm for the case of ethyl ent-threo-2,3-dihydroxyicosanoate. Likewise, Kelley *et al.* showed that some amphiphilic β-hairpin peptides could form ordered periodic nanostructures on mica [50].

The molecular compositions of the monolayer can also be used to control the feature on the water surface. The formation of various types of pattern can be achieved through self-organization processes, such as the growth of condensed-phase domains in an expanded phase at the phase-transition region during micro-phase separation in mixed monolayers. For instance, by using a micro-phase separation in binary mixed Langmuir monolayers of cadmium salts of *n*-alkyl fatty acids and a perfluoropolyether surfactant, which separate into microscopic domains of condensed phase and a surrounding matrix of expanded phase, respectively, it was shown that the pattern shape would depend on the alkyl chain length of *n*-alkyl fatty acids and the temperature of the water surface [51, 52].

Besides the small organic molecules, amphiphilic diblock copolymers represent an important class of materials for pattern formation, by selecting suitable molecular architecture and deposition conditions. The density of the polymer at the surface can also be controlled by the choice of adsorbing block size and deposition conditions, while the properties imparted to the surface can be modified by the choice of free block. For instance, an amphiphilic polyelectrolyte diblock, polystyrene-*b*-poly(4-vinylpyridine) diblock ionomer, can form stable surface structures at the air/water interface. Subsequent transmission electron microscopy (TEM) measurements provided direct evidence of the self-assembly of the diblock copolymers into regular circular surface nanostructures [53] that consisted of a central core of polystyrene chains, from which radiated the ionic poly(vinylpyridium) chains. The distance between nanostructures can be controlled by adjusting the surface pressure. Polyelectrolyte diblocks have also been used to control the spacing between micelles by selection of polymer size, charge, and asymmetry [54]. In addition, nonionic diblock polymers of comparably sized hydrophobic and hydrophilic units, such as polystyrene-poly(*n*-butylmethacrylate), polystyrene-polydimethylsiloxane, and polystyrene-*b*-poly(ethylene oxide) (PS-PEO), can form uniform arrays on solid substrate by LB deposition (Figure 8.5) [55–57].

Similarly, the change in monolayer composition may alter the pattern formation. For instance, when a semifluorinated alkane was blended with a PS-PEO diblock copolymer, a surface nanoscale pattern was obtained which resembled a honeycomb with a hump at the center, with a periodicity of ~40 nm [58]. The same qualitative morphological features were found in all mixed films, independent of the polymer grafting density, while the ordering was increased with the increasing polymer grafting density. These structures arose from the organization of the semifluorinated alkane molecules segregated to the surface of the polymer layer. Other examples included the blends of polystyrene-*b*-poly(ferrocenylsilane) (PS-PF) and polystyrene-*b*-poly(2-vinylpyridine) (PS-P2VP) monolayers, the morphologies of which were distinct from those formed when either of the copolymers was spread alone [59]. Pure PS-P2VP was seen to form a highly ordered hexagonal lattice of spherical

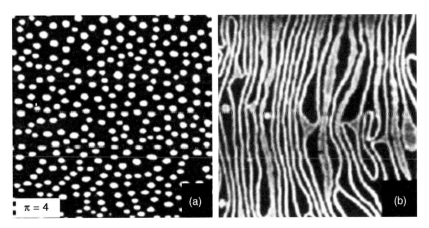

Figure 8.5 The "dots and spaghetti" morphology of a PS-PEO monolayer on a silicon substrate, depending on the transferred conditions by LB deposition. Panel (a) reprinted with permission from Ref. [56]; panel (b) reprinted with permission from Ref. [57].

micelles, whereas pure PS-PF showed three-dimensional (3-D) aggregates with some spherical micelles of irregular size. In the case of blends of these two copolymers, as the fraction of PS-PF increased the morphologies changed from an hexagonal micelle lattice to a cylindrical shape. The application of an electric field in the plane of the air/water interface also caused the structures to compact further and to produce a mesh.

8.3.2
Pattern Formation During LB Transfer

In addition to lateral structures being formed directly at the air/water interface and then transferred onto solid substrates, the LB transfer process itself can be used form patterns close to the three-phase contact line from an homogeneous Langmuir monolayer. As an example, L-α-dipalmitoylphosphatidylcholine (DPPC) (the chemical structure is shown in Figure 8.6) shows how the pattern can be formed during LB transfer, and how the shape, size, and alignment of patterns can be controlled.

DPPC, which constitutes one of the major lipid components of biological membranes, demonstrates the typical phase behavior of a Langmuir monolayer at the air/water interface. This is characterized by a liquid-expanded (LE) phase, a liquid-condensed (LC) phase, and a LE ↔ LC phase transition, as confirmed by the surface pressure–molecular area (π–A) isotherm and BAM images (see Figure 8.6) [35, 36].

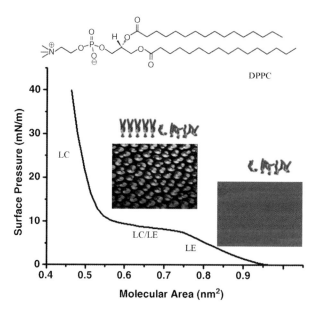

Figure 8.6 Phase behavior of the DPPC monolayer at the air/water interface. Top: Chemical structure of DPPC. Bottom: π–A isotherm of DPPC (∼23 °C) and typical BAM images (430 × 537 μm²) for the LE phases and LE ↔ LC phase transition, along with the corresponding conformations of the DPPC molecules. Reproduced with permission from Ref. [23].

In the LE phase, the DPPC monolayer behaves as a quasi-2-D liquid, with the headgroups of the DPPC molecules being translationally disordered and the chains conformationally disordered. On reducing the molecular areas, however, the DPPC molecules begin to condense such that a coexisting phase of LE and crystalline LC occurs at the plateau region of the isotherm. Finally, a homogeneous well-packed condensed monolayer (the LC phase) appears at smaller molecular areas.

When a solid substrate was used to transfer a homogeneous DPPC Langmuir monolayer at the LE phase, a mesostructure which consisted of alternating stripes about 800 nm wide, separated by channels of about 200 nm width, was observed on the mica surface (Figure 8.7b) [60]. Although it is difficult to observe directly the stripe formation *in situ* at the three-phase contact line in this system, it is possible to imagine the process of stripe pattern formation, as depicted schematically in Figure 8.7a. Here, the height difference between the stripes and channels was about 1 nm, and the stripes were composed of condensed (LC phase) DPPC molecules. Considering that the length of a DPPC molecule is about 2 nm, the material in the channels could be attributed to the expanded (similar to LE phase) DPPC molecules, which have a larger tilt angle compared to condensed DPPC molecules in the stripes, as depicted in Figure 8.7c. The origin of the pattern formation was considered due to phase transitions (i.e., substrate-mediated condensation) close to the three-phase contact line during the LB transfer process [60, 61]. During the transfer, a dewetting instability in the vicinity of the three-phase contact line, or meniscus oscillation, caused a switch of DPPC between the expanded phase (the channels) and the condensed phase (the stripes). One possible mechanism for such a switch upon transfer was an oscillation of the meniscus height (i.e., stick–slip model), which

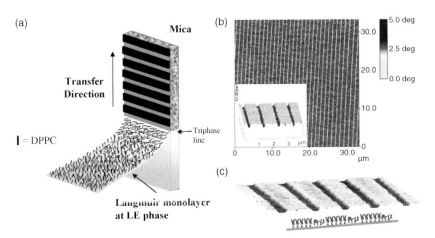

Figure 8.7 (a) Schematic illustration of the process of mesopattern formation; (b) Mesostructures with nanochannels on mica in phase (main figure) and topography (inset) imaging. Experimental conditions: surface pressure 3 mN m^{-1}, transfer velocity 60 mm min^{-1}, temperature 22.5 °C; (c) The composition of DPPC pattern. The DPPC stripe pattern is composed of expanded DPPC molecules in the channels and condensed DPPC molecules in the stripes. Reproduced with permission from Ref. [60].

correlated to the change in interfacial free energies in order to satisfy the Young–Laplace condition [61]. A second possible explanation was a density oscillation in the vicinity of the three-phase contact line.

Importantly, the size and shape of the DPPC patterns can be controlled simply by adjusting the transfer velocity, the surface pressure, the temperature, the substrate chemistry and monolayer composition, and the transfer method. For example, the shape and lateral size of the DPPC stripe pattern from the pure DPPC monolayer depended heavily on the transfer surface pressure and transfer velocity [47, 62]. On mica substrates, at a surface pressure of $3.0\,\mathrm{mN\,m^{-1}}$, a high transfer velocity of $60\,\mathrm{mm\,min^{-1}}$ induced the formation of horizontal DPPC stripes, parallel to the three-phase contact line (Figure 8.8a and d). In contrast, vertical stripes, perpendicular to the three-phase contact line (Figure 8.8c and f), were obtained at a low transfer velocity ($10\,\mathrm{mm\,min^{-1}}$). At a transfer velocity of $40\,\mathrm{mm\,min^{-1}}$, a grid pattern that clearly showed the superposition of horizontal stripes and vertical stripes was observed (Figure 8.8b). In general, the horizontal stripes appeared only at the high transfer velocity ($60\,\mathrm{mm\,min^{-1}}$) with a low transfer surface pressure, whilst the pure vertical stripes appeared only at the low transfer velocity and high transfer surface pressure (still in LE phase). Based on such transfer velocity-dependent pattern formation [62, 63], a simple but novel method – termed *LB rotating transfer* – was

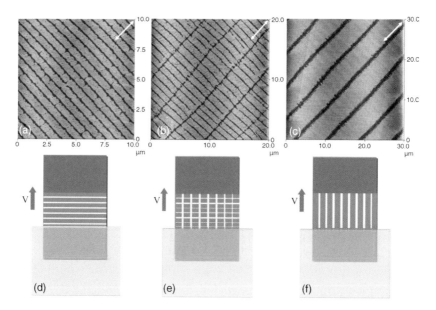

Figure 8.8 The shape and alignment of patterns (pure DPPC) depending on the transfer conditions. (a–c) AFM images of the various pure DPPC patterns on mica surfaces. (a) $60\,\mathrm{mm\,min^{-1}}$ and $3\,\mathrm{mN\,m^{-1}}$; (b) $40\,\mathrm{mm\,min^{-1}}$ and $3\,\mathrm{mN\,m^{-1}}$; (c) $10\,\mathrm{mm\,min^{-1}}$ and $3\,\mathrm{mN\,m^{-1}}$. Double arrows in the AFM images show the axis of film transfer; (d–f) Schematic illustrations for the formation of various patterns during the LB vertical deposition. Reproduced with permission from Ref. [62].

developed to achieve a gradient mesostructure in a well-ordered fashion over large areas [64].

The different hydrophilic substrates can also be used to obtain DPPC mesostructures, although the experimental conditions required for pattern formation will vary due to the different surface properties [65]. One reason for stripe pattern formation is the substrate-mediated condensation of DPPC during the LB transfer; consequently, the molecule–substrate interaction should represent a very important factor in this dynamic self-organization process. For instance, whilst the periodic stripe patterns could be formed on an oxygen plasma-treated silicon surface, the transfer velocity used would need to be slower than that used for transfer onto a mica surface at the same surface pressure and temperature [66].

The addition of a second component to the DPPC monolayer can permit the tuning of DPPC pattern formation, since the miscibility of the various components is important with regard to the phase behavior and stability of the mixed monolayer. For instance, 1,2-di(2,4-octadecadienoyl)-sn-glycero-3-phosphocholine (DOEPC) has been selected as an additive component to study the effects of the second component on DPPC pattern formation during LB deposition. This is based on the fact that DOEPC has a similar molecular structure to DPPC, but forms a fully LE phase at the air/water interface under the same conditions. Compared to the pure DPPC monolayer, pattern formation with the mixed monolayer of DPPC/DOEPC (1:0.1) shifted to lower velocities and higher surface pressures, while the ability to form horizontal stripes was increased [62]. The grid pattern appeared only at a low transfer velocity (1 mm min^{-1}) and high transfer surface pressures. In general, the size of stripes in the mixed DPPC/DOEPC (1:0.1) patterns was about four- to sixfold smaller than that of stripes formed by a pure DPPC monolayer under the same transfer conditions [62]. Other molecules, such as 4-(dicyanomethylene)-2-methyl-6-(4-dimethylaminostyryl)-4H-pyran (DCM) and 2-(12-(7-nitrobenz-2-oxa-1,3-diazol-4-yl)-amino)dodecanoyl-1-hexadecanoyl-sn-glycero-3-phosphocholine (NBD), can also be used to generate regular and tunable luminescent stripes with submicrometer-scale lateral dimensions [67]. These dye molecules are uniformly distributed within the expanded DPPC channels, which are in turn separated by condensed DPPC stripes. The width and periodicity of the luminescent stripes can be controlled by adjusting the ratio of dye to DPPC.

8.4
LB Patterning of Nanomaterials

Recent progress has been reported on the close-packed monolayer fabrication of ligand-stabilized nanomaterials on solid substrates [68–74], as one of the most appealing features of the LB technique is the intrinsic control of the internal layer structure down to a molecular level, and the precise control of the resultant film thickness. Unlike these traditional close-packed nanoparticle monolayers on solid substrates, the LB technique itself represents a means of obtaining regular nanoparticles or nanowire pattern arrays on solid substrates [75].

8.4.1
LB Patterning of Nanoparticles

As an example, Heath and coworkers [76] confirmed the formation of aligned, high-aspect ratio nanowires at a low-density Langmuir monolayer film of alkylthiol-passivated silver nanoparticles during film compression. Prior to monolayer compression (surface coverage ~20%, $\pi \approx 0\,nN\,m^{-1}$), the particles were found to aggregate into circular domains. However, after compression the particle monolayers assembled spontaneously into lamellae or wire-like superstructures with lengths of several micrometers and widths of 20 to 300 nm, which were functions of the solvent and the particle size. The interwire separation distance, as well as the alignment of the wires, could be controlled via compression of the wires. There was, in addition, an agreement between these experimentally acquired data and a computer simulation performed using the standard Metropolis Monte Carlo algorithm [77] (see Figure 8.9). Here, the patterns were described as resulting from competition between an attraction, which makes the particles aggregate, and a longer-ranged repulsion, which limits the aggregation to finite domains. Careful investigations also showed

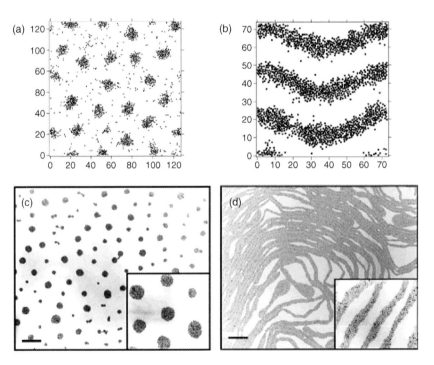

Figure 8.9 Results of the computer simulation (a, b) and the corresponding transmission electron microscopy images (c, d) revealing the spontaneous formation of clusters and stripe-like arrays of alkylthiol-passivated Ag nanocrystals. The solution used to prepare (d) was approximately threefold more concentrated ($\sim$1 mg ml^{-1}) than that used for (c). Scale bar = 0.5 µm. Reproduced with permission from Ref. [77].

that an increase in concentration led to a spontaneous reorganization of the self-assembled domains from circular clusters to stripes, as the repulsions between the aggregates became more important than those between the individual particles within them. This phenomenon was considered to be closely related to the transitions to hexagonal and lamellar phases commonly observed in concentrated surfactant solutions, where the locally preferred curvature of micelles is successively "squeezed out" of the systems as the interaggregate repulsions become dominant and the lower-curvature cylinder and bilayer geometries are found to better minimize the overall interaction free energy.

In contrast to the results of Heath *et al.* [76], where higher-order nanoparticulate structures were formed at the air/water interface before being transferred onto a solid substrate, Schmid and Yang *et al.* found the process of LB transfer also to be an efficient means of obtain regular nanoparticle arrays on solid substrates, with the assistance of dewetting during the LB transfer process [78–80]. Schmid *et al.*, by using the LB technique [80], first successfully obtained parallel rows of $Au_{55}(PPh_3)_{12}Cl_6$ clusters, which are quasi-one-dimensional (1-D) structures of quantum dots of about 10 nm width. A modified LB technique (Figure 8.10a), deposited beneath the monolayer at an angle of $20°$, was used to generate this type of cluster stripe. Pattern formation was shown to depend mainly on the speed at which the substrate was moved; for example, at speeds of about 10 cm min^{-1} the parallel stripes consisted of three to four cluster rows and were separated one from another by 8 nm (Figure 8.10). The formation of such patterns was attributed to oscillation of the water meniscus at

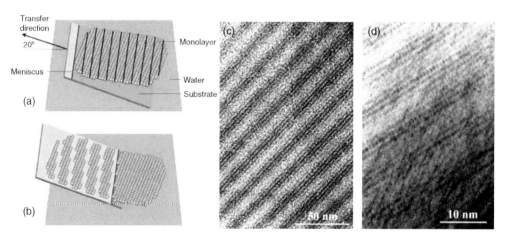

Figure 8.10 (a) Sketch of the formation of cluster stripes from an ordered monolayer. The monolayer is oriented toward the substrate edge and the meniscus, respectively, by a nonpredetermined angle; (b) Owing to the movement of the substrate from the water, and the herewith linked transfer of the monolayer onto the substrate surface, the monolayer is fractured along the black lines due to oscillation of the meniscus. Stripes of three to four rows of clusters lying side by side are formed. The stripes run parallel to the water meniscus; (c) TEM image of cluster stripes consisting of three to four cluster rows; (d) Magnified cutout. The cluster rows consist of equidistantly ordered clusters. Reproduced with permission from Ref. [80].

the substrate, which induced the generation of striped patterns that ran parallel to the meniscus.

Later, Yang *et al.* [79] used the LB technique to generate well-spaced, parallel single particle lines on a substrate from a dilute Langmuir particle monolayer via a stick-slip motion of the water/substrate contact line. In this case, a stick-slip motion was observed *in situ* by optical microscopy, with the three-phase contact line during the transfer process being due to the large interline distance and low density of the Langmuir monolayer at the air/water interface, when compared to the data of Schmid *et al.* [80]. The particle density within the lines could be controlled not only by the particle concentration in the monolayer but also by the pulling speed of the substrate. In this way, lines of a wide variety of materials and sizes, ranging from a few nanometers to a few micrometers, were demonstrated. The ability to assemble nanoparticles into 1-D arrays enables the construction of higher hierarchical device structures. For example, by using gold nanoparticle seeds it is possible to grow vertical single nanowire arrays of silicon, replicating the pattern of single particle lines. The spontaneous formation of ordered gold and silver nanoparticle stripe patterns was identified on dewetting a dilute film of polymer-coated nanoparticles floating on a water surface [78]. However, the difference here was that the nanoparticle stripe patterns were perpendicular to the air/water interface (Figure 8.11), in contrast to the above two examples. The reason for such formation of vertical nanoparticle stripe patterns was considered to be the fingering instability. Taken together, these results showed that the LB technique can provide new avenues for the lithography-free patterning of nanoparticle arrays in a variety of applications, including multiplexed surface-enhanced Raman substrates and the templated fabrication of higher-order nanostructures.

One unique property of the LB technique is that it can control the monolayer composition. To some extent, the morphology of these nanostructures can be controlled by adjusting the parameters that affect the self-assembly process. For example, Hassenkam *et al.* demonstrated the formation of continuous gold nanowires by mixing and spreading the dodecanethiol-capped gold nanoparticles and DPPC at the air/water interface [81]. The unidirectional sintering of particles, which was accompanied by packing into a maze-like structure, was considered due to a template effect of the surfactant at the molecular level. In this case, the amphiphilic DPPC molecules preferred (on an energetic basis) to occupy the entire water surface if left alone, whereas when the hydrophobic gold particles were left alone on the water surface they would form close-packed, floating, 2-D hexagonal rafts. Yet, if a mixture of DPPC and dodecanethiol-capped gold particles were to be placed on the same water surface, the energetic strain between the bare water surface and the hydrophobic particles would be reduced. Since the DPPC molecules can only support single-particle broad lines, this would result in the formation of 1-D aggregates, which is in fact the mechanism of nanowire formation. When Zhang *et al.* described the use of molecular aggregates as templates to assemble water-soluble nanocrystals into branched wire structures at the air/water interface [46], they designed and synthesized a chiral amphiphilic molecule, C12-(L)Cys-(L)Cys-C18, which consisted of two short cysteine peptides as the hydrophilic heads and two hydrophobic alkyl

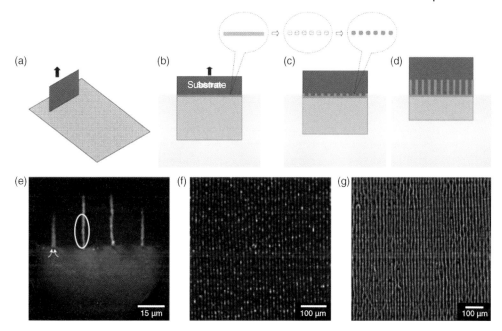

Figure 8.11 Extended stripe pattern formation through dip-coating. (a–d) A schematic drawing illustrating the formation of an aligned gold nanoparticle stripe pattern by vertical deposition (a, b). Only the nanoparticles at the water/substrate contact line (gold dots in b–d) are shown for clarity. The substrate is raised slowly (a, b) so that water is evaporated when a new surface is exposed. The wet contact line containing uniformly dispersed nanoparticles breaks up into aggregates of nanoparticles (b, c), owing to the fingering instability during the initial dewetting stage. These fingertips then guide the further deposition of nanoparticles, finally forming the extended stripe pattern (d); (e) Direct optical microscopy observation of the water front reveals a rapid motion of nanoparticles towards the wet tips (circled area) of the stripes, as indicated by the arrows. This leads to the unidirectional growth of the stripes across the entire substrate as shown in the optical microscopy image in (f); (g) Silver nanoparticle stripes have been obtained in the same fashion. Reproduced with permission from Ref. [78].

chains as the tails, and these formed chiral domains at the air/water interface. This lateral structure, with its chemically active end-groups (thiol groups), was further used for the specific binding of CdTe nanocrystals. After transferring a monolayer of C12-(L)Cys-(L)Cys-C18 via the complexation of CdTe nanocrystals, CdTe nanowires were produced that were 10–15 nm wide, up to several micrometers long, and were branched in a certain fashion.

Polymers may also serve as an important component for fine-tuning the formation of nanoparticle arrays, if there is sufficient attraction between the ligand molecules and the polymer. For instance, poly(vinyl-pyrrolidone) (PVP), which is able to chemisorb $Au_{55}(PPh_3)_{12}C_{16}$ clusters via the phenyl groups in impressive manner, was added into the subphase to tune the nanoparticle array formation [82]. In the absence of PVP, smaller islands of well-ordered Au_{55} were also formed at the air/water phase boundary [83]. The wires (which were 30 nm wide and 1 µm long) were connected by junctions of cluster islands to a complete 2-D network on mica or silicon that had been generated via the LB technique when PVP was added. The pattern of cluster-coated polymer molecules indicated that the nanoparticles had acted partly as linking knots between the polymer chains, so as to generate a stable network. Lu *et al.* [84] also used model electrodes fabricated via nanosphere lithography [85] to connect the nanowires of Au_{55}. In this case, the model electrodes were prepared via metal evaporation through a mask of monodispersed latex beads. At the second stage, the silicon surfaces bearing the model electrodes were used as substrates for transferring nanowires that consisted of Au_{55} and had been prepared via the LB technique on the PVP subphase. In this way, by controlling the structure density on the surface, it was possible to obtain both single connections (as shown in Figure 8.12) and multi-connections.

In addition to linear metal nanoparticle arrays or 2-D networks, ring-like CdSe nanoparticle patterns [86] and tree-like fractal aggregates of CdS nanoparticles in amphiphilic oligomers [87] were also observed. The ring-like structures had diameters ranging from 150 to 1200 nm, and were obtained by transferring a mixed monolayer of amphiphilic copolymer poly[(maleic acid hexadecylmonoamide)-*co*-propylene] and CdSe nanoparticles stabilized with polystyrene-poly(4-vinylpyridine) onto solid substrates, using the LB technique [86]. Due to preferential interactions between the polystyrene-functionalized nanoparticles and the polystyrene block of an amphiphilic PS-PEO block copolymer, a highly stable 1-D nanoparticle/polymer was formed at the air/water interface, via synergistic self-assembly, with surface features that included branched nanowires and nanocables up to 100 µm in length [88].

8.4.2
LB Patterning of Nanowires

One-dimensional nanoscale building blocks, such as nanowires, nanorods, and carbon nanotubes (CNTs), can also be ordered and assembled rationally into

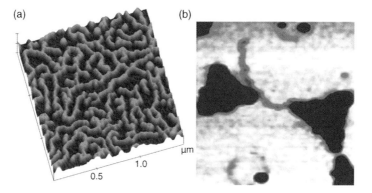

Figure 8.12 Topographical image of network structures of Au_{55} on mica surface ($1.6 \times 1.6\,\mu m^2$) and nanowires of Au_{55} connected with model electrodes ($350 \times 350\,nm^2$). Reproduced with permission from Ref. [84].

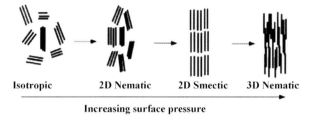

Isotropic   2D Nematic   2D Smectic   3D Nematic

Increasing surface pressure

Figure 8.13 Schematic illustration of the pressure-induced phase transition when the nanorods are compressed at the water/air interface. Reproduced with permission from Ref. [89].

appropriate 2-D architectures using the LB technique. Yang *et al.* supported this proposal by using $BaCrO_4$ nanorods, with a low aspect ratio of $\sim$3–5 : 1 and a typical diameter of approximately 5 nm [89] in the pressure-induction of isotropic-2-D $\rightarrow$ nematic-2-D $\rightarrow$ smectic-3-D nematic phase transitions, as well producing a transformation from monolayer to multilayer nanorod assembly (as shown in Figure 8.13). At low surface pressure, the $BaCrO_4$ nanorods formed raft-like aggregates (i.e., an isotropic state) that comprised generally three to five rods, with the rods aligned side-by-side due to the effects of directional capillary forces and van der Waals attractions. During the process of compression ($<$30 mN m^{-1}) a monolayer of nanorods was formed in a nematic arrangement, with an orientational order parameter S of 0.83, where the directors of the nanorods were aligned qualitatively, presumably dictated by the barrier of the trough. When the surface pressure was raised to about $\sim$35 mN m^{-1}, nanorod assemblies with a smectic arrangement are obtained, whilst when the pressure exceeded 38 mN m^{-1} there was a transition from monolayer (ordered 2-D smectic arrangement) to multilayer (disordered 3-D nematic configuration).

The thiol-capped gold nanorods (diameters $\sim$8 nm) with similar aspect ratios showed a great tendency to form nanorod ribbon superstructures, where many of the gold nanorods are aligned side-by-side [90]. Compression of these nanorod monolayers did not lead to the same phase evolution as seen in the $BaCrO_4$ system, a difference that might be attributed not only to the much more attractive van der Waals forces and directional capillary interaction among gold nanorods when compared to $BaCrO_4$ nanorods, but also to the polydispersity of the available gold nanorods. In contrast, the organization of $BaWO_4$ nanorods (diameter $\sim$10 nm) with a large aspect ratio (150 : 1) again differed significantly from the assembly superstructures of the short $BaCrO_4$ and Au nanorods [91]. Initially, the nanorods were rather dispersed, with the directors of the nanorods being distributed isotropically and no superstructures being observed. After compression, however, the nanorods were readily aligned in roughly the same direction to form a nematic layer such that, with a strong compression they formed bundles that had almost perfect side-by-side alignment between the included nanorods. The preference for a nematic phase formation upon compression proved to be a distinct characteristic of the assembly behavior of nanorods with a large aspect ratio, a situation also identified for the alternative molecular wire system of $Mo_3Se_3^-$ (diameter 0.8 nm, aspect ratio effectively infinite).

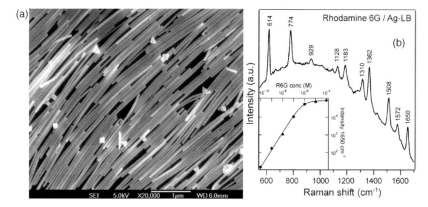

Figure 8.14 (a) Scanning electron microscopy images of the silver nanowire monolayer deposited on a silicon wafer; (b) Surface-enhanced Raman scattering (SERS) spectrum of rhodamine 6G (R6G) on the thiol-capped Ag-LB film (532 nm, 25 mW) after 10 min incubation in a 10^{-9} M R6G solution. The inset shows the linear relationship between the Raman intensity at 1650 cm^{-1} and the R6G concentration. Reproduced with permission from Ref. [92].

Xia and Yang *et al.* also used the LB technique successfully to assemble monolayers (with areas >20 cm^2) of aligned silver nanowires that were ~50 nm in diameter and 2–3 μm long [92]. These nanowires (which had pentagonal cross-sections and pyramidal tips) were close-packed as parallel arrays, with their longitudinal axes aligned perpendicular to the compression direction (see Figure 8.14). The monolayers, which were readily transferred onto any desired substrate, included silicon wafers, glass slides, and polymer substrates, and could serve as simple wire-grid optical polarizers and surface-enhanced Raman spectroscopy (SERS) substrates. The monolayer substrates were shown to behave as major enhancers of electromagnetic fields (factors of 2×10^5 for thiol and 2,4-dinitrotoluene, and of 2×10^9 for Rhodamine 6G), and could be readily used in ultrasensitive, molecule-specific sensing processes by utilizing vibrational signatures. Furthermore, the fact that the observed SERS intensity depended on the polarization direction confirmed the (theoretical) predictions that large electromagnetic fields would be localized within the interstices between adjacent nanowires [93].

Similarly, silicon nanowires can be organized into aligned structures by the LB technique, over large areas [94]. For this, the aligned nanowires were first transferred onto planar substrates via a layer-by-layer process so as to form parallel and crossed nanowire structures (Figure 8.15) that were then transferred onto a substrate. Photolithography was then used to define a pattern over the entire substrate surface, which set the array dimensions and array pitch, after which any nanowires outside the patterned array were removed by gentle sonication. In addition, electrical transport measurements that exhibited linear current versus voltage behavior confirmed that reliable electrical contacts could be made to the hierarchical nanowire arrays prepared via this method. This process offered a flexible pathway for the

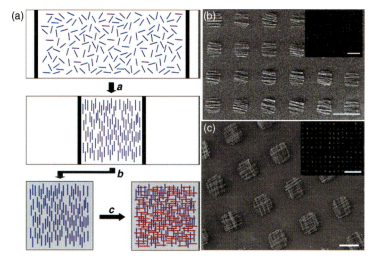

Figure 8.15 (a) Nanowires (blue lines) in a monolayer of surfactant at the air/water interface are compressed (pathway *a*) on a Langmuir–Blodgett trough to a specified pitch. In pathway *b*, the aligned nanowires are transferred to the surface of a substrate to make a uniform parallel array. In pathway *c*, crossed nanowire structures are formed by uniform transfer of a second layer of aligned parallel nanowires (red lines) perpendicular to the first layer (blue lines); (b) Image of patterned 10 μm × 10 μm parallel nanowire arrays. Scale bar = 25 μm. The inset shows a large-area dark-field optical micrograph of patterned parallel nanowire arrays (inset scale bar = 100 μm); (c) Scanning electron microscopy image of patterned crossed nanowire arrays. Scale bar = 10 μm. The inset shows a large-area dark-field optical micrograph of the patterned crossed nanowire arrays (inset scale bar = 100 μm). Reproduced with permission from Ref. [94].

bottom-up assembly of virtually any nanowire material into the highly integrated and hierarchically organized nanodevices required for a broad range of functional nanosystems. For example, crossed nanowires arrays might be used as an addressable nanoscale LED source.

8.5
Application of Structures Formed by LB Patterning

8.5.1
Templated Self-Assembly of Molecules and Nanoparticles

As discussed above, the DPPC pattern is composed of expanded DPPC molecules in the channels, and condensed DPPC molecules in the stripes. This chemically striped pattern shows an anisotropic wetting of 1-phenyloctane [95], due to the different interfacial energies for the channels ($\sim$31 mJ m^{-2}) and stripes ($\sim$23 mJ m^{-2}) [96]. As a result, this type of mesostructured surface can be used as a template to guide the self-assembly of molecules and nanoparticles.

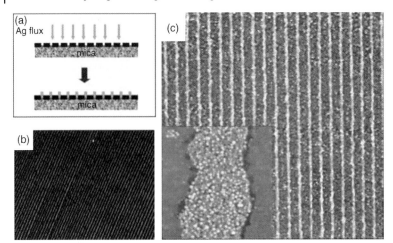

Figure 8.16 (a) Schematic illustration of the process for evaporating silver on structured surface and silver atoms deposit preferably onto channel regions; (b) Optical micrograph representing the regular stripe structure over an area of $80 \times 60\,\mu m^2$. The channels were filled with more silver coating (bright lines), whereas the DPPC stripes appeared dark (less silver); (c) The AFM image ($16 \times 16\,\mu m^2$) indicates that if a small amount of silver is evaporated ($<2\,nm$), then only the channel regions are fully covered, as shown in the inset. Reproduced with permission from Ref. [95].

For example, the $FeCl_3$ molecules which condensed from the vapor phase were adsorbed selectively in the channels, whereas the stripes were not coated when a small droplet of $FeCl_3$ solution was brought onto the structured mica surface. Channels filled with paramagnetic $FeCl_3$ molecules provided a contrast for magnetic force microscopy [60]. In another example, the selective adsorption of thermally evaporated silver ($2–3\,nm$) onto the channels was confirmed using optical microscopy [95] (Figure 8.16). In addition to metals and small molecules that show selective adsorption, Moraille and Badia found that proteins could also be adsorbed selectively onto the nanostriped surface formed by the mixed monolayer of DPPC and L-α-dilauroylphosphatidylcholine (DLPC) [97]. Moraille and Badia confirmed that human blood-plasma proteins (γ-globulin and serum albumin) could be adsorbed selectively to the channels of a nanostructured LB monolayer of DPPC/DLPC, so as to generate well-defined protein and Au nanoparticle/protein patterns. The DPPC mesostructures on oxygen plasma-treated silicon could be used as templates for the directed self-assembly of functional silane molecules to form robust chemical patterns [66]. In this case, a general approach was based on a substitution of the channels and stripes by two different silane molecules (NH_2- and CH_3-terminated silane) that were bound covalently to the surface. As a result, a striped pattern of covalently bound molecules with selective functionality replaced the physisorbed DPPC structure, after which the negatively charged Au_{55} clusters could be adsorbed selectively onto the NH_2-terminated silane stripes, due to an electrostatic interaction [66]. Moreover, the NH_2-terminated silane-striped pattern could be used as a template to assist the electrodeposition of regular arrays of copper nanowires [98].

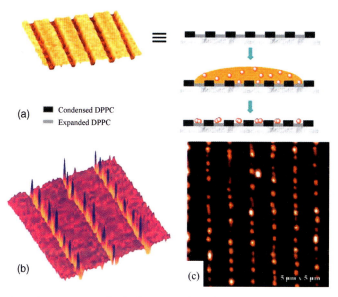

Figure 8.17 (a) Generalized schematic outline of the three steps used to pattern nanoparticles on DPPC stripe pattern. Selective deposition of (b) Au_{55} clusters and (c) CdSe nanocrystals aligned along the channels on a mica surface. Reproduced with permission from Ref. [23].

The DPPC stripe pattern may also serve as a template for the selective deposition of nanoparticles, simply by dropping the 1-phenyloctane solutions of nanoparticles onto the DPPC pattern, as shown in Figure 8.17. The work of adhesion of 1-phenyloctane on the channels was $62.0\,mJ\,m^{-2}$, and greater than that of 1-phenyloctane on the stripes ($53.7\,mJ\,m^{-2}$). As a result, the nanoparticles were found to accumulate in the expanded DPPC channels when the solution was removed from the sample surface after some time. The density of nanoparticle coverage was determined by the concentration of the nanoparticle solution and the duration of exposure to the patterned surface. As an example, quasi 1-D arrays (Figure 8.17b) of Au_{55} clusters stabilized by an organic ligand shell were generated [60]. Semiconductor nanocrystals showed a similar selective adsorption in the channels, as demonstrated by topographic and near-field optical fluorescence measurements (Figure 8.17c) [99, 100]. These examples showed, principally, that nanoparticles could be arranged in 1-D fashion in parallel manner over large areas. Furthermore, the CdSe nanocrystals could be selectively deposited into the green-emitting stripes formed by transferring mixed monolayers of DPPC and 2-(4,4-difluoro-5-methyl-4-bora-3a,4a-diaza-s-indacene-3-dodecanoyl)-1-hexadecanoyl-sn-glycero-3-phosphocholine (BODIPY) (0.5 mol%) onto mica surfaces, for which BODIPY molecules are distributed uniformly within the expanded DPPC channels [101]. Based on the photoinduced enhancement of fluorescence of CdSe nanocrystals and the photobleaching of dyes, a hierarchical luminescence pattern will be generated.

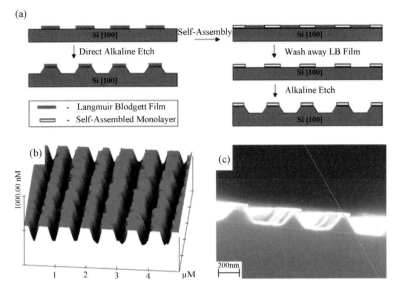

Figure 8.18 (a) Schematic illustration of the chemical-etch process used to transfer LB patterns into topographical features. Groove depth and local periodicity were characterized by (b) AFM, and (c) SEM. Reproduced with permission from Ref. [47].

8.5.2
Pattern Transfer: From Chemical to Topographic Patterns

Both, the self-organized DPPC LB patterns and other LB patterns formed (such as chiral domains) [46, 47] can be used as resistances against wet chemical etching, by employing a very dilute alkaline etchant (e.g., KOH) and a long etching time (~12 h). Such a process, which is referred to as "LB lithography" [47], allows the patterns to be converted into topographic features in silicon (Figure 8.18). In this way, an etch selectivity in excess of 100 (etch depth/resist thickness) can be achieved, while the depth of etching can be controlled at between 20 and 300 nm by varying the etch time.

The topographically patterned silicon obtained with LB lithography can be used as a "master" to generate replicas, by means of nanoimprinting and replica molding (Figure 8.19a) [47, 102]. This is of major interest to certain applications, such as the culturing of biological cells, where it is desirable to mass produce a large number of identical surfaces. In the first step of the process, the silicon master is placed in contact with the polymer under slight pressure, and the system is heated above the glass transition temperature (T_g) of the polymer. After cooling the polymer to below T_g, it is peeled from the master; after which the master can be re-used for the serial production of hundreds of replicas, without any noticeable reduction in quality.

In these studies, surface areas of polystyrene on the order of square centimeters were first topographically patterned using submicrometer-scale grooves, and then used to study the influence of surface texture on the morphology, mobility and differentiation of primary osteoblasts [47, 102]. In this case, cells cultured for 24 h on

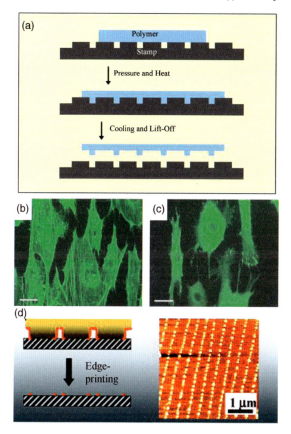

Figure 8.19 (a) Schematic process for pattern transfer from a silicon master to polystyrene. Fluorescence micrographs of osteoblasts aligned on 150 nm-deep grooves, labeled for (b) actin and (c) vinculin. Scale bar = 20 μm; (d) Edge printing of semiconductor nanocrystals by interfacial interaction controlled transport of CdTe nanocrystals. Reproduced with permission from Ref. [23].

grooved polystyrene surfaces with a periodicity of 500 nm were seen to align with the grooves (see Figure 8.19b and c). Notably, the osteoblasts showed a stronger alignment on the deeper grooves, though the numbers of cells attaching to structured surfaces with grooves of different depths (50 nm and 150 nm, and also on a smooth control) seemed to be unaffected by the nanotopography of the surface. Immuno-histochemical staining of the aligned cells confirmed the presence of focal adhesions at opposite ends of the aligned cells. A significant anisotropic migration was observed on both the 50 nm- and 150 nm-deep grooves, though to a greater extent on the deeper grooves [102]. In addition to osteoblasts, other types of cell, including the phyto-pathogenic fungi *Magnaporthe grisea* and *Pucinnia graminis*, were also shown to align on the grooved patterns fabricated by LB lithography [103]. Clearly, the ability to mass produce, on an economic basis, large surface areas patterned with different nanotopographies will create new opportunities to understand the mechanisms behind contact guidance, and to optimize such surfaces for biological applications.

These structured polystyrene surfaces can also be used as masters for the replica molding of polydimethoxysiloxane (PDMS) [104]. This could be achieved by pouring the PDMS precursors over the polystyrene topographies and curing at 60 °C (well below the T_g of polystyrene) for 2 h; the PDMS stamp could then be readily peeled from the polystyrene master. The main benefit of this two-step process is that the PDMS replica molding can be carried out in parallel, thus allowing a simple and rapid fabrication of numerous, low-cost identical copies. The structured PDMS could then be used for microcontact printing (μCP), for example to pattern CdTe nanocrystals on SiO_2/Si surfaces (Figure 8.19d) [104].

Lieber *et al.* developed a new nanolithographic process based on the LB patterning of aligned nanowires that can be used as masks for etching and deposition, so as to fabricate nanometer-scale lines over large areas (Figure 8.20) [105]. For this, the surfactant-stabilized core–shell nanowires with controlled diameter and shell dimensions were first aligned with nanometer- to micrometer-scale pitches, using the LB technique; they were then transferred onto planar substrates to form uniformly ordered parallel arrays. Following such transfer, reactive ion etching (RIE) with CHF_3 was carried out to remove the oxide shell on the sides and tops of the core–shell nanowires, and to transfer the line pattern to the underlying substrate surfaces. Using the same process, metals can be deposited using the aligned nanowires as shadow masks to create arrays of nanoscale wires. Finally, the nanowire masks are removed by isotropic wet etching and sonication so as to expose the etched or deposited parallel line features. When using this method, the feature sizes are comparable to state-of-the-art extreme UV lithography, and also approach the limits of electron-beam lithography and transfer lithography. The width, length, and pitches of the metal lines can be easily controlled via the synthesis of core–shell nanowires

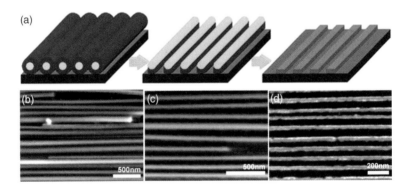

Figure 8.20 (a) Scheme for selective anisotropic etching of the oxide shell of core–shell nanowires and deposition of metal or other materials based on LB patterning nanowires. (b–d) Typical SEM images of (b) close-packed parallel Si-SiO₂ core–shell nanowires on silicon substrate surface; (c) parallel nanowires after selective, anisotropic etching of the SiO₂ shell by reactive ion etching; and (d) 15 nm-thick Cr metal lines following removal of the nanowire mask. Reproduced with permission from Ref. [105].

and a subsequent assembly process. In addition, the nanowires can be assembled in one step over areas of $20\,cm^2$, which is greater than that possible with most other unconventional lithographic methods. Hierarchical parallel nanowire arrays have also been prepared and used as masks to define nanometer pitch lines in $10 \times 10\,\mu m^2$ arrays, repeated with a $25\,\mu m$ array pitch over square-centimeter areas. This nanolithographic method represents a highly scalable and flexible route for defining nanometer-scale lines on multiple length scales, and thus has substantial potential for the fabrication of integrated nanosystems.

Using a similar approach, Choi *et al.* employed the structured Ag nanowire patterns [76] formed by the LB technique as resist masks to fabricate a parallel array of poly(methylmethacrylate) (PMMA) wire patterns [106] that were transferred onto PMMA-coated substrates, using a horizontal deposition method. The pattern was then amplified by immersing the substrate in a solution containing decanedithiol $(HSC_{10}H_{20}SH)$, followed by immersion of the substrate into a hexane/nanoparticle solution. Such amplification caused a slight increase in the width of the wires, and doubled their height to about 8 nm. Subsequently, 50 nm-wide and 10 nm-high PMMA wire patterns were obtained via spatially selective low-energy electron-beam exposure on the Ag nanocrystal wire shadow mask, and development, and a RIE process was then used to obtain 50 nm-wide silicon wires. This method would appear to represent a low-cost, high-throughput technique for the fabrication of semiconductor, nanometer-scale structures.

As an alternative, Meli *et al.* used the surface pattern formed by a PS-P2VP diblock copolymer as a mask to create an extensive array of nanometer-sized features [107] that were later used as stencil masks to generate quasi-hexagonal 2-D arrays of nanoscale gold islands [108]. These ultrathin masks have an intrinsic topology (which depends on the choice of block copolymer), ranging from about 10 to 100 nm in width and spacing. Straightforward argon ion milling of the gold-coated silicon and mica substrates, which had been covered with the ultrathin masks, resulted in arrays of ~25 nm-diameter gold islands, supported on patterned silicon pillars or gold islands that were directly adhered to a mica substrate. In a similar study, Seo *et al.* used this process to fabricate nickel pattern arrays that could be used to separate DNA [12] and, in particular, to eliminate the need for disposable separation media such as gels or polymer solutions that are susceptible to degradation and difficult to load into small devices due to their inherent high viscosity. By conducting molecular dynamics simulations and experiments, it was shown that this method could simultaneously separate a broad band of DNA fragments, ranging from a few hundred base-pairs to mega-base-pairs, without any loss in resolution. Furthermore, the technique required only very low loading amounts and operating voltages, making it amenable for incorporation into chip-based portable detectors or microarrays.

8.5.3
Integration of Nanomaterial Patterning in Nanodevice Fabrication

One fundamental step in the construction of 1-D nanomaterial devices is transfer of the nanomaterials from their stock to the substrate on top of which the device will be built. Hence, the correct alignment and controlled positioning of the 1-D nanomaterials are highly desirable, especially with regards to the large-scale (e.g., on a 10-cm wafer) fabrication of parallel device arrays. The integration of LB patterning with device fabrication fits this technological gap.

A general strategy for the parallel and scalable integration of nanowire devices over large areas, without the need to register individual nanowire-electrode interconnects, has been developed by the group of Lieber and involves a combination of the LB technique and photolithography (Figure 8.21) [109]. In this case, organized nanowires with controlled alignment and spacing over large areas were produced using the LB technique [94], and interconnects between the nanowires and electrodes defined by photolithography, in a statistical manner. Because the separation between nanowires assembled with the LB technique had a defined average value, but varied on the local scale, it was possible to achieve a high yield of metal electrode to nanowire contacts simply by setting the average nanowire separation equal to a value that was comparable to the electrode width. In this way, massive arrays containing thousands of single silicon nanowire field-effect transistors (FETs) were fabricated, and shown to exhibit not only a high performance and unprecedented reproducibility, but also a scalability to at least the 100 nm level. Moreover, scalable device characteristics could be demonstrated by interconnecting a controlled number of nanowires per transistor, in "pixel-like" device arrays. It is likely

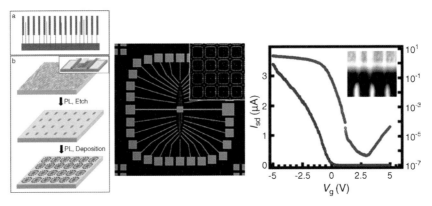

Figure 8.21 Left panel: Parallel and scalable interconnection of nanowire devices without registration. (a) Central electrode region of a single array, emphasizing the high fraction of interconnected nanowires (blue lines) obtained without the registration of individual electrodes; (b) Schematic illustrating key steps of the interconnection approach, including (top) the deposition of aligned nanowires with defined average spacing over the entire substrate, (middle) hierarchical patterning to produce fixed-size and -pitch parallel nanowire arrays, and (bottom) the deposition of a repeating metal electrode array using photolithography. Middle panel: Optical micrograph of integrated metal electrode arrays deposited on top of patterned parallel nanowire arrays defined by photolithography. Right panel: I_{sd} versus gate voltage (V_g) recorded for a typical device plotted on linear (blue) and log (red) scales at a V_{sd} of 1 V. The inset shows SEM images of higher-density nanowire devices, defined by electron-beam lithography. Reproduced with permission from Ref. [109].

that these highly reproducible transistor arrays will find use in many applications, ranging from multiplexed biosensing to information displays. The general applicability of the approach to other nanowire and nanotube building blocks should also enable the assembly, interconnection, and integration of a broad range of functional nanosystems.

In a later report, Dai *et al.* described the creation of densely aligned single-walled carbon nanotubes (SWCNTs), having used the LB technique for device integration [110]. This approach, which enabled the controlled assembly and integration of SWCNTs on a scale far beyond that achieved with an individual SWCNT, will undoubtedly prove important in the future electronics industry. In this procedure, the aligned SWNT monolayers were first transferred onto oxide substrates by the LB technique, followed by the fabrication of arrays of two-terminal devices with a Ti/Au metal source (S) and drain (D) that contacted massively parallel SWNTs in ~10 μm wide S–D regions, with a channel length of ~250 nm (Figure 8.22c and d). Subsequent current versus bias voltage (*I–V*) measurements showed that devices created from Hipco SWNTs were over 25-fold more resistive than similar devices prepared from laser-ablation SWNTs, with currents reaching ~0.13 and ~3.5 mA, respectively, at a bias of 3 V through the collective current carrying of SWNTs in parallel (Figure 8.22e and f). The Hipco SWNT devices also exhibited a greater nonlinearity in their *I–V* characteristics than did the laser-ablation nanotubes (Figure 8.22e). These characteristics were attributed to diameter differences between the Hipco and laser-ablation materials. The same process was also used for the integration of silver nanowires, where both nanowire density and line spacing can be programmed [111].

8.6
Conclusions and Outlook

Today, the fundamental challenge in the development of nanotechnology is the assembly of building blocks into organized nanostructures, albeit in controllable fashion. The use of LB patterning, as one branch of self-assembly and as discussed in this chapter, provides an effective and distinguished solution to the fabrication of high-ordered structures over larger areas. Compared to other assembly technique, such as self-assembly monolayers, layer-by-layer methods and vacuum molecular deposition, LB patterning incorporates certain unique properties. First, it allows the study of how the structural organization of different molecules at interfaces depends on changing various thermodynamic parameters such as temperature, film pressure, the chemical potential through employing different environments, molecular composition (whether single-component or multi-component), subphase composition, or by the controlled manipulation of certain transfer parameters, such as the speeds of transference and compression, and the method of transfer (whether vertical or horizontal). In addition, controlling the shape, size, and distribution of molecular assemblies in self-organized surface patterns will in turn lead to a controlled construction of 2-D supramolecular architectures. Thus, LB patterning can offer

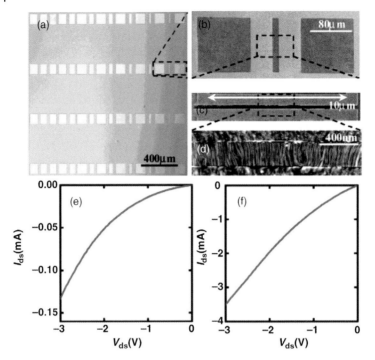

Figure 8.22 Microfabrication patterning and device integration of SWNT LB films. (a) Optical image of a patterned SWNT LB film. The squares and rectangles are regions containing densely aligned SWNTs. Other areas are SiO$_2$ substrate regions; (b) SEM image of a region highlighted in panel (a) with packed SWNTs aligned vertically; (c) SEM image showing a 10 μm-wide SWNT LB film between source and drain electrodes formed in a region marked in panel (b); (d) AFM image of a region in panel (c), showing aligned SWNTs and the edges of the S and D electrodes; (e) Current versus bias (I_{ds}–V_{ds}) curve of a device made from Hipco SWNTs (10 μm channel width and 250 nm channel length); (f) I_{ds}–V_{ds} of a device made from laser ablation SWNTs (10 μm channel width and 250 nm channel length). Reproduced with permission from Ref. [110].

a great opportunity to achieve control over nanoscale assembly by tuning a macroscopic property, whilst linking the LB technique with patterning and fabrication on a solid substrate.

In addition to expanding the types of building block used in LB patterning, including molecules, nanorods, nanotubes, and nanowires, there remain a number of unanswered questions. The first of these questions involves the orthogonal assembly of multicomponent building blocks with different functions into an integrated system, while the second question relates to the combination of LB patterning with other lithographic techniques, such as soft lithography and DPN, so as to enhance the capabilities of LB patterning. Finally, the integration of LB patterning into functional device architectures remains an important issue for practical applications.

References

1 Aizenberg, J., Black, A.J., and Whitesides, G.M. (1999) *Nature*, **398**, 495–498.

2 Kim, S.O., Solak, H.H., Stoykovich, M.P., Ferrier, N.J., de Pablo, J.J., and Nealey, P.F. (2003) *Nature*, **424**, 411–414.

3 Cavallini, M., Biscarini, F., Gomez-Segura, J., Ruiz, D., and Veciana, J. (2003) *Nano Lett.*, **3**, 1527–1530.

4 Jacobs, H.O., Tao, A.R., Schwartz, A., Gracias, D.H., and Whitesides, G.M. (2002) *Science*, **296**, 323–325.

5 Koide, Y., Wang, Q.W., Cui, J., Benson, D.D., and Marks, T.J. (2000) *J. Am. Chem. Soc.*, **122**, 11266–11267.

6 Kataoka, D.E. and Troian, S.M. (1999) *Nature*, **402**, 794–797.

7 Velev, O.D. and Kaler, E.W. (1999) *Langmuir*, **15**, 3693–3698.

8 Michel, R., Lussi, J.W., Csucs, G., Reviakine, I., Danuser, G., Ketterer, B., Hubbell, J.A., Textor, M., and Spencer, N.D. (2002) *Langmuir*, **18**, 3281–3287.

9 Harrison, D.J., Fluri, K., Seiler, K., Fan, Z.H., Effenhauser, C.S., and Manz, A. (1993) *Science*, **261**, 895–897.

10 Delamarche, E., Bernard, A., Schmid, H., Michel, B., and Biebuyck, H. (1997) *Science*, **276**, 779–781.

11 Volkmuth, W.D. and Austin, R.H. (1992) *Nature*, **358**, 600–602.

12 Seo, Y.S., Luo, H., Samuilov, V.A., Rafailovich, M.H., Sokolov, J., Gersappe, D., and Chu, B. (2004) *Nano Lett.*, **4**, 659–664.

13 Fan, Y.W., Cui, F.Z., Hou, S.P., Xu, Q.Y., Chen, L.N., and Lee, I.S. (2002) *J. Neurosci. Methods*, **120**, 17–23.

14 Xu, C.Y., Inai, R., Kotaki, M., and Ramakrishna, S. (2004) *Biomaterials*, **25**, 877–886.

15 Abbott, N.L., Folkers, J.P., and Whitesides, G.M. (1992) *Science*, **257**, 1380–1382.

16 Kramer, S., Fuierer, R.R., and Gorman, C.B. (2003) *Chem. Rev.*, **103**, 4367–4418.

17 Nyffenegger, R.M. and Penner, R.M. (1997) *Chem. Rev.*, **97**, 1195–1230.

18 Chou, S.Y., Krauss, P.R., and Renstrom, P.J. (1996) *Science*, **272**, 85–87.

19 Xia, Y.N. and Whitesides, G.M. (1998) *Annu. Rev. Mater. Sci.*, **28**, 153–184.

20 Park, M., Harrison, C., Chaikin, P.M., Register, R.A., and Adamson, D.H. (1997) *Science*, **276**, 1401–1404.

21 Schaffer, E., Thurn-Albrecht, T., Russell, T.P., and Steiner, U. (2000) *Nature*, **403**, 874–877.

22 Spatz, J.P., Roescher, A., and Moller, M. (1996) *Adv. Mater.*, **8**, 337–340.

23 Chen, X.D., Lenhert, S., Hirtz, M., Lu, N., Fuchs, H., and Chi, L.F. (2007) *Acc. Chem. Res.*, **40**, 393–401.

24 Franklin, B. (1774) *Philos. Trans. R. Soc.*, **64**, 445.

25 Rayleigh, L. (1890) *Proc. R. Soc.*, **47**, 364.

26 Pockels, A. (1891) *Nature*, **43**, 437.

27 Langmuir, I. (1917) *J. Am. Chem. Soc.*, **39**, 1848–1906.

28 Blodgett, K.B. (1935) *J. Am. Chem. Soc.*, **57**, 1007–1022.

29 Gains, L.G. (1969) *Insoluble Monolayers at Liquid-Gas Interfaces*, Interscience Publishers, New York.

30 Roberts, G. (1990) *Langmuir-Blodgett Films*, Plenum Press, New York.

31 Kjaer, K., Alsnielsen, J., Helm, C.A., Laxhuber, L.A., and Mohwald, H. (1987) *Phys. Rev. Lett.*, **58**, 2224–2227.

32 Losche, M. and Mohwald, H. (1984) *Rev. Sci. Instrum.*, **55**, 1968–1972.

33 Henon, S. and Meunier, J. (1991) *Rev. Sci. Instrum.*, **62**, 936–939.

34 Honig, D. and Mobius, D. (1991) *J. Phys. Chem.*, **95**, 4590–4592.

35 McConnell, H.M. (1991) *Annu. Rev. Phys. Chem.*, **42**, 171–195.

36 Mohwald, H. (1990) *Annu. Rev. Phys. Chem.*, **41**, 441–476.

37 Chi, L.F., Anders, M., Fuchs, H., Johnston, R., and Ringsdorf, H. (1993) *Science*, **259**, 213–216.

38 Chi, L.F., Eng, L.M., Graf, K., and Fuchs, H. (1992) *Langmuir*, **8**, 2255–2261.

39 Kato, T., Kameyama, M., Ehara, M., and Iimura, K. (1998) *Langmuir*, **14**, 1786–1798.

40 Trabelsi, S., Zhang, S.S., Zhang, Z.C., Lee, T.R., and Schwartz, D.K. (2009) *Soft Matter*, **5**, 750–758.

41 Fontaine, P., Goldmann, M., Muller, P., Faure, M.C., Konovalov, O., and Krafft, M.P. (2005) *J. Am. Chem. Soc.*, **127**, 512–513.

42 Zhang, G., Marie, P., Maaloum, M., Muller, P., Benoit, N., and Krafft, M.P. (2005) *J. Am. Chem. Soc.*, **127**, 10412–10419.

43 Maaloum, M., Muller, P., and Krafft, M.P. (2002) *Angew. Chem., Int. Ed.*, **41**, 4331–4334.

44 Huang, X., Li, C., Jiang, S.G., Wang, X.S., Zhang, B.W., and Liu, M.H. (2004) *J. Am. Chem. Soc.*, **126**, 1322–1323.

45 Zhang, Y., Chen, P., Jiang, L., Hu, W., and Liu, M. (2009) *J. Am. Chem. Soc.*, **131**, 2756–2757.

46 Zhang, L., Gaponik, N., Muller, J., Plate, U., Weller, H., Erker, G., Fuchs, H., Rogach, A.L., and Chi, L.F. (2005) *Small*, **1**, 524–527.

47 Lenhert, S., Zhang, L., Mueller, J., Wiesmann, H.P., Erker, G., Fuchs, H., and Chi, L.F. (2004) *Adv. Mater.*, **16**, 619–624.

48 Chunbo, Y., Xinmin, L., Desheng, D., Bin, L., Hongjie, Z., Zuhong, L., Juzheng, L., and Jiazuan, N. (1996) *Surf. Sci.*, **366**, L729–L734.

49 Chi, L.F., Jacobi, S., Anczykowski, B., Overs, M., Schafer, H.J., and Fuchs, H. (2000) *Adv. Mater.*, **12**, 25–30.

50 Powers, E.T., Yang, S.I., Lieber, C.M., and Kelly, J.W. (2002) *Angew. Chem., Int. Ed.*, **41**, 127–130.

51 Iimura, K., Shiraku, T., and Kato, T. (2002) *Langmuir*, **18**, 10183–10190.

52 Imae, T., Takeshita, T., and Kato, M. (2000) *Langmuir*, **16**, 612–621.

53 Zhu, J.Y., Eisenberg, A., and Lennox, R.B. (1991) *J. Am. Chem. Soc.*, **113**, 5583–5588.

54 Zhu, J., Eisenberg, A., and Lennox, R.B. (1992) *Macromolecules*, **25**, 6556–6562.

55 Li, S., Hanley, S., Khan, I., Varshney, S.K., Eisenberg, A., and Lennox, R.B. (1993) *Langmuir*, **9**, 2243–2246.

56 Baker, S.M., Leach, K.A., Devereaux, C.E., and Gragson, D.E. (2000) *Macromolecules*, **33**, 5432–5436.

57 Devereaux, C.A. and Baker, S.M. (2002) *Macromolecules*, **35**, 1921–1927.

58 Gamboa, A.L.S., Filipe, E.J.M., and Brogueira, P. (2002) *Nano Lett.*, **2**, 1083–1086.

59 Seo, Y.S., Kim, K.S., Galambos, A., Lammertink, R.G.H., Vancso, G.J., Sokolov, J., and Rafailovich, M. (2004) *Nano Lett.*, **4**, 483–486.

60 Gleiche, M., Chi, L.F., and Fuchs, H. (2000) *Nature*, **403**, 173–175.

61 Spratte, K., Chi, L.F., and Riegler, H. (1994) *Europhys. Lett.*, **25**, 211–217.

62 Chen, X.D., Lu, N., Zhang, H., Hirtz, M., Wu, L.X., Fuchs, H., and Chi, L.F. (2006) *J. Phys. Chem. B*, **110**, 8039–8046.

63 Lenhert, S., Gleiche, M., Fuchs, H., and Chi, L.F. (2005) *ChemPhysChem*, **6**, 2495–2498.

64 Chen, X.D., Hirtz, M., Fuchs, H., and Chi, L.F. (2007) *Langmuir*, **23**, 2280–2283.

65 Hirtz, M., Fuchs, H., and Chi, L.F. (2008) *J. Phys. Chem. B*, **112**, 824–827.

66 Lu, N., Gleiche, M., Zheng, J.W., Lenhert, S., Xu, B., Chi, L.F., and Fuchs, H. (2002) *Adv. Mater.*, **14**, 1812–1815.

67 Chen, X.D., Hirtz, M., Fuchs, H., and Chi, L.F. (2005) *Adv. Mater.*, **17**, 2881–2885.

68 Markovich, G., Collier, C.P., Henrichs, S.E., Remacle, F., Levine, R.D., and Heath, J.R. (1999) *Acc. Chem. Res.*, **32**, 415–423.

69 Brust, M., Stuhr-Hansen, N., Norgaard, K., Christensen, J.B., Nielsen, L.K., and Bjornholm, T. (2001) *Nano Lett.*, **1**, 189–191.

70 Song, H., Kim, F., Connor, S., Somorjai, G.A., and Yang, P.D. (2005) *J. Phys. Chem. B*, **109**, 188–193.

71 Huang, S.J., Tsutsui, G., Sakaue, H., Shingubara, S., and Takahagi, T. (2001) *J. Vac. Sci. Technol. B*, **19**, 115–120.

72 Chen, S.W. (2001) *Langmuir*, **17**, 2878–2884.

73 Tian, Y.C. and Fendler, J.H. (1996) *Chem. Mater.*, **8**, 969–974.

74 Paul, S., Pearson, C., Molloy, A., Cousins, M.A., Green, M., Kolliopoulou, S., Dimitrakis, P., Normand, P., Tsoukalas, D., and Petty, M.C. (2003) *Nano Lett.*, **3**, 533–536.

75 Tao, A.R., Huang, J.X., and Yang, P.D. (2008) *Acc. Chem. Res.*, **41**, 1662–1673.

76 Chung, S.W., Markovich, G., and Heath, J.R. (1998) *J. Phys. Chem. B*, **102**, 6685–6687.

77 Sear, R.P., Chung, S.W., Markovich, G., Gelbart, W.M., and Heath, J.R. (1999) *Phys. Rev. E*, **59**, R6255–R6258.

78 Huang, J.X., Kim, F., Tao, A.R., Connor, S., and Yang, P.D. (2005) *Nat. Mater.*, **4**, 896–900.

79 Huang, J.X., Tao, A.R., Connor, S., He, R.R., Yang, P.D. (2006) *Nano Lett.*, **6**, 524–529.

80 Vidoni, O., Reuter, T., Torma, V., Meyer-Zaika, W., and Schmid, G. (2001) *J. Mater. Chem.*, **11**, 3188–3190.

81 Hassenkam, T., Norgaard, K., Iversen, L., Kiely, C.J., Brust, M., and Bjornholm, T. (2002) *Adv. Mater.*, **14**, 1126–1130.

82 Reuter, T., Vidoni, O., Torma, V., Schmid, G., Lu, N., Gleiche, M., Chi, L.F., and Fuchs, H. (2002) *Nano Lett.*, **2**, 709–711.

83 Chi, L.F., Rakers, S., Hartig, M., Gleiche, M., Fuchs, H., and Schmid, G. (2000) *Colloids Surf. A.*, **17** (1), 241–248.

84 Lu, N., Zheng, J.W., Gleiche, M., Fuchs, H., Chi, L.F., Vidoni, O., Reuter, T., and Schmid, G. (2002) *Nano Lett.*, **2**, 1097–1099.

85 Haynes, C.L. and Van Duyne, R.P. (2001) *J. Phys. Chem. B*, **105**, 5599–5611.

86 Fahmi, A.W., Oertel, U., Steinert, V., Froeck, C., and Stamm, M. (2003) *Macromol. Rapid Comm.*, **24**, 625–629.

87 Li, L.S., Jin, J., Yu, S., Zhao, Y.Y., Zhang, C.X., and Li, T.J. (1998) *J. Phys. Chem. B*, **102**, 5648–5652.

88 Cheyne, R.B. and Moffitt, M.G. (2005) *Langmuir*, **21**, 10297–10300.

89 Kim, F., Kwan, S., Akana, J., and Yang, P.D. (2001) *J. Am. Chem. Soc*, **123**, 4360–4361.

90 Yang, P.D. and Kim, F. (2002) *ChemPhysChem*, **3**, 503–506.

91 Kwan, S., Kim, F., Akana, J., and Yang, P.D. (2001) *Chem. Commun.*, 447–448.

92 Tao, A., Kim, F., Hess, C., Goldberger, J., He, R.R., Sun, Y.G., Xia, Y.N., and Yang, P.D. (2003) *Nano Lett.*, **3**, 1229–1233.

93 Tao, A.R. and Yang, P.D. (2005) *J. Phys. Chem. B*, **109**, 15687–15690.

94 Whang, D., Jin, S., Wu, Y., and Lieber, C.M. (2003) *Nano Lett.*, **3**, 1255–1259.

95 Gleiche, M., Chi, L.F., Gedig, E., and Fuchs, H. (2001) *ChemPhysChem*, **2**, 187–191.

96 Berger, C.E.H., Vanderwerf, K.O., Kooyman, R.P.H., Degrooth, B.G., and Greve, J. (1995) *Langmuir*, **11**, 4188–4192.

97 Moraille, P. and Badia, A. (2002) *Angew. Chem., Int. Ed.*, **41**, 4303–4306.

98 Zhang, M.Z., Lenhert, S., Wang, M., Chi, L.F., Lu, N., Fuchs, H., and Ming, N.B. (2004) *Adv. Mater.*, **16**, 409–413.

99 Lu, N., Chen, X.D., Molenda, D., Naber, A., Fuchs, H., Talapin, D.V., Weller, H., Muller, J., Lupton, J.M., Feldmann, J., Rogach, A.L., and Chi, L.F. (2004) *Nano Lett.*, **4**, 885–888.

100 Naber, A., Molenda, D., Fischer, U.C., Maas, H.J., Hoppener, C., Lu, N., and Fuchs, H. (2002) *Phys. Rev. Lett.*, **89**, 210801.

101 Chen, X.D., Rogach, A.L., Talapin, D.V., Fuchs, H., and Chi, L.F. (2006) *J. Am. Chem. Soc.*, **128**, 9592–9593.

102 Lenhert, S., Meier, M.B., Meyer, U., Chi, L.F., and Wiesmann, H.P. (2005) *Biomaterials*, **26**, 563–570.

103 Lenhert, S., Semsa, A., Hirtz, M., Chi, L.F., Fuchs, H., Wiesmann, H.P., Osbourn, A.E., and Moerschbacher, B.M. (2007) *Langmuir*, **23**, 10216.

104 Wu, X.C., Lenhert, S., Chi, L.F., and Fuchs, H. (2006) *Langmuir*, **22**, 7807–7811.

105 Whang, D., Jin, S., and Lieber, C.M. (2003) *Nano Lett.*, **3**, 951–954.

106 Choi, S.H., Wang, K.L., Leung, M.S., Stupian, G.W., Presser, N., Chung, S.W., Markovich, G., Kim, S.H., and Heath, J.R. (1999) *J. Vac. Sci. Technol. A*, **17**, 1425–1427.

107 Meli, M.V., Badia, A., Grutter, P., and Lennox, R.B. (2002) *Nano Lett.*, **2**, 131–135.

108 Meli, M.V. and Lennox, R.B. (2003) *Langmuir*, **19**, 9097–9100.

109 Jin, S., Whang, D.M., McAlpine, M.C., Friedman, R.S., Wu, Y., and Lieber, C.M. (2004) *Nano Lett.*, **4**, 915–919.

110 Li, X.L., Zhang, L., Wang, X.R., Shimoyama, I., Sun, X.M., Seo, W.S., and Dai, H.J. (2007) *J. Am. Chem. Soc.*, **129**, 4890–4891.

111 Huang, J.X., Fan, R., Connor, S., and Yang, P.D. (2007) *Angew. Chem., Int. Ed.*, **46**, 2414–2417.

9
Surface-Supported Nanostructures Directed by Atomic- and Molecular-Level Templates

Dingyong Zhong, Haiming Zhang, and Lifeng Chi

9.1
Introduction

Shrinking the size of devices to nanoscale, and discovering new phenomena of objects at the nanoscale, represent the two main goals of nanotechnology in both academia and industry. Unfortunately, the traditional photolithographic techniques that have been used widely to create patterns of characteristic size in the micrometer scale, encounter bottlenecks when attempts are made to further reduce the size to the nanoscale, due to the diffractive effect of light. Many so-called "top-down" methods of fabrication, which include electron-beam lithography (EBL), imprinting, contact printing, and scanning probe lithography, have been developed during the past two decades. Whilst such techniques have the advantage of producing patterns with sizes that, characteristically, are smaller than 100 nm, their low throughput and/or poor reproducibility limits their application.

In contrast to the top-down techniques, "bottom-up" techniques utilize the self-assembly of nanosized objects such as atoms, molecules and nanoparticles, from which ordered structures in the nanoscale are built. Moreover, by adjusting the interactions between the nanosized objects and certain kinetic parameters, such as the growth temperature and rate, the process of self-assembly can easily be controlled to produce final phases with desired architectures. The characteristic sizes of these self-assembled architectures, which range from a few nanometers to tens of nanometers, are below the limitations of traditional patterning techniques. Nonetheless, although routine industrial applications might still be a long way off, patterning techniques based on self-assembly continue to show much promise, based on their ability to control the utilization of small entities such atoms, molecules, or nanoparticles.

Self-assembly processes directed by surface-supported templates are widely used to build architectures of functional materials. For this technique, the substrate surfaces are pre-patterned in order to modulate – either thermodynamically or kinetically – the aggregation of certain nanosized objects at specific sites and/or orientations. One type of natural template with an atomic order is the crystalline surface (Figure 9.1), where the atomic periodicities of an original surface are several angstroms, whilst reconstructions and reconstruction-induced patterns have a

Nanotechnology, Volume 8: Nanostructured Surfaces. Edited by Lifeng Chi
Copyright © 2010 WILEY-VCH Verlag GmbH & Co. KGaA, Weinheim
ISBN: 978-3-527-31739-4

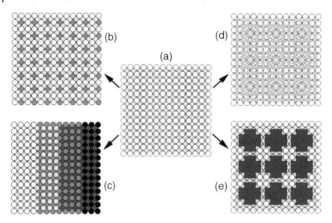

Figure 9.1 Atomic and molecular level templates on surfaces. (a) Original surface with 2-D lattice; (b) Reconstructed surface; (c) Vicinal surface; (d) Strain-relief epitaxial layer; (e) Supramolecular network.

periodicity of several nanometers. Furthermore, the vicinal surfaces with a periodic succession of terraces and steps may have a periodicity ranging from several nanometers to tens of nanometers. These natural templates, as well as self-assembled supramolecular structures and strain-relief epitaxial layers on surfaces, are used to direct the formation of further surface-supported nanostructures.

Scanning tunneling microscopy (STM) is a powerful tool that can be used to visualize nanostructured surfaces. In this process, a sharp conductive tip is positioned near the surface of a conductive sample. With a typical gap of 0.5–1 nm, the electron wave functions of the tip and the surface overlap, such that a tunneling current is created when a voltage bias is applied between the tip and the sample. The tunneling current is relevant to the local density of states on the surface, and is also very sensitive to the gap width. By keeping the current constant and varying the height of the tip, with the help of a piezoelectric system and feedback electronics, the tip is allowed to scan the sample surface such that a topographic image of the surface is obtained with ∼0.1 nm lateral resolution, and ∼0.01 nm height resolution.

For simplicity, this chapter contain two parts detailing two-dimensional (2-D) atomic- and molecular-level templates, and nanostructure formation as directed by the templates. Initially, the different types of template, including reconstructed surfaces, vicinal surfaces, strain-relief epitaxial layers and supramolecular assemblies, will be introduced, after which the formation of surface-supported nanostructures guided by the templates will be discussed. Throughout the chapter, emphasis will be placed on organic and organic–inorganic hybrid nanostructures.

9.2
Atomic- and Molecular-Level Templates on Surfaces

The root of atomic- and molecular-level templates is the periodic arrangement of atoms and molecules in crystalline structures. Such periodic arrangement is reflected by the 2-D lattices of single crystalline surfaces. In order to template the formation of nanostructures, a "clean" surface is required under a well-controlled environment, for example under ultra-high-vacuum (UHV) conditions, or in specific solutions. Methods to obtain ordered and clean surfaces include the cleavage of certain crystals (notably layered materials such as graphite, mica and MoS_2), sputtering–annealing cycles for metals, and high-temperature flashing for semiconductors, such as silicon.

9.2.1
Surface Reconstructions and Reconstruction-Related Patterns

Similar to the structure in the bulk, the atomic periodicities of an original surface are several angstroms. However, due to the absence of neighboring atoms on one side of a surface, the first few layers of atoms beneath the surface will be reorganized so as to achieve an equilibrium state with lower surface free energy, and this will result in surface reconstruction. Several well-known surface reconstructions, including Si(111)-7 $\times$ 7, Au(111)-22 $\times \sqrt{3}$ and Cu(110)-(2 $\times$ 1)O, are briefly introduced in the following subsections.

9.2.1.1 Si(111)-7 $\times$ 7

The Si(111)-7 $\times$ 7 was the first surface reconstruction to be visualized by STM [1]. To prepare the Si(111)-7 $\times$ 7 reconstruction, the Si(111) surface is etched with HF solution to remove the native oxide layer on the surface. The Si(111) surface is then heated repeatedly to about ~1200 K under UHV conditions, which causes the atoms of the outermost atomic layers to reorganize and to form a structure with a hexagonal unit cell, the lattice constant of which is 2.7 nm. The surface atoms are rearranged in such a way that the number of dangling bonds is minimized. The unit cell of the reconstruction contains 12 adatoms, nine dimers, and a stacking fault layer based on the DAS model proposed by K. Takayanagi *et al.* [2, 3].

9.2.1.2 Au(111)-22 $\times \sqrt{3}$ and the Herringbone Pattern

In the Au(111)-22 $\times \sqrt{3}$ reconstruction, the first hexagonally arranged atomic layer of Au(111) is compressed with 23 atoms stacked on 22 bulk lattice sites along the [01-1] direction. As a result, alternative stripes of domains with face-centered cubic (*fcc*) and hexagonal-close-packed (*hcp*) stacking styles running along the perpendicular [−211] direction are formed (Figure 9.2). The two types of domain are gradually transited with a height difference of 0.02 nm. The reconstruction has a rectangle unit cell with a periodicity in [01-1] of 6.34 nm and in [−211] of 0.416 nm. Corresponding to the threefold symmetry of the Au(111) surface, there are three equivalent orientations of the stripes by 120° rotation. The orientational domains coexist, and their boundaries merge in such a way that transition from one domain to another occurs through a correlated periodic bending of the parallel stripes, and this results in a zigzag or "herringbone" pattern. The herringbone structure changes the orientation over distances of up to 25 nm as a result of long-range elastic lattice strain [4, 5].

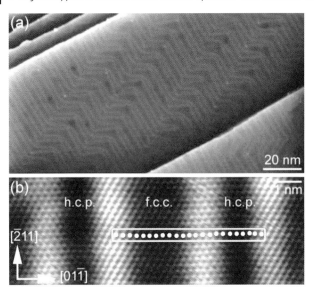

Figure 9.2 Au(111) 22 × √3 reconstruction. (a) Large-scale STM image showing the herringbone pattern; (b) High-resolution STM image showing the *hcp* and *fcc* regions. The unit cell of the reconstruction is denoted by the rectangle.

9.2.1.3 Cu(110)-(2 × 1)O and the Stripe Pattern

Although no reconstruction exists at a clean Cu(110) surface, the controlled condensation of oxygen atoms on the surfaces results in a 2 × 1 added-row reconstruction. The O atoms are chemisorbed on the surface, while the Cu adatoms evaporate from steps and diffuse across the terraces of the substrate surface [6, 7]. In this construction, Cu atom rows are added along the [001] direction with a distance of 0.51 nm, and O atoms are adsorbed at the long-bridge sites in the rows (Figure 9.3a). Depending on the O atom coverage, full or partial coverage of the adsorbate-induced reconstruction can be obtained. By exposing a clean Cu(110) surface to 4–6 Langmuir (1 Langmuir = 10^{-6} Torr·s) of oxygen at 625 K, the stripe pattern with alternating stripes of bare Cu and (2 × 1)O reconstructed regions along the [001] direction are obtained, as shown in Figure 9.3b and c [8, 9]. The dimensions of the stripe structure may be adjusted by controlling the oxidation process; that is, the temperature and exposure dose. The width and distance of the stripes are increased when the process temperature is increased, whereas an increase in exposure will result in narrower stripes. For instance, stripe patterns with long-range order on the length scale of several hundred nanometers consisting of bare Cu troughs 2.0 ± 0.3 nm wide, separated by Cu–O regions 5 ± 2 nm wide have been obtained (Figure 9.3b and c).

9.2.2
Strain-Relief Epitaxial Layers

In heteroepitaxial systems exhibiting large lattice mismatch, the substrate lattice is not strictly followed by the epitaxial layer, and this results in the generation of dense

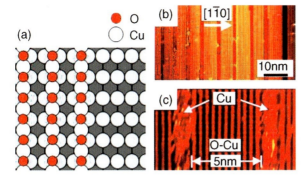

Figure 9.3 Cu(110)-(2 × 1)O: Nanostripes of Cu(110) and Cu(110)-(2 × 1)O reconstruction regions. (a) Schematic of the oxygen-induced added-row reconstruction; (b, c), STM images of the stripe patterns containing alternative bare Cu(110) regions and oxygen-induced 2 × 1 reconstruction regions, respectively [8].

dislocations to relieve large strain in the systems. Due to interactions between the epitaxial layer and the substrate lattice, and the high mobility of dislocations located at the surfaces, the dislocations quite often arrange into highly ordered periodic patterns. In other words, the epitaxial layer prefers to form a large superstructure that is commensurate with the substrate. Such superstructures, showing periodicities of several nanometers, will further modulate surface processes such as adsorption, diffusion, and the nucleation of adatoms or molecules deposited onto the strain-relief epitaxial layers.

9.2.2.1 Boron Nitride Nanomesh

Analogous to carbon solids, covalent-bonded boron nitride exists in a variety of structures, including graphitic hexagonal boron nitride (h-BN) and diamond-like cubic boron nitride (c-BN). Ultrathin h-BN films are formed on certain metallic surfaces by chemical vapor deposition (CVD). For example, large terraces of h-BN films with monolayer thickness are formed on Ni(111), which shows a lattice mismatch of 0.4% with the h-BN layer [10]. The honeycomb-structured h-BN films show little corrugation with the N atoms located on top of the outermost Ni atoms and the B atoms on *fcc* adsorption sites of the Ni(111) surface. In case of substrates with large lattice misfit, an obvious corrugation appears in the epitaxial h-BN film, resulting in ordered superstructures with a periodicity of several nanometers [11, 12]. By exposing a Rh(111) surface kept at a temperature of 1070 K to a borazine (HBNH)$_3$ vapor pressure of 3×10^{-7} mbar for about 2 min (40 L), an h-BN film with a regular nanomesh would be formed (as shown in Figure 9.4) [11]. The hexagonal nanomesh has a periodicity of 3.22 nm, with pores of 2 nm diameter; this corresponds to a commensurate lattice of (13 × 13) h-BN units on a (12 × 12) Rh lattice spacing. The mismatch between the h-BN layer (0.248 nm) and the Rh(111) surface (0.269 nm) plays a key role in the nanomesh formation. Based on experimental results and density functional theory (DFT) calculations, it has been proposed that the nanomesh would consist of one layer of h-BN that would be

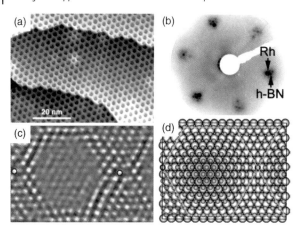

Figure 9.4 Hexagonal boron nitride (h-BN) nanomesh. (a) Large-area constant-current STM image (−1.0 V, 2.5 nA, at room temperature) of the boron nitride nanomesh formed by high-temperature decomposition of borazine on a Rh(111) surface; (b) Low-energy electron diffraction (LEED) pattern from h-BN nanomesh (40-L exposure) on Rh(111). The principal diffraction spots of the Rh(111) surface and h-BN (arrowed) are accompanied with satellite nanomesh superlattice spots. Electron energy: 92 eV; (c) Low-frequency filtered STM image (−2 mV, 1 nA, at 77 K) showing the atomic corrugation. Bright protrusions indicate N atoms; (d) Atomic structures of the h-BN nanomesh on Rh(111) (Green: N; orange: B; gray: Rh) [11, 14].

strongly corrugated due to mismatch with the substrate [13, 14]. The N atoms of the h-BN layer in holes occupy the on-top sites, which are the energetically favorable sites for h-BN grown on a metal surface, whereas the locations of the N atoms from the surrounding of holes will deviate from the on-top sites, owing to the large lattice misfit (6.7%) (see Figure 9.4d). Besides Rh(111), similar nanomesh has been observed on Ru(0001) [12].

9.2.2.2 Ag/Pt(111)

The double atomic-layer of Ag on Pt(111) is another example of superstructures induced by mismatched epitaxy. Since the lattice constant of Ag is 4.3% larger than that of Pt, the first commensurate monolayer of Ag on Pt(111) is coherently strained. The second monolayer of Ag, on the other hand, forms an ordered trigonal network of dislocations to partially relieve the compressive strain. Domains with *fcc* and *hcp* stacking coexist in the second monolayer. The unit cell of the superstructure with trigonal symmetry has an average periodicity of 4.5 nm consisting of a large quasi-hexagon (*fcc* stacking) and two triangles with opposite orientation (*hcp* stacking) [15, 16]. The strained stacking styles in the epitaxial Ag film show effect on certain processes such as surface diffusion, nucleation, and reaction activity [15, 17]. The stability of the strain-relief pattern is enhanced by removing about 0.1 mono-loayer (ML) of the Ag top layer of this surface structure by He- or Ar-ion sputtering. As a result, a hexagonally well-ordered, room-temperature-stable array of 1 ML-deep holes with a tunable size of about 4 nm² and a fixed spacing of 7 nm was fabricated [18]. In this process, the *hcp*-stacked Ag atoms in the triangle-shaped domains were removed. A similar hole array has been obtained by exposing a strained monolayer-thick Ag layer on Ru(0001), in which a superstructure with a periodicity of about 4–6 nm was formed due to the 7% lattice mismatch, to sulfur at room temperature. In this way, the Ag atoms at dislocated regions could be selectively replaced by S atoms [19, 20].

9.2.3
Vicinal Surfaces

Vicinal surfaces (also known as "high-index surfaces") on which a periodic succession of terraces and steps of monoatomic height exist, are obtained by cutting crystals along a plane that deviates by a small angle from a low-index plane. Such structural anisotropy may be represented in macroscopic physical proper-ties [21]. In comparison to a low-index surface, the high step density increases the surface energy and makes the vicinal surfaces metastable, and tends towards to faceting with the formation of macroscopic low-index surfaces in low-temperature limits. Nevertheless, the stepped vicinal surfaces may be available at low tempera-tures if the kinetics of reordering is too slow (owing to the reduced temperatures), so as to allow a transition from a stepped-back to a faceted morphology. At high temperature, the entropy of the steps provides a substantial contribution to the balance of free energy, and the formation of an ordered vicinal surface may minimize the total surface free energy. The entropy, which provides a mechanism for step–step repulsion, also plays an important role in the regularity of the step arrangement on a vicinal surface [22]. However, a roughing transition may take place if the temperature exceeds a critical transition point, which is variable for different systems. For instance, the transition temperature is 290 K for vicinal Cu $(11n)$ $(n = 13, 19, 79)$ surfaces [23] and 465 K for Ag(115) surfaces [24]. To an annealing temperature above 900 K, faceting takes place on a Pt(997) vicinal surface [25].

Besides the step–step interactions, the surface morphology of vicinal surfaces is affected by thermal kink creation energies [26]. For example, highly ordered step arrays are obtained on a vicinal Si(111) surface about $1°$ miscut toward $[-1\,-1\,2]$. As the kink width is half a 7×7 unit cell (2.3 nm), the energy barrier for creating a kink is very high and the step edges are atomically straight up to 2×10^4 lattice sites [27]. Furthermore, adsorbate-induced faceting takes place on certain vicinal surfaces. The adsorption of O on a vicinal Ag(110) misoriented $2°$ toward [001] or $[3 -3\,1]$ induces faceting of the surface, with the formation of large (110) facets and step-bunching [28]. Step-doubling takes place on a Pt(997) surface by annealing the surface to 700 K at an oxygen atmosphere for a few minutes [25].

9.2.3.1 Vicinal Au(111) Surfaces
The vicinal Au(111) surfaces are briefly introduced as an example in this section (for detailed discussions, see Ref. [30]). Two types of steps running along $[0 -1\,1]$, with {111} and {100} microfacets, are obtained by miscutting toward $[-2\,1\,1]$ and $[2 -1\,-1]$,

respectively. Among these vicinal surfaces misoriented with an angle up to 12°, the (322), (755), and (233) surfaces are stable with unreconstructed terraces, while the (788) and (11 12 12) surfaces are stable with reconstructed terraces. However, some vicinal surfaces, including (455), (577), and (12 11 11), are unstable and undergo faceting with "hill-and-valley" morphology. As a result, facets with two or more stable orientations coexist on the surface may be self-organized into a larger periodicity from 10 nm to a few hundreds of nanometers. The Au(788) and Au(11, 12, 12) surfaces, which are misoriented by 3.5° and 2.3° with respect to the (111) towards the [−211] direction, are regularly stepped surfaces with monoatomic {111} microfacets and reconstructed terraces, which are 3.9 and 5.8 nm in width, respectively (Figure 9.5). In this way, a very narrow terrace width distribution with a 0.85 nm full width at half-maximum (FWHM) has been obtained [30]. The discommensuration lines on the terraces run perpendicular to the step edges. Due to the partial release of the stress by the steps, the reconstruction along the steps is greater on the vicinal area than that on wide Au(111) terraces. Meanwhile, the discommensuration lines are disturbed by the steps and no longer run perpendicular to the close-packed direction, forming a "V" shape (see Figure 9.5d). The *fcc* domain width decreases when approaching the upper part of the step, and this is consistent with the fact that the *fcc* domain should be larger near the bottom of the step, since it is the bulk stacking of gold. Although the periodicity along the [−211] direction – that is, the terrace width – is dependent on the miscutting angle, the periodicity along the [0 −1 1] direction originated from the reconstruction, 7.2 nm, is almost invariant.

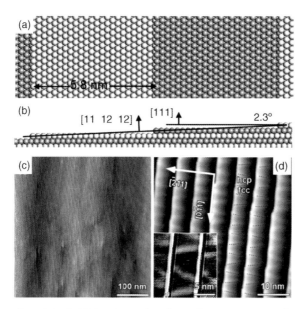

Figure 9.5 Au(11 12 12) vicinal surface with 2.3° miscut towards [−211] with respect to (111) surface. (a) Top view and (b) cross-section of Au(11 12 12); (c, d) STM images of Au(11 12 12) surface. The inset in panel (d) shows a zoomed image [29].

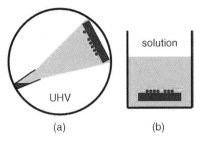

Figure 9.6 Preparation techniques for supramolecular templates. (a) Organic molecular beam deposition (OMBD) under UHV conditions; (b) Liquid-phase deposition in solution.

9.2.4
Surface-Supported Organic Supramolecular Assemblies

The above-discussed templates are either covalent-bonded or metal-bonded inorganic surfaces. Hence, organic supramolecular architectures that are self-assembled on surfaces bound by noncovalent interactions, will be introduced in the following subsections.

9.2.4.1 Preparation Techniques
Two methods are used for preparing surface-supported supramolecular architectures, namely organic molecular-beam deposition (OMBD) under UHV conditions, and liquid-phase deposition at solid–liquid interfaces (see Figure 9.6).

In OMBD, the organic compound is loaded into a crucible under UHV conditions and heated to temperatures at which the organic molecules will either sublime or evaporate onto the substrate surfaces. This technique has the following advantages:

High purity: Prior to OMBD growth, a high purity of organic materials is achieved by thermal gradient sublimation. For this, both the organic source and substrate are maintained under UHV with a background vacuum (typically on the order of 10^{-10} mbar) so that contamination from the environment is avoided.

Well-controlled kinetics: Both, the energetic parameters (i.e., the intermolecular and molecule–substrate interactions) and the kinetic parameters (including growth temperature and deposition rate) play key roles in determining the final structure of the supramolecular assembly. Notably, these kinetic parameters are adjustable during the deposition process.

Multicomponent deposition: Supramolecular structures consisting of multiple components may easily be produced by using more than one source in the UHV chamber. In addition, the temperatures of the sources can be controlled independently, such that it is possible to deposit different organic molecules or metal atoms at the same time or in sequence.

Combination with various characteristic methods: In addition to STM, other surface-analysis techniques, such as low-energy electron diffraction, photoemission spectroscopy and electron energy loss spectroscopy (EELS) are useful when investigating the structure and properties of surface-supported supramolecular assemblies. These surface-analysis techniques can be integrated with the OMBD preparation chamber.

When using OMBD it is necessary to use sublimable or vaporizable molecules with a vapor pressure of $\sim 10^{-8}$ mbar at a temperature in the range from 60 to 600 °C, although this limits the application of OMBD to molecules that do not sublime, nor are thermally stable. In contrast, for liquid-phase deposition the molecules are deposited from solutions onto the substrate surfaces, which are themselves immersed in a solution of the molecules. Liquid-phase deposition is easier to use than OMBD; moreover, in biological systems it is also possible to mimic the environment when investigating biological molecules. Nonetheless, inert substrates such as highly oriented pyrolitic graphite (HOPG) and Au(111) will be required when using this technique, and the kinetic processes cannot be well controlled.

9.2.4.2 0-D and 1-D Nanostructures

The formation of molecular structures, ranging from single molecules to few-molecule aggregates, linear wires, extended 2-D compact layers and open networks up to 3-D architectures, on surfaces is dependent on the intermolecular interactions and the growth parameters. Well-defined zero-dimensional (0-D) and one-dimensional (1-D) structures are normally obtained using a submonolayer regime via OMBD, under UHV. At low temperature, the surface diffusion ability of molecules will be inhibited such that aggregation processes which originate from certain attractive interactions (e.g., van der Waals forces) are prevented, and this results in the presence of isolated molecules on the surfaces. Such aggregation processes are also prevented in the case of molecule–substrate systems by repulsive interactions, such as charge transfer [32–34]. The assembly of molecules with directed and selective noncovalent interactions, such as H-bonding and metal–ligand coordination coupling, is determined by the specific anisotropic feature of the interactions. A careful placement of functional groups that are capable of participating in directed noncovalent interactions will allow the rational design and construction of a wide range of supramolecular architectures assembled on surfaces. Few-molecule aggregates will be formed if the active interaction sites are self-saturated [31] (also D.Y. Zhong, unpublished results), whilst linear supramolecular wires will be formed in the case that the molecules possess two active interaction sites with anti-parallel directions. When molecules possess three or more active interaction sites in plane, 2-D networks will be formed.

Figure 9.7 shows the STM study of substituted porphyrin molecules adsorbed on a Au(111) surface. Cyanophenyl substituents, which possess directed dipole–dipole and H-bonding interactions, are used to control the molecular aggregation. Isolated single molecules, trimers and tetramers are observed when depositing the substituted porphyrin molecules without, with one, and with two cyanophenyl groups at the *cis* sites, respectively. However, when depositing the molecules with two cyanophenyl groups substituted at the *trans* sites, the anti-parallel configuration between the cyanophenyl substituents results in a linear arrangement and the formation of supramolecular wires [31].

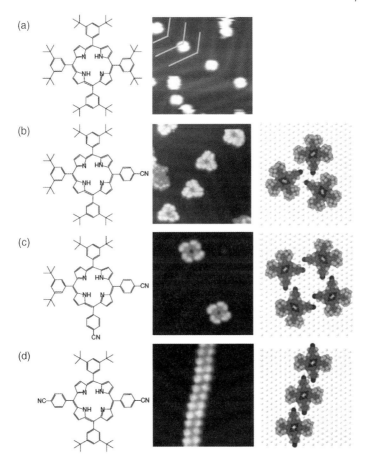

Figure 9.7 0-D and 1-D molecular nanostructures. (a) Monomers of the porphyrin derivative without cyanophenyl substituent; (b) Trimers of the porphyrin derivative with one cyanophenyl substituent; (c) Tetramers of the porphyrin derivative with two *cis* cyanophenyl substituents; (d) 1-D molecular wire of the porphyrin derivative with two *trans* cyanophenyl substituents. STM image area $= 20 \times 20\,\mathrm{nm}^2$ [31].

The formation of supramolecular wires is also directed by H-bonding and metal–ligand coordination [35–45]. The formation of double-row molecular assembly of 4-[*trans*-2-(pyrid-4-yl-vinyl)]benzoic acid (PVBA), on a Ag(111) surface results from the head-to-end OH...N bonding, as well as the CH...OH bonding between the rows [35, 45]. A similar coupled double-row architecture has been observed on the assembly of L-methionine on a Ag(111) surface [38, 39]. Here, the regular molecular gratings, which are formed at intermediate coverage with tunable periodicity at the nanometer scale by varying the methionine surface concentration, can serve as a template to guide the formation of metal atom lines via surface-state confinement at the Ag(111) surface [38]. In general, by optimizing the growth parameters, molecules with strong anisotropic interactions – including H-bonding, dipole–dipole coupling, metal–ligand coordination, as well as van der Waals interactions – prefer to form 1-D structures. Yet, the strong anisotropy may induce the formation of 1-D chains that extend for over several hundred nanometers [40].

9.2.4.3 **2-D Molecular Patterns**

The self-assembly of organic molecules on surfaces is determined by the subtle balance between intermolecular and molecule–substrate interactions. In general, close-packed configurations are favorable for supramolecular assembly on surfaces due to the attractive van der Waals interactions between molecules, and between molecules and substrates. The latter effect is dominant in some cases, even though the molecules may possess repulsive interactions, the reason being that those configurations with more molecules adsorbed onto the surfaces will reduce the system total energy. However, by introducing certain directional and selective noncovalent interactions, such as H-bonding and metal–ligand coordination, it is possible to form open networks with voids of substrates. These porous networks attract intrigue in host–guest chemistry, since by combining the different noncovalent interactions with various strengths it is possible to form complicated structures that include hierarchical or multilevel architectures. Moreover, besides the energetic consideration of the systems, certain growth parameters – including growth temperature, rate and coverage, as well as the concentration in liquid-phase deposition – will play important roles, with such experimental parameters affecting the diffusion–aggregation and adsorption–desorption processes of adsorbed molecules. As the polymorphic feature is a common property of most molecule–substrate systems, different metastable structures are attained, depending on the growth parameters.

Molecular Design Due to the large variety of organic molecules, it is relatively easy to alter the supramolecular structures by molecular design. By adjusting the intermolecular and molecule–substrate interactions, it is possible to tune the final supramolecular structures which are at energetic minimum states by self-assembly under quasi-equilibrium conditions. On the basis of this concept, there are two main routes: (i) to alter the geometry of the molecules, and also the packing behaviors of the molecules adsorbed on surfaces via long-range and nondirectional van der Waals interactions; and (ii) to introduce directional and/or selective noncovalent interactions, such as H-bonds and metal–ligand coordination coupling. In this case, different H-bonds, including OH...O [46–49], OH...N [50, 51], NH...O [42, 43, 52–59], NH...N, [52–61], and CH...O [37, 50, 51, 62, 63], can be introduced in surface-supported supramolecular assemblies. Frequently, more than one H-bond is formed on each molecule, whilst a cooperative effect may enhance the binding between molecules [52]. Coordination coupling between transition metals and organic ligands is also used to adjust the supramolecular architectures on the surfaces [64, 65], such that the metal atoms or ions are either codeposited on the surface [66–75], from thermally activated diffusing adatoms on a metal substrate [36, 76–78], or from the solution in the case of liquid-phase deposition [41, 79].

Among these molecules, benzoic acid and its derivatives have been investigated intensely as model systems. Although the carboxyl group exhibited abundant

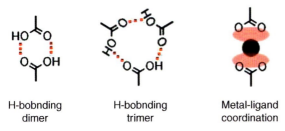

H-bobnding   H-bobnding   Metal-ligand
   dimer   trimer   coordination

Figure 9.8 Noncovalent interactions of (deprotonated) carboxyl groups.

behaviors in the self-assembly process (Figure 9.8), it is also possible to form H-bonds between the carboxyl groups, and between the carboxyl groups and benzene rings. In this way, dimers or trimers are formed with either two or three H-bonds between two or three carboxyl groups, respectively. According to DFT calculations, hydrogen bonds in the cyclic dimer of benzoic acid, as are present in the "chicken-wire" network, are $1.5\,\mathrm{kcal\,mol}^{-1}$ stronger than those in the cyclic trimer in the gas phase, as are present in the "flower" structure [80]. On the other hand, the deprotonated species of carboxyl (carboxylate) act as ligands to coordinate with transition metal atoms.

The adsorption of benzoic acid (Figure 9.9, **1a**), which contains one carboxyl group substituting one of the six H atoms on a benzene ring, prefers an upright config-uration at high coverage; that is, with the benzene ring perpendicular to the surface [81–85]. On $TiO_2(110)$ surfaces, the oxygen atoms of the deprotonated species (benzoate) are bonded with the fivefold-coordinated Ti^{4+} cations to form an ordered overlayer, which is mainly determined by the relatively strong adsorba-te–substrate interaction. Attractive interactions between the aromatic rings of the benzoates lead to the formation of dimerized benzoate rows along the [001] direction [81–85]. The flat-down configuration (with the benzene ring parallel to the surface) only exists at a very low coverage [81–85]. Similarly, on Cu(110) surfaces, H-bonded flat-down dimers are formed at a temperature below 150 K, while deprotonation takes place at a temperature above 150 K and benzoate dimers coordinating with a Cu atom in between are formed. At saturation coverage, however, the adsorption of benzoic acid on Cu(110) between 300 and 350 K results in benzoate species which is oriented perpendicular to the surface with a $c(8 \times 2)$ periodicity [83].

Increasing the number of substituting carboxyl group on the benzene ring, or substituting the benzene ring with a pyridine ring [iso-nicotinic acid (INA); **1b** in Figure 9.9], will have a dramatic influence on the assembly. In this case, it is possible to form more H-bonds in the flat-down configuration with a reduced system total energy, which makes the flat-down configuration more favorable than the upright configuration. By introducing the pyridine ring, the molecular self-assembly of INA on Ag(111) adopts a head-to-tail hydrogen-bond configuration from ring nitrogen atom to hydroxyl hydrogen, with the aromatic rings parallel to the surface plane [86]. Here, there are two sets of H-bonds: the primary head-to-tail H-bonds (OH...N) link molecules into long chains along the Ag[11-2], while the secondary hydrogen-bonding interactions link the carbonyl oxygen of one INA chain with the aromatic

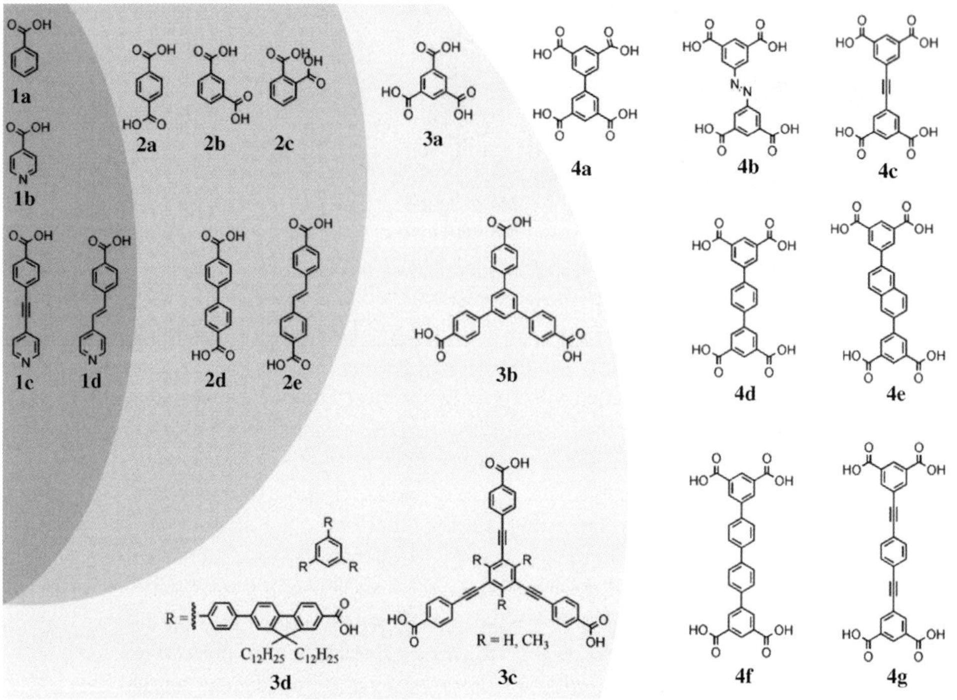

Figure 9.9 Benzoic acid derivatives. 1a–1d, 2a–2e, 3a–3d, and 4a–4g contain one, two, three, and four carboxyl groups, respectively. Abbreviations and references: 1a [81–85]; 1b (INA) [86]; 1c (PEBA) [50]; 1d (PVBA) [50, 87]; 2a (TPA) [69, 72, 73, 88–94]; 2b [90]; 2c [90]; 2d (BDA) [63, 73, 74, 87, 88, 95]; 2e (SDA) [63, 75]; 3a (TMA) [36, 46, 48, 49, 51, 68, 76, 80, 92, 93, 96–101]; 3b (BTB) [99]; 3c [102]; 3d [47]; 4a [103]; 4b (NN4A) [104]; 4c [103]; 4d (TPTC) [105]; 4e [106]; 4f [106]; 4g [103].

hydrogen on an adjacent chain. The benzoic acid derivatives containing two carboxyl groups have three isomers, depending on the two substitution sites: terephthalic acid (TPA; 2a in Figure 9.9), iso-phthalic acid (2b in Figure 9.9) and phthalic acid (2c in Figure 9.9). The self-assembly of TPA on the Au(111) surface at room temperature under UHV conditions forms a highly ordered, close-packed layer at high coverage. The head-to-tail hydrogen bonds between the carboxyl groups of neighboring molecules are the dominant interactions in the molecular monolayers, and result in linear molecular chains, analogous to the bulk structure [91]. However, the length of the H-bridges exceeds that in the TPA bulk phase due to modulation of the substrate surface. A similar structure, with linear molecular chains stabilized by H-bonds, is formed by the assembly of TPA at liquid/solid interfaces [90, 91]. By comparison, the assembly of iso-phthalic acid molecules results in the zigzag configuration owing to H-bond formation. No ordered structure has been found for the assembly of phthalic acid [90, 91].

The assembly behaviors are changed by further increasing the number of carboxyl groups. Two coexisting phases – the "chicken-wire" and "flower" structures, both of

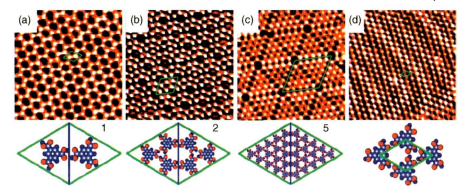

Figure 9.10 1,3,5-Benzenetricarboxylic (trimesic) acid (TMA) on Au(111). The distance of the pores increases by increasing the coverage. (a) "Chicken-wire" structure with only dimeric H-bonding; (b) "Flower" structure with mixed dimeric and trimeric H-bonding; (c) Porous structure similar to the "flower" structure, but with a larger distance between the pores; (d) Close-packed structure with only trimeric H-bonding. STM image area = 16.5 × 16.5 nm² [46].

which are induced by directional hydrogen bonding – are formed by the adsorption of 1,3,5-benzenetricarboxylic (trimesic) acid (TMA; **3a** in Figure 9.9) to graphite or Au (111) surfaces under UHV conditions [49]. In the "chicken-wire" structure (Figure 9.10a), all molecules are connected by dimeric H-bonds (two H-bonds involving two carboxyl groups), to form sixfold molecular rings. In contrast to the "chicken-wire" structure, the "flower" structure can be seen as a closed packing of the sixfold rings (Figure 9.10b). Within the rings, the hydrogen bonds are formed in the same way as in the "chicken-wire" structure, whilst between the neighboring sixfold rings trimeric H-bonds are formed that involve three molecules. In both structures, all of the H-bonds have a length about 3 Å, which is well within the range of OH...O bonds (2.7–3.1 Å).

Consider, then, the situation in which the symmetry of TPA and TMA molecules is retained, while the molecular size is increased. The molecule 4,4′-biphenyl dicarboxylic acid (BDA; **2d** in Figure 9.9) shows the same twofold symmetry as TPA, but with two phenyl rings as the backbone. The behavior of BDA molecules assembled on Au(111) surface is similar to that of TPA, forming linear molecular chains stabilized by head-to-tail H-bonding between the carboxyl groups of neighboring molecules [95]. The case with threefold rotational symmetry as TMA is 4,4′,4″-benzene-1,3,5-triyl-tribenzoic acid (BTA), in which three 4′-benzoic acid groups are arranged around the central benzene core. In this case, 2-D supramolecular honeycomb networks of BTA with cavities of a larger internal diameter of 2.95 nm are formed by self-assembly on a Ag(111) surface at room temperature [51]. The configuration of the networks is similar to the "chicken-wire" structure of TMA self-assembled on graphite [49]. The symmetry rule is obeyed in the assembly of even more complicated molecules [47].

The benzoic acid derivatives with four carboxyl groups can form both a parallel network and a Kagomé network on the surfaces (Figure 9.11) [103, 105, 106]. In the

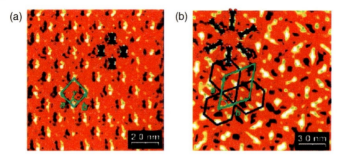

Figure 9.11 Tetra-acids self-assembled on HOPG (deposition from heptanoic acid solution, −1.5 V, 50 pA). (a) Parallel configuration of **4a** (see Figure 9.9); (b) Kagomé network of **4g** (see Figure 9.9) [103].

parallel network, each molecule forms four double H-bonds with four neighboring molecules at the corners, and all molecules show the same orientation. In the Kagomé network, three molecules, which are rotated ±60° with respect to each other, are H-bonded head-to-tail with a triangle-like feature. The molecules with short (e.g., biphenyl, **4a** of Figure 9.9) and long (e.g., four phenyl rings, **4f** of Figure 9.9) backbones adopt single configurations with long-range periodic order, while those with intermediate backbone lengths, such as *p*-terphenyl-3,5,3′,5′-tetracarboxylic acid (three phenyl rings, **4d** of Figure 9.9) and 5,5′-(1,2-ethynediyl)bis(1,3-benzenedicarboxylic acid) on graphite form mixed networks coexisting both parallel and Kagomé configurations [103, 105]. The specific molecular lengths allow their growth of one polymorph to be interrupted by a smooth transition to the alternative polymorph, without necessarily introducing defects in which molecular building blocks are missing, improperly oriented, or unable to form the optimal number of hydrogen bonds with neighbors [103]. As a result, a random, nonperiodic, entropically stabilized, rhombus tiling is formed in a 2-D molecular network of *p*-terphenyl-3,5,3′,5′-tetracarboxylic acid adsorbed onto graphite [105]. Similar 2-D nonperiodic tiling has been observed in the self-assembly of rubrene molecules in supramolecular pentagons, hexagons, and heptagons on a Au(111) surface [107].

In addition to the H-bond-dominated supramolecular assembly of benzoic acid derivatives described above, another important intermolecular interaction is that of metal–ligand interaction. The deprotonated species of carboxyl groups is able to form metal–ligand coordination with certain transition metal atoms and, in the presence of such interactions, the assembly of organic molecules on surfaces may be changed. Except for the H-bonded "chicken-wire" and "flower" patterns of TMA self-assembled on graphite and Au(111) [46, 76], the deposition of TMA on Cu(100) surfaces at 300 K results in the formation of cloverleaf-shaped Cu(TMA)$_4$ complexes, which are organized into a regular array at high coverage (Figure 9.12). The four deprotonated TMA molecules are bonded with the centered Cu atom through the carboxylate groups. The carboxylate ligands of TMA do not point directly towards the central Cu atom, and the oxygen atoms in the respective COO$^-$ moieties are not equivalent, which indicates a unidentate coordination of the Cu atom [76]. For comparison, the

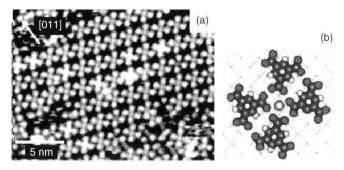

Figure 9.12 Cu(TMA)$_4$ complex formed by depositing TMA on Cu(100) at 300 K. (a) Regular array of Cu(TMA)$_4$ complex; (b) Model of the complex showing the coordination of the carboxylate groups of four TMA molecules with the central Cu atom [76].

deposition of TMA on a Cu(110) surface results in 1-D metal–organic coordination chains of TMA and Cu atoms, owing to the anisotropy of the substrate [36]. Dicarboxylic acids containing one (TPA), two (TDA) and three (DBA) phenyl rings show similar behaviors as TMA. Although these molecules, when self-assembled on Au(111) surface, adopt a H-bonded head-to-tail configuration [91, 95], porous coordination networks of TPA or TBA and iron atoms with variable cavity sizes are formed on the Cu(100) surface [72]. The codeposition of DBA molecules and Mo atoms, followed by annealing to 400 K, results in carboxylate–Mo coordination and the formation of rectangular-shaped or ladder-like networks, depending on the ratios of the deposited amounts of BDA molecules and Mn atoms [74]. In addition, the coordination interaction between the O atoms of carboxylate groups and Fe atoms has been confirmed by comparing the chemical shift of O 1s and Fe 3p peaks in X-ray photoelectron spectroscopy (XPS) measurements with various Fe : TPA ratios [69].

When compared to H-bonds and metal–ligand coupling, van der Waals interactions – which exhibit an indispensable effect on multilevel structures of biomolecules – are much weaker. In some cases, the van der Waals interactions have a dramatic influence on supramolecular assembly, even in those systems where H-bonds or coordination coupling are predominant. For example, a slight variation of a submolecular alkyl group, which is not involved directly in the hydrogen bonding, may have a pronounced effect on the self-assembled surface nanostructures, thus causing a change in the molecular nanostructures obtained, from extended periodic rows to localized chains and polygonal clusters. This change is attributed to subtle differences in van der Waals interactions between the alkyl side chains found on some of the compounds, an insight that can be employed to control the formation of self-assembled molecular surface nanostructures when multifunctional groups are involved in the molecular building blocks [108]. Similarly, the 2-D pattern formation of hydrogen-bonding iso-phthalic acid derivatives at the liquid/solid interface has been investigated by using STM. By varying the location and nature of the alkyl substituents on the aromatic core, in combination with the intrinsic hydrogen-bonding properties of the iso-phthalic acid units, the 2-D supramolecular ordering has been controlled, leading to several different motifs [59].

Complicated supramolecular structures may occur in the systems with only van der Waals interactions. In such systems, subtle intermolecular and molecule–substrate interactions result in a superstructure with several and/or up to several tens of molecules, the relative orientation and positions of which are different from each other. A long-range orientational order of C_{60} monolayers on Au(111) has been observed with a unit cell comprised of 49 molecules adopting 11 different orientations [109]. In this case, intermolecular interactions play a major role in stabilizing the superlattice, while the substrate induces minute changes in the orientation of the C_{60} molecules. Diferrocene molecules, which contains two ferrocenyl groups bridged by an alkyl chain, show van der Waals intermolecular interactions and are weakly bound on certain surfaces, such as Cu(110). The assembly of diferrocenes on Cu(110) exhibits 2-D multilevel structures up to quaternary, resulting from the subtle balance of intermolecular and molecule–substrate interactions that have comparable strength, as well as the mismatch of the molecular packing and the surface atomic periodicity. In such a multi-periodicity modulated system, neither the intermolecular nor molecule–substrate interactions solely dominate the molecular assembly, and this results in complicated supramolecular architectures. The multilevel assemblies demonstrate site-selective properties for the adsorption of guest molecules (D.Y. Zhong, unpublished results).

Substrate Effects   Substrates are not only the support for the assembly of organic molecules, but also play a key role in supramolecular assembly. On the one hand, the surface atomic potential with specific periodicities will affect the arrangement of adsorbed molecules. The molecule–substrate interactions include long-range van der Waals interactions, dipole–dipole interactions, and covalent bonding in some cases, which cause the molecules to prefer specific adsorption sites and orientations. On the other hand, molecule–substrate interactions will alter the features of molecules themselves, such as their structure, conformation, and electronic state. For example, charge transfer and substrate-induced dissociation are common phenomena in molecule-on-surface systems. The substrate-induced modification of molecules will further influence intermolecular interactions, and finally the supramolecular assembly. The assembly of BDA (**2d** of Figure 9.9) on Au(111) and Cu(100) surfaces are compared in Figure 9.13. On the Au(111) surface, linear molecular chains are formed at room temperature, with H-bonding between the carboxyl groups of neighboring molecules, analogous to PBA [95]. On a more reactive Cu(100) surface, however, the carboxyl groups are deprotonated owing to the strong molecule–substrate coupling, and this results in a square-type structure through the H-bonds between the carboxylate and the benzene ring, with the molecules alternatively 90° rotated [63].

Growth Parameters   The *temperature* of the molecular assembly, including that during growth and post-growth annealing, represents one of the most important experimental factors to directly affect the supramolecular assembly on surfaces [51, 110, 111]. The temperature affects not only the diffusion ability of molecules on surfaces, but also the ability of conformation change and bond dissociation [112]. In this case, 2-D supramolecular honeycomb networks of BTA with cavities of internal

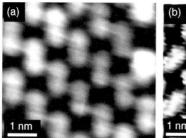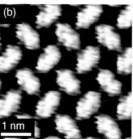

Figure 9.13 Substrate effect: BDA on Au(111) and Cu(100). (a) Linear molecular chains of DBA on Au(111); (b) Orthogonal configuration of deprotonated DBA molecules on Cu(100) [63, 95].

diameter 2.95 nm are formed on a Ag(111) surface at room temperature, in analogy to the "chicken-wire" structure of TMA self-assembled on graphite. However, annealing to a higher temperature results in two sequential phase transformations into closer-packed supramolecular arrangements, which are associated with a stepwise deprotonation of the carboxylic acid groups.

Coverage is another factor which affects molecular self-assembly [46, 60, 113]. As noted above, 0-D and 1-D nanostructures are both formed at lower coverage. However, by varying the coverage from 0.3 up to 1 ML, when TMA is assembled on an Au(111) surface under UHV conditions it forms a series of supramolecular structures, among which "chicken-wire" and "flower" are two special cases (see Figure 9.10). All observed assembling structures formed hexagonal porous networks that are well-described by a unified model in which the TMA molecules inside the half-unit cells (equilateral triangles) are bound via trimeric H-bonds, and all half-unit cells are connected to each other via dimeric hydrogen bonds. These porous networks possess pores of 1.1 nm diameter, and the interpore distance is tunable from 1.6 nm at a step size of 0.93 nm [46].

Solvent Effects In the case of molecular systems self-assembled at liquid–solid interfaces, the solvent concentration should be considered [99, 114–120]. A systematic study on the concentration-dependent formation of surface-confined 2-D networks at the interface of HOPG and 1,2,4-trichlorobenzene shows the competition of two polymorphs. Here, the building blocks are alkoxylated dehydrobenzo[12]annulenes (DBAs), which form 2-D porous networks when the alkoxy chain is less than 12 carbon atoms long [115], and preferentially form close-packed linear structure DBAs with longer alkoxy chains. By adjusting the DBA concentration in solution, the ratio of the two polymorphs can be controlled such that either a regular 2-D porous honeycomb network (at low concentrations) or a dense-packed linear network (at high concentrations) is formed [114]. The competition is related to the chemical potentials of the two surface phases and solution.

Multicomponent Assembly Supramolecular assemblies containing more than one component can be prepared by both OMBD and liquid-phase deposition [98, 99, 121, 122]. In this case, bicomponent and multicomponent assemblies usually result in

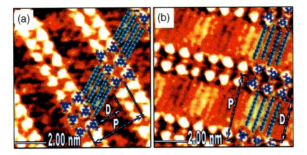

Figure 9.14 STM images of bicomponent assembly of TMA and normal aliphatic alcohols at the heptanoic acid solution/HOPG interface. These architectures contain alternative hydrophilic tapes and hydrophobic inter-tape spaces with adjustable dimensions. (a) TMA and 1-hexadecanol (−1.4 V, 200 pA). Distance between two successive tapes D = 1.7 nm; periodicity of the pattern P = 3.4 nm; (b) TMA and heptadecanol (−1.1 V, 200 pA). D = 2.4 nm, P = 4.1 nm [98].

architectures that differ from the structures assembled from single components. The complexity of the supramolecular structures is dramatically increased, which makes it more feasible to obtain desired structures by the careful molecular design of each component participating in the assembly.

The hydrogen bond-associated assembly of TMA and a variety of normal aliphatic alcohols have been studied [98]. The motif of the mixed assembly (Figure 9.14), which consists of alternative double-row TMA molecular tapes and aliphatic chains running parallel to each other, is distinctly different from the hexagonal patterns normally favored by TMA itself [49]. Its periodicity is proportional to the length of the alcohol, and thus can be modulated with high predictability by changing a readily available component. Very different properties of the tapes (hydrophilic) and inter-tape spaces (hydrophobic) create an opportunity to guide the position-specific adsorption of other atoms and molecules [98].

The coadsorption of benzenetribenzoic acid and trimesic acid at the liquid–solid interface in two different solvents (heptanoic and nonanoic acid) results in six nondensely packed monolayer phases with different structures and stoichiometries stabilized by intermolecular hydrogen bonding between the carboxylic acid functional groups, depending on the concentrations in the binary solutions. Moreover, phase transitions of the monolayer structures, accompanied by an alteration in the size and shape of cavity voids in the 2-D molecular assembly, could be achieved by *in situ* dilution. The emergence of the various phases could be described by a simple thermodynamic model [99, 121].

9.2.4.4 Porous Networks

Surface-supported porous networks are related to the supramolecular architectures with ordered separated voids where the substrate surface is exposed. Due to the different physical and chemical reactivities at the nanosized voids and molecule links, such porous networks offer a platform to perform site-selective physical and chemical processes at molecular scale. A detailed discussion of porous networks combined with nanostructure fabrications using the porous networks as template will be discussed in Section 9.4.2. A review of supramolecular nanoporous networks self-assembled on surfaces has recently been produced [123].

9.3
Surface-Supported Nanostructures Directed by Atomic-Level Inorganic Templates

The formation of nanostructures guided by inorganic templates, including surface reconstructions, stepped surfaces, and strain-relief patterns is discussed in the following subsections. Supramolecular network-related nanostructures will be discussed in Section 9.4.

9.3.1
Reconstruction

Au(111)-22 $\times \sqrt{3}$ Herring-Bone Pattern   Ordered arrays of Ni nanodots are formed due to preferential nucleation on the elbow sites of the Au(111) herring-bone reconstruction patterns [124]. Associated by the ordered arrays of transition metal nanodots, complicated organic–inorganic hybrid nanostructures have been fabricated on reconstructed Au(111) surfaces [125–129]. Meanwhile, single-molecule or few-molecule aggregates can also be anchored on the elbow sites of the herring-bone patterns, without metal nanodots [130–132]. Depending on the geometry and the intermolecular interactions, the elbow sites and the *fcc* regions may serve as the active sites for the growth of organic nanostructures. Écija *et al.* have investigated the crossover of site-selectivity in the adsorption and self-assembly of phenyl-C61-butyric acid methyl ester (PCBM) on the herringbone-reconstructed Au(111) surface as a function of the coverage (Figure 9.15) [133]. Initially, the molecules nucleated at the elbow sites, but with increasing coverage long, parallel, isolated zigzag 1-D wires were formed exclusively at the *fcc* regions. However, a compact arrangement of molecules with double-molecular rows was formed and the site-selectivity lost when the coverage was further increased.

Cu(110)-(2 $\times$ 1)O and the Stripe Pattern   In comparison to the oxygen-adsorbed regions, the bare Cu(110) regions are normally more active in adsorbing organic molecules. The template effect of the stripe pattern for the fabrication of 1-D organic nanostructures has been demonstrated by Besenbacher and coworkers [8], with well-ordered arrays of long molecular chains of "Single Lander" molecules being self-assembled on the Cu(110) stripes. By controlling the width of the nanotemplate, it was possible to select the adsorption orientation of the molecules, and thereby steer their alignment along the specific direction of the template (Figure 9.16). A similar template effect of the stripe patterns has been also applied for the assembly of α-quinquethiophene [134], rubrene [135], and *para*-Sexiphenyl [136].

Si(111)-7 $\times$ 7   The use of semiconductor substrates is more attractive than metal substrates for potential applications in the field of nanoelectronics. The Si(111)-7 $\times$ 7

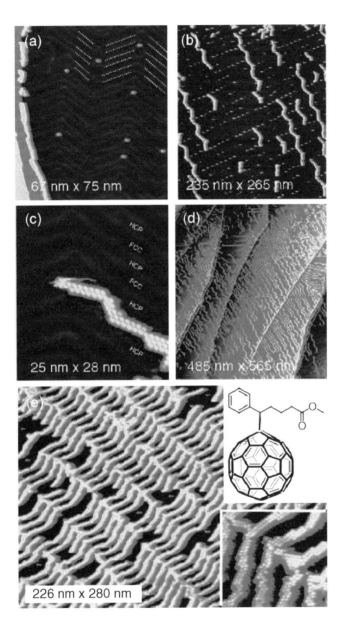

Figure 9.15 Nanostructures of PCBM guided by Au(111) herringbone template with different coverages. (a) <0.1 ML; (b) 0.1 ML; (c) A zigzag structure formed at the *fcc* region; (d) 0.3 ML; (e) 0.4 ML. Upper inset shows the molecular formula of PCBM; Lower inset shows high-resolution image of 2-D network of PCBM molecules (refer to Figure 9.2 for clean Au(111) surface) [133].

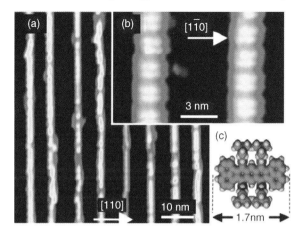

Figure 9.16 Molecular chains formed by the deposition of a "Single Lander" molecules on Cu (110)-(2 × 1)O stripe pattern. Molecules adsorb exclusively on the bare Cu stripes. (a, b) STM images; (c) Model of the "Single Lander" molecule with a polyaromatic hydrocarbon central board and four 3,5-di-*tert*-butylphenyl substituents [8].

is a well-known reconstruction with a surface lattice constant of 2.7 nm. By carefully controlling the kinetic parameters, including the growth temperature and the flux, well-ordered indium nanocluster arrays with identical size could be formed [137]. However, the template effect of the Si(111)-7 × 7 surface cannot simply be applied to the assembly of organic nanostructure, due to the strong interactions of the Si dangling bonds with organic molecules [138]. The diffusion ability of the deposited molecules is also restricted by the surface reaction, such that the molecules are normally immobilized before they move to an energetically favorable site. For example, the deposition of C_{60} molecules on the Si(111) surface resulted in a disordered first layer [139, 140], despite the faulted half and unfaulted half being the most favorably adsorbed sites in the case of a single molecule [141].

One way to avoid adsorbate–surface interactions on Si(111)-7 × 7 surfaces is to use zwitterionic molecules; these are neutral, but carry formal positive and negative charges on different atoms. The negative site of a zwitterionic molecule acts as a electrostatic shield to prevent any reaction of the electron-deficient Si adatoms with the electron-rich carbon atoms of the organic molecules [142]. This strategy has been verified by Makoudi *et al.*, who chose 4-methoxy-4′-(3-sulfonatopropyl)stilbazolium (MSPS) as a model zwitterionic molecule. The MSPS molecules are terminated by a negatively charged SO_3^- group, which acts as an electrostatic shield that protects the organic molecules against the dangling bonds of the surface. At low coverage, the molecules prefer to adsorb at the faulted half cells with a star-shaped configuration (containing three MSPS molecules), indicating a more or less site-selectivity of the reconstructed surface [142, 143].

The reactive surface may also be passivated by silver or boron atoms, although in most cases passivation of the reactive surface may result in a loss of site-selectivity [139, 144, 145]. When Xu and coworkers demonstrated the feasibility of controllable growth of ordered molecular nanostructures on passivated Si(111)-7×7 surfaces, ordered 2-D Cu clusters were first formed at the faulted half-cells, before the deposition of organic molecules. The thiophene molecules were shown to bind preferentially to the copper clusters through the S–Cu interaction, and this resulted in large-scale 2-D thiophene molecular nanostructures that followed the ordered Cu cluster pattern [146].

9.3.2
Strain-Relief Epitaxial Layers

The dislocations in strain-relief layers grown on lattice-mismatched surfaces often repel adsorbates diffusing over the surface, such that they may serve as templates for the confined nucleation of nanostructures from adsorbed atoms or molecules. Highly ordered, 2-D Fe and Ag nanostructure arrays are fabricated on the strain-relief patterns of double layers of Ag on the Pt(111) surface [15]. At a reduced growth temperature (110 K), the Ag atoms are preferentially nucleated within the *fcc* areas (distorted hexagons), owing to a stronger binding to the *fcc* areas than to the *hcp* areas [147]. The ordered nucleation is accompanied by an enhanced size uniformity. The repulsive nature of the dislocations and the attraction towards specific sites within the unit cell represent the key properties for transferring the periodicity of the dislocation network to a highly ordered 2-D island superlattice.

The application of the same templates to organic materials was achieved by Aït-Mansour *et al.* [18, 148], who deposited C_{60} molecules on strain-relief patterns induced by two monolayers of Ag on Pt(111). At room temperature, nucleation of the C_{60} islands took place on both the *fcc* and *hcp* domains of the template. Moreover, the C_{60} molecules were sufficiently mobile on the template surface to cross the dislocations and to self-assemble into large, hexagonally close-packed 2-D islands [148]. The loss of site-selectivity for C_{60} implied that the well-established repulsive character of the crossing dislocations was not sufficiently strong to prevent significant molecule diffusion across the discommensuration lines from *fcc* sites into *hcp* sites at room temperature. In order to organize the organic molecules to a regular structure that followed the strain-relief pattern, a technique was developed to fabricate a new type of nanotemplate surface that consisted of a well-ordered hexagonal array of one monolayer-deep holes, with a tunable size of about $4\,nm^2$ and a fixed spacing of 7 nm, based on the strain-relief trigonal network formed in the 2 ML Ag on Pt(111) system [18]. The removal of about 0.1 ML of the Ag top layer of this surface structure by He- or Ar-ion sputtering, led to the formation of nanoholes at specific domains of the trigonal network, which were stable at room temperature. The regularly distributed C_{60} nanoclusters trapped in the holes, replicating the periodicity and hexagonal symmetry of the nanohole template surface, were formed by the deposition of about 0.1 ML of C_{60} molecules at room temperature.

Another important strain-relief pattern, which shows a template effect for organic molecules, is the boron nitride nanomesh grown on Rh(111) and Ru(0001) surfaces. Single molecules such as copper phthalocyanine (CuPc) can be trapped in holes of such nanopatterned surfaces, without the formation of strong covalent bonds. The

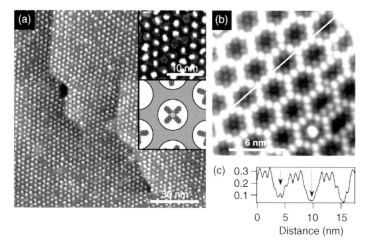

Figure 9.17 Organic molecules on BN nanomesh. (a) Nc molecules located at the center of the holes. The insets show a zoomed STM image (top) and model (bottom). The arrows show two holes with one molecule and empty, respectively; (b) C_{60} molecules decorated on the BN nanomesh; (c) Profile along the line in panel (b) [11, 14].

holes were identified as regions of low work function, with the trapping potential being localized at the rims of the holes [149]. The deposition of planar naphthalo-cyanine (Nc) molecules (the diameter of which at 2 nm was comparable to that of the nanomesh pores) onto the nanomesh at room temperature resulted in well-ordered arrays with the same periodicity as the nanomesh (3.22 nm) (Figure 9.17) [14]. In analogy to CuPc, the individual Nc molecules became trapped inside the pores with high site-selectivity, such that the molecule–substrate interactions dominated the adsorption behavior and the intermolecular interactions were relatively weak. The trapped molecules exhibited a very low mobility at room temperature, with only rare hopping to a neighboring pore, indicating a rather high trapping potential. In the case of C_{60}, however, the centers of the holes were the least stable adsorption sites [11]. Following the room-temperature deposition of approximately 1 ML of C_{60} molecules, the mesh wires were decorated by lines of individual molecules, and either six or seven molecules were adsorbed inside the holes, while the hole centers remained almost empty and were rarely occupied by one C_{60} molecule. Nevertheless, the periodicity of the mesh supercell was retained. This different behavior of C_{60} on the BN nanomesh might result from its relatively stronger intermolecular interaction compared to CuPc and Nc.

9.3.3
Vicinal Surfaces

Vicinal surfaces as natural templates for the fabrication of 1-D nanostructures have been investigated intensively during the past decades. The systems studied have included the growth of metal nanowires and nanodots [22, 150–154], wide-band-gap materials such as CaF_2, NaCl, MgO [155], and the alignment of carbon nanotubes (CNTs) [156]. Recently, organic nanostructures guided by vicinal surfaces have been prepared; by carefully controlling the arrangement of kinks on a vicinal surface [22], or with a combination of surface reconstruction patterns, it is possible to obtain ordered 2-D arrays of nanosized objects.

Form an energetic point of view, the step edges are active sites for the nucleation of adsorbates, due to the higher coordinates and/or density of states of electrons. However, the kinetic parameters, including the growth temperature, growth rate and coverage, are also important for controlling the nanostructures. During the growth of metal wires on vicinal metallic or semiconducting surfaces, for example, the optimized growth temperatures should be sufficiently high as to ensure a smooth wire formation, but sufficiently low as to avoid any interlayer diffusion of adatoms [151]. Yet, the surface alloy effect should also be taken account [22]. The solid-state reaction between Fe and Si takes place even at room temperature [157] and, depending on the amount of deposition, either single- or double-row chains of Au and Ag can be grown on the vicinal Si(5 5 12) surface [152].

Vicinal gold surfaces have been used as substrates to grow organic materials [29, 158–162]. In this case, the template effect depends heavily on the chemical and geometric features of the molecules, which determine the interactions with the substrates. It has been reported that C_{60} molecules can recognize the substrate template of Au(433), [159] Au(11 12 12), [29] and Au(788), [158], but that there is no site selectivity on the Au(788) surface for perylene-3,4,9,10-tetracarboxylic-dianhydride (PTCDA) [163].

Xiao *et al.* reported the formation of a regular C_{60} nanochain lattice with long-range order on vicinal Au(11 12 12) surfaces (Figure 9.18a and b) [29]. Here, the C_{60} molecules were sublimated from a Kundsen-cell-type evaporator on the surface at room temperature such that, with a coverage of 0.1 ML ($\sim$0.1 nm^{-2}), well-ordered arrays of short molecular chains containing between two and six C_{60} molecules in each chain were formed. The periodicities of the array were unique to the rectangle superstructure of the vicinal Au(11 12 12) surface; that is, 5.8 nm in the $[-2 1 1]$ direction and 7.2 nm in the $[0–11]$ direction. The chains were located at the lower step edges of the *fcc* domains, where the molecules were preferentially nucleated. The template effect of the surface was lost when increasing the coverage up to 1 ML, however, at which close-packed ordered layer of C_{60} molecules were formed over the entire surface, accompanied by small islands of the second layer.

In the case of the Au(788) surface, a similar template effect has been investigated by Berndt and coworkers (Figure 9.18c and d) [158]. At close to 1 ML coverage, rather than a continuous close-packed molecular layer a well-ordered rectangle array of small single layer noncoalescing islands was observed. The islands, which consisted of approximately 20 molecules, were located at the *fcc* regions of the reconstructed surface, across the step edges. The different ML behavior on the two vicinal surfaces might be attributed to the width of the terraces (see Section 9.2.3). Meanwhile, it was clear that preparation parameters such as deposition rate should also be taken into account. Notably, a smaller deposition rate normally results in more ordered structures due to the efficient diffusion of adsorbates and a full relaxation of the

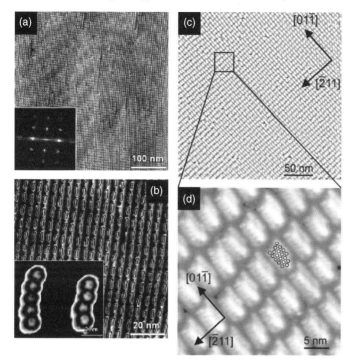

Figure 9.18 C$_{60}$ nanostructures on vicinal Au (11 12 12) and Au(788). (a, b) Highly regular 2-D superlattice of C$_{60}$ nanochains on the Au (11 12 12) template surface after deposition of ∼0.1 ML at room temperature. The inset in panel (a) shows the Fourier power spectrum. The inset in panel (b) shows a high-resolution STM image of the nanochains. (c, d) Periodic C$_{60}$ nanomesh on Au(788) at a coverage about 0.9 ML, deposited at room temperature [29, 158].

deposited layer, whereas an increase in the deposition rate might result in a loss of long-range order.

As discussed in Section 9.2.3, faceting takes places on unstable vicinal surfaces, and this results in stable facets with different surface atomic structures and different orientations. In some cases, the facets may be regularly organized, but by carefully selecting the molecules they may show selectivity for the separation of different molecules, due to differences in the binding energies. This concept has been realized by the coadsorption of PTCDA and 2,5-dimethyl-*N,N'*-dicyanoquinonediimine (DMe-DCNQI) on the (111) and (221) facets of a Ag(775) substrate [164]. The selectivity was shown to depend on the deposition sequence. When PTCDA was first deposited at room temperature the molecules were adsorbed onto both facets, though with an ordered structure on only the (221) facets. The subsequent deposition of DMe-DCNQI led to a disappearance of the ordered structure. Finally, annealing at 330 K resulted in only PTCDA on the (111) facets, with a mixture of both molecules on the (221) facets. In the second sequence, however, the molecules were deposited in reverse order. When DMe-DCNQI was deposited first at room temperature, no ordered structures were found by low-energy electron diffraction (LEED), but when

PTCDA was deposited next the system was annealed at 340 K. The final result showed ordered monolayers of PTCDA exclusively on (111) facets and DMe-DCNQI exclusively on (221) facets. with LEED analysis at different energies confirming the ordered structures on the two facets. In a final experiment, only DMe-DCNQI was deposited, and the sample was annealed at 318 K; this led to the molecule being adsorbed exclusively on the (221) terraces. Subsequent DFT calculations indicated that the PTCDA was bound more strongly on the (111) facet than on the (221) facet (0.54 versus 0.22 eV). DMe-DCNQI formed even stronger bonds on either of the facets, with a small preference for the stepped (221) facet (1.46 versus 1.36 eV). In fact, the stepped (221) facet proved to be favorable for DMe-DCNQI bonding with N atoms at the step edges, but unfavorable for planar PTCDA, which was longer than the narrow terraces so that the O terminators could not reach the step for extra bonding and the bonding was weakened by the presence of the step.

It is well known that the adsorption of certain species may induce the faceting of surfaces, due to an interplay between the molecules and the substrates [165–170]. Regular nanostructures may be obtained on faceted surfaces induced by adsorbates. A sequence of (115) and (001) nanofacets may be formed on the vicinal Cu(119) by the deposition of pentacene at room temperature, followed by annealing to 150–190 °C [171]. The faceted surface appears as a regular sequence of parallel stripes running along the [−110] direction for up to several tens of nanometers, and consists of a sequence of (115) and (001) facets tilted a few degrees off the (119) plane. The opposite tilt angle of the two facets gives rise to V-shape ripples at the surface, with dimensions in the range 2–5 nm. On (115) facets, the molecules are organized into parallel regular chains, with the long axis aligned along the [−110] direction, while on (001) facets about 50% of the molecules are aligned perpendicular to the [−110] direction. The faceting transition induced by the adsorption of pentacene molecules is thermally activated, and the annealing process is preliminary. Without annealing, long-range-ordered pentacene chains assembled on the Cu(119) vicinal surface have been obtained [172]. Pentacene aligns on the step edges of the Cu(119) vicinal surface, resulting in the formation of a long-range-ordered layer of unidirectional molecular chains. The planar molecule adopts a flat adsorption geometry, with the long molecular axis aligned along the steps, and the benzene units centered on the copper hollow site.

Stepped surfaces are also used as templates for directing the growth of organic–inorganic hybrid nanostructures. For example, PTCDA molecules deposited on a vicinal Ag(10 8 7) surface induce faceting, with the formation of (111) regions and step-bunched regions. The molecules are selectively adsorbed onto the step-bunched region, leaving the (111) region free. However, following the further deposition of about 1.1 ML iron on the striped structure, the iron atoms are adsorbed exclusively onto the PTCDA covered facets and small disk-shaped islands with a diameter of 4–6 nm and height of 0.5 nm are formed [173]. Arrays of iron nanowires have been fabricated by Lin *et al.* in a three-step process [174] where first, a silicon template with a regular array of straight steps was prepared by annealing vicinal Si(111) in a specific temperature sequence. Continuous CaF_2 stripes were then grown on top of a CaF_1/Si (111) surface, after which Fe nanowires in the CaF_1 trenches between the CaF_2 stripes were formed via the selective adsorption of ferrocene and photolysis into Fe. This method has been observed for a variety of other molecules, and is today emerging as a general technique for growing 1-D nanostructures of transitional metals and other materials using CVD [175].

9.4
Surface-Supported Nanostructures Directed by Supramolecular Assemblies

9.4.1
Polymerization

The 2-D polymerization of organic molecules represents a possible means of fabricating stable, surface-supported nanostructures. These polymerized structures (especially linear structures) may have potential applications in molecular electronics as a form of candidate for nanowires to connect various switching elements. Moreover, polymerized organic thin films have huge potential as materials for use as field-effect transistors (FETs), rectifiers, photoconductors and light-emitting diodes (LEDs) [176, 177]. Studies on the polymerization of organic monomers on single crystal surfaces would be valuable for understanding the formation, propagation, and properties of the polymerized structures. On the basis of its ability to provide unprecedented atomic-resolved information, and to initiate local polymerization by applying a pulsed sample bias, STM has become a powerful tool in studies of low-dimensional polymerization. In the following subsections, attention will be focused on STM studies of 2-D polymerization on single-crystal surfaces.

9.4.1.1 Polymerization of Diacetylenes
The polymerization of diacetylenes is a typical and early reported example of the fabrication of linear polymerized structures on an atomic flat substrate. The critical condition of this reaction is the relative orientation and distance between the adjacent diacetylene monomer units (Figure 9.19). In 1997, Grim *et al.* showed that the polymerization of diacetylenes could be induced at the liquid/substrate interface following the irradiation with UV light of monolayers of diacetylenes containing an isophthalic acid derivative [178]. Monolayers of the isophthalic acid derivative were first prepared on HOPG surfaces, in which the diacetylene functional groups were packed close to each other, with the desired orientation. When, following UV irradiation (254 nm), the monolayers were reinvestigated using STM, some domains in the monolayers were seen to be replaced by polymerized structures, but not *entire* monolayers. This effect was confirmed by the increase in distance between the isophthalic acid groups, and also by the change in contrast of the polydiacetylene region (Figure 9.20).

This type of surface-supported polymerization was also observed by others [179–181]. For example, the groups of both Okawa and Wan reported the polymerization of diacetylenes in the self-assembled monolayers (SAMs) of 10,12-pentacosadiynoic acid on HOPG surfaces after UV irradiation [182, 183]. One interesting

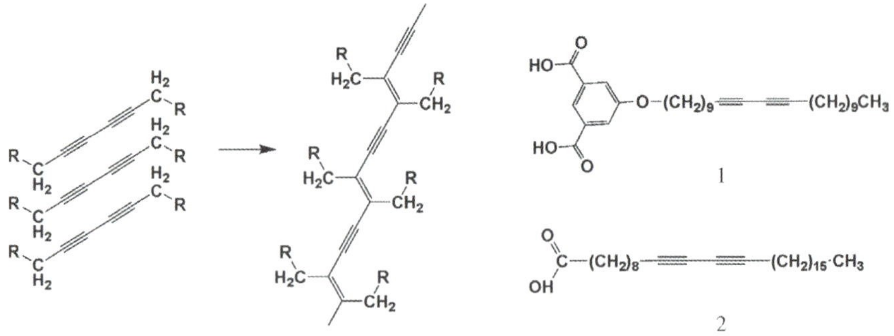

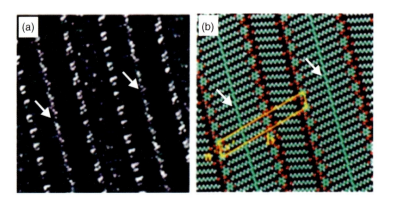

Figure 9.19 Polymerization of diacetylenes. Compounds 1 and 2 are two derivatives of diacetylenes which have been successfully observed after polymerization on single-crystal surfaces.

observation reported by Okawa's group was the controlled behavior of polymerization when using a STM tip [182, 184]. In this case, a negative-pulsed sample bias (-4 V in height, 5 us in width) was applied via the STM tip at a special point on top of the diacetylene groups. STM measurements subsequently demonstrated the presence of a polymerized line that highlighted an enhanced tunneling probability compared to the remainder of the SAMs. This line started from the point where the pulsed sample bias was applied, and terminated at an artificial defect made by a positive-pulsed sample bias (5 V in height, 10 us in width) (Figure 9.21).

In addition to studies on the polymerization of diacetylenes, the electronic properties of the resultant polydiacetylene nanowires on different substrates have been reported recently [185]. Kelly *et al.* revealed that polydiacetylene (PDA) nanowires exhibit intriguing substrate-dependent electronic effects when probed at varying sample bias voltage conditions on HOPG and molybdenum disulfide (MoS_2). On HOPG surfaces, the PDA nanowires exhibited a decreased tunneling probability as the bias voltage was reduced. The height of the PDA nanowires, when measured at

Figure 9.20 STM image of the polymerization of diacetylenes on HOPG. (a) STM image of the polymerization of compound 1. The enhanced tunneling probability in the middle of the molecules marked by white arrows shows the evidence of the polymerized structures; (b) Molecular model of the polymerized structures [179–181].

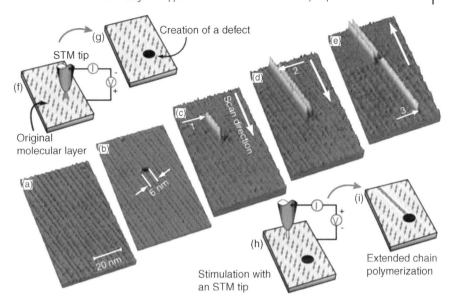

Figure 9.21 STM images and diagrams, showing the controlled polymerization by STM tip. (a) The original SAMs of compound 2p; (b) Artificial defect made by STM tip; (c) First chain polymerization, initiated at arrow (1); (d) Second chain polymerization, initiated at arrow (2); (e) Third chain polymerization, initiated at arrow (3); (f, g) Diagrams showing the creation of an artificial defect; (h, i) Diagrams showing initiation of chain polymerization with an STM tip, and termination of the polymerization at the artificial defect [185].

negative voltages, was substantially higher than that measured at positive voltages. On MoS_2, the PDA nanowires appeared with a much higher contrast on HOPG when imaged under the same negative bias conditions, but could not be visualized under positive bias conditions on MoS_2, despite it being possible still to image the unpolymerized molecules. The authors attributed these phenomena to certain substrate-dependent effects, such as substrate doping, screening, or surface dipole effects

9.4.1.2 Polymerization by Electrochemical Methods

Electrochemistry represents a conventional technique for synthesizing polymerized structures on electrodes. A reliance on *in situ* electrochemical scanning tunneling microscopy (EC-STM), and the formation and propagation of linear polymerized structures on single-crystal surfaces, has been revealed at the single-molecule level [186–189]. Yao *et al.* reported the polymerization of an aniline monolayer on a Au(111) electrode in 0.1 M sulfuric acid containing 30 mM aniline [189]. In this case, the ordered aniline monolayer was observed between 0.47 and 0.9 V, versus the reversible hydrogen electrode (RHE). Shifting the potential from 0.9 to 1.05 V led to the polymerization of aniline (see Figure 9.22). Here, the polymerized aniline (PAN) lines were found to propagate preferentially along $\langle 112 \rangle$ directions, while the height

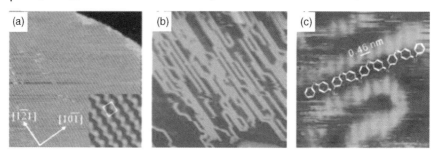

Figure 9.22 Polymerization of aniline on Au(111). (a) *In situ* STM images recorded at 0.9 V; (b) The polymerized aniline structures observed 20 min after the shift of potential from 0.9 to 1.05 V; (c) High-resolution STM image showing the detailed structures of the polymerized aniline [188].

of the polymerized lines was seen to be 0.1–0.4 nm higher than the molecular rows of aniline monomers. According to the high-resolution STM image and the periodic distance of the PAN, the authors proposed that the PAN consisted of aniline molecules linked in a head-to-tail manner (Figure 9.22c).

Other types of electrochemical method have also been reported for producing a single conjugated-polymer wire on a single-crystal electrode. For example, Saka-guchi *et al.* reported the technique of "electrochemical epitaxial polymerization," by which they observed the nucleation and propagation of high-density arrays of single conjugated-polymer wires as long as 75 nm on Au(111) surfaces [188]. In these studies, thiophene derivatives, including 3-butoxy-4-methylthiophene (BuOMT), 3-octylthiophene, 3,3-dibutyl-3,4-dihydro-2*H*-thieno[3,4-b]-[1,4]dioxepine (DBuP-DOT) and 3-[(S)-2-methylbutoxy]-4-methylthiophene (MBuOMT), were selected to investigate electrochemical polymerization in an iodine-containing electrolyte solution. The electrochemical growth of single-conjugated polymer wires was achieved by applying a given number of positive-voltage pulses (1.4 V, 150 ms, versus Pt) to the Au (111) surfaces. Under the oxidation potential of 1.4 V, the monomer of thiophene derivatives was oxidized to the cation radical, which was the reaction source for the propagation of conjugated polymer. Both, the length and density of single-poly-thiophene wires were found to depend on the number of pulses of the applied voltage. The application of 15 pulses led to the Au(111) surfaces being almost fully covered by the conjugated polymer, while the iodine-covered Au(111) surfaces acted as a form of molecular template to guide the propagation of the conjugated polymer, as the polythiophene wires appeared along three specific directions (Figure 9.23).

The same method was also reported available for preparing heterojunctions of conjugated copolymers on iodine-covered Au(111) surfaces [187]. For this, two types of thiophene monomer – 3-octyloxy-4-methylthiophene (C8OMT) and 3-octyl-4-methylthiophene (C8MT) – were used as building blocks to create heterowires. Cyclic voltammography showed the oxidation potential of C8OMT to be about 0.4 V lower than that of C8MT, which makes available a multistep electrochemical epitaxial polymerization (ECEP) to prepare the heterowires of conjugated polymers. Several linkage types, including diblock, triblock, and multiblock have been observed using

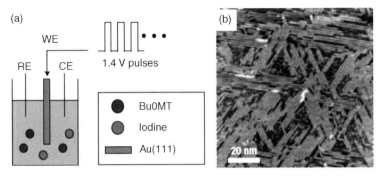

Figure 9.23 (a) Experimental set-up of electrochemical epitaxial polymerization; (b) STM image of the resulting structures after applying 15 voltage pulses (1.4 V, 150 ms) in the BuOMT (10 mM) iodine (0.1 mM) NBu$_4$PF$_6$ (0.1 M) DCM solution [187].

STM. Subsequent scanning tunneling spectroscopy (STS) studies of the heterowires showed the HOMO–LUMO gaps of each polymer to be the same as those of the wires of each homopolymer.

9.4.1.3 Polymerization by Thermal Activation

Thermally initiated polymerization has been used traditionally for the industrial synthesis of polymers. With thermal treatment, reactive radicals can be derived either from the monomer itself or from a small amount of additives, such as organic peroxides. During recent years, thermally initiated polymerization has been applied to the synthesis of covalent connected networks on single-crystal surfaces under UHV conditions [162, 190–192], the aim being to create stable molecular networks with a controlled shape and an efficient electron transport. The critical step in thermally initiated polymerization is the generation of sufficient radicals, and for this two types of method have been reported by Grill and coworkers: (i) where the radicals are produced on the substrate when the sample is heated; or (ii) where they are produced directly in the evaporator [191]. Both methods have been used successfully for the polymerization of molecules containing carbon–halogen bonds.

As shown in Figure 9.24, one type of porphyrin derivative, tetra (4-bromophenyl) porphyrin (Br$_4$TPP), was selected because: (i) the central part of the molecule is chemically stable, and it is easy to form ordered structures on metal surfaces; and (ii) the radicals may be derived by breaking chemical bonds between bromine and the phenyl group, in a controlled manner. When the evaporator temperature was below 550 K, normal close-packed structures of intact Br$_4$TPP molecules were found as a result of self-assembly, although covalent connected networks were found on the Au (111) surfaces when the evaporator temperature was higher than 590 K. The pattern of covalent connected structures may be controlled by adjusting the position of the Br substituent. Three types of structure – dimers, chains, and networks – were identified on the surfaces; these corresponded to the self-assembly of one Br substituent, to two *trans*-Br substituents, and to four Br substituents.

Another successful polymerization reaction was reported by Lipton-Duffin and coworkers, who selected 1,4-diiodobenzene and 1,3-diiodobenzene as building

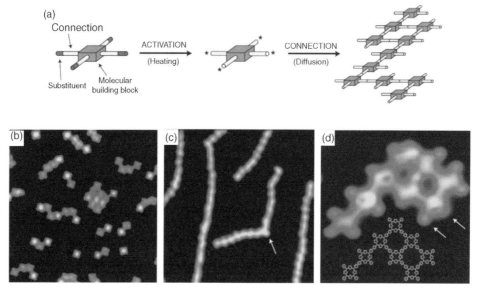

Figure 9.24 (a) Diagram of the polymerization by activated building blocks; (b–d) STM images exhibiting the polymerized structures of dimers, chains and networks, corresponding to the self-assembly of one Br substituent (b), two trans-Br substituents (c), and four Br substituents (d) [192].

blocks [192]. Polymerization reactions were performed on Cu(110) surfaces, as copper may catalyze breaking of the C−I bond. Compared to the bonding strength of the C−Br bond, the weaker C−I bond was easier to break and this allowed the reaction to occur at a relatively lower temperature (ca. 500 K). Subsequent STM studies demonstrated the presence of two types of polymer chain, namely straight and zigzag, which corresponded to the polymerization of 1,4-diiodobenzene and 1,3-diiodobenzene, respectively.

9.4.2
Host–Guest Systems

The host–guest phenomenon is at the origin of supramolecular chemistry. Guest entities (ions, molecules) may be selectively recognized and accommodated by host systems through noncovalent interactions. Recently, these concepts have been introduced for the fabrication of 2-D nanostructures on single-crystal surfaces [72, 193–199], targeting the building of complex ordered structures with nanometer precision. The guest entities, which range from tiny metallic cations [195] to complex organic-molecule-protected metal clusters [200, 201], have been applied to build host–guest structures on the prefabricated molecular template. An overview of recent efforts related to the preparation of molecular templates will be provided in the following subsections, with emphasis placed on the inclusion of guest entities when designing the template.

9.4.2.1 Molecular Template with Porous Networks

A molecular template with porous networks is widely used when studying host–guest systems, as the periodic pores may provide sufficient space for the inclusion of guest entities. The sizes and properties of the pores may be adjusted by changing the molecular structures of the building blocks. Until now, three variant methods have been described for building porous networks on single-crystal surfaces:

- Planar organic molecules with potential to form lateral hydrogen bonds are selected to build hydrogen-bond-connected networks. The pore size may be adjusted by changing the length of the building molecule.
- Under UHV conditions, metal–organic coordination networks may be built by the sequential deposition of organic ligands and metal atoms on preheated substrates.
- At liquid/solid interfaces, using specially synthesized building blocks to self-assemble the porous networks. In this case, the building block consists of a rigid core to ensure the shape of the pore, and lateral length-tunable alkyl chains to adjust the size of the pore.

Hydrogen-Bond-Connected Networks Hydrogen bonding interactions between molecules may cause a remarkable increase in molecule–molecule interactions, increasing the stability of the SAMs. By relying on the selectivity and directionality of the H-bonds, many examples of H-bond-directed molecular templates have been reported, including 1-D lines [35, 50] and 2-D porous networks [49, 193, 202]. As with the porous networks, hexagonal structures are commonly found, and the pore size can be adjusted by changing the building molecules.

The self-assembly of trimesic acid (TMA, **3a** in Figure 9.9) is one the earliest reported examples of forming H-bond-directed 2-D porous networks on single-crystal surfaces [46, 49]. The dimeric H-bonding of the TMA molecules may result in the formation of cavities of diameter about 1.7 nm, which is large enough to accommodate guest molecules such as trimesic acid itself [49], coronene [203], and C_{60} [96]. On the basis of hydrogen bond formation between carboxylic groups, porous networks with larger cavity diameters have been observed by the self-assembly of tetracarboxylic acids (**4e** and **4f** in Figure 9.9) [106] and a tetra-acidic azobenzene molecule (**4b** in Figure 9.9) [104]. However, with increasing molecular length, these larger hexagonal porous networks tend to collapse. As with the self-assembly of tetracarboxylic acids, the molecules prefer to form close-packed structures rather than porous networks on HOPG surfaces [106]. Interestingly, the participation of a guest molecule of coronene significantly enhances the stability of porous networks over the close-packed parallel structures, though this might be attributed to a form of guest molecule-guided template. However, it also shows that the hydrogen bonds between the carboxylic acid are not strong enough to ensure the formation of porous networks. The phase transition, such as from oblique to hexagonal, was also observed in the SAMs of 1,3,5-benzenetribenzoic acid (BTB, **3b** in Figure 9.9) in different solvents at the liquid/substrate interface [116]. This solvent-dependent phase transition implicates the versatility of the SAMs directed by carboxylic hydrogen bonds.

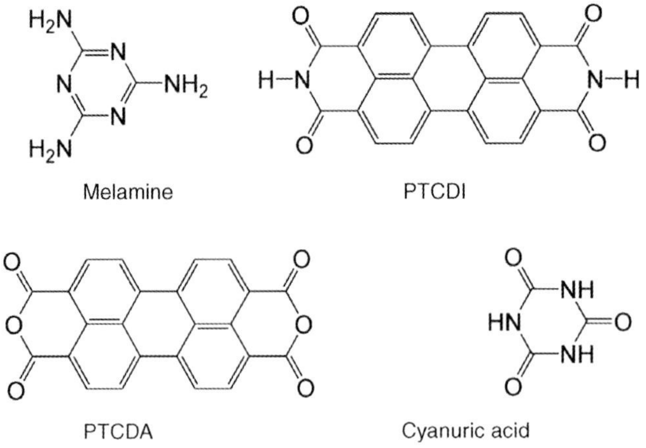

Melamine

PTCDI

PTCDA

Cyanuric acid

Figure 9.25 Chemical structures of compounds used for building porous networks directed by hydrogen bonds.

To ensure the formation of porous networks, other types of molecule with potential to form stronger hydrogen bonds should be considered. The melamine molecule represents an ideal candidate that may form triple hydrogen bonds with perylene tetracarboxylic diimide (PTCDI) [53, 204–210], perylene tetracarboxylic dianhydride (PTCDA) [211] and cyanuric acid [55, 57, 212], as shown in Figure 9.25. The threefold symmetry of melamine molecule and the strength of the lateral hydrogen bonds (e.g., $15 \, kcal \, mol^{-1}$ between a melamine and a cyanuric acid) [212, 213] ensure the formation of hexagonal porous networks. Robust H-bond-directed porous networks formed by the coadsorption of melamine and PTCDI have been reported both under UHV conditions on silver-covered Si(111) surfaces [204] and on Au(111) surfaces at the liquid/substrate interface [214]. The porous networks formed by melamine and PTCDI were found not only to be capable of accommodating fullerene molecules under UHV conditions [204], but also of patterning the structures of chemisorbed SAMs, such as thiols [214]. Three types of thiol, namely adamantane thiols (ASH), ω-(4′-methylbiphenyl-4-yl) propane thiol (BP3SH) and dodecane thiol (C12SH), were successfully filled in the pores of the networks by forming S–Au bonds. Interestingly, these combined structures, thiols and H-bond-directed networks survived even after the underpotential deposition of copper atoms on the Au substrate, thus demonstrating the adequate stability of the H-bond-directed networks to act as templates in subsequent processes (Figure 9.26).

Porous Networks Directed by Metal–Organic Coordination Bonds   The strength of a typical single hydrogen bond is about $5 \, kcal \, mol^{-1}$, but when multiple hydrogen bonds are formed between self-assembled molecules the molecular interactions will increase correspondingly, giving rise to an enhanced stability of the derived open networks. Compared to metal–organic coordination bonds, however, even multiple hydrogen bonds may be considered only as medium strength interactions, as the typical bond energy of a metal–organic coordination bond amounts to

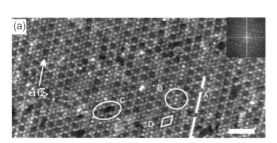
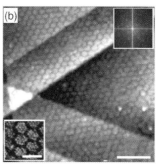

Figure 9.26 (a) STM image showing hexagonal networks formed by melamine and PTCDI; (b) Filled networks by accommodation of guest thiols of ASH [214].

$10–30\,kcal\,mol^{-1}$ per interaction [215]. It may be reasonably anticipated that porous networks directed by metal–organic coordination bonds will possess a greater stability and increased functionality.

The first example of a metal–organic coordination network (MOCN) was reported by the group of Kern, on Cu(100) surfaces under UHV conditions [66]. Here, organic ligands of 1,2,4-benzenetricarboxylic acid (TMLA) and Fe atoms were deposited sequentially onto preheated Cu(100) surfaces (400 K). The structures of the MOCNs could be adjusted by increasing the adsorbate coverage ratio of Fe/TMLA from 1 : 1 to 2 : 1. By using the same method, other organic ligands with carboxylic groups, such as trimesic acid [68], 1,4-dicarboxylic benzoic acid (TPA) and 4,1′,4′,1″-terphenyl-1,4″-dicarboxylic acid (TDA) [72], have been selected to build MOCNs, exhibiting features of chirality and an ability to accommodate guest molecules such as C_{60} [72]. The MOCNs prepared by this method proved to be stable at temperatures up to 500 K under vacuum conditions, which allowed for annealing experiments to investigate the binding strength of the guest molecules. The reversible inclusion of guest molecules, such as cystine, L,L-diphenylalanine (Phe-Phe) and fullerene C_{60}, has been examined by using cavities of MOCNs formed by TMA and Fe as receptors [216] (Figure 9.27).

Those MOCNs formed by the chelation of Fe and carboxylic group often possess twofold or fourfold symmetry. Hexagonal coordination networks may be prepared either from iron centers with linear 4,4′-biphenol ligands, or from cobalt centers with linear 1,4′;4′,1″-terphenyl-4,4″-dicarbonitrile ligands on Cu(100) or Ag(111) surfaces [67]. The fact that the symmetry of the hexagonal structures is independent of the symmetry of the substrate indicates that the strong molecule–molecule interactions predominate over the substrate influences, while the size of the hexagonal pore can be tuned simply by lengthening the size of the ligands. A series of organic linkers (abbreviated NC-Ph$_n$-CN, where n may be three, four, or five) has been synthesized and used to prepare hexagonal networks with Co atoms on Ag(111) surfaces [217]. In this case, hexagonal porous structures were observed with a tunable pore size that ranged from $10\,nm^2$ ($n = 3$) to $20\,nm^2$ ($n = 5$). Very recently, the largest size of hexagonal cavity reported when using this method was $24\,nm^2$, by the

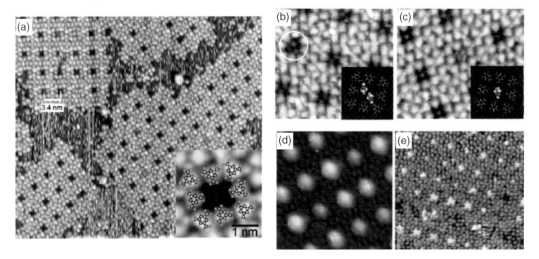

Figure 9.27 (a) Porous networks formed by organic ligands of trimesic acid and metal atoms of Fe; (b) STM image showing two guest cystine molecules anchored in one pore; (c) Upon 430 K annealing, the nanocavities typically accommodate a single cystine guest at the center; (d, e) STM images showing the host–guest system by binding of single C_{60} molecules (d) and Phe-Phe molecules (e) in the cavities [67].

coordination of NC-Ph_6-CN and Co atoms on Ag(111) surfaces [70]. A large area of a single domain was found to cover terraces over μm^2 areas, with a low defect concentration. Under UHV conditions, these hexagonal porous networks have been selected as the template to direct the deposition and the shape of small Fe and Co clusters [218]. These small metal clusters were adsorbed preferentially on top of the organic ligands, for deposition temperatures ranging from 90 to 130 K.

Porous Networks Directed by Van der Waals Forces The porous networks directed by H-bonds and metal–organic coordination bonds usually form rigid structures, due to the properties of molecular interactions. In contrast to rigid porous networks, a type of soft porous network may be prepared at liquid/substrate interfaces by the self-assembly of specially synthesized molecules. Those molecules often have a rigid core to maintain the shape of the networks, and several length-tunable legs (alkyl chains) to adjust the pore size [115, 219–221]. The largest pore prepared in this way was reported to be 7 nm in diameter, and capable of accommodating a giant molecular spoked wheel [222]. In the SAMs of those molecules, the molecular interactions were mainly van der Waals forces. Although the strength of typical van der Waals interactions is less than 1 kcal mol^{-1} between small molecules, adequate molecular interactions to ensure the stability of the SAMs may be obtained by an elongation of the alkyl chains. As the van der Waals interactions are less directional than H-bonds and metal–organic coordination bonds, many factors – such as solvent [115], concentration [114] and guest molecules [223] – may influence the structures of the SAMs.

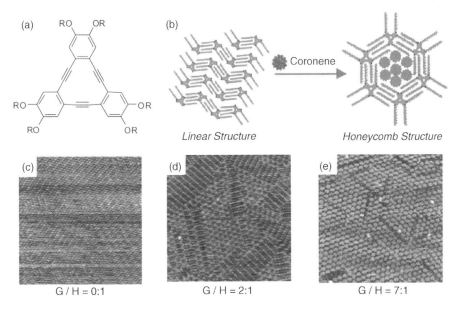

Figure 9.28 (a) Chemical structure of dehydrobenzo[12]annulene (DBA) derivatives; (b) Tentative models of the surface patterns of DBA derivatives with alkyl chain length of C_{14}. Left: linear structure without coronene; right: honeycomb structure capturing at most seven coronene molecules. (c–e) Large STM images of the network structures with or without coronene: (c) guest–host = 0 : 1; (d) guest–host = 2 : 1; (e) guest–host = 7 : 1 [115].

Figure 9.28a shows a molecular building block of dehydrobenzo[12]annulene (DBA) derivatives. The self-assembly of DBA derivatives with alkyl chain length from C_{10} to C_{18} on HOPG surfaces reveals that the structural transformation from honeycomb to a linear structure is related to the length of the alkyl chains [115]. The honeycomb structure predominates in the SAMs of DBA derivatives containing shorter alkyl chains of C_{10}, whereas only the linear structure was found for compounds with chain lengths of C_{14}, C_{16}, and C_{18}. Both, the honeycomb and the linear structure coexist in the SAMs of compounds with alkyl chains of C_{12}. Interestingly, upon the addition of a tenfold excess of guest coronene molecules dissolved in 1,2,4-trichlorobenzene (TCB) to the already-formed linear-type pattern at the liquid/substrate interface, the structures of SAMs formed by compounds with chain lengths of C_{14} were completely converted from the linear structure into the honeycomb structure [223]. Other guest molecules, including hexakis(phenylethy-nyl) benzene (HPEB), fullerene, 9,10-diphenylanthracene (DPA), chrysene, hexalo-dobenzene (HIB), and phthalocyanine (PC), have been checked to explore the phase transition of the host template. Only those planar guest molecules with large π-conjugated cores, such as HPEB and PC, led to the formation of honeycomb networks, whereas the small π-conjugated molecules such as HIB and chrysene, as well as the nonplanar molecules such as DPA and fullerene, had no influence on the linear structure [223]. On the basis of the template for the DBA derivatives, more complex host–guest systems have been observed by adding guest molecules of coronene, TMA and isophthalic acid (ISA) into the liquid at the 1-octanoic acid/ HOPG interface [224]. One coronene molecule with six surrounded ISA molecules was seen to assemble to a complex guest entity that could be accommodated by the molecular template of DBA derivatives, to form a three-component host–guest system.

Those porous networks directed by van der Waals interactions may be prepared at the liquid/substrate interface, which allows for the exploration of the selectivity of the host template by simply adding guest molecules into the liquid. Porous networks formed by the self-assembly of 1,3,5-tris [(E)-2-(3,5-didecyloxyphenyl)-ethenyl]- benzene at the interface of HOPG and 1-phenyloctane may selectively accommodate guest molecules, such as benzo[*rst*] perylene (BPL), coronene, benzo[*rst*]pentaphene (BPP), hexabenzocoronene(HBC), and pentacene [220]. Due to their very large size, only the pentacene molecules were unable to adsorb into the pores of the template at any concentration up to saturation.

9.4.2.2 SAMs of Functional Molecules

The recognition and accommodation of guest molecules on a molecular template with porous networks depend mainly on the structures of the template in space, while the guest entities are restricted to those molecules which can fit into the pores. Besides those porous molecular template, other types of template have been reported to accommodate guest entities, such as metal ions [195], ionic molecules [225], biomolecules [226], C_{60} [227–231] and HBC [232], relying on the properties of the building blocks.

The self-assembly of alkane and alkane derivatives on single-crystal surfaces have been realized for twenty years. At the liquid/substrate interface, these molecules may form spontaneously ordered lamellar structures, with the width of the lamellae being adjustable simply by altering the length of the carbon chains. The well-ordered lamellar structures may be used as molecular templates when the molecules are modified by the functionalized groups [194], The SAMs of fatty acid, such as $C_{19}H_{39}COOH$, were found capable of acting as molecular templates following the addition of guest urea [226]; the molecules of the latter were adsorbed along the boundary of the lamellae by forming hydrogen bonds with carboxylic groups. Other alkane derivatives, such as those modified by amino acid, have been reported to behave in similar fashion when accommodating guest molecules of urea [226]. Besides the interactions between functional groups of the template and the guest molecules, the interactions between alkyl chains may also be utilized to accommodate any guest entities that possess similar structures [200]. This idea originated from the biological proposal that large proteins, when supplied with a long alkyl chain, may be incorporated into the lipid bilayer, during which process the alkyl chain acts as a type of anchor. Based on this strategy, Au_{55} clusters decorated by $C_{18}H_{37}SH$ were prepared as guest entities, whereby a droplet of a mixture containing $C_{14}H_{29}COOH$ and decorated Au_{55} clusters was used to investigate the packing of the Au_{55} cluster on the HOPG substrate. The molecular template of $C_{14}H_{29}COOH$ guided the packing of Au_{55} clusters, leading to strands of linearly packed nanostructures (Figure 9.29) [200].

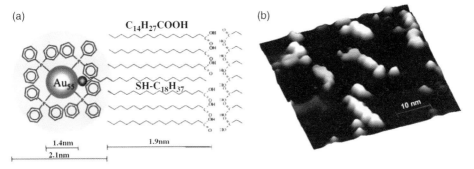

Figure 9.29 (a) Scheme of the exchange mechanism to couple the cluster core with an anchor molecule for the incorporation into a template of tetradecanoic acid; (b) STM image showing the strands of Au_{55} clusters co-adsorbed between $C_{14}H_{29}COOH$ rows [200].

A host template capable of recognizing and accommodating metal ions may be prepared by the self-assembly of functionalized molecules containing a crown ether, such as 15-crown-5-ether-substituted cobalt(II) phthalocyanine (CoCRPc). It has been found that the functional group of 15-crown-5-ether is able to accommodate guest ions such as K^+ and Ca^{2+} in solution. However, the SAMs of CoCRPc prepared on Au(111) and Au(100) surfaces showed different behaviors in the capture of Ca^{2+} ions. In the presence of Ca^{2+}, the SAMs of CoCRPc on Au(111) may capture Ca^{2+} ions in two diagonally located 15-crown-5-ether moieties, whereas the SAMs on Au(100)-(1 × 1) were unable to capture Ca^{2+} ions. These results suggested that the relationship between the crown moieties and the underlying Au lattice plays an important role in the accommodation of guest ions [195].

Molecules such as 15-crown-5-ether may be considered as a form of "molecular container" the SAMs of which, by relying on their chemical properties, can be used to capture guest entities to form complex host–guest systems. The bowl-shaped calyx [8] arene derivative (Figure 9.30a), OBOCMC8 ($C_{104}H_{128}O_{24}$), is one such type of

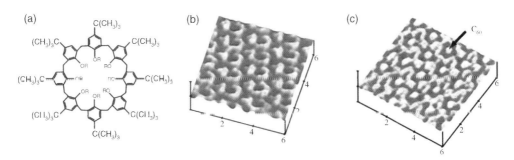

Figure 9.30 (a) Chemical structures of calyx[8] arene derivative (OBOCMC8); (b) STM image showing the SAMs of OBOCMC8. Well-ordered dark depressions are observed which represent the cavities of the OBOCMC8; (c) STM image showing the SAMs of OBOCMC8/C_{60}. The cavities of the OBOCMC8 are filled by guest fullerene molecules, showing bright spots in the center of the cavities [227].

molecular container [227], where the ring size is large enough to accommodate large molecules such as fullerene. In an electrochemical environment, the SAMs of OBOCMC8 were observed when the potential of the Au(111) surfaces was held at 0.6 V (versus RHE), as shown in Figure 9.30b. Here, well-ordered dark depressions were observed that may have been associated with the cavities of the OBOCMC8. Under the same preparation and imaging conditions, the SAMs of OBOCMC8/C_{60} showed different patterns from the SAMs of OBOCMC8. Figure 9.30c shows the high-resolution STM image of the SAMs of OBOCMC8/C_{60}, in which the cavities of the OBOCMC8 were filled by guest fullerene molecules that appeared as bright spots in the center of the cavities. However, not all molecular containers preferentially capture guest entities in the position of the cavities. For example, the molecular template of fully conjugated cyclo[12]thiophene (C[12]T) demonstrated an ability to capture fullerene molecules preferentially on the rim of the C[12]T [233], as a result of the attractive donor–acceptor interactions. Although the guest fullerene molecules might occasionally be captured in the cavities, the interaction between the fullerene and the host C[12]T was found to be very weak, and the fullerene molecules captured in the cavities were easily desorbed during scanning.

9.4.2.3 Two-Dimensional Chiral Template

In chemistry, chirality is a concept involving molecular structures, and describes a molecule that cannot be superposed on its mirror image. It is only very recently that the concept of chirality has been introduced to the 2-D building of chiral templates on surfaces. Various types of molecule, including chiral molecules, prochiral molecules and even achiral molecules, have been reported to be successful in the building of 2-D chiral patterns on single-crystal surfaces. The building of chiral templates, and their selective inclusion of guest molecules, will be introduced briefly in the following subsection. More detailed discussions on surface chirality are available in other reviews [234–237].

On occasion, the self-assembly of chiral molecules may cause chirality to be transferred directly from the molecule to SAMs. The forces required to direct such chiral self-assembly include hydrogen-bonding interactions, such as the self-assembly of L(D)-cysteine on Au(110) [238–240], and van der Waals forces, an example being the SAMs of (M)-or (P)-[7]-Helicene on Cu(111) [237, 241, 242]. In differing from chiral molecules, the self-assembly of prochiral molecules can create enantiomers on surfaces, but only when the adsorption of a molecule breaks its symmetry element [45, 50, 243, 244]. The aggregation of pure enantiomers gives rise to the formation of homochiral domains. Besides the self-assembly of chiral and prochiral molecules, chiral packing structures may also be observed, where chiral adsorption geometry is introduced by the adsorbate–substrate interactions, such as the chiral structures observed in the SAMs of normal alkanes [235] and star-shaped molecules [245], although the adsorption of achiral molecules never results in the creation of enantiomers. Achiral molecules can also form chiral structures when several molecules form rotating structures under the directional interactions of hydrogen bonds or metal–organic coordination bonds [63, 67, 207, 212, 246, 247].

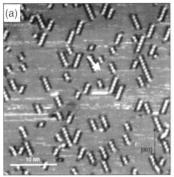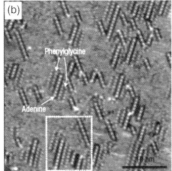

Figure 9.31 Selective adsorptions of guest molecules on basis of chiral structures. (a) STM image of Cu(110) surface with submonolayer coverage of adenine, showing chiral packing molecular chains aligned along [±1,2] directions; (b) STM image of the selective attachment of guest S-phenylglycine which were found to adsorb preferentially near the chains aligned along the [1,2] direction [248].

Although many 2-D chiral templates have been realized recently, very few reports have been made on the selective inclusion of guest molecules on basis of the prefabricated chiral template [248]. Molecular dimer chains formed by the self-assembly of adenine on Cu(110) exhibit chiral features due to the preferential adsorption of adenine molecules along [±1,2] directions with respect to the Cu (110) surfaces, as shown in Figure 9.31a. These dimer chains show significant chiral selectivity to the inclusion of guest amino acid molecules. In this case, guest molecules of S-phenylglycine were found to adsorb near the chains aligned along the [1,2] direction (see Figure 9.31b), whereas R-phenylglycine only attached to the chains aligned along the [−1,2] direction. According to the results of DFT calculations, the coulombic repulsion between the phenylglycine amino group and the DNA base was considered to be responsible for the chiral recognition. The substrate-mediated charge transfer played a critical role in chiral selectivity, whereas the direct molecular interactions such as hydrogen bonds did not [249].

9.5
Summary and Outlook

In this chapter, the recent progress on surface-supported nanostructures directed by atomic- and molecular-level templates has been reviewed, with attention focused on those nanostructured systems that are mainly organic-related and involve organic molecules as either templates or as objects, the organization of which is directed by nanostructured templates. The subject of surface-supported nanostructures that can serve as templates for the further fabrication of nanosized objects was introduced, whereby nanostructures – including surface reconstructions and reconstruction-related patterns, strain-relief epitaxial layers, vicinal surfaces, and surface-supported organic supramolecular assemblies – may serve as naturally formed templates on the atomic and molecular scale. The organization of nanosized objects directed by templates was then discussed. Despite being unable to include the details of many other reported studies, it is hoped that the present review will provide the reader with basic information regarding recent investigations in this field. Further data are available in other reviews on surface-supported supramolecular assembly [250], and the controlled assembly of organic molecules on 2-D nanotemplates [250, 251].

The size scales that can be approached by either self-assembly or so-called "bottom-up" techniques are far beyond the limit of "top-down" lithographic techniques. The former has the advantage of precisely controlling the position and orientation of nanosized objects. Although knowledge regarding self-assembly continues to be unveiled, there remain major challenges for scientists and engineers to blend the findings of the basic research conducted at academic institutions with applications in industry. For device fabrication, the robust nature of self-assembled nanostructures is vital, since molecules in surface-supported supramolecular architectures, which usually are prepared under UHV or at liquid/solid interfaces, are bound only weakly to the surface and to each other. The ability to improve the stability of these nanostructures during fabrication under ambient conditions remains a major problem; whereas, for electronic devices an insulating substrate is required, the substrates used widely today for supramolecular assembly are crystalline metals or semiconductors. Thus, the expansion of a supramolecular assembly onto an insulating or even amorphous substrate represents a major challenge.

References

1 Binnig, G., Rohrer, H., Gerber, C., and Weibel, E. (1983) *Phys. Rev. Lett.*, **50**, 120.

2 Takayanagi, K., Tanishiro, Y., Takahashi, S., and Takahashi, M. (1985) *Surf. Sci.*, **164**, 367.

3 Takayanagi, K., Tanishiro, Y., Takahashi, M., and Takahashi, S. (1985) *J. Vac. Sci. Technol. A.*, **3**, 1502.

4 Vanhove, M.A., Koestner, R.J., Stair, P.C., Biberian, J.P., Kesmodel, L.L., Bartos, I., and Somorjai, G.A. (1981) *Surf. Sci.*, **103**, 189.

5 Barth, J.V., Brune, H., Ertl, G., and Behm, R.J. (1990) *Phys. Rev. B*, **42**, 9307.

6 Kuk, Y., Chua, F.M., Silverman, P.J., and Meyer, J.A. (1990) *Phys. Rev. B*, **41**, 12393.

7 Coulman, D.J., Wintterlin, J., Behm, R.J., and Ertl, G. (1990) *Phys. Rev. Lett.*, **64**, 1761.

8 Otero, R., Naitoh, Y., Rosei, F., Jiang, P., Thostrup, P., Gourdon, A., Laegsgaard, E., Stensgaard, I., Joachim, C., and Besenbacher, F. (2004) *Angew. Chem., Int. Ed.*, **43**, 2092.

9 Kern, K., Niehus, H., Schatz, A., Zeppenfeld, P., George, J., and Comsa, G. (1991) *Phys. Rev. Lett.*, **67**, 855.

10 Auwarter, W., Kreutz, T.J., Greber, T., and Osterwalder, J. (1999) *Surf. Sci.*, **429**, 229.

11 Corso, M., Auwarter, W., Muntwiler, M., Tamai, A., Greber, T., and Osterwalder, J. (2004) *Science*, **303**, 217.

12 Goriachko, A., He, Y.B., Knapp, M., Over, H., Corso, M., Brugger, T., Berner, S., Osterwalder, J., and Greber, T. (2007) *Langmuir*, **23**, 2928.

13 Laskowski, R., Blaha, P., Gallauner, T., and Schwarz, K. (2007) *Phys. Rev. Lett.*, **98**, 106802.

14 Berner, S., Corso, M., Widmer, R., Groening, O., Laskowski, R., Blaha, P., Schwarz, K., Goriachko, A., Over, H., Gsell, S., Schreck, M., Sachdev, H., Greber, T., and Osterwalder, J. (2007) *Angew. Chem., Int. Ed.*, **46**, 5115.

15 Brune, H., Giovannini, M., Bromann, K., and Kern, K. (1998) *Nature*, **394**, 451.

16 Brune, H., Roder, H., Boragno, C., and Kern, K. (1994) *Phys. Rev. B*, **49**, 2997.

17 Brune, H., Bromann, K., Roder, H., Kern, K., Jacobsen, J., Stoltze, P., Jacobsen, K., and Norskov, J. (1995) *Phys. Rev. B*, **52**, 14380.

18 Ait-Mansour, K., Buchsbaum, A., Ruffieux, P., Schmid, M., Groning, P., Varga, P., Fasel, R., and Groning, O. (2008) *Nano Lett.*, **8**, 2035.

19 Pohl, K., Bartelt, M.C., de la Figuera, J., Bartelt, N.C., Hrbek, J., and Hwang, R.Q. (1999) *Nature*, **397**, 238.

20 Thurmer, K., Hwang, R.Q., and Bartelt, N.C. (2006) *Science*, **311**, 1272.

21 Jaloviar, S.G., Lin, J.L., Liu, F., Zielasek, V., McCaughan, L., and Lagally, M.G. (1999) *Phys. Rev. Lett.*, **82**, 791.

22 Kuhnke, K. and Kern, K. (2003) *J. Phys. Condens. Matter*, **15**, S3311.

23 Giesenseibert, M., Schmitz, F., Jentjens, R., and Ibach, H. (1995) *Surf. Sci.*, **329**, 47.

24 Hoogeman, M.S., Klik, M.A.J., Schlosser, D.C., Kuipers, L., and Frenken, J.W.H. (1999) *Phys. Rev. Lett.*, **82**, 1728.

25 Hahn, E., Schief, H., Marsico, V., Fricke, A., and Kern, K. (1994) *Phys. Rev. Lett.*, **72**, 3378.

26 Barbier, L., Masson, L., Cousty, J., and Salanon, B. (1996) *Surf. Sci.*, **345**, 197.

27 Viernow, J., Lin, J.L., Petrovykh, D.Y., Leibsle, F.M., Men, F.K., and Himpsel, F.J. (1998) *Appl. Phys. Lett.*, **72**, 948.

28 Ozcomert, J.S., Pai, W.W., Bartelt, N.C., and Reuttrobey, J.E. (1994) *Phys. Rev. Lett.*, **72**, 258.

29 Xiao, W.D., Ruffieux, P., Ait-Mansour, K., Groning, O., Palotas, K., Hofer, W.A., Groning, P., and Fasel, R. (2006) *J. Phys. Chem. B*, **110**, 21394.

30 Rousset, S., Repain, V., Baudot, G., Garreau, Y., and Lecoeur, J. (2003) *J. Phys. Condens. Matter*, **15**, S3363.

31 Yokoyama, T., Yokoyama, S., Kamikado, T., Okuno, Y., and Mashiko, S. (2001) *Nature*, **413**, 619.

32 Fernandez-Torrente, I., Monturet, S., Franke, K.J., Fraxedas, J., Lorente, N., and Pascual, J.I. (2007) *Phys. Rev. Lett.*, **99**, 176103.

33 Stadler, C., Hansen, S., Kroger, I., Kumpf, C., and Umbach, E. (2009) *Nat. Phys.*, **5**, 153.

34 Yokoyama, T., Takahashi, T., Shinozaki, K., and Okamoto, M. (2007) *Phys. Rev. Lett.*, **98**, 206102.

35 Barth, J.V., Weckesser, J., Cai, C.Z., Gunter, P., Burgi, L., Jeandupeux, O., and Kern, K. (2000) *Angew. Chem., Int. Ed.*, **39**, 1230.

36 Classen, T., Fratesi, G., Costantini, G., Fabris, S., Stadler, F.L., Kim, C., de Gironcoli, S., Baroni, S., and Kern, K. (2005) *Angew. Chem., Int. Edit.*, **44**, 6142.

37 Pawin, G., Solanki, U., Kwon, K.Y., Wong, K.L., Lin, X., Jiao, T., and Bartels, L. (2007) *J. Am. Chem. Soc.*, **129**, 12056.

38 Schiffrin, A., Reichert, J., Auwarter, W., Jahnz, G., Pennec, Y., Weber-Bargioni, A., Stepanyuk, V.S., Niebergall, L., Bruno, P., and Barth, J.V. (2008) *Phys. Rev. B*, **78**, 035424.

39 Schiffrin, A., Riemann, A., Auwarter, W., Pennec, Y., Weber-Bargioni, A., Cvetko, D., Cossaro, A., Alberto, M., and Barth, J.V. (2007) *Proc. Natl Acad. Sci. USA*, **104**, 5279.

40 Schnadt, J., Rauls, E., Xu, W., Vang, R.T., Knudsen, J., Laegsgaard, E., Li, Z., Hammer, B., and Besenbacher, F. (2008) *Phys. Rev. Lett.*, **100**, 046103.

41 Surin, M., Samori, P., Jouaiti, A., Kyritsakas, N., and Hosseini, M.W. (2007) *Angew. Chem., Int. Ed.*, **46**, 245.

42 Klappenberger, F., Canas-Ventura, M.E., Clair, S., Pons, S., Schlickum, U., Qu, Z.R., Brune, H., Kern, K., Strunskus, T., Woll, C., Comisso, A., De Vita, A., Ruben, M., and Barth, J.V. (2007) *ChemPhysChem*, **8**, 1782.

43 Trixler, F., Market, T., Lackinger, M., Jamitzky, F., and Heckl, W.M. (2007) *Chem. Eur. J.*, **13**, 7785.

44 Ciesielski, A., Schaeffer, G., Petitjean, A., Lehn, J.M., and Samori, P. (2009) *Angew. Chem., Int. Ed.*, **48**, 2039.

45 Weckesser, J., De Vita, A., Barth, J.V., Cai, C., and Kern, K. (2001) *Phys. Rev. Lett.*, **87**, 096101.

46 Ye, Y.C., Sun, W., Wang, Y.F., Shao, X., Xu, X.G., Cheng, F., Li, J.L., and Wu, K. (2007) *J. Phys. Chem. C*, **111**, 10138.

47 Ma, Z., Wang, Y.Y., Wang, P., Huang, W., Li, Y.B., Lei, S.B., Yang, Y.L., Fan, X.L., and Wang, C. (2007) *ACS Nano*, **1**, 160.

48 Ishikawa, Y., Ohira, A., Sakata, M., Hirayama, C., and Kunitake, M. (2002) *Chem. Commun.*, 2652.

49 Griessl, S., Lackinger, M., Edelwirth, M., Hietschold, M., and Heckl, W.M. (2002) *Single Molecules*, **3**, 25.

50 Barth, J.V., Weckesser, J., Trimarchi, G., Vladimirova, M., De Vita, A., Cai, C.Z., Brune, H., Gunter, P., and Kern, K. (2002) *J. Am. Chem. Soc.*, **124**, 7991.

51 Ruben, M., Payer, D., Landa, A., Comisso, A., Gattinoni, C., Lin, N., Collin, J.P., Sauvage, J.P., De Vita, A., and Kern, K. (2006) *J. Am. Chem. Soc.*, **128**, 15644.

52 Otero, R., Schock, M., Molina, L.M., Laegsgaard, E., Stensgaard, I., Hammer, B., and Besenbacher, F. (2005) *Angew. Chem., Int. Ed.*, **44**, 2270.

53 Silly, F., Shaw, A.Q., Porfyrakis, K., Briggs, G.A.D., and Castell, M.R. (2007) *Appl. Phys. Lett.*, **91**, 253109.

54 Silly, F., Shaw, A.Q., Briggs, G.A.D., and Castell, M.R. (2008) *Appl. Phys. Lett.*, **92**, 023102.

55 Perdigao, L.M.A., Champness, N.R., and Beton, P.H. (2006) *Chem. Commun.*, 538.

56 Llanes-Pallas, A., Palma, C.A., Piot, L., Belbakra, A., Listorti, A., Prato, M., Samori, P., Armaroli, N., and Bonifazi, D. (2009) *J. Am. Chem. Soc.*, **131**, 509.

57 Staniec, P.A., Perdigao, L.M.A., Rogers, B.L., Champness, N.R., and Beton, P.H. (2007) *J. Phys. Chem. C*, **111**, 886.

58 Gesquiere, A., Jonkheijm, P., Hoeben, F.J.M., Schenning, A., De Feyter, S., De Schryver, F.C., and Meijer, E.W. (2004) *Nano Lett.*, **4**, 1175.

59 De Feyter, S., Gesquiere, A., Klapper, M., Mullen, K., and De Schryver, F.C. (2003) *Nano Lett.*, **3**, 1485.

60 Stohr, M., Wahl, M., Galka, C.H., Riehm, T., Jung, T.A., and Gade, L.H. (2005) *Angew. Chem., Int. Ed.*, **44**, 7394.

61 Silly, F., Shaw, A.Q., Castell, M.R., Briggs, G.A.D., Mura, M., Martsinovich, N., and Kantorovich, L. (2008) *J. Phys. Chem. C*, **112**, 11476.

62 Pawin, G., Wong, K.L., Kwon, K.Y., and Bartels, L. (2006) *Science*, **313**, 961.

63 Stepanow, S., Lin, N., Vidal, F., Landa, A., Ruben, M., Barth, J.V., and Kern, K. (2005) *Nano Lett.*, **5**, 901.

64 Lin, N., Stepanow, S., Ruben, M., and Barth, J.V. (2009) *Top. Curr. Chem.*, **287**, 1.

65 Stepanow, S., Lin, N., and Barth, J.V. (2008) *J. Phys. Condens. Matter*, **20**, 184002.

66 Dmitriev, A., Spillmann, H., Lin, N., Barth, J.V., and Kern, K. (2003) *Angew. Chem., Int. Ed.*, **42**, 2670.

67 Stepanow, S., Lin, N., Payer, D., Schlickum, U., Klappenberger, F., Zoppellaro, G., Ruben, M., Brune, H., Barth, J.V., and Kern, K. (2007) *Angew. Chem., Int. Ed.*, **46**, 710.

68 Spillmann, H., Dmitriev, A., Lin, N., Messina, P., Barth, J.V., and Kern, K. (2003) *J. Am. Chem. Soc.*, **125**, 10725.

69 Tait, S.L., Wang, Y., Costantini, G., Lin, N., Baraldi, A., Esch, F., Petaccia, L., Lizzit, S., and Kern, K. (2008) *J. Am. Chem. Soc.*, **130**, 2108.

70 Kuhne, D., Klappenberger, F., Decker, R., Schlickum, U., Brune, H., Klyatskaya, S., Ruben, M., and Barth, J.V. (2009) *J. Am. Chem. Soc.*, **131**, 3881.

71 Schlickum, U., Decker, R., Klappenberger, F., Zoppellaro, G., Klyatskaya, S., Ruben, M., Silanes, I., Arnau, A., Kern, K., Brune, H., and Barth, J.V. (2007) *Nano Lett.*, **7**, 3813.

72 Stepanow, S., Lingenfelder, M., Dmitriev, A., Spillmann, H., Delvigne, E., Lin, N., Deng, X.B., Cai, C.Z., Barth, J.V., and Kern, K. (2004) *Nat. Mater.*, **3**, 229.

73 Langner, A., Tait, S.L., Lin, N., Rajadurai, C., Ruben, M., and Kern, K. (2007) *Proc. Natl Acad. Sci. USA*, **104**, 17927.

74 Zhang, Y.F., Zhu, N., and Komeda, T. (2008) *Surf. Sci.*, **602**, 614.

75 Zhang, Y.F., Zhu, N., and Komeda, T. (2007) *J. Phys. Chem. C*, **111**, 16946.

76 Lin, N., Dmitriev, A., Weckesser, J., Barth, J.V., and Kern, K. (2002) *Angew. Chem., Int. Ed.*, **41**, 4779.

77 Tait, S.L., Langner, A., Lin, N., Stepanow, S., Rajadurai, C., Ruben, M., and Kern, K. (2007) *J. Phys. Chem. C*, **111**, 10982.

78 Pawin, G., Wong, K.L., Kim, D., Sun, D.Z., Bartels, L., Hong, S., Rahman, T.S., Carp, R., and Marsella, M. (2008) *Angew. Chem., Int. Ed.*, **47**, 8442.

79 Zhang, H.M., Zhao, W., Xie, Z.X., Long, L.S., Mao, B.W., Xu, X., and Zheng, L.S. (2007) *J. Phys. Chem. C*, **111**, 7570.

80 Nath, K.G., Ivasenko, O., MacLeod, J.M., Miwa, J.A., Wuest, J.D., Nanci, A., Perepichka, D.F., and Rosei, F. (2007) *J. Phys. Chem. C*, **111**, 16996.

81 Lennartz, M.C., Atodiresei, N., Muller-Meskamp, L., Karthauser, S., Waser, R., and Blugel, S. (2009) *Langmuir*, **25**, 856.

82 Guo, Q., Cocks, I., and Williams, E.M. (1997) *Surf. Sci.*, **393**, 1.

83 Frederick, B.G., Chen, Q., Leibsle, F.M., Lee, M.B., Kitching, K.J., and Richardson, N.V. (1997) *Surf. Sci.*, **394**, 1.

84 Dougherty, D.B., Maksymovych, P., and Yates, J.T. (2006) *Surf. Sci.*, **600**, 4484.

85 Chen, Q., Perry, C.C., Frederick, B.G., Murray, P.W., Haq, S., and Richardson, N.V. (2000) *Surf. Sci.*, **446**, 63.

86 Li, H., Xu, B., Evans, D., and Reutt-Robey, J.E. (2007) *J. Phys. Chem. C*, **111**, 2102.

87 Lin, N., Stepanow, S., Vidal, F., Barth, J.V., and Kern, K. (2005) *Chem. Commun.*, 1681.

88 Langner, A., Tait, S.L., Lin, N., Chandrasekar, R., Ruben, M., and Kern, K. (2008) *Angew. Chem., Int. Ed.*, **47**, 8835.

89 Yang, Y.L., Deng, K., Zeng, Q.D., and Wang, C. (2006) *Surf. Interface Anal.*, **38**, 1039.

90 Lackinger, M., Griessl, S., Markert, T., Jamitzky, F., and Heckl, W.M. (2004) *J. Phys. Chem. B*, **108**, 13652.

91 Clair, S., Pons, S., Seitsonen, A.P., Brune, H., Kern, K., and Barth, J.V. (2004) *J. Phys. Chem. B*, **108**, 14585.

92 Kampschulte, L., Griessl, S., Heckl, W.M., and Lackinger, M. (2005) *J. Phys. Chem. B*, **109**, 14074.

93 Lackinger, M., Griessl, S., Kampschulte, L., Jamitzky, F., and Heckl, W.M. (2005) *Small*, **1**, 532.

94 Sheerin, G. and Cafolla, A.A. (2005) *Surf. Sci.*, **577**, 211.

95 Zhu, N., Osada, T., and Komeda, T. (2007) *Surf. Sci.*, **601**, 1789.

96 Griessl, S.J.H., Lackinger, M., Jamitzky, F., Markert, T., Hietschold, M., and Heckl, W.M. (2004) *J. Phys. Chem. B*, **108**, 11556.

97 Li, Z., Han, B., Wan, L.J., and Wandlowski, T. (2005) *Langmuir*, **21**, 6915.

98 Nath, K.G., Ivasenko, O., Miwa, J.A., Dang, H., Wuest, J.D., Nanci, A., Perepichka, D.F., and Rosei, F. (2006) *J. Am. Chem. Soc.*, **128**, 4212.

99 Kampschulte, L., Werblowsky, T.L., Kishore, R.S.K., Schmittel, M., Heckl, W.M., and Lackinger, M. (2008) *J. Am. Chem. Soc.*, **130**, 8502.

100 Su, G.J., Zhang, H.M., Wan, L.J., Bai, C.L., and Wandlowski, T. (2004) *J. Phys. Chem. B*, **108**, 1931.

101 Dmitriev, A., Lin, N., Weckesser, J., Barth, J.V., and Kern, K. (2002) *J. Phys. Chem. B*, **106**, 6907.

102 Gutzler, R., Lappe, S., Mahata, K., Schmittel, M., Heckl, W.M., and Lackinger, M. (2009) *Chem. Commun.*, 680.

103 Zhou, H., Dang, H., Yi, J.H., Nanci, A., Rochefort, A., and Wuest, J.D. (2007) *J. Am. Chem. Soc.*, **129**, 13774.

104 Li, M., Deng, K., Lei, S.B., Yang, Y.L., Wang, T.S., Shen, Y.T., Wang, C.R., Zeng, Q.D., and Wang, C. (2008) *Angew. Chem., Int. Ed.*, **47**, 6717.

105 Blunt, M.O., Russell, J.C., Gimenez-Lopez, M.D., Garrahan, J.P., Lin, X., Schroder, M., Champness, N.R., and Beton, P.H. (2008) *Science*, **322**, 1077.

106 Blunt, M., Lin, X., Gimenez-Lopez, M.D., Schroder, M., Champness, N.R., and Beton, P.H. (2008) *Chem. Commun.*, 2304.

107 Pivetta, M., Blum, M.C., Patthey, F., and Schneider, W.D. (2008) *Angew. Chem., Int. Ed.*, **47**, 1076.

108 Xu, W., Dong, M.D., Gersen, H., Rauls, E., Vazquez-Campos, S., Crego-Calama, M., Reinhoudt, D.N., Laegsgaard, E., Stensgaard, I., Linderoth, T.R., and Besenbacher, F. (2008) *Small*, **4**, 1620.

109 Schull, G., and Berndt, R. (2007) *Phys. Rev. Lett.*, **99**, 226105.

110 Lin, F., Zhong, D.Y., Chi, L.F., Ye, K., Wang, Y., and Fuchs, H. (2006) *Phys. Rev. B*, **73**, 235420.

111 Kong, X.H., Deng, K., Yang, Y.L., Zeng, Q.D., and Wang, C. (2007) *J. Phys. Chem. C*, **111**, 9235.

112 Stepanow, S., Strunskus, T., Lingenfelder, M., Dmitriev, A., Spillmann, H., Lin, N., Barth, J.V., Woll, C., and Kern, K. (2004) *J. Phys. Chem. B*, **108**, 19392.

113 Zhong, D.Y., Lin, F., Chi, L.F., Wang, Y., and Fuchs, H. (2005) *Phys. Rev. B*, **71**, 125336.

114 Lei, S.B., Tahara, K., De Schryver, F.C., Van der Auweraer, M., Tobe, Y., and De Feyter, S. (2008) *Angew. Chem., Int. Ed.*, **47**, 2964.

115 Tahara, K., Furukawa, S., Uji-i, H., Uchino, T., Ichikawa, T., Zhang, J., Mamdouh, W., Sonoda, M., De Schryver, F.C., De Feyter, S., and Tobe, Y. (2006) *J. Am. Chem. Soc.*, **128**, 16613.

116 Kampschulte, L., Lackinger, M., Maier, A.K., Kishore, R.S.K., Griessl, S., Schmittel, M., and Heckl, W.M. (2006) *J. Phys. Chem. B*, **110**, 10829.

117 Lackinger, M., Griessl, S., Heckl, W.A., Hietschold, M., and Flynn, G.W. (2005) *Langmuir*, **21**, 4984.

118 Mamdouh, W., Uji-i, H., Ladislaw, J.S., Dulcey, A.E., Percec, V., De Schryver, F.C., and De Feyter, S. (2006) *J. Am. Chem. Soc.*, **128**, 317.

119 Yang, Y.L. and Wang, C. (2009) *Curr. Opin. Colloid Interface Sci.*, **14**, 135.

120 Florio, G.M., Ilan, B., Muller, T., Baker, T.A., Rothman, A., Werblowsky, T.L., Berne, B.J., and Flynn, G.W. (2009) *J. Phys. Chem. C*, **113**, 3631.

121 Palma, C.A., Bonini, M., Breiner, T., and Samori, P. (2009) *Adv. Mater.*, **21**, 1383.

122 Palma, C.A., Bonini, M., Llanes-Pallas, A., Breiner, T., Prato, M., Bonifazi, D., and Samori, P. (2008) *Chem. Commun.*, 5289.

123 Kudernac, T., Lei, S.B., Elemans, J., and De Feyter, S. (2009) *Chem. Soc. Rev.*, **38**, 402.

124 Chambliss, D.D., Wilson, R.J., and Chiang, S. (1991) *Phys. Rev. Lett.*, **66**, 1721.

125 Clair, S., Pons, S., Fabris, S., Baroni, S., Brune, H., Kern, K., and Barth, J.V. (2006) *J. Phys. Chem. B*, **110**, 5627.

126 Clair, S., Pons, W., Brune, H., Kern, K., and Barth, J.V. (2005) *Angew. Chem., Int. Ed.*, **44**, 7294.

127 Jensen, S. and Baddeley, C.J. (2008) *J. Phys. Chem. C*, **112**, 15439.

128 Mendez, J., Caillard, R., Otero, G., Nicoara, N., and Martin-Gago, J.A. (2006) *Adv. Mater.*, **18**, 2048.

129 Trant, A.G., Jones, T.E., and Baddeley, C.J. (2007) *J. Phys. Chem. C*, **111**, 10534.

130 Gao, L., Liu, Q., Zhang, Y.Y., Jiang, N., Zhang, H.G., Cheng, Z.H., Qiu, W.F., Du, S.X., Liu, Y.Q., Hofer, W.A., and Gao, H.J. (2008) *Phys. Rev. Lett.*, **101**, 197209.

131 Wang, Y.F., Ge, X., Schull, G., Berndt, R., Bornholdt, C., Koehler, F., and Herges, R. (2008) *J. Am. Chem. Soc.*, **130**, 4218.

132 Zhong, D.Y., Blömker, T., Wedeking, K., Chi, L.F., Erker, G., and Fuchs, H. (2009) *Nano Lett.*, **9**, 4387.

133 Ecija, D., Otero, R., Sanchez, L., Gallego, J.M., Wang, Y., Alcami, M., Martin, F., Martin, N., and Miranda, R. (2007) *Angew. Chem., Int. Ed.*, **46**, 7874.

134 Cicoira, F., Miwa, J.A., Melucci, M., Barbarella, G., and Rosei, F. (2006) *Small*, **2**, 1366.

135 Cicoira, F., Miwa, J.A., Perepichka, D.F., and Rosei, F. (2007) *J. Phys. Chem. A*, **111**, 12674.

136 Oehzelt, M., Grill, L., Berkebile, S., Koller, G., Netzer, F.P., and Ramsey, M.G. (2007) *ChemPhysChem*, **8**, 1707.

137 Li, J.L., Jia, J.F., Liang, X.J., Liu, X., Wang, J.Z., Xue, Q.K., Li, Z.Q., Tse, J.S., Zhang, Z.Y., and Zhang, S.B. (2002) *Phys. Rev. Lett.*, **88**, 066101.

138 Suto, S., Sakamoto, K., Wakita, T., Harada, M., and Kasuya, A. (1998) *Surf. Sci.*, **404**, 523.

139 Nakaya, M., Nakayama, T., Kuwahara, Y., and Aono, M. (2006) *Surf. Sci.*, **600**, 2810.

140 Wang, X.D., Hashizume, T., Shinohara, H., Saito, Y., Nishina, Y., and Sakurai, T. (1992) *Jpn. J. Appl. Phys. 2*, **31**, L983.

141 Wang, H.Q., Zeng, C.G., Li, Q.X., Wang, B., Yang, J.L., Hou, J.G., and Zhu, Q.S. (1999) *Surf. Sci.*, **442**, L1024.

142 Makoudi, Y., Arab, M., Palmino, F., Duverger, E., Ramseyer, C., Picaud, F., and Cherioux, F. (2007) *Angew. Chem., Int. Ed.*, **46**, 9287.

143 Makoudi, Y., El Garah, M., Palmino, F., Duverger, E., Arab, M., and Cherioux, F. (2008) *Surf. Sci.*, **602**, 2719.

144 Stimpel, T., Schraufstetter, M., Baumgartner, H., and Eisele, I. (2002) *Mater. Sci. Eng., B - Solid*, **89**, 394.

145 Makoudi, Y., Palmino, F., Arab, M., Duverger, E., and Cherioux, F. (2008) *J. Am. Chem. Soc.*, **130**, 6670.

146 Zhang, Y.P., Yong, K.S., Lai, Y.H., Xu, G.Q., and Wang, X.S. (2004) *Appl. Phys. Lett.*, **85**, 2926.

147 Ratsch, C., Seitsonen, A.P., and Scheffler, M. (1997) *Phys. Rev. B*, **55**, 6750.

148 Ait-Mansour, K., Ruffieux, P., Xiao, W., Groning, P., Fasel, R., and Groning, O. (2006) *Phys. Rev. B*, **74**, 195418.

149 Dil, H., Lobo-Checa, J., Laskowski, R., Blaha, P., Berner, S., Osterwalder, J., and Greber, T. (2008) *Science*, **319**, 1824.

150 Wang, S.C., Yilmaz, M.B., Knox, K.R., Zaki, N., Dadap, J.I., Valla, T., Johnson, P.D., and Osgood, R.M. (2008) *Phys. Rev. B*, **77**, 115448.

151 Gambardella, P., Blanc, M., Brune, H., Kuhnke, K., and Kern, K. (2000) *Phys. Rev. B*, **61**, 2254.

152 Ahn, J.R., Kim, Y.J., Lee, H.S., Hwang, C.C., Kim, B.S., and Yeom, H.W. (2002) *Phys. Rev. B*, **66**, 153403.

153 Lipton-Duffin, J.A., Mark, A.G., MacLeod, J.M., and McLean, A.B. (2008) *Phys. Rev. B*, **77**, 125419.

154 Jalochowski, M. and Bauer, E. (2001) *Prog. Surf. Sci.*, **67**, 79.

155 Tegenkamp, C. (2009) *J. Phys. Condens. Matter*, **21**, 013002.

156 Ismach, A., Segev, L., Wachtel, E., and Joselevich, E. (2004) *Angew. Chem., Int. Ed.*, **43**, 6140.

157 Wawro, A., Suto, S., Czajka, R., and Kasuya, A. (2003) *Phys. Rev. B*, **67**, 195401.

158 Neel, N., Kroger, J., and Berndt, R. (2006) *Adv. Mater.*, **18**, 174.

159 Neel, N., Kroger, J., and Berndt, R. (2006) *Appl. Phys. Lett.*, **88**, 163101.

160 Vladimirova, M., Stengel, M., De Vita, A., Baldereschi, A., Bohringer, M., Morgenstern, K., Berndt, R., and

Schneider, W.D. (2001) *Europhys. Lett.*, **56**, 254.

161 Kroger, J., Jensen, H., and Neel, N. (2007) *Surf. Sci.*, **601**, 4180.

162 Treier, M., Ruffieux, P., Schillinger, R., Greber, T., Mullen, K., and Fasel, R. (2008) *Surf. Sci.*, **602**, L84.

163 Kroger, J., Neel, N., Jensen, H., Berndt, R., Rurali, R., and Lorente, N. (2006) *J. Phys. Condens. Matter*, **18**, S51.

164 Du, S.X., Gao, H.J., Seidel, C., Tsetseris, L., Ji, W., Kopf, H., Chi, L.F., Fuchs, H., Pennycook, S.J., and Pantelides, S.T. (2006) *Phys. Rev. Lett.*, **97**, 156105.

165 Zhong, D.Y., Wang, W.C., Dou, R.F., Wedeking, K., Erker, G., Chi, L.F., and Fuchs, H. (2007) *Phys. Rev. B*, **76**, 205428.

166 Jones, T.E., Baddeley, C.J., Gerbi, A., Savio, L., Rocca, M., and Vattuone, L. (2005) *Langmuir*, **21**, 9468.

167 Chen, Q. and Richardson, N.V. (2003) *Prog. Surf. Sci.*, **73**, 59.

168 Chen, Q., Frankel, D.J., and Richardson, N.V. (2001) *Langmuir*, **17**, 8276.

169 Zhao, X.Y., Wang, H., Zhao, R.G., and Yang, W.S. (2001) *Mater. Sci. Eng., C Biomim.*, **16**, 41.

170 Leibsle, F.M., Haq, S., Frederick, B.G., Bowker, M., and Richardson, N.V. (1995) *Surf. Sci.*, **343**, L1175.

171 Fanetti, M., Gavioli, L., and Sancrotti, M. (2006) *Adv. Mater.*, **18**, 2863.

172 Gavioli, L., Fanetti, M., Sancrotti, M., and Betti, M.G. (2005) *Phys. Rev. B*, **72**, 035458.

173 Ma, X., Meyerheim, H.L., Barthel, J., Kirschner, J., Schmitt, S., and Umbach, E. (2004) *Appl. Phys. Lett.*, **84**, 4038.

174 Lin, J.L., Petrovykh, D.Y., Kirakosian, A., Rauscher, H., Himpsel, F.J., and Dowben, P.A. (2001) *Appl. Phys. Lett.*, **78**, 829.

175 Rauscher, H., Jung, T.A., Lin, J.L., Kirakosian, A., Himpsel, F.J., Rohr, U., and Mullen, K. (1999) *Chem. Phys. Lett.*, **303**, 363.

176 Garnier, F., Horowitz, G., Peng, X.H., and Fichou, D. (1990) *Adv. Mater.*, **2**, 592.

177 Sirringhaus, H., Brown, P.J., Friend, R.H., Nielsen, M.M., Bechgaard, K., Langeveld-Voss, B.M.W., Spiering,

A.J.H., Janssen, R.A.J., Meijer, E.W., Herwig, P., and de Leeuw, D.M. (1999) *Nature*, **401**, 685.

178 Grim, P.C.M., De Feyter, S., Gesquiere, A., Vanoppen, P., Rucker, M., Valiyaveettil, S., Moessner, G., Mullen, K., and De Schryver, F.C. (1997) *Angew. Chem., Int. Ed.*, **36**, 2601.

179 Takami, T., Ozaki, H., Kasuga, M., Tsuchiya, T., Mazaki, Y., Fukushi, D., Ogawa, A., Uda, M., and Aono, M. (1997) *Angew. Chem., Int. Ed.*, **36**, 2755.

180 Nishio, S., I-i, D., Matsuda, H., Yoshidome, M., Uji-i, H., and Fukumura, H. (2005) *Jpn. J. Appl. Phys. 1*, **44**, 5417.

181 Okawa, Y. and Aono, M. (2001) *Nature*, **409**, 683.

182 Okawa, Y. and Aono, M. (2001) *J. Chem. Phys.*, **115**, 2317.

183 Wan, L.J. (2006) *Acc. Chem. Res.*, **39**, 334.

184 Takajo, D., Okawa, Y., Hasegawa, T., and Aono, M. (2007) *Langmuir*, **23**, 5247.

185 Giridharagopal, R. and Kelly, K.F. (2008) *ACS Nano*, **2**, 1571.

186 Wen, R., Pan, G.B., and Wan, U.J. (2008) *J. Am. Chem. Soc.*, **130**, 12123.

187 Sakaguchi, H., Matsumura, H., Gong, H., and Abouelwafa, A.M. (2005) *Science*, **310**, 1002.

188 Sakaguchi, H., Matsumura, H., and Gong, H. (2004) *Nat. Mater.*, **3**, 551.

189 Yang, L.Y.O., Chang, C., Liu, S., Wu, C., and Yau, S.L. (2007) *J. Am. Chem. Soc.*, **129**, 8076.

190 Matena, M., Riehm, T., Stohr, M., Jung, T.A., and Gade, L.H. (2008) *Angew. Chem., Int. Ed.*, **47**, 2414.

191 Grill, L., Dyer, M., Lafferentz, L., Persson, M., Peters, M.V., and Hecht, S. (2007) *Nat. Nanotechnol.*, **2**, 687.

192 Lipton-Duffin, J.A., Ivasenko, O., Perepichka, D.F., and Rosei, F. (2009) *Small*, **5**, 592.

193 Lu, J., Lei, S.B., Zeng, Q.D., Kang, S.Z., Wang, C., Wan, L.J., and Bai, C.L. (2004) *J. Phys. Chem. B*, **108**, 5161.

194 Lei, S.B., Wang, C., Fan, X.L., Wan, L.J., and Bai, C.L. (2003) *Langmuir*, **19**, 9759.

195 Yoshimoto, S., Suto, K., Tada, A., Kobayashi, N., and Itaya, K. (2004) *J. Am. Chem. Soc.*, **126**, 8020.

196 Yoshimoto, S., Tsutsumi, E., Fujii, O., Narita, R., and Itaya, K. (2005) *Chem. Commun.*, 1188.

197 Bonifazi, D., Spillmann, H., Kiebele, A., de Wild, M., Seiler, P., Cheng, F.Y., Guntherodt, H.J., Jung, T., and Diederich, F. (2004) *Angew. Chem., Int. Ed.*, **43**, 4759.

198 Spillmann, H., Kiebele, A., Stohr, M., Jung, T.A., Bonifazi, D., Cheng, F.Y., and Diederich, F. (2006) *Adv. Mater.*, **18**, 275.

199 Bonifazi, D., Kiebele, A., Stohr, M., Cheng, F.Y., Jung, T., Diederich, F., and Spillmann, H. (2007) *Adv. Funct. Mater.*, **17**, 1051.

200 Hoeppener, S., Chi, L.F., and Fuchs, H. (2002) *Nano Lett.*, **2**, 459.

201 Lei, S.B., Wang, C., Yin, S.X., Wan, L.J., and Bai, C.L. (2003) *ChemPhysChem*, **4**, 1114.

202 Kong, X.H., Deng, K., Yang, Y.L., Zeng, Q.D., and Wang, C. (2007) *J. Phys. Chem. C*, **111**, 17382.

203 Griessl, S.J.H., Lackinger, M., Jamitzky, F., Markert, T., Hietschold, M., and Heckl, W.A. (2004) *Langmuir*, **20**, 9403.

204 Theobald, J.A., Oxtoby, N.S., Phillips, M.A., Champness, N.R., and Beton, P.H. (2003) *Nature*, **424**, 1029.

205 Perdigao, L.M.A., Perkins, E.W., Ma, J., Staniec, P.A., Rogers, B.L., Champness, N.R., and Beton, P.H. (2006) *J. Phys. Chem. B*, **110**, 12539.

206 Perdigao, L.M.A., Saywell, A., Fontes, G.N., Staniec, P.A., Goretzki, G., Phillips, A.G., Champness, N.R., and Beton, P.H. (2008) *Chem. Eur. J.*, **14**, 7600.

207 Silly, F., Shaw, A.Q., Castell, M.R., and Briggs, G.A.D. (2008) *Chem. Commun.*, 1907.

208 Saywell, A., Magnano, G., Satterley, C.J., Perdigao, L.M.A., Champness, N.R., Beton, P.H., and O'Shea, J.N. (2008) *J. Phys. Chem. C*, **112**, 7706.

209 Weber, U.K., Burlakov, V.M., Perdigao, L.M.A., Fawcett, R.H.J., Beton, P.H., Champness, N.R., , J.H., Briggs, G.A.D., and Pettifor, D.G. (2008) *Phys. Rev. Lett.*, **100**, 156101.

210 Silly, F., Shaw, A.Q., Porfyrakis, K., Warner, J.H., Watt, A.A.R., Castell, M.R., Umemoto, H., Akachi, T., Shinohara, H.,

and Briggs, G.A.D. (2008) *Chem. Commun.*, 4616.

211 Swarbrick, J.C., Rogers, B.L., Champness, N.R., and Beton, P.H. (2006) *J. Phys. Chem. B*, **110**, 6110.

212 Zhang, H.M., Xie, Z.X., Long, L.S., Zhong, H.P., Zhao, W., Mao, B.W., Xu, X., and Zheng, L.S. (2008) *J. Phys. Chem. C*, **112**, 4209.

213 Xu, W., Dong, M.D., Gersen, H., Rauls, E., Vazquez-Campos, S., Crego-Calama, M., Reinhoudt, D.N., Stensgaard, I., Laegsgaard, E., Linderoth, T.R., and Besenbacher, F. (2007) *Small*, **3**, 854.

214 Madueno, R., Raisanen, M.T., Silien, C., and Buck, M. (2008) *Nature*, **454**, 618.

215 Leininger, S., Olenyuk, B., and Stang, P.J. (2000) *Chem. Rev.*, **100**, 853.

216 Stepanow, S., Lin, N., Barth, J.V., and Kern, K. (2006) *Chem. Commun.*, **2006**, 2153.

217 Schickum, U., Decker, R., Klappenberger, F., Zoppellaro, G., Klyatskaya, S., Ruben, M., Silanes, I., Arnau, A., Kern, K., Brune, H., and Barth, J.V. (2007) *Nano Lett.*, **7**, 3813.

218 Decker, R., Schlickum, U., Klappenberger, F., Zoppellaro, G., Klyatskaya, S., Ruben, M., Barth, J.V., and Brune, H. (2008) *Appl. Phys. Lett.*, **93**, 243102.

219 Furukawa, S., Uji-i, H., Tahara, K., Ichikawa, T., Sonoda, M., De Schryver, F.C., Tobe, Y., and De Feyter, S. (2006) *J. Am. Chem. Soc.*, **128**, 3502.

220 Schull, G., Douillard, L., Fiorini-Debuisschert, C., Charra, F., Mathevet, F., Kreher, D., and Attias, A.J. (2006) *Adv. Mater.*, **18**, 2954.

221 Schull, G., Douillard, L., Fiorini-Debuisschert, C., Charra, F., Mathevet, F., Kreher, D., and Attias, A.J. (2006) *Nano Lett.*, **6**, 1360.

222 Tahara, K., Lei, S., Mossinger, D., Kozuma, H., Inukai, K., Van der Auweraer, M., De Schryver, F.C., Hoger, S., Tobe, Y., and De Feyter, S. (2008) *Chem. Commun.*, 3897.

223 Furukawa, S., Tahara, K., De Schryver, F.C., Van der Auweraer, M., Tobe, Y., and De Feyter, S. (2007) *Angew. Chem., Int. Ed.*, **46**, 2831.

224 Lei, S., Surin, M., Tahara, K., Adisoejoso, J., Lazzaroni, R., Tobe, Y., and De Feyter, S. (2008) *Nano Lett.*, **8**, 2541.

225 Tahara, K., Lei, S., Mamdouh, W., Yamaguchi, Y., Ichikawa, T., Uji,-I H., Sonoda, M., Hirose, K., De Schryver, F.C., De Feyter, S., and Tobe, Y. (2008) *J. Am. Chem. Soc.*, **130**, 6666.

226 Hoeppener, S., Wonnemann, J., Chi, L.F., Erker, G., and Fuchs, H. (2003) *ChemPhysChem*, **4**, 490.

227 Pan, G.B., Liu, J.M., Zhang, H.M., Wan, L.J., Zheng, Q.Y., and Bai, C.L. (2003) *Angew. Chem., Int. Ed.*, **42**, 2747.

228 Zhang, H.L., Chen, W., Chen, L., Huang, H., Wang, X.S., Yuhara, J., and Wee, A.T.S. (2007) *Small*, **3**, 2015.

229 Zeng, C.G., Wang, B., Li, B., Wang, H.Q., and Hou, J.G. (2001) *Appl. Phys. Lett.*, **79**, 1685.

230 Huang, H., Chen, W., Chen, L., Zhang, H.L., Sen Wang, X., Bao, S.N., and Wee, A.T.S. (2008) *Appl. Phys. Lett.*, **92**, 023105.

231 Xu, B., Tao, C.G., Cullen, W.G., Reutt-Robey, J.E., and Williams, E.D. (2005) *Nano Lett.*, **5**, 2207.

232 Schmaltz, B., Rouhanipour, A., Rader, H.J., Pisula, W., and Mullen, K. (2009) *Angew. Chem., Int. Ed.*, **48**, 720.

233 Mena-Osteritz, E. and Bauerle, P. (2006) *Adv. Mater.*, **18**, 447.

234 De Feyter, S. and De Schryver, F.C. (2003) *Chem. Soc. Rev.*, **32**, 139.

235 Humblot, V., Barlow, S.M., and Raval, R. (2004) *Prog. Surf. Sci.*, **76**, 1.

236 Barlow, S.M. and Raval, R. (2003) *Surf. Sci. Rep.*, **50**, 201.

237 Ernst, K.H. (2006) *Supramolecular Chirality*, vol. 265, Springer-Verlag Berlin, Berlin, p. 209.

238 Kuhnle, A., Linderoth, T.R., and Besenbacher, F. (2003) *J. Am. Chem. Soc.*, **125**, 14680.

239 Kuhnle, A., Linderoth, T.R., Hammer, B., and Besenbacher, F. (2002) *Nature*, **415**, 891.

240 Kuhnle, A., Linderoth, T.R., and Besenbacher, F. (2006) *J. Am. Chem. Soc.*, **128**, 1076.

241 Fasel, R., Parschau, M., and Ernst, K.H. (2003) *Angew. Chem., Int. Ed.*, **42**, 5178.

242 Parschau, M., Romer, S., and Ernst, K.H. (2004) *J. Am. Chem. Soc.*, **126**, 15398.

243 Vidal, F., Delvigne, E., Stepanow, S., Lin, N., Barth, J.V., and Kern, K. (2005) *J. Am. Chem. Soc.*, **127**, 10101.

244 Cortes, R., Mascaraque, A., Schmidt-Weber, P., Dil, H., Kampen, T.U., and Horn, K. (2008) *Nano Lett.*, **8**, 4162.

245 Schock, M., Otero, R., Stojkovic, S., Hummelink, F., Gourdon, A., Laegsgaard, E., Stensgaard, I., Joachim, C., and Besenbacher, F. (2006) *J. Phys. Chem. B*, **110**, 12835.

246 Schlickum, U., Decker, R., Klappenberger, F., Zoppellaro, G., Klyatskaya, S., Auwarter, W., Neppl, S.,

Kern, K., Brune, H., Ruben, M., and Barth, J.V. (2008) *J. Am. Chem. Soc.*, **130**, 11778.

247 Mu, Z.C., Shu, L.J., Fuchs, H., Mayor, M., and Chi, L.F. (2008) *J. Am. Chem. Soc.*, **130**, 10840.

248 Chen, Q. and Richardson, N.V. (2003) *Nat. Mater.*, **2**, 324.

249 Blankenburg, S. and Schmidt, W.G. (2007) *Phys. Rev. Lett.*, **99**, 196107.

250 Furukawa, S. and De Feyter, S. (2009) *Top. Curr. Chem.*, **287**, 87.

251 Cicoira, F., Santato, C., and Rosei, F. (2008) *STM and AFM Studies on (Bio) Molecular Systems: Unravelling The Nanoworld*, vol. 285, Springer-Verlag Berlin, Berlin, p. 203.

10
Surface Microstructures and Nanostructures in Natural Systems

Taolei Sun and Lei Jiang

10.1
Introduction

Biosystems in Nature have evolved for billions of years, with their structures and functions having reached an optimized state during the evolutionary process. Natural biomaterials obtained from animals or plants normally exhibit certain unique properties that are far superior to those of artificial biomaterials. On closer examination, however, these properties are found to be determined not only by the intrinsic properties of the materials but, more importantly, they are related to the well-designed topological structures at both the micro level and nano level. The details of some delicate surface nanostructures present in natural systems, based on their contributions to different surface properties, are discussed in the following subsections.

10.2
Surface Nanostructures and Special Wettability

Wettability is a fundamental property of a material surface, and plays important roles in many aspects of human activities. Recently, special wettability has aroused much interest because its great advantages in applications [1]. For example, a superhydrophilic surface with a water contact angle (CA) of about $0°$, generated by ultraviolet (UV) irradiation has been used successfully as a transparent coating with antifogging and self-cleaning properties [2]. Likewise, various phenomena that include contamination, snow sticking, erosion, and even the conduction of an electrical current, would be expected to be inhibited on superhydrophobic surfaces [3–6] with a CA larger than $150°$ and a sliding angle (SA) less than $10°$ [7]. In Nature, many interesting phenomena occur that are relevant to the special wettability that proves to be highly convenient for the lives of plants and animals. Examples include the self-cleaning effect on the lotus leaf, the super water-repellent force of the water strider's legs, and the anisotropic wetting and dewetting properties of the rice leaf. Yet, various studies have indicated that these phenomena are contributed to not only by the chemical

Nanotechnology, Volume 8: Nanostructured Surfaces. Edited by Lifeng Chi
Copyright © 2010 WILEY-VCH Verlag GmbH & Co. KGaA, Weinheim
ISBN: 978-3-527-31739-4

properties of the surface, but more importantly, are governed by the special structural effects at the microlevel and nanolevel.

Although the chemical compositions [8, 9] determine the surface free energy, and thus have a major influence on wettability, the system has certain limitations. For example, a $-CF_3$-terminated surface was reported to possess the lowest free energy and the best hydrophobicity whereas, on flat surfaces, the maximum CA achieved was only about 120° [10]. One other important factor that influences wettability is the surface topographic structure, as described by Wenzel's equation [11]:

$$\cos \theta' = r \cos \theta \tag{10.1}$$

where θ' is the apparent CA on a rough surface, θ is the intrinsic CA on a flat surface, and the surface roughness (r) can enhance both the hydrophilicity and hydrophobicity of the surfaces. Thus, the modified Cassie's equation becomes [12]:

$$\cos \theta' = f \cos \theta - (1-f) \tag{10.2}$$

in which f is the fraction of solid/water interface, while $(1-f)$ is that of the air/water interface. This indicates that when a rough surface comes into contact with water, air trapping in the trough area may occur, which would contribute greatly to the increase in hydrophobicity, and help to achieve superhydrophobicity with a CA larger than 150°. These are the most important mechanisms for the special wettability phenomena in Nature.

However, the structural effect has a much greater role, as it may also alter the properties of the solid/water/air triple contact line (TCL), thus greatly influencing the dynamic aspects of wettability. The wettability also shows a distinct size effect for the nanostructures, and this plays important roles not only in the mesoscale assembly of the bio-units but also the stability of the biostructures.

10.2.1
Self-Cleaning Effect on the Lotus Leaf

The self-cleaning effect exists widely in Nature on the surface of plant leaves, with perhaps the best-known example being that of the lotus leaf (Figure 10.1a); indeed, the "lotus effect" is so-named for this very reason! The effect involves two main aspects: (i) superhydrophobicity (CA > 150°) of the surface; and (ii) a strong anti-adhesive effect towards water (i.e., a small SA). Although initially, Barthlott and Neihuis [13] considered the lotus effect to be induced by the coexistence of wax compounds and micrometer-scale papillae structures on the surface, recent studies have indicated that nanostructures still occur in the micropapillae (Figure 10.1b), with diameters of about 5–9 μm. As shown in Figure 10.1c, each papilla is composed of further nanofibrous structures with an average diameter of about 120 nm, and these are also found on the lower part of the leaf. The static CA and the SA on this surface are about $161 \pm 3°$ and less than 3°, respectively.

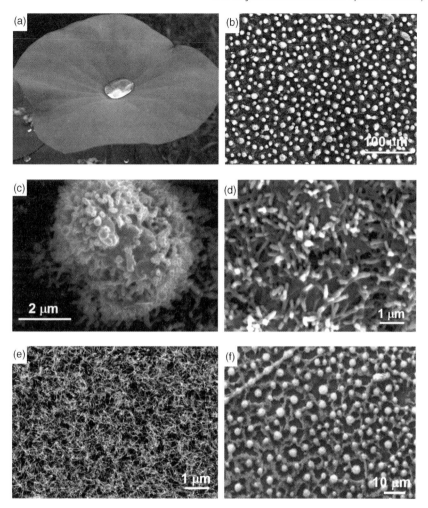

Figure 10.1 Microstructures and nanostructures on the lotus leaf. (a) The lotus leaf; (b) Large-scale scanning electron microscopy (SEM) image of the lotus leaf. Each epidermal cell forms a papilla, and has a dense layer of epicular waxes superimposed on it; (c) Magnified image of a single papilla of panel (b);
(d) SEM image on the lower surface of the lotus leaf; (e) Densely packed ACNT film with pure nanostructure (top view); (f) Lotus-like ACNT film with multilevel microstructures and nanostructures. Panels (b–f) adapted from Ref. [4].

According to Adamson and Gast [14], a theoretical model can be built for the relationship between the superhydrophobicity and the multilevel surface structure. In this model, the multilevel structures on lotus leaf can be described as a fractal structure that is similar to the Koch curve [15], where the fractal dimension (D) was used to characterize the roughness of the surface. According to Wenzel's formula [see Eq. (10.1)] and Cassie's equations [Eq. (10.2)], the relationship between the CA

(θ_f) on the rough surface and that (θ_0) on the corresponding smooth surface can be described as:

$$\cos\theta_f = f_s\left(\frac{L}{l}\right)^{D-2}\cos\theta_0 - f_v \tag{10.3}$$

where $(L/l)^{D-2}$ is the roughness factor of the surface, and L and l represent the maximum and minimum sizes, respectively, for surface structures with the fractal behavior. For the lotus leaf surface, these correspond to the diameters of the micro-papillae and the nanofibers in each micro-papilla, respectively. In the Koch curve, D is about 2.282, and (L/l) is 3^n, where n is an integer determined by the exact fractal structure. An increase in n illustrates a corresponding increase in the surface roughness. f_s and f_v ($f_s + f_v = 1$) represent the fractions of the solid/water and air/water interfaces when the surface contacts with water. Thus, a relationship between θ_f on the surface of lotus leaf and the value of n can be obtained, as shown in Figure 10.1d. By using the above results, it is possible to calculate the theoretical diameter of the nanofibers that corresponds to a CA value of about 160°; a value of 128 nm is very close to the experimental value. This analysis shows clearly why Nature would select multiscale structures to achieve a superior self-cleaning effect, but not only microstructures or nanostructures [16].

In order to identify the role of the hierarchical structures in the self-cleaning effect, the present authors' group synthesized aligned carbon nanotube (ACNT) films with and without hierarchical structures, for comparison. The ACNT film [17] with a pure nanostructure (Figure 10.1e) was fabricated using a chemical vapor deposition (CVD) method on a silica substrate with homogeneous catalyst distribution, and demonstrated superhydrophobicity with a CA of about $158 \pm 2°$; however, the fact that the SA was greater than 30° indicated a relatively large CA hysteresis and a strong adhesion to water. When the ACNT film was fabricated using the same CVD method on a silica substrate, but with a heterogeneous catalyst distribution, similar hierarchical micro-structures and nanostructures were seen (Figure 10.1f) as on the lotus leaf, but the CA on the surface was about 166° and the SA only about 3°. A further honeycomb-like ACNT film [18] with a hierarchical structure was also fabricated that showed a large CA of about 163° and a small SA of <5°. A subsequent comparison of the data obtained with these films confirmed that the hierarchical structure not only further improved the hydrophobicity but, most importantly, also provided a small SA.

Similar phenomena are also observed on many other plant leaves, such as Indian Cress or Lady's Mantle (*Alchemilla vulgaris* L.). However, following extensive in-vestigations of the mechanisms involved, these phenomena were shown to be relevant to special microstructures and nanostructures on the leaves, despite differences in the shape and arrangement of the structures, and the corresponding mechanisms. On the basis of these findings, superhydrophobicity and other more specialized properties of wettability have been demonstrated on a variety of artificial functional surfaces [19–22], using several methods. Two examples of artificial superhydrophobic surfaces prepared by the present authors' group are shown in Figure 10.2a and b [23, 24]. Moreover, when a functional surface was combined with well-designed microstructures and nanostructures, a reversible switching between

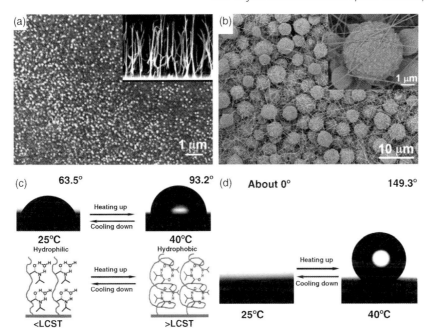

Figure 10.2 Artificial surfaces with special wettability. (a) An aligned polyacrylonitrile (PAN) nanofiber film (top view) with superhydrophobicity. The inset shows a side view; (b) Superhydrophobic polystyrene film with microsphere/nanofiber composite structure; (c) Temperature-sensitive wettability of a poly(N-isopropylacrylamide) film on a flat substrate; (d) Reversible switching between superhydrophilicity and superhydrophobicity on a structured substrate. LCST = lowest critical solution temperature (of the responsive polymer). Adapted from Refs [23], [24], and [25].

superhydrophobicity and superhydrophilicity (Figure 10.2c and d) could be conveniently achieved, using a variety of methods that included thermal treatment [25], light irradiation [26, 27], and solvent treatment [28]. Ultimately, the results of such studies opened up a novel research field for biomimetic materials, and greatly extended the application domains of specialized wettability.

10.2.2
Multifunctional Surfaces of Insect Wings with a Self-Cleaning Effect

In addition to plant leaves, self-cleaning effects may also be observed on the wings of many insects, including dragon fly, honeybee, cicada, and moths, where the main benefit is to protect against the wings being wetted by the dew. Notably, the self-cleaning effects of insect wings differs from that of surfaces, in that it is normally accompanied by various other extraordinary functions.

In the case of the cicada (see Figure 10.3a, inset), which lives either in the soil or on trees, the wings show excellent superhydrophobicity, with a CA >160° and superior dewetting properties that are of great convenience to the insect. When investigating the relationship between the wettability and nanostructures located on the cicada wings [29, 30] (see Figure 10.3a), a well-arranged nanopillar structure with a feature size of approximately 100 nm was identified on the insect wings. Whilst the tops of the nanopillars were of dissimilar heights, and showed an uneven arrangement, the operating principle was seen to be somewhat similar to the multilevel structures on the lotus leaf. This guaranteed a repellent force that prevented water droplets from contacting the surface (as per Wenzel's equation), while simultaneously causing an efficient reduction in the contact area between the water droplet and the surface, and also in the total TCL length. This resulted in a discontinuous TCL arrangement whereby the nanopillar structure and uneven arrangement of the nanopillars, together with the wax components on the wing surface, resulted not only in an outstanding superhydrophobicity but also an anti-adhesive effect against water. The cicada wing is also famous for its ultra-transparency, which results from its excellent anti-reflective properties that have been shown to result from the nanostructure's periodic arrangement. In order to monitor this effect, the present authors' group used a template-based "rolling press" technique to create well-patterned nanopillars (Figure 10.3b) on a polymer surface, thus mimicking the nanostructures on the cicada wings. Subsequently, a remarkable similarity was observed for the nanostructures (see Figure 10.3a and b), while the as-prepared film also showed a similar superhydrophobic property on its surface.

Another example of low-reflective properties can be found in the compound eyes of moths [31], mosquitoes, butterflies, or other insects. In the case of moths, this makes them difficult to be detected by their natural enemies whilst, at the same time, providing perfect antifogging and dewetting properties [32] that help to maintain clear vision in a humid environment. The reason for these benefits also relate to the special nanostructures on the eyes, with studies on mosquito compound eyes having shown the duplex functions to have originated from the papilla structure on the micrometer scale, and from the hexagonally arranged nanostructures on its surface [32].

In summary, both microstructures and nanostructures on the surface of organisms can help to integrate several peculiar functions into a simple system. This in turn provides much insight into the development of novel functional devices. An example was shown in a biomimetic study conducted by Gao *et al.*, who fabricated artificial compound eyes using a soft-lithographic technique and then discussed the

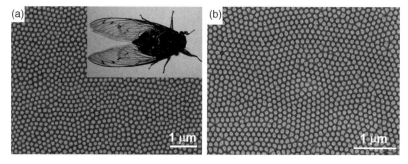

Figure 10.3 Nanostructure (a) of the cicada wing and (b) of the artificial simulation by a template-based method. Adapted from Ref. [29].

influence of the microstructures and nanostructures on the eyes' properties. Gu *et al.* [33] were also successful in creating functional nanomaterials with both coloration properties and superhydrophobicity. Taken together, these results have provided an important theoretical and practical background for the exploration of other biomimetically functional materials.

10.2.3
The Anisotropic Dewetting Property on Plant Leaves

Whilst, on a lotus leaf, water is able to roll freely in any direction over the entire surface, on the rice leaf an anisotropic dewetting property is observed, whereby the water droplet can roll freely in only *one* direction. The scanning electron microscopy (SEM) images in Figure 10.4a and b indicate a hierarchical structure on the rice leaf [16] that is similar to the lotus leaf; accordingly, the surface is superhydrophobic. A different situation arises, however, in the case of the papillae, which are arranged in one-dimensional (1-D) order parallel to the edge of the leaf (arrows 'a' in Figure 10.4). This means that the water drop can roll off freely along this direction, but will move with greater difficulty along the perpendicular direction (arrow 'b' in Figure 10.4). The SAs in these two directions are about 3–5° and 9–15°, respectively. Such a phenomenon is also considered relevant to the anisotropic TCL arrangement. In the case of the rice leaf, the density of the micro-papillae in the parallel direction of the leaf edge is significantly less than in the perpendicular direction, and this will result in an anisotropic arrangement of the TCLs; this is in contrast to the isotropic arrangement on the lotus leaf, which is due to the homogeneous distribution of the papillae. In an attempt to mimic this phenomenon, the present authors' group prepared a rice-like ACNT film (Figure 10.4b) by controlling the surface distribution of the catalyst on which the micro-level ACNT arrays; this was achieved by patterning with different spacings in mutually orthogonal directions. A similar anisotropic dewetting phenomenon was also observed on this film.

An anisotropic dewetting phenomenon also exists on the feathers of water-fowls [34]. These birds live in water and while their feathers are waterproof, any

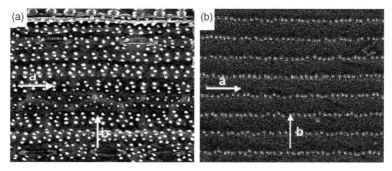

Figure 10.4 Anisotropic structures on a rice leaf (a) and an artificial ACNT film (b). Adapted from Ref. [16].

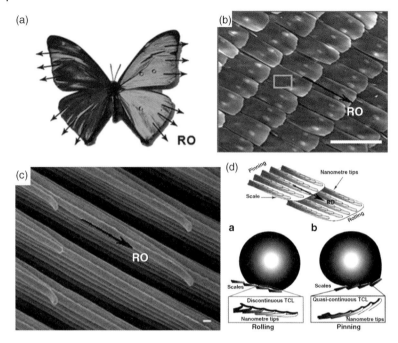

Figure 10.5 (a) Hierarchical anisotropic microstructures and nanostructures on butterfly wings; (b, c) Scanning electron microscopy images of the periodic arrangement of overlapping microscales on the wings and fine lamella-stacking nanostripes on the scales; (d) Schematic diagram of the mechanism of the anisotropic dewetting property on butterfly wings. Adapted from Ref. [35], with permission.

adhered water droplets can be easily removed simply by the bird shaking its wings. This special function is also due to the anisotropically aligned strip-like microstructures and nanostructures of the feather, which can provide an excellent hydrophobicity and water-repellent properties, whilst at the same time helping to preserve a good permeability against the air.

Recently, details were reported of the anisotropic rolling properties of water drops on the wings of the butterfly *Morpho aega* (Figure 10.5a) [35]; in this case, the wings were found to have well-defined multilevel microstructures and nanostructures. Figure 10.5b shows the SEM image of the first level of the overlapping micro-scales with a width of about 40–50 μm on the wings, which are composed of nanostripes (see Figure 10.4c) with a width of about 100 nm. Further lamellar-stacking nanotip structures (Figure 10.5c) for each nanostripe can be observed in the magnified image. This periodic stripe structure and the multilevel structures produce not only beautiful colors (known as "structural colors"; see Section 10.3.2) to the butterfly, but also bring about unique anisotropic dewetting properties. The static CA on the butterfly's wings was found to be $152 \pm 2°$, which indicated the wing to have superhydrophobic properties. Perhaps more interestingly, however, whilst the water drop could roll along the outer direction of the microscales, it would stop in the opposite direction, even if the wings were stood vertically. Such a property could be highly beneficial to protect the insect body against being wetted by water. The mechanism for this effect is shown in Figure 10.5d. Here, when the wing is tilted down, the oriented nanotips on the nanostripes and microscales become separated from one another; this causes any water droplets deposited on the wing to form a discontinuous TCL, which shows a small SA of about 9°. However, when the wing is tilted upwards the nanotips take on a close arrangement so as to form a continuous TCL with the water drop.

10.2.4
The Super Water-Repellent Force of the Water Strider's Legs

The water strider (Figure 10.6a) is an insect which lives in water but can run and jump both rapidly and freely on the water's surface, without wetting its legs. This interesting phenomenon has long attracted much attention, with many investigations being conducted to determine the dynamic reasons that permit the water strider to act in this way [36, 37]. By using a high-speed camera, Bush et al. [38] showed that the insect's leg movement created a vortex in the water that in turn created a rapid leg movement on the water's surface. However, these studies failed to meet the crux of the problem, namely, what forces prevented the water strider's legs from piercing the water surface?

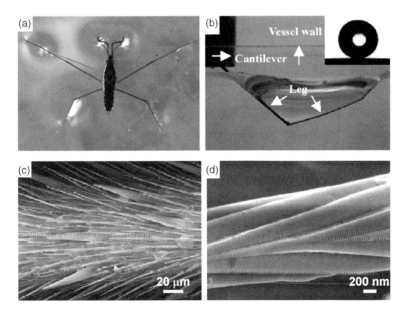

Figure 10.6 Hierarchical microstructures and nanostructures on the legs of a water spider (a); (b) Side view of the maximal dimple just before the leg pierces the water surface. The inset shows the profile of a water drop in the contact angle measurement for the superhydrophobic leg surface; (c) Scanning electron microscopy image of the leg surface, showing numerous oriented spindly microsetae; (d) Nanoscale groove structure on a seta. Adapted from Ref. [39], with permission.

A recent study conducted by Jiang's and coworkers provided some fundamental answers to these questions [39], when it shown that a large water-repellent force (Figure 10.6b) was produced by nanostructures on the water strider's legs. On examination, the surfaces of the legs were shown to bear numerous bristles that had diameters of about 1–3 μm and were arranged to lie in the same direction (see Figure 10.6c). On the surface of each bristle was a further well-defined spiral groove structure (Figure 10.6d). The nanostructure was shown capable of trapping air within the grooves, and this resulted in an excellent superhydrophobicity (see inset of Figure 10.6b) with a static CA >160° on the leg surface. In contrast, according to the relationship between the force provided by the surface tension (γ) at the border of the interface and the length of the border, the water-repellent force (f_r) provided by a leg could be written as:

$$f_r = \gamma \cos \theta_0 \cdot \sum_i l_i \cos \beta_i \qquad (10.4)$$

where l_i is the length of the TCL provided by each bristle on the leg, β_i is the angle between the direction of each bristle and the vertical direction of water surface, γ is the surface tension of water, and θ_0 is the intrinsic CA of the wax material on the surface of the bristles. This shows that microbristles, and the nanostructures on them, can greatly increase the total length of the TCL, resulting in a large water-repellent force such that each leg could support about 15 times the insect's body weight. In fact, the load capacity was so high that it could assure the free activities of the water strider on water surfaces, even within some complicated environments. In time, such an effect might bring inspiration to the development of novel water robots or other devices.

10.2.5
Extraordinary Water-Harvesting Ability of the Desert Beetle's Wings

The desert is very dry, yet some insects have developed unique methods to locate water. A typical example is the *Stenocara* beetle [40] (Figure 10.7a), which lives in the Nambi Desert in South Africa. This desert supports a unique sand-dune fauna, and normally experiences high winds, extreme daytime temperatures and dense, early-morning fog, yet with a rainfall that is very low and almost negligible. Yet, in this extremely dry environment, the *Stenocara* beetle is able to collect water droplets from the fog, with assistance from the wind blow. Moreover, the water drops which form on the top elytra (wing cover) subsequently roll down the beetle's outer surface towards its mouthparts.

In examining this phenomenon, Parker and Lawrence [40] reported the existence of two types of randomly distributed arrays of bumps on the beetle's carapace; these are located 0.5–1.5 mm apart, and each bump is about 0.5 mm in diameter (Figure 10.7b). The peaks of the bumps are smooth at the microscopic level and are without any covering; thus, they are highly hydrophilic. In contrast, in the trough area the surface is covered by microstructures coated in wax (Figure 10.7c). These microstructures consist of hexagonally arranged flattened hemispheres with

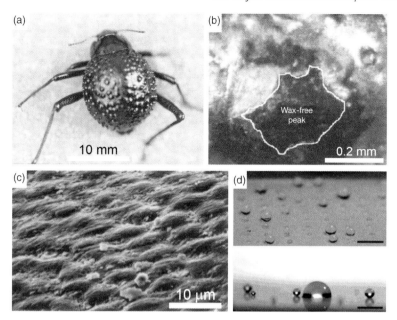

Figure 10.7 The water-capturing surface of the fused overwings (elytra) of the desert beetle. (a) Adult female beetle, dorsal view; (b) A "bump" on the elytra; (c) Scanning electron microscopy image of the textured surface of the suppressed areas; (d) Artificial simulation of the water-capturing process on the alternate hydrophobic/hydrophilic surface pattern. Panels (a–c) adapted from Ref. [40]; Panel (d) adapted from Ref. [41], with permission.

a diameter of about 10 μm, are reminiscent of those on the lotus leaf, and result in these areas having superhydrophobic properties. During foggy weather, tiny water droplets contained in the fog are able to gather on the hydrophilic peak area, where they rapidly form a larger drop. Water coming into contact with the hydrophobic grooves will also be collected by these hydrophilic regions. The water droplets then coalesce until their weight is sufficient to overcome the binding force between the water and the surface, at which point they flow down to the beetle's mouth under the action of wind blow.

This "fog-catching ability" of the *Stenocara* beetle, which is based on an alternative design of the hydrophilic and hydrophobic domains, brings important insights to the development of highly efficient water-harvesting devices that might have numerous applications in the future. For example, synthetic films could be fabricated onto polymer sheets and attached to buildings and tents so as to harvest water vapor, perhaps to serve refugee camps. A similar process might also help in the capture and recycling of water vapor from cooling towers, which would in turn lead to reductions in energy costs. With these possibilities in mind, Zhai *et al.* [41] created hydrophilic patterns on superhydrophobic surfaces by using water/isopropanol solutions of a polyelectrolyte, the aim being ultimately to produce surfaces with an extreme hydrophobic contrast. These surfaces perfectly mimicked the water-capturing mechanism on the back of the *Stenocara* beetle, and could be used to capture very small drops of water and convert them to larger drops (Figure 10.7d). By using the same technique, it might also be possible to create superhydrophilic canals by applying superhydrophilic multilayers onto hydrophilic stripes on the superhydrophobic surface. These structures might find broader applications in other domains, such as microfluidic devices.

10.3
Structure-Related Special Optical Phenomena in Nature

When a substance is illuminated with white light, a specific color is observed because only a particular range of wavelength of light is reflected and is visible to the eye. There are two ways to eliminate the other wavelengths of light [42]. The first approach is for the substance to absorb the light, and this is the mechanism normally employed when coloring with by pigments [43, 44]. Whilst this is the main route taken by Nature to generate colors, there are many cases where Nature prefers to select structural colors to present its beauty. This is a purely physical process that depends on interactions between the light and the elaborate periodic submicro- or nanostructures with scales that are comparable to the light's wavelength [45, 46]. Compared to pigments, the structural colors have not only a much greater stability (amongst other advantages), but can also help to achieve certain special functionalities such as supertransparency and ultra-low reflection. They are, therefore, very useful in modern materials science, and have attracted much interest during recent decades.

10.3.1
Photonic Crystal Structures in Opal and Opal Analogues

The periodic submicro- or nanostructures that show special optical properties are termed "photonic crystals." Similar to semiconductor crystals, photonic crystals also show an energy band structure that influences the propagation of light (which is also an electromagnetic wave). Photons propagate through these structures, or not, depending on their wavelength. As the basic physical phenomenon is based on diffraction, the periodicity of the photon crystal structure should be of a similar length scale as the half of light wavelength in order for the material to exhibit specific colors.

One representative example in Nature is that of *opals*, which are a natural mineral that has a well-known range of beautiful colors and glosses. Opals are mineraloid gels that are composed of silica nanospheres with different sizes and arrangements. The diverse periodic arrangements of the nanostructures give rise to the changeable colors and glosses associated with opals [47]. With this in mind, a variety of artificial nanostructures have been created (Figure 10.8) that display structural colors and other functionalities [33, 48].

The opal analogue has also been found on scales of certain beetles. For example, Parker *et al.* [49] reported a beetle, *Pachyrhynchus argus* (Figure 10.9a), which was found in the forests of northeastern Queensland, Australia and has a metallic coloration that is visible from any direction. According to the studies conducted,

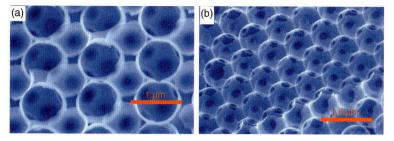

Figure 10.8 Typical scanning electron microscopy images for an artificial inverse opal structure. (a) 110 facet; (b) 111 facet. Adapted from Ref. [48], with permission.

the unique optical property that distinguishes this beetle from others is due to the photonic crystal structure that is analogous to that of opal. The beetle is seen to be covered by scales of about 0.1 mm (Figure 10.9b), which are individually flat, lie parallel with the body, and consist of an outer shell and an inner structure. Both SEM and transmission electron microscopy (TEM) images have shown that the inner structure of the scales is composed of a solid array of transparent spheres, each with a diameter of 250 nm. The nanospheres are arranged precisely in a hexagonal close-packing fashion (Figure 10.9c), thus forming a photonic crystal structure that is very

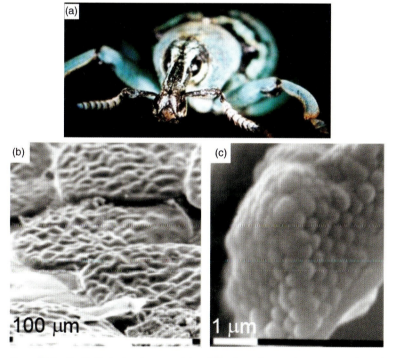

Figure 10.9 Beetle *Pachyrhynchus argus* (a) and the photonic crystal structures on its scales (b, c). Adapted from Ref. [49], with permission.

similar to the common nanostructure found in opal. As the lattice parameter of the structure is close to the half-wavelength of the visible light, the single scale acts as a three-dimensional (3-D) diffraction grating, and this allows the reflection of a narrow range of wavelengths over a wide range of incident angles. In transmitted white light, the scales appear as the negative of the reflected color: yellow-green in reflected light, and purple in transmitted light from most directions. In the spectroscopic analysis results, with white light incident at 20° to the normal direction of the scale surface, the peak reflection occurred at a wavelength of 530 nm, at an angle of 20° to the other side of the normal direction. As shown in Figure 10.9c, the photonic crystal structure is a 3-D structure; however, when compared to the similar 2-D photonic structure that was reported on the sea mouse (*Aphrodita* sp.) [50], it can provide an omnidirectional optical property to the beetles, and this may bring about important insights for the design of novel, high-performance display devices.

10.3.2
Structural Colors in Biological Systems

Almost 300 years ago, Newton [51] noted that the brilliant colors of peacock feathers (Figure 10.10a) were not caused by pigments, but rather were due to a thin-film interference mechanism. Recently, when Zi *et al.* [52] further studied the detailed mechanism, they found the coloration strategy for peacock feathers to be very delicate, to originate mainly from the periodic nanostructures of the cortex layer on barbules. As shown in Figure 10.10b, a barbule of a peacock feather consists of a medullar core of ~3 μm enclosed by a cortex layer. Interestingly, the cortex of all different-colored barbules contains a 2-D photonic crystal structure (Figure 10.10c

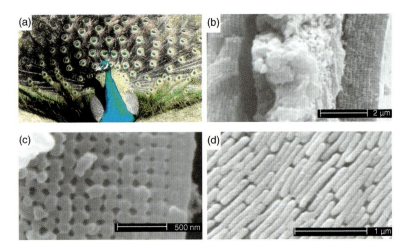

Figure 10.10 Scanning electron microscopy images of the barbule structures on a peacock's feathers (a); (b) Transverse cross-section of a green barbules; (c) Magnification of the image in panel (b); (d) Longitudinal cross-section of a green barbule with the surface layer removed. Adapted from Ref. [52], with permission.

and d), composed of melanin rods connected by keratin. Moreover, the photonic crystal structures in the differently colored barbules were quite similar, whereas the lattice constants and the number of periods varied widely. According to the analysis made by Zi *et al.*, the 2-D photonic crystal structure showed a strong reflection for the light with specific wavelengths along the direction of cortex layer, thus generating colors which were regulated by the lattice constants and the number of periods. The different colors were due to the different lattice constants, which increased regularly for the blue, green, yellow, and brown barbules. The Fabry–Perot interference effect has also been found for the brown barbules, in which the periodic number is the smallest. Due to this effect, an extra blue color was generated and contributed to the final brown color of the barbules.

For the wings of butterflies [53, 54], the periodic structure appears in different ways, and Vukusic *et al.* have undertaken several systematic investigations in this aspect. As has been shown previously [55, 56], the broad wings of butterflies are invariably covered with well-arranged arrays of minute scales, each of which is a thin, flattened, cuticular evagination from an individual cell in the wing epithelium. The scales overlap with each other, much as do roof tiles, and this functions as a quarter-wave interference device by presenting a series of alternating lucent and dense layers. The scales are composed further of complicated, delicately arranged nanostructures (see Figure 10.11), but this differs very much among the butterfly species. The diverse

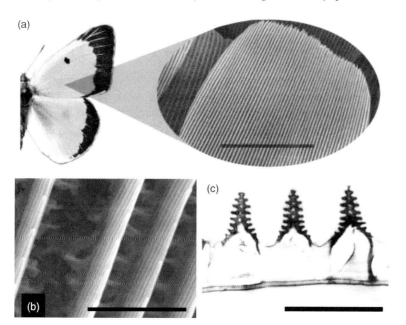

Figure 10.11 Microstructures and nanostructures on the wings of the butterfly *Colias eurytheme*. (a) Scanning electron microscopy (SEM) image of a single scale; (b) Magnified SEM image showing the ridges in close-up; (c) Transmission electron microscopy image of a cross-section through the scale, indicating the horizontal lamellae borne on the vertical scale ridges. Adapted from Ref. [58], with permission.

shapes and arrangement of these nanostructures provide butterflies with richer colors than peacocks, as well as other interesting optical properties on their wings. For example, the discrete multilayers of the cuticle and air on iridescent blue *Morpho rhetenor* butterflies [57] give rise to an ultralong-range visibility of up to 800 m, to the photonic structures of reduced dimensions that are present in certain *Colias* butterflies [58], and also effect an intense UV visibility. The orientational adjustments of such multilayers produces a highly angle-dependent iridescence that provides a high-contrast color flicker, with minimal wing movement.

Structural colors are also observed in plants, and normally mediated by the 1-D multilayer structure. These structures give rise to vivid colors and iridescence in vascular leaves, fruits and marine algae, which not only makes them beautiful but also greatly affects the development of the plant. For example, iridescence in leaves is believed to produce particular intensity ratios of incident radiation bands that can penetrate to phytochrome centers. In fruit skin, this can reduce post-maturation discoloration and ultimately improve dispersal.

10.3.3
The Directional Fluorescence Emission Property in *Papilio* Butterflies

Vukusic *et al.* also studied in detail the directionally controlled fluorescence emission properties in *Papilio* butterflies (*Princeps nireus* group) [59]. These butterflies have dark wings with bright blue or blue-green dorsal wing bands or patches. Interestingly, the studies of Vukusic *et al.* showed that nanostructures on the wings perfectly matched the design of high-efficiency light-emitting-diode (LED) devices that use 2-D photonic-crystal geometries to enhance the extraction efficiency of light, and also distributed Bragg reflectors (DBRs) to control emission direction. As shown in Figure 10.12a, the wing scales from their colored regions make up a nanostructure that is characterized by a ∼2 μm-thick 2-D photonic crystal slab (PCS) of hollow air cylinders, with a mean diameter of about 240 nm and a spacing of about 240 nm in a medium of solid cuticle (Figure 10.12b). The PCS is infused exclusively with

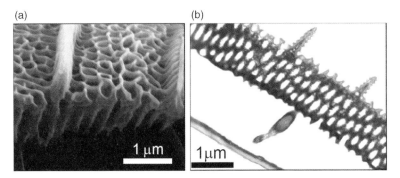

(a)   (b)

Figure 10.12 (a) Scanning electron microscopy image of the air cylinder nanostructure on the scale of butterfly *P. nireus*; (b) Transmission electron microscopy image of a section through the scale. Adapted from Ref. [59], with permission.

a highly fluorescent pigment, which rests parallel to and ~1.5 μm above a three-layer, cuticle-based DBR and forms the base of the scale. The DBRs reflect upwardly the downward-emitted fluorescence from the nanostructure, concurrent with nonabsorbed longer wavelengths that pass through the PCS. In this way it is possible to realize a directional emission of the bright blue-green color, which enhances signaling and is important in communication between different butterfly individuals.

10.3.4
Super Anti-Reflection Structures of Lepidopteran Eyes and Wings

Although most photonic structures in Nature are associated with bright colors or broad angle reflectivity, a specific type of nanostructure can minimize the reflectivity over broad angles or frequency ranges. In Nature, this effect is normally observed in the ommateum of moths or other lepidoptera [60], and shows that a super anti-reflection property can improve the light sensitivity of light-craving moths and help them not to be detected by natural enemies at night. Hence, this is also termed the "moth-eye effect." The effect is commonly achieved by the incorporation of arrays of tapered elements, also described as nipple arrays (Figure 10.13a–c). When light is

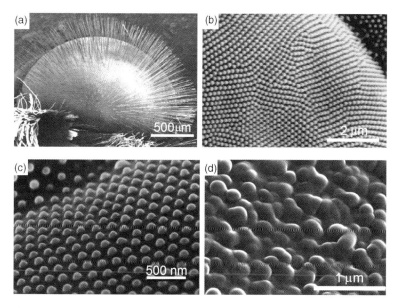

Figure 10.13 Scanning electron microscopy images of nipple arrays in the compound eye of butterflies and on the wings of a dragonfly. (a) The whole compound eye of butterfly *Inachis io*; (b) The detailed nanostructure in one facet lens of the compound eye; (c) Nipple array structure in compound eyes of another type of butterfly, *Polygonia c-aureum*; (d) Nipple array structure on wings of the dragonfly *Aeshna cyanea*. Panels (a–c) adapted from Ref. [60]; Panel (d) adapted from Ref. [61], with permission.

projected onto a transparent medium, the sharp change in refractive index at two sides of the interface will result in a partial reflection of the light. However, the feature size of the nipple arrays, and the distance between neighboring nipples on the ommatidial surface (which are normally within 250 nm) are less than the wavelength of the visible light. This induces a continuous change for the apparent refractive index along the depth direction, such that the structure will gradually match the optical impedance of one medium with its neighbor, and this can cause a significant reduction in reflection at the interface.

According to different materials and usages, the moth-eye effect can be used to achieve different superior properties. On an opaque material surface, the structure may result in a super-black color or cause a notable increase in the adsorption of light. This effect has already found broad applications in solar energy utilization and other fields, such as solar cells and solar water heaters.

Another important property related to such structure is the ultra-transparency that has been widely observed on the wings of many insects, including cicadas (see above; Figure 10.3a) and dragonflies [61]. The nipple array structure has also been identified on the wings of these insects; the well-aligned nanonipple arrays on a dragonfly's wings are shown in Figure 10.13d. These structures are composed of wax, which may help to achieve super water-repellent properties while efficiently preventing the wings from being wetted, when combined with the nanostructure (see Section 10.2).

10.3.5
Unusual Bright Whiteness in Ultrathin Beetle Scales

Whilst many things in life are white – snow, milk, paper, and so on – none of these can be compared to the whiteness of the *Cyphochilus* beetle (Figure 10.14a), a genus of beetle with an unusually brilliant white body that is found in Southeast Asia. According to Vukusic *et al.* [62], the exceptional whiteness and brilliance of the *Cyphochilus* beetle's body was not augmented by either pigments or fluorescence, but rather resulted from a 3-D photonic solid in the scales.

The scales (Figure 10.14b) that imbricate the beetle's body are about 5 μm thick, 250 μm, and 100 μm wide, and their interiors are composed of a random network of interconnecting cuticular filaments with diameters of about 250 nm (Figure 10.14c and d). However, unlike conventional photonic crystal structures there is no well-defined periodicity of the nanostructure. According to Vukusic *et al.*, the 5 μm-thick scales can provide standard whiteness and brightness values of 60 and 65, respectively. In synthetic systems where whiteness is desirable, a far more substantial structure is necessary. For example, an ultrawhite paper to which optical brightening agents have been added can reach similar brightness and whiteness for a thickness which is about 25-fold greater than the beetle scales. Detailed studies have indicated that the cuticular filament network is the origin of the extraordinary whiteness and brightness properties, in a thickness as low as 5 μm. On the one hand, an intrascale cuticle occupation rate of about 70% can optimize scattering intensity by maximizing the scattering center number, but on the other hand the aperiodicity will efficiently assure that scattering occurs over the whole wavelength range.

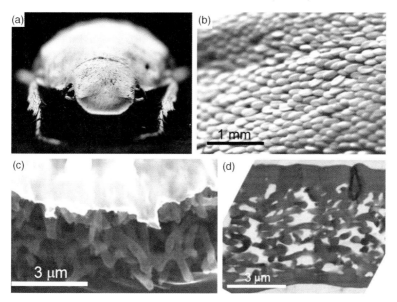

Figure 10.14 *Cyphochilus* beetle (a) with super whiteness and the nanostructures of its scales; (b) Large-scale SEM image of the scales; (c) Magnified SEM image of the scale nanostructure; (d) TEM image of the nanostructure. Adapted from Ref. [62], with permission.

10.3.6
Photosensitivity in Brittlestar (*Ophiuroidea*)

Photosensitivity is normally considered to be a chemical process that is induced by specific chemical-based photoreceptors. This phenomenon is frequently observed in Nature – chameleons and frogs can change their skin colors according to the color and light of their environment. However, in some cases – and especially in the case of echinoderm animals – the special arrangement of microstructures and nanostructures of the skeleton may also act as a component of the specialized photosensory organs, conceivably with the function of compound eyes.

Echinoderms (starfish), especially the brittlestars (*Ophiuroidea*) [63], generally exhibit a wide range of responses to light intensity. Whilst some show almost no response to environmental light (e.g., *Ophiocoma pumila*), others – such as *Ophiocoma wendtii* (Figure 10.15a) – can change their colors markedly when the light intensity of their environment changes. Another interesting behavior of *O. wendtii* is that it can detect shadows and rapidly escape from predators; this is unexpected for such animals because they have no photosensory organs such as eyes. This sensitivity to light appears to be contributed by to the specialized skeletal structure of the dorsal arm plates, which protect the upper part of each joint in brittlestar arms (Figure 10.15b). Recent SEM analyses have disclosed elaborate regular arrays of the spherical microstructures (Figure 10.15c and d) for the skeletal structure of the dorsal arm plates. The skeletal elements of echinoderms are each composed of a single

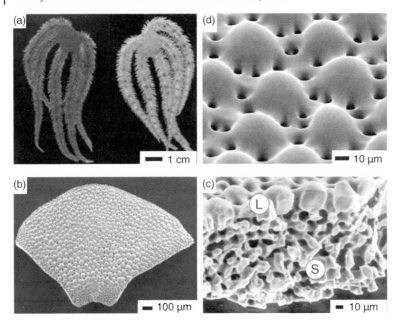

Figure 10.15 Photosensitive brittlestar *Ophiocoma wendtii* (a) and the microstructures of its bones; (b) A dorsal arm plate (DAP) of *O. wendtii*; (c) Cross-section of a fractured DAP, showing the typical calcitic stereom (S) and the enlarged lens structures (L); (d) Peripheral layer of a DAP enlarged lens structures. Adapted from Ref. [63] with permission.

crystal of oriented calcite shaped into a unique, 3-D mesh, although in the case of *O. wendtii* the structure has a remarkably regular double-lens design. Aizenberg *et al.* have shown that such structures can guide and focus the light inside the tissue, and this coincides with the location of the nerve bundles, which act as the primary photoreceptors. A special design of the lens array was also found to minimize spherical aberration and birefringence, and to allow the detection of light from a specific direction. These structures represent examples of biomaterials that perform simultaneous mechanical and optical functions, and may shed light on the design of multifunctional artificial materials.

10.4
The High Adhesive Force of Gecko Foot-Hairs

In biological systems, microstructures and nanostructures also contribute to superior mechanical and dynamic properties. Typical examples include porous structures in bones, wood, and pith, which bestow the materials with maximum strength at the lowest density [64–66]. In tooth materials [67], the dense arrangement of the nanostructures that is combined intimately with proteins provides sufficient strength and toughness at the same time. For surface materials, the nanostructure brings some unique properties that differ from those in the bulk materials.

The gecko is capable of climbing rapidly and freely along vertical walls, or even on the ceiling. Since this phenomenon was first noted almost 100 years ago, much effort has been expended to determine the origin of the high adhesive force between the gecko foot and the underlying surface. Experimental analyses [68, 69] have indicated that each gecko foot (Figure 10.16a) has about 5000 setae (Figure 10.16b) per mm^2, and can produce 10 N with approximately 100 mm^2 pad area; in other words, each seta should produce an average force of about 20 μN, and an average stress of 0.1 N mm^2 (1 atm). However, this force might be greatly underestimated as only a small number of setae would contact the surface simultaneously.

Full *et al.* [70] measured the exact force of a single seta using a micro-electro-mechanical system (MEMS) cantilever that attached with the seta. This showed that one seta could provide a force that, when parallel to the surface, might be as large

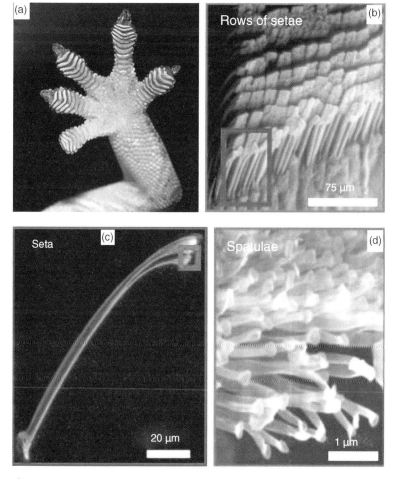

Figure 10.16 Nanostructures on a high-adhesive gecko's foot (a); (b) Rows of setae on the foot; (c) A single seta; (c) Nanospatulae structure of a single seta. Adapted from Ref. [70], with permission.

as $194 \pm 25\,\mu N$ – almost tenfold greater than the estimated value. This indicates that, if all the setae were to be attached simultaneously to the surface, a single gecko foot could provide a 100 N adhesive force (10 atm), which is several hundred-fold the gecko's own body weight. Subsequent SEM studies showed that the terminal of each seta (Figure 10.16c) was further composed of smaller branches (Figure 10.16d) termed *spatulae*, each about 200 nm in size. Results reported by Full *et al.* revealed that the intermolecular forces (e.g., van der Waals forces, etc.) between the spatulae and the surface were the origin of the high adhesive force. Whilst the gecko's feet contain about one billion spatulae, providing a large contact area with the surface, the spatulae are soft and thin and can deform easily so as to fit the complicated local surface topology, thus guaranteeing sufficient surface contact.

More interestingly, the gecko's feet possess good anti-adhesive properties to dust [71], while simultaneously exhibiting a high adhesive force to the substrate. In other words, as the gecko walks about, its sticky feet will always be clean and free from dust contamination, but will not require grooming as they will retain their stickiness for months. In fact, geckos with dirty feet have been shown to recover their ability to cling to vertical surfaces after only a few steps. By using an array of setae isolated from geckos, it was possible to demonstrate the self-cleaning process and to show, using contact mechanical models, that the self-cleaning occurred via an energetic disequilibrium between the adhesive forces that attract dirt to the substrate and those that attract the same particle to the setae. In this process, the setal nanostructure plays a crucial role.

Similar to the gecko, spiders and some beetles can also creep in inverted fashion along almost any type of surface. The study of Kesel *et al.* [72] showed the feet of spiders to be covered with setae nanostructures, very similar to the gecko. Figure 10.17a–c are SEM images of the setae structure and the further densely packed setule structures on each seta, at different magnifications. According to Kesel's experiments and calculations, each nanosetule can provide an adhesive force in excess of 40 nN, with all of the setae on a spider's feet providing a total adhesive force of about 170-fold its own body weight. A similar nanostructure was observed in the case of the beetle *Hemisphaerota cynea* [73], as shown in Figure 10.17d–f.

On the basis of this recognition, much effort has been made to mimic the gecko foot artificially, by using elastic polymers or other materials [74, 75]. In a typical study conducted at the University of Dayton and Georgia Institute of Technology [76], ACNT arrays were used (Figure 10.18b and c) to mimic the binding-on and lifting-off behaviors of gecko foot setae as the gecko walked. The devices fabricated could provide adhesive forces (Figure 10.18a) of about 100 N per cm^2, which was about 10-fold that of the gecko foot, and almost equal to the theoretical value that all setae attach close to the surface. The shear adhesive force was shown to be much stronger than the normal adhesive direction, which ensured a strong binding along the shear direction. This effect was found to be caused by a shear-induced alignment of the nonaligned nanotube top layer, which caused a dramatic enhancement of the line contact with the surface, similar to the operating function of the gecko setae.

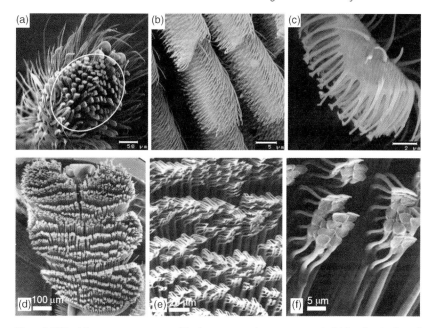

Figure 10.17 Microsetae structure and further nanosetule structure on the high-adhesive feet of a spider (a–c) and a beetle *Hemisphaerota cynea* (d–f), with different magnifications (see scale bars). Adapted from Refs [72] and [73], with permission.

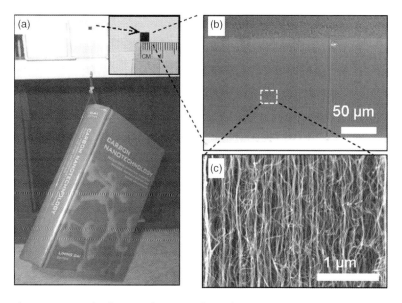

Figure 10.18 High-adhesive carbon nanotube film. (a) A book of 1480 g in weight suspended from a glass surface with use of ACNT supported on a silicon wafer; (b, c) Scanning electron microscopy images of ACNT arrays at different magnifications (see scale bars). Adapted from Ref. [76], with permission.

10.5
Summary and Outlook

During billions of years of evolution, biosystems in Nature have developed diverse and elegant microstructures and nanostructures on their surfaces that play important roles in the special functions and properties of organisms, including superhydrophobicity, anti-contamination, optical properties, and dynamic and mechanical properties. Yet, learning from Nature provides much inspiration to combine these structural effects with conventional artificial materials, so as produce superior properties, the essence of which is the cooperative effect on the microscale and nanoscale. Indeed, in recent years the deep and broad investigation of this effect has become one of the most important aspects of biomimetics, and will surely provide tremendous insights into the design of novel artificial materials and devices for use in a wide variety of domains that includes industry, medicine, agriculture, and general lifestyle.

References

1 Sun, T., Feng, L., Gao, X., and Jiang, L. (2005) *Acc. Chem. Res.*, **38**, 644.

2 Wang, R., Hashimoto, K., Fujishima, A., Chikuni, M., Kojima, E., Kitamura, A., Shimohigoshi, M., and Watanabe, T. (1997) *Nature*, **388**, 431.

3 Chen, W., Fadeev, A.Y., Hsieh, M.C., Öner, D., Youngblood, J., and McCarthy, T.J. (1999) *Langmuir*, **15**, 3395.

4 Feng, L., Li, S., Li, Y., Li, H., Zhang, L., Zhai, J., Song, Y., Liu, B., Jiang, J., and Zhu, D. (2002) *Adv. Mater.*, **14**, 1857.

5 Blossey, R. (2003) *Nature Mater.*, **2**, 301.

6 Lafuma, A. and Quéré, D. (2003) *Nature Mater.*, **2**, 457.

7 Nakajima, A., Fujishima, A., Hashimoto, K., and Watanabe, T. (1999) *Adv. Mater.*, **11**, 1365.

8 Woodward, J.T., Gwin, H., and Schwartz, D.K. (2000) *Langmuir*, **16**, 2957.

9 Sun, T., Song, W., and Jiang, L. (2005) *Chem. Commun.*, 1723.

10 Nishino, T., Meguro, M., Nakamae, K., Matsushita, M., and Ueda, Y. (1999) *Langmuir*, **15**, 4321.

11 Wenzel, R.N. (1936) *Ind. Eng. Chem.*, **28**, 988.

12 Cassie, A.B.D. and Baxter, S. (1944) *Trans. Faraday Soc.*, **40**, 546.

13 Barthlott, W. and Neinhuis, C. (1997) *Planta*, **202**, 1.

14 Adamson, A.W. and Gast, A.P. (1997) *Physical Chemistry of Surfaces*, John Wiley & Sons, New York.

15 Mandelbrot, B.B. (1982) *The Fractal Geometry of Nature*, Freeman, San Francisco, CA.

16 Feng, L., Li, S., Li, Y., Li, H., Zhang, L., Zhai, J., Song, Y., Liu, B., Jiang, L., and Zhu, D. (2002) *Adv. Mater.*, **14**, 1857.

17 Li, H., Wang, X., Song, Y., Liu, Y., Li, Q., Jiang, L., and Zhu, D. (2001) *Angew. Chem., Int. Ed.*, **40**, 1743.

18 Liu, H., Li, S., Zhai, J., Li, H., Zheng, Q., Jiang, L., and Zhu, D. (2004) *Angew. Chem., Int. Ed.*, **43**, 1146.

19 Erbil, H.Y., Demirel, A.L., Avci, Y., and Mert, O. (2003) *Science*, **299**, 1377.

20 Li, S., Li, H., Wang, X., Song, Y., Liu, Y., Jiang, L., and Zhu, D. (2002) *J. Phys. Chem. B*, **106**, 9274.

21 Li, H., Wang, X., Song, Y., Liu, Y., Li, Q., Jiang, L., and Zhu, D. (2001) *Angew. Chem., Int. Ed.*, **40**, 1743.

22 Marmur, A. (2004) *Langmuir*, **20**, 3517.

23 Feng, L., Li, S., Li, H., Zhai, J., Song, Y., Jiang, L., and Zhu, D. (2002) *Angew. Chem., Int. Ed.*, **41**, 1221.

24 Jiang, L., Zhao, Y., and Zhai, J. (2004) *Angew. Chem., Int. Ed.*, **43**, 4338.

25 Sun, T., Wang, G., Feng, L., Liu, B., Ma, Y., Jiang, L., and Zhu, D. (2004) *Angew. Chem., Int. Ed.*, **43**, 357.

26 Feng, X., Feng, L., Zhai, J., Jiang, L., and Zhu, D. (2004) *J. Am. Chem. Soc.*, **126**, 62.

27 Liu, H., Feng, L., Zhai, J., Jiang, L., and Zhu, D. (2004) *Langmuir*, **20**, 5659.

28 Minko, S., Müller, M., Motornov, M., Nitschke, M., Grundke, K., and Stamm, M. (2003) *J. Am. Chem. Soc.*, **125**, 3896.

29 Guo, C., Feng, L., Zhai, J., Wang, G., Song, Y., Jiang, L., and Zhu, D. (2004) *ChemPhysChem*, **5**, 750.

30 Zhang, G., Zhang, J., Xie, G., Liu, Z., and Shao, H. (2006) *Small*, **2**, 1440.

31 Stavega, D.G., Foletti, S., Palasantzas, G., and Arikawa, K. (2006) *Proc. R. Soc. B*, **273**, 661.

32 Gao, X., Yan, X., Yao, X., Xu, L., Zhang, K., Zhang, J., Yang, B., and Jiang, L. (2007) *Adv. Mater.*, **19**, 2213.

33 Gu, Z., Uetsuka, H., Takahashi, K., Nakajima, R., Onishi, H., Fujishima, A., and Sato, O. (2003) *Angew. Chem., Int. Ed.*, **42**, 894.

34 Kennedy, R.J. (1970) *Nature*, **227**, 736.

35 Zheng, Y., Gao, X., and Jiang, L. (2007) *Soft Matter*, **3**, 178.

36 Keller, J.B. (1998) *Phys. Fluids*, **10**, 3009.

37 Sun, S.M. and Keller, J.B. (2001) *Phys. Fluids*, **13**, 2146.

38 Hu, D.L., Chan, B., and Bush, J.W.M. (2003) *Nature*, **424**, 663.

39 Gao, X. and Jiang, L. (2004) *Nature*, **432**, 36.

40 Parker, A.W. and Lawrence, C.R. (2001) *Nature*, **414**, 33.

41 Zhai, L., Berg, M.C., Cebeci, F., Kim, Y., Milwid, J.M., Rubner, M.F., and Cohen, R.E. (2006) *Nano Lett.*, **6**, 1213.

42 Kinoshita, S., Yoshioka, S., and Miyazaki, J. (2008) *Rep. Prog. Phys.*, **71**, 076401.

43 Rüdiger, W. and Thümmler, F. (1991) *Angew. Chem., Int. Ed.*, **30**, 1216.

44 Britton, G. (1995) *FASEB J.*, **9**, 1551.

45 Vukusic, P. and Sambles, J.R. (2003) *Nature*, **424**, 852.

46 Istrate, E. and Sargent, E.H. (2006) *Rev. Modern Phys.*, **78**, 455.

47 Fritsch, E., Gaillou, E., Rondeau, B., Barreau, A., Albertini, D., and Ostroumov, M. (2006) *J. Non-Cryst. Solids*, **352**, 3957.

48 Blanco, A., Chomski, E., Grabtchak, S., Ibisate, M., John, S., Leonard, S.W., Lopez,

C., Meseguer, F., Migues, H., Mondia, J.P., Ozin, G.A., Toader, O., and van Driel, H.M. (2000) *Nature*, **405**, 437.

49 Parker, A.R., Welch, V.L., Driver, D., and Martini, N. (2003) *Nature*, **426**, 786.

50 Parker, A.R., McPhedran, R.C., McKenzie, D.R., Botten, L.C., and Nicorovici, N.-A.P. (2001) *Nature*, **409**, 36.

51 Newton, I. (1730) *Optics*, 4th edn, reprinted by Dover Publications, New York, p. 252.

52 Zi, J., Yu, X., Li, Y., Hu, X., Xu, C., Wang, X., Liu, X., and Fu, R. (2003) *Proc. Natl Acad. Sci. USA*, **100**, 12576.

53 Srnivasarao, M. (1999) *Chem. Rev.*, **99**, 1935.

54 Vukusic, P. (2006) *Curr. Biol.*, **16**, R621.

55 Vukusic, P., Sambles, J.R., and Lawrence, C.R. (2000) *Nature*, **404**, 457.

56 Vukusic, P., Sambles, J.R., Lawrence, C.R., and Wootton, R.J. (2001) *Nature*, **410**, 36.

57 Plattner, L. (2004) *J. R. Soc. Interface*, **1**, 49.

58 Kemp, D.J., Vukusic, P., and Rutowski, R.L. (2006) *Funct. Ecol.*, **20**, 282.

59 Vukusic, P. and Hooper, I. (2005) *Science*, **310**, 1151.

60 Stavenga, D.G., Foletti, S., Palasantzas, G., and Arikawa, K. (2006) *Proc. R. Soc. B*, **273**, 661.

61 Hooper, I.R., Vukusic, P., and Wootton, R.J. (2006) *Opt. Express*, **14**, 4891.

62 Vukusic, P., Hallam, B., and Noyes, J. (2007) *Science*, **315**, 348.

63 Aizenberg, J., Tkachenko, A., Weiner, S., Addadi, L., and Hendler, G. (2001) *Nature*, **412**, 819.

64 Gibson, L.J. and Ashby, M.F. (1982) Mechanics of 3-dimensional cellular materials. *Proc. R. Soc. London A*, **382**, 43.

65 Fan, H., Hartshorn, C., Buchheit, T., Tallant, D., Assink, R., Simpson, R., Kissel, D.J., Lacks, D.J., Torquato, S., and Brinker, C.J. (2007) *Nat. Mater.*, **6**, 418.

66 Tai, K., Dao, M., Suresh, S., Palazoglu, A., and Ortiz, C. (2007) *Nat. Mater.*, **6**, 454.

67 Meyers, M.A., Chen, P.-Y., Lin, A.Y.-M., and Seki, Y. (2008) *Prog. Mater. Sci.*, **53**, 1.

68 Ruibal, R. and Ernst, V. (1965) *J. Morphol.*, **117**, 271.

69 Irschick, D.J., Austin, C.C., Petren, K., Fisher, R.N., Losos, J.B., and Ellers, O. (1996) *J. Linnaen Soc.*, **59**, 21.

70 Autumn, K., Liang, Y.A., Hsieh, S.T., Zesch, W., Chan, W.P., Kenny, T.W., Fearing, R., and Full, R.J. (2000) *Nature*, **405**, 681.

71 Hansen, W.R. and Autumn, K. (2005) *Proc. Natl Acad. Sci. USA*, **102**, 385.

72 Kesel, A.B., Martin, A., and Seidl, T. (2004) *Smart Mater. Struct.*, **13**, 512.

73 Eisner, T. and Aneshansley, D.J. (2000) *Proc. Natl Acad. Sci. USA*, **97**, 6568.

74 Sitti, M., Fearing, R.S., and Adhes, J. (2003) *Sci. Technol.*, **17**, 1055.

75 Geim, A.K., Dubonos, S.V., Grigorieva, I.V., Novoselov, K.S., Zhukov, A.A., and Shapoval, S.Yu. (2003) *Nat. Mater.*, **2**, 461.

76 Qu, L., Dai, L., Stone, M., Xia, Z., and Wang, Z.-L. (2008) *Science*, **322**, 238.

Index